This standard and internationally known reference manual for the identification of medically important bacteria, *Cowan and Steel*, occupies an essential place at the bench of all medical microbiologists. The material in this new edition, which follows the successful pattern of previous editions, has been extensively revised, and is suitable for use in all medical bacteriology laboratories using traditional diagnostic methods.

The core of the manual is the series of diagnostic tables which, with the accompanying descriptive text and definitions, give the characteristics of all bacteria likely to be encountered in public health laboratories, and in medical and veterinary practice. This edition contains new sections on rapid and mechanized test methods and on the laboratory applications of computers to the identification of bacteria. The importance of laboratory quality control and proficiency procedures is emphasized throughout.

The Appendices give details of laboratory methods and media for all the recommended diagnostic tests, and provide abstracts of the official guidelines for bacterial nomenclature. As in previous editions, the text contains comprehensive and up to date references.

Cowan and Steel's manual for the identification of medical bacteria

The following titles, originally published by the Public Health Laboratory Service, might also be of interest and these are now available from Cambridge University Press

Quality Control – Principles and Practice in the Microbiology Laboratory (1991) Edited by J. J. S. Snell, I. D. Farrell & C. Roberts

Current Topics in Clinical Virology (1991) Edited by P. Morgan-Capner

Multipoint Methods in the Clinical Laboratory (1991) M. Faiers, R. George, J. Jolly & P. Wheat

ELISA in the Clinical Microbiology Laboratory (1990) Edited by T. G. Wreghitt & P. Morgan-Capner

Anaerobic Infections: Clinical and Laboratory Practice (1988) A. Trevor Willis & Kenneth D. Phillips

Making Monoclonals: A Practical Beginners' Guide to the Production and Characterisation of Monoclonal Antibodies Against Bacteria and Viruses (1988) D. G. Newell, B. W. McBride and S. A. Clark

COWAN AND STEEL'S
Manual for the identification of medical bacteria

THIRD EDITION

EDITED AND REVISED BY

G. I. BARROW
M.D., F.R.C.Path., Dip. Bact.
formerly Consultant Medical Microbiologist,
Public Health Laboratory Service
and Director, Public Health Laboratory, Truro, Cornwall

and

R. K. A. FELTHAM
B.Sc., Ph.D., M.I.Biol.
formerly Principal Microbiologist and Director
ACT Medisys Ltd, Edgbaston, Birmingham,
and Senior Microbiologist, Public Health Laboratory, Leicester

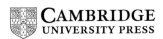
CAMBRIDGE
UNIVERSITY PRESS

Published by the Press Syndicate of the University of Cambridge,
The Pitt Building, Trumpington Street, Cambridge CB2 1RP
40 West 20th Street, New York, NY 10011–4211, USA
10 Stamford Road, Oakleigh, Victoria 3116, Australia

First published 1965
Second edition 1974
Third edition 1993

Printed in Great Britain at the University Press, Cambridge

A catalogue record for this book is available from the British Library

Library of Congress cataloguing in publication data
Cowan and Steel's manual for identification of medical bacteria –
3rd ed. / edited and rev. by G.I. Barrow and R.K.A. Feltham.
p. cm.
Includes bibliographical references.
Includes index.
ISBN 0 521 32611 7
1. Diagnostic bacteriology – Handbooks, manuals, etc. I. Cowan,
S.T. (Samuel Tertius) II. Steel, K.J. (Kenneth John)
III. Barrow, G.I. IV. Feltham, R.K.A. V. Title: Manual for the
identification of medical bacteria.
[DNLM: 1. Bacteria – classification.
QW 15 C874]
QR67.2.C68 1993
616.014 – dc20 90-2511 CIP

ISBN 0 521 32611 7 hardback

Contents

Foreword

For over 25 years now, medical bacteriologists all over the world have turned to 'Cowan and Steel' as their first reference book when they encountered an unfamiliar bacterial isolate. A generation of laboratory workers has grown up with it. They turned to it not only because there was clear information on how to examine isolates, with concise details of culture media and test methods that were applicable to the great majority of bacteria of medical importance, but also because of the famous successive tables that led from genera with their minidefinitions to species with their characters. These were combined with practical hints on where one might go wrong, and succinct information on the pathogenic species. The tables contained carefully chosen data in just the right amount for a useful laboratory manual on the identification of medically important bacteria.

In the years since the last edition, test methods and the variety of bacteria of medical interest have both grown considerably. Not only have poorly studied areas like the 'diphtheroids' been much clarified, but a number of newly recognized pathogens such as legionellae have become important. Medical and other workers will therefore welcome this new edition, which follows closely the emphasis and style of its predecessors. The contributors and editors are to be congratulated on their labours in bringing a complex field to the concise summary that is contained here, often in the face of difficulties in finding convenient diagnostic tests for the newer taxa.

Some new features in this edition will greatly help users. The chapters on theory and practice in bacterial taxonomy, on computer identification and on bacterial nomenclature will be especially welcomed. The further emphasis on quality control and proficiency assessment procedures, both within laboratories and between them, will also be most useful. It is a pleasure to be able to recommend this *Manual* wholeheartedly to those concerned with medical and associated bacteriology everywhere.

Leicester   *P.H.A. Sneath*

Preface to the first edition

Our 'Diagnostic Tables for the Common Medical Bacteria' were originally published in the *Journal of Hygiene*. The tables seemed to fill a need and the demand for reprints was so great that Cambridge University Press reprinted them in pamphlet form.

Many inquired about the technical methods, and there were constant complaints that the methods were not described and that the text lacked details of the taxonomic problems. We resolved, therefore, to expand the original paper and to prepare a book which would give sufficient detail of media and methods to justify its description as a laboratory manual.

Although designed for medical workers we hope that others will use it.

The value of a laboratory manual was impressed on one of us in 1935 at the British Postgraduate Medical School. Dr A. A. Miles had prepared a loose-leaf mimeographed manual to supplement (and improve on) a popular laboratory handbook. With this example in mind a manual suited to the special needs of the National Collection of Type Cultures was prepared, and contributions were made by other members of the Collection staff, particularly Mrs P. H. Clarke, Miss H. E. Ross, Miss C. Shaw, and Mr C. S. Brindle. The National Collection Manual in turn became the basis for the appendices to the present *Manual*.

In compiling the tables we sought information from various sources, including authoritative works such as the Reports of the Enterobacteriaceae Subcommittee of the International Committee on Bacteriological Nomenclature, and monographs such as Kauffmann's (1954) *Enterobacteriaceae*, Edwards & Ewing's *Identification of Entero-bacteriaceae* (1962), and Smith, Gordon & Clark's (1952) *Aerobic Sporeforming Bacteria*. We found large gaps in published works, and in many instances our own data have been the only source of information. While we have taken great care in compiling and checking the tables, we are sure that the *Manual* is unlikely to be free from error. When such errors are detected we hope that the finders will let us know. We will also welcome data to fill up the few gaps in the tables.

It is with pleasure that we acknowledge our indebtedness to many friends and colleagues at home and abroad for facts and discussions that have helped to clarify ideas. It is impossible to name them all, but we could not have planned or written the *Manual* without the help of Dr R. E. Gordon, Dr P. R. Edwards, Dr W. H. Ewing, Dr T. Gibson, Dr Joan Taylor, Mrs P. H. Clarke, Miss C. Shaw, and Miss H. E. Ross. We also wish to thank Miss B. H. Whyte and Miss A. Bowman, the Colindale librarians, Miss M. I. Hammond who dealt skilfully with the manuscript, and Mr W. Clifford who made the figures.

London   S.T.C.
1964   K.J.S.

POSTSCRIPT

My colleague, Dr K. J. Steel, died suddenly on 25 September 1964, between the completion of the manuscript and the proof stage of the book. His death at the age of 34 is a great loss for he seemed destined to reach the highest branches of bacteriology. In this *Manual* he was responsible for the whole of Appendices A to D and F and for much of Chapter 3; and he played a big part in revising and recasting the tables that form the heart of our work. I hope that the book will serve as a fitting memorial to a great collaborator and friend.

London   S.T.C.
1965

Preface to the second edition

The first edition of this *Manual*, judged by its spread around the world, seems to have been useful to hospital bacteriologists. It was translated into Japanese by Dr Riichi Sakazaki, who will also translate this edition.

It has not been easy to prepare a worthy successor; not only have I been unable to discuss and argue every sentence with my colleague, but I have missed the ready access to libraries that one has when working in a large research institution. However, I have been greatly helped by the Librarians at Colindale (Miss B. H. Whyte) and the Royal Society of Medicine (Mr P. Wade) and their staffs.

In this edition Chapter 2 and Appendices A, B, C and E, originally written mainly by Dr Steel, are little changed; most of the other chapters have been completely rewritten. Chapters 8 and 9 are entirely new, as are Appendices D, F, G and H. I must thank Mr A. Waltho, of the Medical Research Council's Central Store, who gave me great help in preparing the list of firms which supply media and chemicals (Appendix H) and, together with Dr O. M. Lidwell, suggested and drafted what became Table 2.1.

I am also grateful to many other colleagues who gave me information and advice; while it is impossible to mention all by name, I am particularly indebted to G. I. Barrow, W. B. Cherry, E. A. Dawes, N. E. Gibbons, R. E. Gordon, R. M. Keddie, S. P. Lapage, H. Lautrop, J. Midgeley, M. J. Pickett, R. Sakazaki, R. Whittenbury and S. A. Wright.

On behalf of the Executive Committee of the International Association of Microbiological Societies (IAMS), Dr N. E. Gibbons gave permission for the reproduction of the Introduction to the proposed revision of the Bacteriological Code (Appendix G), and I should like to express my thanks to the IAMS Executive.

In a book with so many tables and cross-references it is inevitable that some errors and inconsistencies are still undetected; I hope that these will be drawn to my attention so that corrections can be made in later impressions.

For the proof reading I am grateful for help from former colleagues, Miss H. E. Ross, Dr G. I. Barrow and Dr A. F. B. Standfast. Checking the numerous and large tables in the manuscript and proof stages has been an onerous task which I could not have done without the co-operation of my wife, who also helped to check the references, which must now number about a thousand.

With all this help, I hope the book will continue to be a worthy memorial to my much missed young colleague, Dr K. J. Steel.

Queen Camel   S.T.C.
1973

Preface to the third edition

The demand for a new edition of this *Manual* has been enormous. We hope that we have done justice to it and that it will prove a fitting tribute to the late Sam Cowan. He not only obtained every paper he cited in the references but personally perused and annotated each one. We cannot alas say the same. It is now beyond the scope of one person or even of two persons to cover the entire and seemingly ever-changing fields of bacterial classification, nomenclature and taxonomy, especially with the range of 'medical' bacteria expanding with the advancement of biotechnology and modern medicine to include many environmental organisms. For this third edition we have therefore sought the help of the experts listed on pages xv and xvi for various groups of organisms and we gratefully acknowledge all their contributions to this *Manual*. The opinions expressed are mostly theirs though the final responsibility is ours. We hope that together they will provide enlightenment and understanding of a subject which, though not everyone's 'cup of tea', is nevertheless at the heart of diagnostic medical bacteriology.

In outline, this edition follows that of the two previous ones. We have received numerous suggestions for change but have resisted many of them, preferring to regard continuity as more important. We have also retained references to some methods and equipment which may be regarded as 'old-fashioned' or not quite reaching the current acme of absolute safety, but we are conscious that not all diagnostic laboratories are equally endowed; we know for example that, despite their limitations, manually operated autoclaves are still used frequently and apparently satisfactorily throughout the world. Apart from extensive updating of the text, tables and appendices, we have added new Sections: on rapid methods and test kits; on the theory and use of computers for bacterial iden-

tification; on the principles of the Bacteriological Code and the *Approved Lists of Bacterial Names*; and on the reconciliation of different approaches to bacterial systematics. Unlike previous editions, we have not listed 'sources of information' separately in Chapters 6 and 7 but have included all references in the text. Also, in this edition we have omitted the Appendix listing some of the manufacturers of media, reagents and other laboratory supplies as the international names are now well known and we think it would be invidious to select arbitrarily from the many others. For reference purposes we have included the type strain of the type species in the minidefinitions, but we emphasize that they should not be regarded as necessarily 'typical' in all respects of the species.

In a book such as this with so much material and so many cross-references we know that there are bound to be some errors and inconsistencies that we have missed; moreover with the increasing scope and application of genetic and other techniques, some of the taxonomic information will probably be out of date already. We should be glad therefore if readers would draw such occurrences to our attention for subsequent correction.

Professor P. H. A. Sneath, who has himself contributed much to bacterial systematics and taxonomy, has kindly written a Foreword. On behalf of the International Union of Microbiological Societies Professor S. W. Glover gave permission to reproduce the Introduction from the *International Code of Nomenclature of Bacteria* and from the *Approved Lists of Bacterial Names*, and also the text of the *Report of the Ad Hoc Committee on the Reconciliation of Approaches to Bacterial Systematics*. We wish to express our thanks to him and to the IUMS executive. For proof-reading and checking so many tables, we express our sincere thanks to Dr Joan M. Davies and, in particular to Dr B. Holmes who also contributed a large part of Chapter 7 on the Gram-negative bacteria and made many useful suggestions as did Dr Dorothy Jones. We also thank our many other colleagues, too numerous to name, for their help in many if unspecified ways. As before, Dr R. Sakazaki will translate this edition into Japanese and we are grateful to him for this. Last but not least we thank our wives and the staff of Cambridge University Press for their forbearance and support in what proved to be a long and arduous task. We hope that this new edition will be at least as useful as the previous two seem to have been.

Salisbury   G.I.B.
Leicester   R.K.A.F.
1992

Contributors

G. Colman

Division of Hospital Infection, Central Public Health Laboratory, 61 Colindale Avenue, London NW9 5HT.

E. Fox[†]

Public Health Laboratory, Leicester Royal Infirmary, Leicester LE1 5WW.

R. J. Gross

Division of Enteric Pathogens, Central Public Health Laboratory, 61 Colindale Avenue, London NW9 5HT.

B. Holmes

Identification Services Laboratory, National Collection of Type Cultures, Central Public Health Laboratory, 61 Colindale Avenue, London NW9 5HT.

P. A. Jenkins

PHLS Mycobacterium Reference Unit, University Hospital of Wales, Heath Park, Cardiff CF4 4XW.

Dorothy M. Jones

Department of Microbiology, Medical Sciences Building, University of Leicester, University Road, Leicester LE1 9HN.

J. V. Lee

PHLS Environmental Microbiology Reference Unit, Public Health Laboratory, Queen's Medical Centre, Nottingham NG7 2UH.

R. R. Marples

Division of Hospital Infection, Central Public Health Laboratory, 61 Colindale Avenue, London NW9 5HT.

F. G. Priest

Department of Biological Sciences, Heriot-Watt University, Riccarton, Edinburgh EH14 4AS.

[†] deceased

Geraldine M. Schofield

Unilever Research Laboratory, Colworth House, Sharnbrook, Bedford MK44 1LQ.

M. W. Scruton

Sterilization R&D Unit, PHLS Centre for Applied Microbiology & Research, Porton Down, Salisbury, Wiltshire SP4 0JG.

M. B. Skirrow

Public Health Laboratory, Gloucester Royal Hospital, Gloucester GL1 3NN.

Mary P. E. Slack

Department of Bacteriology, John Radcliffe Hospital, Headington, Oxford OX3 9DU.

J. J. S. Snell

Quality Assurance Laboratory, Division of Microbiological Reagents and Quality Control, Central Public Health Laboratory, 61 Colindale Avenue, London NW9 5HT.

A. T. Willis

Public Health Laboratory, Luton & Dunstable Hospital, Lewsey Road, Luton LU4 0DZ.

Introduction

It is assumed that the reader of this *Manual* has some knowledge and experience of bacteriology and of elementary chemistry and that the basic principles including those of laboratory safety are understood. Thus, though many other essential details are given in the Appendices, how to determine the pH value of a medium, or how to make a normal or molar solution, is not described; nor are details given about how to use anaerobic jars or microscopes. Serology is not discussed but methods commonly used in the preparation of extracts for grouping streptococci are described as the Lancefield serological groups are referred to in Table 6.3*b*. Details of sterilization temperatures and times are also given as these so-called standard procedures still vary from one laboratory to another.

This *Manual* is intended to help those who have isolated a bacterium and want to identify it. The methods used by clinical bacteriologists to isolate organisms from specimens sent to the laboratory are not described as to do so would be to enter ever-changing fields, and our recommendations might well be out of date. We stress, however, that before identification of any organism is attempted, it must be obtained in pure culture. Some advice on how to recognize that a culture is impure, and on the steps to be taken to purify it, is therefore given.

The tables for identification of medical bacteria developed in phases: the original tables of Cowan & Steel (1961) were based mainly on the results of tests carried out on strains in the National Collection of Type Cultures (NCTC) between 1948 and 1960. For the tables in the first edition of this *Manual*, the NCTC information was supplemented by surveys of the literature up to 1963; the second edition included the results of further literature surveys up to 1972; and for the present (third) edition, the literature up to 1990 has been reviewed by individual experts for each of the principal bacterial groups; where possible, new genera subsequently accepted, such as *Enterococcus* and *Helicobacter*, have been included. Each expert was asked to provide identification tables and methods suitable for use in routine diagnostic laboratories. It follows that in this edition we are less often able to indicate the relative value of the different technical methods used to obtain the characters shown in the tables. Once again, discrepancies occurred between the results of different workers – probably due more often to differences in methods than to variation between strains of the same species. To try to cover every possibility in the tables would be self-defeating, for either we multiply the columns (species or varieties) or we increase the number of equivocal or doubtful entries (d or D) equivalent to words like 'often', 'some(times)', or 'not infrequently', so that a clear positive or negative character would become rare and the tables thus confusing and unhelpful. We were tempted to use the percentage of positive results, as utilized for computer-assisted identification, but after careful consideration we felt that this would complicate the tables unnecessarily and be helpful only to a minority of readers. We have tried therefore to be definite and have treated descriptions such as 'occasionally', 'occasional strains' and 'a few strains' as exceptions not worthy of note. The tables are therefore not perfect as there are exceptions to all rules: it is the user who must be realistic and bear in mind that the bacteria they are trying to identify may not conform to the expected norm.

Intelligent use of the tables demands technical skill and sensitive but specific methods for the individual tests. As in all determinative bacteriology, true identification must be based on careful work, and the tables will not help those who are in too much of a hurry to carry out the basic tests needed, though this does not necessarily mean every test in a table. We considered cutting down the tables to show only those characters that had immediate value in distinguishing one species from others in the tables, but we decided against this because conditions vary considerably in different laboratories and in different countries. We do not expect all the tests in the tables to be carried out; each bacteriologist has individual preferences and dislikes; and not all laboratories are equally well equipped. For these reasons many more characters than are necessary for identification have been included. We considered indicating the more important characters in bold type, but as this would merely reflect our own preferences we decided against it. Bacteriologists must choose those tests that seem to them to be most discriminating and use those that can be performed with the equipment and media available. As the tables are constructed from information from many sources, particular methods are not stipulated, but those given in the Appendices should be satisfactory. In this edition we have omitted many of the micromethods described in the first edition; those retained are included in Appendix C, together with methods using larger volumes (and often taking a longer time).

Three points should be emphasized about the tables. (i) They should not be considered in isolation; other evidence that cannot be included in them such as colony form, experimental pathogenicity, chromatographic profiles, chemotaxonomy and DNA hybridization results should also be taken into account. (ii) The tables do not characterize an organism; they are intended to focus attention on tests and characters most valuable in differentiation. (iii) The tables do not form part of any classification system, but they may draw attention to bacterial similarities and relationships that are not otherwise apparent. We have not been able to avoid taxonomic terms completely but a brief glossary of those in current use is included at the end of this *Manual*; for further information, Cowan's *Dictionary of microbial taxonomy* (Hill, 1978) should be consulted.

Names of species are not shown in the table headings but as numbered footnotes, and these include common synonyms so that, with the Index, it should be possible to find the main characters of many named species. The definitive names given in the

new *Approved Lists of Bacterial Names* (Skerman, McGowan & Sneath, 1980) including validated changes and additions subsequently published in the *International Journal of Systematic Bacteriology* (IJSB), are used throughout. The older generic name 'Bacterium' is not included and the term *Bacillus* is restricted to aerobic spore-formers.

In general, the tables allow identification of species that can often be further differentiated into serotypes, biotypes or phage types. However, users of the *Manual* will seldom have all the sera needed for detailed antigenic analysis of the species they isolate; this is a task for a reference laboratory. Those who aspire to do such work themselves should consult the excellent practical manual by Edwards & Ewing (1962, 1972) which highlights the problems and, for the Enterobacteriaceae, gives the essential details.

The tables seldom mention sensitivity or resistance to antibiotics although sometimes such tests are of practical differential value. In the present era, however, apart from selection pressure, the genetic effects of antibiotic therapy and usage are known to affect bacterial characters, including sensitivity or resistance to antibiotics, by transfer of plasmids.

We have tried to refer readers to pertinent literature in which fuller details of methods are given; in this way we have kept the *Manual* free from unnecessary detail and from the more theoretical aspects of taxonomy and nomenclature. We have, however, tried to retain where possible some of the nomenclatural life stories of many organisms, lest they be forgotten.

In plan, the *Manual* falls into two parts: the first, divided into chapters, is discursive; the second, made up of appendices, is instructive and written tersely with free use of scientific abbreviations (Ellis, 1971), chemical formulae, and prescription-like recipes for media. The essence of the book is in Chapters 6 and 7, which comprise the diagnostic tables and notes on the different genera. In this edition we include more little-known genera, many of them incompletely defined. It may seem that we have sometimes strayed outside the medical field, but many environmental organisms are now becoming important as opportunist pathogens especially with the widespread use of immunosuppressive therapy and the advent of AIDS and the Human Immunodeficiency Virus.

A practical example is given of the application of the diagnostic tables to punched cards for easy sorting and bacterial identification. Reference is also made to the use of computers for rapid comparison and identification of isolates. In addition, the *Manual* now includes a short chapter on the quality control of laboratory procedures and reagents as well as on quality assessment, both within and between laboratories, with simulated material of known but undisclosed content.

1

Classification and nomenclature

Taxonomy is not every man's meat, but neither is it everyone's poison. It can be likened to a cocktail: a skilful blend in which it is not easy to discern the individual ingredients. In taxonomy the ingredients are (i) *classification*, or the orderly arrangement of units, (ii) *nomenclature*, the naming or labelling of the units, and (iii) *identification* of the unknown with a unit defined and named by (i) and (ii). The subdivisions should be taken in the order indicated, for without adequate classification it is impossible to name rationally, and without a system of labelled units it is impossible to identify others with them or to communicate the results.

1.1   Classification

Before discussing the identification of bacteria, the principles of classification and nomenclature must first be dealt with briefly. Since this book is essentially a practical manual, theoretical speculations about the validity of bacterial species (Lwoff, 1958; Cowan, 1962a; Lapage et al., 1975) are not considered.

For this *Manual*, the concept of bacterial species is therefore accepted as a convenient unit. However, as it so obviously has different values in different groups of bacteria, no attempt is made to define it, or to analyse the qualities that distinguish one species from another. Nor is any attempt made to determine whether a taxonomic group (taxon) is a species, a variety or a subspecies; or to estimate the value or importance of different kinds of bacterial characters (Cowan, 1968, 1970b). We dislike the idea of subspecies and prefer to recognize subdivisions of species either as varieties (biotypes) or as serotypes. We do not accept the contention of Kauffmann (1959a, b; 1963b) that the serotypes or phage types of the various members of the Enterobacteriaceae

should be equated with species. However, the collection of similar species into larger groups (genera), and similar though not necessarily related genera into families, are convenient and generally accepted groupings. But they should not be regarded as phylogenetic groups; thus to combine families into even larger groups (orders) would be artificial and highly speculative. The different kinds of bacteria are not separated by sharp divisions but by slight and subtle differences in characters so that they seem to blend into each other and resemble a spectrum (Fig. 1.1a, b). This spectrum-like intergrading of different kinds of bacteria is confirmed by other methods of grouping, such as the base composition of the deoxyribonucleic acid (DNA) of the bacterial cell (Vendrely, 1958). The DNA composition varies among different groups of bacteria but it should be homogeneous within a group. Marmur, Falkow & Mandel (1963), Hill (1966) and Brenner (1978) collected the results of numerous workers and summarized in tables the DNA-base composition and DNA homology of many bacteria. These techniques are not applicable in day-to-day diagnostic work but the results are of fundamental importance to the taxonomist; the essential aspects are considered in a recent Report (Wayne et al., 1987) on the reconciliation of different approaches to bacterial systematics. The recent introduction of cloned DNA as probes in diagnostic bacteriology is not only very exciting but may well revolutionize diagnostic bacteriology as currently practised. Indeed, diagnostic DNA probes have already been developed for many of the pathogenic bacteria as well as for several viruses.

A theoretical classification scheme divides the higher ranks into two or more kinds of a lower rank; for example, earlier editions of *Bergey's Manual of Determinative Bacteriology* (1923–57) divided the

1

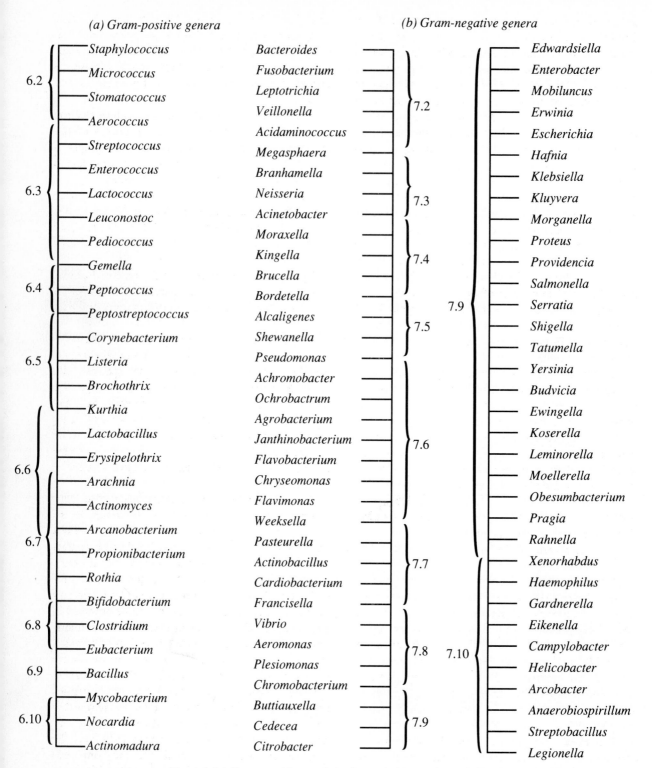

Fig. 1.1 *(a)* Gram-positive *and (b)* Gram-negative genera dealt with in this manual.

kingdom Bacteria into orders and continued the breakdown through families, tribes, genera, and species; however, neither the last (8th) edition (1974) nor the current volumes of *Bergey's Manual of Systematic Bacteriology* (1984, 1986, 1989) attempt to produce a complete hierarchy. We suggest, as in previous editions of this *Manual*, that a pragmatic classification should be built up from the basal unit (species); basal units which share a number of characters are combined to form the next higher unit (genus) so that the common characters become those which are important in the definition or characterization of the genus. The emphasis on certain characters – which are regarded as important because they are significant in identification – differs from the Adansonian concept now referred to as numerical taxonomy (Sneath, 1957a), in which each character has equal merit in the eyes of the taxonomist.

What are called 'important characters' may be of three kinds: (i) *specific,* such as the ability to produce coagulase by *Staphylococcus aureus*; (ii) *distinguishing* characters which, though not specific, are useful in separating organisms that are otherwise very similar (for example, indole production by *Proteus vulgaris* is one of the characters that distinguishes it from *P. mirabilis*); (iii) characters *shared* by all members of a group; thus, acid-fastness is an important character of mycobacteria since all members are acid-fast, but not of the nocardias only some of which are acid-fast. Needless to say, there are degrees of importance and it would be feasible to continue the list; but enough has been said to illustrate the point that characters can have an importance in a pragmatic scheme that are denied to them in numerical (Adansonian) classification.

Taxonomists use and put much weight on what are called 'fermentation tests' without paying too much attention to the way in which carbohydrate is broken down; this breakdown is characteristic of an organism and of great informative value for classification. In this *Manual* the terms 'oxidative' and 'fermentative' are used though it is not at all certain that they describe accurately what is happening in the Oxidation–Fermentation (OF) test of Hugh & Leifson (1953).

A practical classification should preferably be based on characters that are easily determined; consequently features that demand difficult techniques or special apparatus should not be used. Thus, bacterial components such as cell walls, septa, nuclei, and fimbriae are excluded from our scheme despite their importance, though to add them would increase the weight of our argument and support our general conclusions.

Again, because it is difficult, even with an electron microscope, to obtain accurate pictures of the arrangement of flagella on bacteria, little weight is placed on this character though it is very important in all except the most rigid numerical taxonomy.

The scheme used in this *Manual* is built on a wide range of characters; the identification of each unit is based on the same characters and it is not necessary to make the hypothetical and sometimes absurd assumptions of classical taxonomy.

By omitting any reference to the type of flagellation, there is no need to postulate that *Shigella* species, if they had any, would have peritrichous flagella.

We do not use any formal classification scheme in this *Manual* but, because of the need to label recognizable taxonomic units, usually at the species level, advantage is taken of the specific epithets and generic names that are already part of formal systems. Labelling is discussed more fully in Chapter 8; only the problems that immediately concern the identification of bacteria, and how the organisms are to be described in reports to clinicians and health officials, are mentioned here.

It is convenient to divide bacteria into two large groups based on the reactions of the organisms to Gram's method of staining, though latinized names are not given to these groups. In formal schemes most genera consist of bacteria that are either Gram-positive or Gram-negative, so that each genus can be allocated according to the Gram reaction of the majority of species it contains. The genera can be arranged in some order so that adjacent ones show some similarities but the more distant genera have less in common (Fig. 1.1a, b); the arrangement resembles two series of pigeon-holes – one for Gram-positive and the other for Gram-negative organisms – where the partitions between the individual pigeon-holes are removable so that the contents of adjacent holes will be in contact with each other. But although bacteria may be regarded as a series of gradually merging forms and likened to a spectrum, we do not imply that the sequences shown in Fig. 1.1a, b are the best that can be devised to show relationships, if present, between the genera. The sequences have some merit in that they do not violate too severely the order that might be presented in a classification made on orthodox lines. We stress therefore that the lists of names in Fig. 1.1a, b are those of taxa that are normally regarded as having generic rank; they are not an attempt at classification. Most of the names have been in use for a long time and are generally accepted.

With some bacteria the Gram reaction is regarded as variable, indeterminate, and occasionally misleading. Many cocci and some rods may be Gram-positive in young cultures and become negative as the culture ages; in such cases it is usual to regard the reaction of the young culture as correct. Occasionally the reverse sequence occurs: *Acinetobacter* strains for example may become somewhat Gram-positive in cultures several days old and some workers (e.g. Thornley, 1967) describe them as Gram-variable; this is a phenomenon better known outside the medical field, as in the genus *Arthrobacter*. Strains of *Gemella* are unusual in that when stained they seem to be Gram-negative, but in the chemical nature of the cell wall they resemble the Gram-positive bacteria. Although cell wall analysis is far from a routine procedure, we have placed the genus *Gemella* in Fig. 1.1a among the Gram-positive bacteria but show the characters of the species in tables dealing with both Gram-positive (Table 6.3a, b) and Gram-negative (Table 7.3) cocci.

Because we do not start with an orthodox classification in a hierarchical system, it may be argued that the identifying characteristics of bacteria cannot be presented in a logical manner. However, by avoiding a formal classification we believe that the characters can be displayed in a manner that is both logical and orderly; that similarities and differences shown by the tables will point the way to a more orderly arrangement of the different taxa; and, as orderly arrangements are the essence of all classifications, the tables may thus lead to a logical classification.

It is essential that the reader should understand that there is no single classification ordained by God or by Nature but numerous different classifications, all made by man, each with a particular purpose in mind. The main difficulty without a classification relates to the labelling of the taxa; this difficulty is overcome in our tables by using the names(s) by which each taxon (usually a species) is generally known, irrespective of the rightness of the name(s) in terms of the *International Code of Nomenclature of Bacteria*. The taxa listed in Fig. 1.1a, b are groups approximating to genera and the components of these groups will be species whose characters are shown in the secondary and tertiary tables in Chapters 6 and 7. Usually the acceptable name for a group will be obvious and well known.

The Gram-positive and Gram-negative bacteria can each be considered as a continuous series. Some of the genera shown in Fig. 1.1a, b are dealt with only summarily in this *Manual* but they are mentioned because they may be met either as contaminants or as suspected pathogens. Organisms such as *Leptospira* and other spirochaetes that are identified on morphological and serological grounds, or by their pathogenicity for various animals, do not fit into the scheme in this *Manual*. Neither do mycoplasmas, though they are referred to briefly in Section 7.10.10. Our purpose is to identify bacteria isolated in medical laboratories, commonly, if incorrectly, called the medical bacteria. They are derived mainly from clinical material (hospital laboratories) but may come from apparently healthy individuals (public health laboratories), or from water, sewage, foodstuffs and other environmental sources. Apparently identical bacteria may produce infection in animals other than man, so our survey must include the fields of medical and veterinary science, and it will necessarily impinge on plant pathology and industrial processes.

1.2 Nomenclature

In this *Manual*, emphasis is placed on the characterization of organisms, for it is a waste of time to work out carefully the characters of the unknown and then compare these with vague descriptions. We do not make a great point about nomenclature, believing that a simple label, as long as it is unique, is adequate for communication though we abide by the *Approved Lists of Bacterial Names* (Skerman, McGowan & Sneath, 1980). In the tables in Chapters 6 and 7, the columns of characters of a taxon are numbered and the name(s) by which the taxon is known will be found in numbered footnotes. The first name, usually in bold type, is generally regarded as the most acceptable name; this is usually, but not necessarily, the nomenclaturally correct name. It is important that everyone concerned – the bacteriologist, the clinician, and the health official – should all understand fully the nature of the organism reported. The nomenclaturally correct name often means little outside the laboratory and those in charge of patients may still be blissfully unaware of the implications; on the other hand, the common name in English may be understood more readily. In the tables we give, for good measure, other names used in English- and American-speaking countries; these synonyms appear in the footnotes without further explanation. Latin and latinized names in the text are avoided as far as possible.

In this chapter, the problems and principles of nomenclature are not discussed, but we must point out now that, as nomenclature is dependent on classification, there may be more than one correct name for a bacterium. Nomenclature is subject to the rules of the *International Code of Nomenclature of Bacteria*, usually referred to as the *Bacteriological Code* (1976 revision); there are not, and never can be, any rules for classification. Classification is subjective and a matter of opinion, and it is within the rights (if not the competence) of each worker to classify bacteria as he or she will. The classification adopted determines the names to be appended to the organisms, and the rules of nomenclature should be a guide to the choice of correct names. If a worker believes that all rod-shaped organisms are to be grouped together in one genus, *Bacillus*, he is entitled to name the diphtheria organism '*Bacillus diphtheriae*', but if he thinks that rod-shaped bacteria can be split into different groups he can use a name such as *Corynebacterium diphtheriae*; each name is correct within its own taxonomic scheme or classification, and would be wrong in the other scheme. Regrettably, the application of the rules of the *Bacteriological Code* is still subjective and different workers may draw quite different conclusions from reading the rules and may interpret them in contrasting and even conflicting ways.

One of the aims of the *Bacteriological Code* was to stabilize nomenclature; but this is an impossibility for nomenclature is itself dependent on ever-changing ideas on classification. The rediscovery and application of an old or the development of a new

technique may indeed act as a stimulus.

Sometimes, an organism remains unclassified for decades after its discovery and characterization. Morgan's no. 1 bacillus (Morgan, 1906) needed the insight of Rauss (1936) and the discovery that under the right conditions it could be made to swarm to establish it as a species of *Proteus*. It was the rediscovery and application of the phenylalanine test that made Singer & Bar-Chay (1954) realize that Stuart's 29911 (Stuart, Wheeler & McGann, 1946) or Providence group was also a species of *Proteus*. With the advent of DNA hybridization techniques, both these organisms have now been reclassified and placed in the genera *Morganella* and *Providencia* respectively.

It is often easier to create a new genus or species than to do the comparative work necessary to put an organism into its rightful place in an existing genus or species. The temptation to designate a new genus or species should be resisted, as it would be if it was appreciated that taxonomic ability is judged as inversely proportional to the number of new taxa created.

Many workers use common names (in the vernacular language of their own country) in preference to scientific names that may be subject to change. Since English is now the language of science, common English names are widely understood, but French or German equivalents may present difficulty to English-speaking people (e.g. bacteridie de charbon = der Milzbrandbazillus = the anthrax bacillus = *Bacillus anthracis*). The great advantage of the latinized binomial name is that it is accepted throughout the world and the same words should have the same meaning everywhere. Although printed in the same way, even in journals using pictorial characters, the sound and pronunciation can, however, differ considerably.

Nomenclature often presents difficulties because a change in name may be necessary when an organism is moved from one group to another. Sometimes the nomenclatural difficulties arose because the rules in the *Bacteriological Code*, first published in 1948 (Buchanan, St John-Brooks & Breed, 1948), revised and annotated in 1958 (Buchanan *et al.*, 1958) and revised again in 1966, were made retroactive. This meant applying the rules to names first used in the last century, long before a bacteriological code was thought of, and in some instances, before the organism named had been isolated and characterized. Fortunately, following initial proposals by Lapage *et al.*, (1973) the rules in the *Bacteriological Code* were revised and simplified in 1975 (1976 revision) by the International Committee on Systematic Bacteriology which also reviewed bacterial nomenclature critically and published *Approved Lists of Bacterial Names* in 1980. This will do much to avoid petty squabbles on the priority of names in future.

Another source of confusion is due to the well-intentioned efforts of workers to give a meaning to the specific epithet, and to make the epithet appropriate. For example, an ill-conceived attempt was made about 50 years ago to apply the epithet '*pyogenes*' to the generic name *Staphylococcus* because the legitimate epithet '*aureus*' was inappropriate for strains that produced white colonies. More recently Foster & Bragg (1962) suggested that various specific epithets for *Klebsiella*, correctly proposed by the old Rules, should be transposed (which would greatly add to confusion) because, as originally proposed, they seemed to them to be inappropriate.

Yet another source of confusion is the re-use of a discarded name for a newly described genus or species. An example was the use of '*Aerobacter*' (a later synonym for *Klebsiella*) for a group of motile organisms which share several characters in common with non-motile organisms then named '*Aerobacter aerogenes*'. This confusion was later remedied by its authors (Hormaeche & Edwards, 1960) who withdrew their proposal and substituted the new generic name *Enterobacter*. Unfortunately so many authors continued to use the name *Aerobacter* for both motile and non-motile organisms that the problem was submitted (Carpenter *et al*, 1970) to the Judicial Commission of the International Committee on Systematic Bacteriology for an Official Opinion on the validity of the name *Aerobacter*; the Commission ruled (Opinion 46, 1971) against the use of the generic name *Aerobacter* because its application was uncertain. This kind of situation should not occur with the *Approved Lists of Bacterial Names* (Skerman, McGowan & Sneath, 1980) provided the rules are followed carefully and thoughtfully. We do, however, recommend caution in applying the results of new techniques such as DNA hybridization to the reclassification of existing species. A new name, although perhaps valid for DNA relatedness, is of little use if the same organism cannot be readily differentiated from close neighbours by routine clinical laboratory methods.

6

2
Culture media: constituents and sterilization

In the introduction to a *Good Food Guide* for bacteria, Miles (1965) described most culture media formulations as 'kitchen recipes, written ... by increasingly sophisticated cooks'. There are two entirely different kinds of media: those of defined composition and those of undefined composition, usually containing peptone. Defined media have disadvantages for identification because the characters of organisms grown in them may differ from those developed in undefined media (Meynell & Meynell, 1965). In general, published descriptions of bacteria refer to those characters found after growth in complex, undefined media, and because of this the results of biochemical tests do not always correspond with those obtained in defined media.

Media preparation seldom receives the attention it deserves; moreover, the media room is often overcrowded and understaffed, and the conditions in which media-makers work are often among the worst in the laboratory. Complaints about media, whether commercial or home-prepared, are still common and many laboratories have therefore set up internal quality control and assessment procedures (see Chapter 11); others have also made formal arrangements for supervision of media preparation.

In this chapter we discuss the general aspects of media making; formulae for the different media will be found in Appendix A. The majority of the commonly used culture media are now available commercially as dehydrated products, in either powder or tablet form, which are reconstituted by the addition of distilled water and then sterilized in the conventional manner. The manufacturers' directions for reconstitution should aways be followed for the best results. The advantages of dehydrated media include: ease of preparation usually without the necessity for pH adjustment or phosphate removal; batch to batch uni-

formity, which is often greater than with laboratory-prepared media; convenience for the preparation of small quantities; ease of storage; and economy especially in saving time and labour. Against these must be set certain disadvantages. Most of the dehydrated products are hygroscopic but this is usually overcome by the use of plastic or foil sachets containing sufficient for one batch of medium. Dehydration is not suitable for media containing blood, other thermolabile components, or egg. Another consideration where dehydrated media are widely used is that technical staff may not receive adequate training in the principles of media preparation.

Although ordinary media may be used for the growth of obligate anaerobes, better growth usually occurs if the redox potential (E_h) of the medium is reduced before inoculation. Ideally, reduction should be made during preparation of the media, the reduced conditions being maintained during storage and, as far as possible, during inoculation. The specialized techniques used for such 'pre-reduced anaerobically sterilized (PRAS) media' are described fully by Holdeman, Cato & Moore (1977). There are three essential steps in the preparation of PRAS media: (i) driving off dissolved oxygen by boiling, (ii) addition of cysteine, and (iii) flushing with oxygen-free gas and storing in stoppered tubes or bottles containing oxygen-free gas. These media contain an $E_{(h)}$ indicator (resazurin) which is colourless when reduced; if oxidation occurs, it becomes pink, indicating that the medium should not be used. Cysteine inhibits some proteolytic enzymes, and so should not be added to media for tests of this property.

There is little doubt that roll-tube techniques such as those described by Hungate (1969) and Moore (1966) provide one of the best methods for the isolation and study of organisms which are highly sensitive to oxygen. PRAS media prepared in roll-tubes are inoculated in the complete absence of oxygen, and all subsequent manipulations are performed in a stream of sterile oxygen-free gas. The value of this method in some non-clinical areas of anaerobic bacteriology is beyond dispute but it is not universally used in clinical work in the UK, mainly because of the special apparatus and techniques required.

2.1   Media for different purposes

Not all media are intended to encourage the growth of all bacteria; some media are tailored to suit the organism(s) they are able to encourage, and others are deliberately made unsuitable in order to inhibit the growth of certain (specified) organisms.

2.1.1   Isolation media. These may be simple nutrient media containing all essential constituents for growth; in medical laboratories the commonest general purpose medium is Blood Agar, but Chocolate Agar may often be more successful in the isolation of fastidious bacteria. The nature of the specimens received for examination is usually known and, with intelligent anticipation of the probable bacterial flora, media are chosen to suit the nutritional requirements of the organisms which can reasonably be expected to be present. For some bacteria the medium is made from constituents of known composition (that is, a defined medium) but most organisms isolated from clinical material are exacting and need the basal nutrient medium to be enriched or supplemented by substances such as serum, blood, haemin and vitamin K. Thus, media used in medical and veterinary laboratories are rich in unspecified proteins, and they encourage the growth of both wanted and unwanted organisms.

2.1.2   Selective or inhibitory media. When the specimen is from a part of the body (skin, throat, mouth, nose, intestine, vagina) with a natural microbial flora, growth of the normal inhabitants may be inconveniently profuse and the bacteriologist will want to limit or suppress such commensals but at the same time encourage growth of the invaders which, in clinical pathology, are the 'wanted' organisms. For this, selective or inhibitory media are used and as the inhibitory properties may be specific, the media must

be chosen with some particular organism (or group of organisms) in mind. There is no medium exclusively or universally selective for all pathogens, and it might seem that success in isolation depends on accurate prediction of which bacteria are to be inhibited and what requirements are needed for those that are to be encouraged. Since prediction is usually difficult, most workers increase the chances of isolating the organisms wanted by using several kinds of selective media.

2.1.3   Enrichment media. Usually both selective and inhibitory, these are liquid media into which swabs or specimens are placed; after incubation for 6 and 18 hours, subcultures are made to plates of (i) selective, and (ii) non-inhibitory nutrient media (Nutrient Agar, Blood Agar). After incubation these plates are examined and selected colonies subcultured to non-inhibitory media. This second plating is an important step in the isolation process; without it the colonies first subcultured may well yield a mixture of wanted and unwanted organisms. Whenever possible, selective media should be avoided; repeated plating on non-inhibitory media is preferable, although this is a council of perfection seldom satisfied in practice.

2.1.4   Media for the maintenance of cultures. These are simple and should not encourage luxurious growth; Nutrient Agar (in its many formulations) is the commonest (see Lapage, Shelton & Mitchell, 1970). For the preservation of serological characters, Dorset Egg, in spite of its imperfections, seems to be the medium of choice. Robertson's Cooked Meat medium is a good all-round maintenance medium, especially for clostridia.

Simple media, such as Nutrient Broth, containing glycerol, can be used for freezing bacteria at temperatures as low as $-76\,°C$ (Feltham et al., 1978).

2.1.5   Media for determining nutritional requirements or ability to use a single substrate are now being used increasingly in diagnostic work. To avoid chemical contaminants, agar of the highest purity should be used for solid media. When the nutritional requirements of an organism are unknown, omission of one component at a time and substitution of another may be used to identify which substrates

are essential for growth and which can be replaced by others. This is a time-consuming process not used in routine work. But in a simplified form, as in Koser's Citrate medium, a test for the ability to use citrate as a source of carbon is a useful characterizing test for enteric bacteria.

For non-exacting bacteria, a basal medium inadequate for growth of the organism is used and one substrate at a time added to find out whether the organism can use the substrate as a source of carbon or nitrogen. A suitable mineral base of this kind was described by Owens & Keddie (1969) and Cure & Keddie (1973). For the value of these tests, see Snell & Lapage (1973).

Chemically clean glassware is essential for tests used to determine the nutritional requirements of an organism. Dirty glassware can provide nutrients; it may also be contaminated by substances inhibitory to growth (see Appendix A1.1).

2.1.6   Media for bacterial characterization generally consist of a simple but nutritionally adequate base to which the substrate under test has been added. Sometimes an indicator is included to show that a change in reaction has occurred; in other cases reagents are added after a specified period of incubation.

2.1.7   Screening media. These are intended to show at a glance the reactions obtained with several substrates, hence the term multitest media; they can be relied upon only when pure cultures are used. For this reason, the Knox (1949) plate, described as a screening plate, cannot be used for the original specimen but only for subcultures. Some multitest media are better used as a standard, relatively insensitive method for one of the reactions, as with TSI for H₂S production by enterobacteria.

2.1.8   Media for microbiological assay of vitamins and amino acids need stringent control during preparation to ensure freedom from impurities; such media are available from commercial sources. The assay of antibiotics and the sensitivity testing of microorganisms do not need media of such rigid specification and can usually be carried out on ordinary nutrient media, with or without indicator.

2.1.9   Non-nutrient basal media. Occasionally a clear solidifying medium without nutrient properties is useful. Such a medium is needed for the top layer of Chitin Agar, the insoluble chitin being suspended in Water or Salt Agar.

Saline Agar has other uses. Physiological saline solidified with agar may be used to line tubes for the collection of rabbit blood. After the blood has clotted, the agar lining retracts with the clot, and the serum, expressed through the agar, is water-clear. Such serum is anticomplementary.

Non-nutrient media are widely used for transport purposes.

2.2   Media constituents

A fuller account of the derivation and properties of peptone, meat extract, yeast extract, gelatin, agar and bile salts is given in the Special Report of the Society for General Microbiology on constituents of bacteriological culture media (Report, 1956a); the design and formulation of media were reviewed by Bridson & Brecker (1970).

2.2.1   Agar can be obtained as shreds, flakes, granules or powder and is made from certain types of seaweed. The usefulness of its unusual gelling properties for bacteriological work was recognized by Frau Hesse, who suggested its use to her husband, Walther Hesse, an early colleague of Robert Koch (Bulloch, 1938; Hitchens & Leikind, 1939).

When mixed with cold water, agar does not go into solution; it can therefore be washed to free it from soluble impurities. The concentration for use depends on the geographic source of species of seaweed from which the agar is made, and on the purpose for which the medium is intended (Appendix A, Table A5). In this *Manual*, the concentration of agar given in the formulae for media relates to the product derived from Japanese seaweed.

In addition to the agar concentration, other factors affect gel strength; for example, repeated melting of the medium or prolonged sterilization especially at a low pH value will decrease it.

2.2.2   Peptone is a product of varying composition made by acid or enzymic hydrolysis of animal or vegetable protein, from material such as muscle,

9

liver, blood, milk, casein, lactalbumin, gelatin and soya bean. The exact composition depends on the raw material and the method of manufacture.

No two batches of peptone are exactly alike, but commercial firms try to produce peptones in which the measurable constituents are present within certain defined limits. For many kinds of media the make or type of peptone is immaterial, but for certain tests a particular type may be specified. This does not mean that all other types are unsuitable; more often than not it means that other peptones may not have been tried. Certain batches of peptone, however, may be quite unsuitable for a particular purpose, and before general use a peptone should be tested. In the section on media control (Appendix A3) we discuss this problem in more detail and give examples of fallacious results due to the use of unsuitable peptones. Most peptones from reputable commercial sources are equally good.

2.2.3 Meat. Beef heart, muscle, and liver are commonly used but calf brain, veal, spleen, and placenta also have a place in media preparation. The quality of meat and other tissues varies with the age and health of the animal and with the conditions under which it was slaughtered. To minimize variations the preparation of meat media requires extensive quality control, and this may be impracticable for small laboratories. In these circumstances, commercial meat extracts or dehydrated meat media are often more convenient. When meat media are to be used as the basis for fermentation studies, they should be tested for the absence of fermentable carbohydrate.

2.2.4 Meat extract. Commercial meat extracts contain soluble organic bases, protein degradation products, vitamins and minerals. As these extracts are readily available and easy to use they have largely superseded fresh meat infusions, which are both time-consuming to prepare and variable in quality.

2.2.5 Yeast extract is made from bakers' or brewers' yeast and is a rich source of amino acids and vitamins of the B-complex. In culture media it is used to supplement or replace meat extracts. Meat extract (1%) can be replaced by yeast extract (0.3%) in Nutrient Broth without significant change in the growth-promoting capacity.

2.2.6 Blood. The choice of blood is often a matter of convenience and may depend on the animals kept by a laboratory. Horse blood from commercial sources is commonly used, but the blood of other species (man, cow, goat, rabbit, sheep) may be necessary for special purposes; they should be free from antimicrobial agents. Sheep Blood Agar can be used for detecting the different haemolysins of staphylococci and streptococci although bovine blood may give stronger reactions; haemolysis of sheep and human blood may be used also in the identification and biotyping of some species of *Vibrio*. Sodium citrate is inhibitory to staphylococci (Rammell, 1962) as is Liquoid to some anaerobic cocci and *Streptobacillus* (Holdeman & Moore, 1972). In general, defibrinated horse blood is preferable; it should be relatively fresh and should not be used if haemolysed. Blood must be stored in a refrigerator but should not be allowed to freeze; all blood products must be tested for sterility as well as for inhibitory substances such as citrates.

2.2.7 Plasma is used for demonstrating coagulase activity. In medical bacteriology laboratories, human plasma is usually preferred but rabbit plasma may be used. As some bacteria utilize citrate, oxalated plasma is better but citrated plasma may be used when heparin is added (Harper & Conway, 1948). Plasma may be obtained by removing the supernatant of the blood–anticoagulant mixture after the red cells have settled. Blood samples obtained for biochemical examination and containing sodium fluoride or ethylenediaminetetra-acetic acid (EDTA or 'sequestric acid') are to be avoided. Liquid plasma is an unstable product liable to coagulate or to form particles which cause a turbidity or deposit. It should not be filtered. Plasma should be stored in a refrigerator but should not be frozen. Dehydrated plasma is available commercially.

2.2.8 Serum is prepared from blood, collected without addition of an anticoagulant, by removal of the liquid that separates when the clot contracts. Alternatively it may be obtained from citrated plasma clotted by the addition of calcium. Serum should be sterilized by filtration. Horse serum may contain a maltase and an amylase and it is essential that these be inactivated by heat before addition to maltose- or starch-containing media (Goldsworthy, Still & Dumaresq, 1938). Hendry (1938) reported that the maltase was inactivated at 75 °C for 30 minutes but not at 55 °C for 4 hours; Goldsworthy, Still & Dumaresq (1938) recommended heating serum at 65 °C for 1 hour. Horse serum kept at 0–4 °C for a month or longer may show a deposit, believed to contain calcium, lipids and protein (Roche & Marquet, 1935) and this deposit may be mistaken for bacterial contamination.

2.2.9 **Ascitic** and **hydrocele** fluids are preferred to serum by some workers in hospitals. Most laboratories do not use them because they are not generally available.

2.2.10 **Bile** contains several bile acids as compounds conjugated with amino acids; bile acids can also form addition compounds with higher fatty acids and other substances. Bile also contains the pigments bilirubin and biliverdin. Fresh ox bile (ox gall) has been superseded by bile extract, dehydrated bile or bile salts. Bile extract, a dark yellowish-green material, is prepared by concentration of fresh bile, extraction with 90% ethanol, and evaporation of the ethanolic extract. A 10% solution of the dehydrated product is equivalent to fresh bile.

2.2.11 **Bile salts.** Commercial bile salts are prepared by extracting dried ox or pig bile with ethanol, decolorizing the extract with charcoal, and precipitating the bile salts with ether to form a water-soluble yellowish-brown hygroscopic powder. When prepared from ox bile the salts consist mainly of sodium taurocholate and sodium glycocholate with smaller amounts of the sodium salts of taurodeoxycholic and glycodeoxycholic acids. The bile acid conjugates may be hydrolysed by alkali, and it is possible to prepare sodium cholate or deoxycholate in this way, but these substances are not chemically pure. Several workers (Mair, 1917; Downie, Stent & White, 1931) showed that, in selective culture media, deoxycholic acid is the most active component of bile; its effects were studied by Leifson (1935).

2.2.12 **Gelatin** is the protein obtained by extraction of collagenous material from animal tissues, and is available as sheets, shreds, granules or powder. A gelatin of pharmaceutical or edible quality should be used for culture media. When immersed in water below 20 °C, gelatin does not dissolve but swells and imbibes 5–10 times its volume of water. Solution is effected by heating and the solution gels on cooling to about 25 °C. Gelatin has little nutritive value but is used in culture media as a substrate for detecting gelatinase activity. As with agar gels, excessive heating is detrimental and destroys the setting properties.

2.2.13 **Carbohydrates.** Carbohydrates, collectively called 'sugars', are usually used to enrich media to promote growth or pigmentation, and to determine whether organisms can produce acid or acid and gas from them. The carbohydrates generally used are listed in Table A2 (Appendix A), which also includes glycosides and polyhydric alcohols, with concentrations of aqueous solutions suitable for addition to media. The concentration of carbohydrate in oxidation and fermentation studies is usually 0.5–1%; 1% carbohydrate is preferable as reversion of the reaction is then less likely. Some carbohydrate solutions may be sterilized by autoclaving whereas with others decomposition may occur. Durham (1898) recommended steaming for 'sugars' but Mudge (1917) found that maltose and lactose suffered greater hydrolysis when steamed for 30 minutes on each of three days than when autoclaved at 121 °C for 15 minutes. Smith (1932) showed the adverse effect of heat and the accelerated decomposition of glucose and maltose in the presence of phosphate.

Although Whittenbury (1963) found that some lactic acid bacteria differed in oxygen requirements for fermentation in media (i) made up with carbohydrate before sterilization, and (ii) with filtered or autoclaved carbohydrate solutions added to previously autoclaved basal medium, he could not detect any significant difference in the ability of the organisms to utilize the substrate sterilized by the different methods. Such sugar solutions are often sterilized by momentary autoclaving or by steaming but for most purposes it is better to sterilize them by filtration.

We have deliberately omitted dextrin from the list of carbohydrates. White dextrin is generally prepared by heating starch moistened with a small volume of dilute nitric acid and dried at 100–120 °C; it contains up to 15% of starch, the remainder consisting of erythrodextrin. Inferior grades are prepared by roasting starch without acid at 150–250 °C, and have a yellow colour; they are hydrolysed to a greater extent than white dextrin and may contain appreciable quantities of maltose. Because of its variable composition, we do not recommend the use of dextrin. Soluble starch is prepared by treating potato starch with dilute hydrochloric acid until, after washing, it forms a limpid, almost clear solution in hot water; it is insoluble in cold water.

2.2.14   Defined media for studies of bacterial nutrition and carbon source utilization (CSU) tests comprise solutions of mineral salts to which the substrate to be tested is added. For nutritionally exacting organisms, as for example some coryneforms, media such as Mineral Salts Medium E (Owens & Keddie, 1969) may need to be supplemented with 0.02% yeast extract and 2 µg vitamin B_{12} per litre.

2.3   Indicators

Indicators are incorporated in some culture media to give visual evidence of pH or other changes occurring during the growth of bacteria. Indicators for this purpose must be non-toxic in the concentrations used; for example, some batches of neutral red may inhibit growth of *Escherichia coli* in MacConkey Broth or Agar (Childs & Allen, 1953). With some bacteria (e.g. *Actinomyces israelii*), media containing an ethanolic solution of indicator may give better growth than media with aqueous indicator, thus suggesting that the solvent is used as a more readily available carbon source. Where the indicator is prepared as its sodium salt it is preferable to use water as the solvent. Table A1 of Appendix A lists the pH indicators commonly used; the amounts recommended are for the addition of concentrated indicator solutions to culture media and are not necessarily suitable for the colorimetric determination of pH values.

Indicators of oxidation–reduction potential (redox indicators) have limited use in culture media. Examples are methylene blue or resazurin in thioglycollate media and methylene blue in milk (Ulrich, 1944).

The use of tetrazolium compounds such as TTC (2,3,5-triphenyltetrazolium chloride) as indicators of bacterial growth has been advocated, for example, in motility media (Kelly & Fulton, 1953) and in KCN Broth (Gershman, 1961). With bacterial growth, the

colourless reagent is reduced to an insoluble red formazan.

2.4   Sterilization

Sterility implies freedom from all viable micro-organisms including spores so that the term sterilization is strictly a misnomer in relation to the processes to which media or their constituents are subjected. For example, the heat applied during steaming is sufficient to kill only vegetative bacteria; media that appear to be sterile may therefore still contain viable spores of thermophiles that do not grow at the temperatures at which 'sterility' tests are usually carried out (37 °C); and labile constituents of media that are normally kept at about 4 °C may contain organisms that can grow at room temperature but not at 37 °C. Even autoclaving does not provide an absolute guarantee of sterility as the exponential nature of the survival curve means that, during heating, the proportion of organisms surviving per unit of time is constant. The microbiological concept of sterility, however, is well understood and we do not therefore intend to define or qualify the term 'sterilization' other than to say that for culture media the particular method chosen should take account of (i) the likely initial bacterial (and spore) concentration, (ii) the confidence level required for 'sterility' of the final product, and (iii) the need to preserve heat-sensitive constituents.

In contrast, for reasons of laboratory safety, all cultures for discard (including those from environmental samples), as well as infected glassware and plastic containers must be sterilized in the strict sense of the term even though some of the material will ultimately be destroyed by incineration. The use of chemical disinfectants for the disposal of cultures and infected materials should not be permitted; it should be an inviolable rule that all discarded cultures are sterilized by autoclaving.

The lethal action of heat on bacteria depends on both the temperature and the time for which it is applied: the higher the temperature, the shorter the time needed. Sporing bacteria are more resistant to heat than vegetative bacteria but all sporing forms, including different strains of the same species as well as different organisms of the same strain, are not equally resistant (Stumbo, 1973). Some, such as the spores of *Bacillus subtilis*, are killed by a short exposure to 100 °C; others, such as those of *B. stearother-mophilus*, can resist boiling for hours or survive conventional laboratory autoclaving for short times and for this reason have been used as indicators of the efficacy of steam (though not dry-heat) sterilization. To ensure adequate heat-penetration and the destruction of discarded culture, autoclaving must be maintained either for longer times or at temperatures higher than those used for sterilizing culture media. In practice, for sterilization of discarded cultures we use a time–temperature combination of 20 minutes at 121 °C (1.06 kgf/cm^2). Alternatively, 10 minutes at 126 °C (1.41 kgf/cm^2) as sensed within the load is satisfactory for modern autoclaves with 'make-safe' cycles.

2.4.1   Autoclaving. An autoclave is a pressure vessel which must be regarded as a potential hazard and protective clothing should be worn when opening it for unloading. During autoclaving, a temperature above 100 °C is achieved with steam under pressure, the latent heat released in condensation rapidly heating the load to the temperature of the surrounding steam. When all the air has been expelled and the autoclave chamber is filled with saturated steam there is a direct relationship between temperature and pressure (Table 2.1); if any air is present, the temperature will often be lower than that corresponding to the steam pressure.

Overheating is detrimental to most culture media, but autoclaving is the most satisfactory method of sterilizing material or media that will withstand temperatures over 100 °C, the usual temperature–time combinations for most microbiological media being either 115 °C (0.69 kg/cm^2) for 20 minutes or 121 °C (1.06 kg/cm^2) for 15 minutes. As the rate of heat penetration into large containers is slow, especially if they contain agar, small volumes (less than 1 litre) are preferable; when the volume does exceed 1 litre, the time but not the temperature should be increased to aid heat penetration. Containers such as test tubes, flasks and bottles should be of a capacity sufficient to allow a generous head space; containers of Stuart's (1959) transport medium, which should be filled completely, are an exception. For consistent autoclave results, the temperatures within media in standard loads should be established and the loading patterns adhered to strictly. The temperature inside

Table 2.1 *Relation between temperature and pressure of saturated steam at some commonly used autoclaving temperatures*

Temperature	Pressure above standard atmosphere*		
°C	bar	kgf/cm^2	lbf/in^2
100	0	0	0
105	0.21	0.20	3.1
110	0.43	0.43	6.2
115	0.69	0.69	10.0
120	0.98	0.99	14.2
121	1.05	1.06	15.2
125	1.32	1.33	19.1
126	1.39	1.41	20.2
130	1.70	1.72	24.7
134	2.04	2.10	29.6

* 14.7 lbf/in^2 at sea level.
NOTE: 1 lbf/in^2 = 0.0689 bar = 0.07 kgf/cm^2

the autoclave should be allowed to fall to 100 °C before it is vented to the atmosphere and then to 80 °C or below before the door is opened to remove the contents.

The detrimental effects of heat on media begin at about 60 °C and include the decomposition of growth factors; caramelization of sugars; the Maillard reaction between sugars and amino compounds; and pH changes (Peer, 1971). As the lethal effect of heat on bacterial spores increases about tenfold compared with twofold for chemical effects with each rise of 10 °C in temperature, a higher temperature for a shorter time should cause fewer chemical changes in media than a lower temperature for a longer time. Similarly, during cooling, the chemical effects reduce twofold and the lethal effect on spores tenfold for each fall of 10 °C in temperature. These effects thus emphasize the importance of minimizing the heating and cooling times of the autoclave cycle; if possible, steam should be admitted at a high temperature for rapid sterilization and the autoclave cooled to below 80 °C as quickly as possible. Media in small containers (less than 1 litre) will contribute to the speed of heating and cooling (Everall & Morris, 1975).

2.4.2   Momentary autoclaving. A high-temperature, short time (HTST) procedure represents a compromise between sufficient reduction in the number

13

of microorganisms present and the limitation of undesirable side-effects. The heat or steam is turned off as soon as the autoclave reaches the required temperature (e.g. 121 °C) chosen from experience with known media and uniform loads. The valve is opened to vent the chamber to the atmosphere when the temperature in the bottles falls to 100 °C, and the autoclave is unloaded below 80 °C.

2.4.3 Steaming, including Tyndallization,

consists of exposing the medium to the vapour of boiling water in a non-pressurized vessel, though the medium itself seldom reaches 100 °C. Sterilization by steaming may be carried out once only, or on three successive days, when it is a high temperature form of fractional sterilization known as 'Tyndallization'. Sterilization by boiling or steaming may be necessary when media cannot be autoclaved without detriment to their constituents, for example those containing selenite or tetrathionate which are sometimes referred to as 'self-sterilizing'. Many of those that cannot be sterilized by autoclaving are enrichment or selective media used for isolating particular organisms from a mixed flora; in these circumstances, sterility is not always essential.

Tyndallization has limited use in the media department and is suitable only for nutrient media in which spores, if present, can germinate during the intervals between successive steaming. It was originally used for Litmus Milk medium, which was heated at 80 °C for one hour on three successive days. It is a time consuming procedure which has been superseded by autoclaving at 115 °C for 10 minutes.

2.4.4 Inspissation

is a fractional sterilization procedure carried out at a temperature sufficiently high to coagulate serum or other heat-labile constituents such as egg-white and it consists of heating them at 75–80 °C for one hour on three successive days.

An alternative method of inspissation using older autoclaves is described for Dorset Egg medium in Appendix A, but it is not suitable for modern autoclaves fitted with temperature-sensed door-release mechanisms. Other methods for inspissation were described by Levin (1943), Foster & Cohn (1945), Spray & Johnson (1946) and Brown (1959).

2.4.5 Other methods of 'heat' sterilization.

These include the use of dry heat, ultra-violet light, microwave ovens and gamma irradiation, though they each have practical limitations for the sterilization of media. For apparatus and glassware, sterilization in the strict sense can be achieved by dry heat in a hot air oven provided the temperature is raised to and maintained at 160 °C for at least one hour; a higher temperature will char paper and cotton wool.

2.4.6 Sterilization by filtration

Sterilization by filtration has the advantage that it is a process suitable for solutions of thermolabile materials; its disadvantages include the possibility of hidden defects in the filtration apparatus, the need for sterilization of the apparatus before use, the possibility of selective adsorption from dilute solutions and of pH changes, and difficulty in cleaning certain filters after use. Filtration is not just a mechanical sieve-like action depending on porosity and thickness of the filter but is also a complex physico-chemical procedure involving the ionic charge on the filter and the pH of the solution.

Bacterial filters may be made of porous porcelain, kieselguhr (diatomite), sintered glass, or cellulose esters. Doulton and Pasteur–Chamberland candles or cylinders are made of porous porcelain and are available in varying porosities, not all of which are suitable for bacterial filtration. Berkefeld and Mandler filters are made from kieselguhr. Porcelain and kieselguhr filters carry a negative charge.

Sintered or frittered glass filters are available in varying porosities, no. 5 being suitable for bacterial filtration; it is usually available as a 5/3 combination consisting of a no. 5 filter supported on a no. 3 filter for mechanical strength. Sintered metal filters are not widely used in bacteriology as they are not completely inert to the action of materials likely to be found in culture media.

Collodion and asbestos filters have largely been replaced by the more convenient membrane filters composed of cellulose esters, nylon or polytetrafluoroethylene (PTFE), which are stored in the dry state; although cellulose filters are somewhat brittle, they all have good wet strength and may be sterilized by autoclaving.

3
Principles of isolation

3.1   Isolation methods

Isolation begins with the collection of the specimen. Normally the clinician takes the specimen and sends it to the laboratory, but there are occasions when the bacteriologist should go to the patient or *vice versa*, so that fresh material can be examined while 'hot'.

3.1.1   Direct microscopy. Since amoebic and bacillary dysentery cannot be distinguished clinically, it is essential when amoebic dysentery is endemic or is suspected, to examine a freshly passed stool on a warmed microscope stage to see the characteristic movements of vegetative *Entamoeba histolytica*; even better specimens may be obtained at sigmoidoscopy. Only by seeing the movement of *E. histolytica* can it be distinguished from *Entamoeba coli*; the differences between the encysted forms are not sufficiently great or constant to be diagnostic. The serous fluid of a primary chancre collected in a capillary tube can also be examined unstained by microscopy for spirochaetes. Stained material from leprosy lesions usually shows abundant organisms which, as yet, defy the usual cultural methods.

It is usually unrewarding to stain blood films for bacteria, but in hot countries bacteria are not the only causes of fever; malaria parasites and other blood-borne protozoa should therefore always be sought. Pus, cerebrospinal fluid (centrifuged deposit), pleural effusions, and other transudates may show bacteria or other microorganisms when stained by Gram's method; if none is seen, a film stained by the Ziehl–Neelsen (ZN) method may reveal acid-fast rods. Failure to find bacteria is not conclusive and, like other negative results, may indicate simply that the method used was not sensitive enough; Corper (1928) estimated that 100 000 acid-fast bacilli per millilitre

of sputum was the minimum concentration that could be detected by direct microscopy. However Tazir *et al.* (1979) suggested that 90–96% of specimens containing between 30 000 and 50 000 acid-fast bacilli per millilitre and 50–58% of those containing between 2 000 and 5 000 bacilli per millilitre give positive Ziehl–Neelsen stained smears. A negative microscopic result could indicate that the infecting agent was a virus or a mycoplasma. Urethral smears, on the other hand, may be more successful than cultures, and after seeing Gram-negative diplococci, treatment can be started before the results of culture are available. When treatment is started before the specimen is taken, cultures are unlikely to yield growth of gonococci.

To summarize: microscopic examination of all specimens except blood (in temperate climates), faeces, and rectal swabs are always worth making but prolonged and exhaustive microscopic examination for tubercle bacilli does not justify the effort expended on them.

3.1.2   Fluorescent microscopy. The use of fluorescent and immunofluorescent techniques for the detection of particular organisms or bacterial antigens has increased rapidly and greatly improved the chances of early diagnosis. These methods are outside the scope of this *Manual* and the reader should consult, for example, *Fluorescent Protein Tracing* by Nairn (1976).

3.1.3   Cultural methods. With knowledge of the site of origin of the specimen and from examination of stained smears, the clinical bacteriologist is able to anticipate the kinds of organism likely to be present so that the culture media can be matched to the

15

organism(s) expected. Knowledge of the nature of likely contaminating and therefore unwanted organisms is also essential, although it is often true that what is looked for is isolated but the unexpected or unsought organism is missed. Anaerobes should not be regarded as special cases and should be sought in most specimens.

In considering isolation procedures the strategy must start from the nature of the specimen; it is important to know whether it is likely to contain only one kind of organism as in cerebrospinal fluid; several significant species as in many anaerobic infections; or whether, as in material from the oropharynx, gastrointestinal tract and lower female genital tract, the specimen will yield a background of bacteria from which the relevant pathogens have to be distinguished and separated. Specimens from blood and tissues that are normally sterile are inoculated on rich, non-inhibitory media, to isolate all kinds of organisms present. And bearing in mind that not all bacteria grow in air, replicate plates should be made for incubation with added CO_2 and under anaerobic conditions. The specialized techniques used for isolating anaerobes are described in detail in several monographs which give useful laboratory tips based on years of experience (Holdeman, Cato & Moore, 1977; Willis, 1977; Sutter, Citron & Finegold, 1980; Willis & Phillips, 1983, 1988).

In clinical laboratories anaerobic jars provide the usual means of obtaining an oxygen-free atmosphere for the culture of obligate anaerobes. Modern anaerobic jars operate by catalytic removal of oxygen from the internal atmosphere by palladium in the presence of excess hydrogen. A variety of jars is available commercially for both evacuation–replacement methods and internal gas generation. Anaerobic bacteria vary widely in their sensitivity to oxygen and the choice of technique depends to some extent on the aerotolerance of the species sought and on the numbers of organisms present. Many of the anaerobes commonly implicated in human infections are not extremely oxygen-sensitive and are often present in clinical specimens in predominant numbers. Thus, provided careful attention is paid to operational techniques, the anaerobic jar can be relied upon for the isolation of most anaerobic species of clinical significance.

An anaerobic cabinet, equipped with glove ports and a rigid airlock for transfer of materials, provides an oxygen-free environment in which conventional bacteriological techniques can be applied to the isolation and manipulation of obligate anaerobes in conditions of strict and continuous anaerobiosis. Such a continuity of anaerobiosis is intrinsically more efficient than the cyclic operation of multiple anaerobic jars.

A few organisms, notably some of the pathogenic mycobacteria, grow slowly and are best cultivated in screw-capped containers to prevent the medium drying out. *Mycobacterium leprae* does not grow on culture media and knowledge of its presence in tissues depends on microscopical evidence. The leprosy organism will grow in the footpad of the mouse or the nine-banded armadillo; the latter has provided the material for a vaccine.

Although bacteriological culture methods will not isolate viruses, *Mycoplasma* species in specimens will grow from time to time on media containing blood or serum in a closed – but not necessarily anaerobic – jar. When the presence of mycoplasmas is suspected, special media (the so-called PPLO media) should be used for their isolation and propagation; such media are available commercially.

Specimens from areas or sites that have a normal microbial flora cannot be treated so cavalierly. Look at the specimen with an appreciative eye, for it must be inoculated onto appropriate selective media; for example, a loose watery stool and faeces with flecks of blood and mucus should be inoculated onto a number of different media. Experience is the best guide but in its absence several selective media should be used, including the less inhibitory media such as MacConkey or Eosin Methylene Blue (EMB) Agar for faeces from adults and children; for stools from babies use Blood Agar on which the enteropathogenic strains of *Escherichia coli* can be successfully isolated and identified. For enrichment, a large inoculum of the specimen (usually faeces) is placed in about 10 ml of medium such as Tetrathionate or Selenite Broth; after incubation for a few hours subcultures are made to selective (inhibitory) media such as Deoxycholate Citrate Agar (DCA) or Salmonella-Shigella (SS) and to basal or only slightly inhibitory media (MacConkey or EMB Agar). After incubation overnight the plates are examined and colonies selected for subculture to non-inhibitory media. This selection of colonies is not the end of the isolation process as further plating on non-inhibitory media may be necessary to obtain a pure culture suitable for characterization tests. In the absence of good growth on the first plates subcultured from the enrichment medium, further subcultures are made after longer incubation. Enrichment media such as Tetrathionate Broth can also be used as transport media for faeces.

A few points need special attention.

(i) Blood should usually be inoculated into large volumes (at least ten times that of the specimen) of broth containing 0.03 to 0.05% sodium polyanethol sulphonate (Liquoid) or other anticoagulant; incubation should be continued for at least 7–10 days and the broth subcultured at intervals to detect growth. Liquoid may inhibit growth of some anaerobic cocci; Holdeman & Moore (1972) recommend that blood cultures should be inoculated into media with and without Liquoid.

(ii) On first isolation most bacteria grow better in an atmosphere containing 5–10% CO_2 but CO_2-inhibited mutants of *Escherichia coli* and *Salmonella typhimurium* do occur occasionally (Roberts & Charles, 1970). CO_2 is either essential or stimulatory for the growth of many anaerobes and is a well-established supplement to an anaerobic atmosphere. A precise concentration is probably not critical for growth but may be important when a controlled atmosphere is required, as for example in antibiotic sensitivity tests.

(iii) Specimens from patients with suspected gonorrhoea or meningitis should be inoculated on to freshly poured (and undried) Chocolate and Blood Agar plates; when the inoculation of plates cannot be made speedily, the swab or specimen should be put into transport medium (Stuart, 1959).

(iv) Some pathogenic mycobacteria grow slowly and usually not on the standard media used for pyogenic pathogens. Lowenstein–Jensen Egg medium is widely used for the growth of mycobacteria but in some countries Middlebrook Agar (Difco) is preferred. The growth of *Mycobacterium bovis* is enhanced by the presence of sodium pyruvate (Stonebrink, 1961) and *M. johnei* requires an iron chelating agent, mycobactin, which can be supplied by incorporating killed *M. phlei* in the medium (Francis *et al.*, 1953). As incubation will continue for

several weeks the medium should be in screw-capped containers and have plenty of water of condensation (synæresis).

Specimens containing mycobacteria often have a mixed bacterial flora; to isolate the more slowly growing mycobacteria the specimen must first be treated (with acid or alkali, to which mycobacteria are usually resistant) to destroy the more rapidly growing, and less acid- or alkali-resistant, bacteria. After treatment for a short time (usually about fifteen minutes) the acid or alkali can be neutralized before the specimen is inoculated onto appropriate media.

3.2   Importance of pure cultures

Many difficulties in identification are due to the use of an impure culture as starting material. Before an organism can be identified it must be obtained in what we glibly describe as a 'pure culture'. By this we mean the descendants of a single colony obtained after plating the material in such a way that much of the growth consists of well-isolated colonies; it is only an assumption that these have developed from a single organism or a single clump of similar organisms. In routine diagnostic bacteriology a single plating may have to suffice but replating can always be made with advantage, and, as explained below, is essential when highly selective and inhibitory media are used for the primary culture.

A 'pure culture' is one that generally breeds true; this means that when replated, the majority of the daughter colonies will be like the parent, though occasionally (perhaps once in several million times) a bacterial cell will mutate and the colony developing from it will consist of organisms that have changed a character. A 'pure culture' retains its original characters because the chances are, on an ordinary nutrient medium, millions to one against subculturing the mutant, and also because once satisfied that the culture is pure we no longer choose isolated colonies (lest, perchance, the mutant is picked) but subculture from a sweep (or pool) of several colonies.

When two organisms grow together as in an impure culture, one of four things may happen: (i) each organism may grow independently; (ii) one may produce a substance that will enable the other to grow or grow better in the particular medium (synergy);

(iii) one may produce a substance (bacteriocin) that inhibits the growth of the other (antagonism); or (iv) one may grow faster than the other and deprive the second of some essential part of its food supply. In (i) and (ii) characterization of the impure culture would probably yield a summation of characters unless for example one organism produces acid and the other an equivalent amount of alkali to neutralize it. In (iii) and (iv) the characterization will be that of the organism which grows at the expense of the other. In (i) and (ii) an organism A (characterized as X+, Y–, Z–) growing with B (X–, Y+, Z–) in mixed culture (A+B), might be characterized as X+, Y+, Z–, which might be characteristic of a third organism C, and the mixture would inevitably be misidentified.

Often bacteriologists look for a particular organism, such as a shigella in faeces or *Corynebacterium diphtheriae* in a throat swab, and isolations are usually made on selective or differential media which contain substances that inhibit the growth of some (unwanted) organisms. The inhibitory substance(s) does not kill the unwanted organism but merely suppresses or retards its growth on that medium; when an unwanted organism inhibited in this way forms part of a colony made up mainly of the suspected pathogen, subculture to another medium will result either in further suppression of growth, or, in the absence of the inhibitory substance, a resumption of growth in competition with the pathogen sought. From an inoculum of faeces on Deoxycholate Citrate Agar medium a colourless colony (indicating a lactose non-fermenter) is likely to be made up of lactose non-fermenters and a few suppressed lactose fermenters. Subculture to Lactose Peptone Water will allow the lactose fermenters to grow and produce acid from the lactose and, unless the colony is replated on a non-inhibitory medium, the presence of the lactose non-fermenters may be overlooked. A working routine should be developed so that, before a culture is assumed to be pure, colonies from a selective medium are replated on a non-inhibitory and preferably differential medium. Until a culture is known to be pure, it is a waste of time to attempt any characterization tests.

The reader may think that we have laboured the presence of mixed colonies, but experience has shown that many of the cultures difficult to identify are, in fact, mixed and came from colonies on inhibitory media. We cannot stress too strongly the importance of obtaining a pure culture before attempting to identify it. While inhibitory media are the main source of impure cultures, other causes are sufficiently common to warrant mention here. The presence of a 'spreader' on a plate may be difficult to detect; this spreading growth will also cover any discrete colonies on the plate. The most troublesome spreading organisms are members of two genera, *Proteus* and *Clostridium*, and different methods must be used to purify cultures contaminated by them.

Proteus species grow readily on most media but swarming can be inhibited by bile salts and by substances in some of the selective and inhibitory media on which *Proteus* organisms produce discrete colonies. Thus, a culture contaminated by a *Proteus* species can be plated on MacConkey Agar; if, however, the organism sought will not grow on this medium, the contaminated culture should be spread on plates of a richer nutrient medium in which the agar concentration has been increased to 7% (Hayward & Miles, 1943).

It is much more difficult to purify a culture contaminated by a *Clostridium* species. This difficulty of freeing a culture from a clostridial contaminant applies also to separating one *Clostridium* species from another and explains why it takes so long to identify many of them. Since more than one species of this genus may occur in the same material, it is not surprising that the original descriptions of many so-called species of *Clostridium* were based on mixtures of two or more species.

The separation of *Clostridium* species may entail a long series of platings and selection of colonies unless one of the mixture is a pathogen with invasive properties. Such an organism might be isolated from a remote site (e.g. the surface of the liver) when an animal dies after subcutaneous or intramuscular inoculation of the mixed culture in a hind limb. Separation may also be achieved when the spores of the strains in the mixture differ in their resistance to heat or when one of the strains is motile and the other non-motile. The separation of two pathogens may depend on the ability of the bacteriologist to recognize which species (or even which toxin types) are present. Much information can be obtained from *in vitro* tests, such as lecithinase production on Egg-Yolk medium, before going on to *in vivo* tests in animals.

18

The contamination of bacterial cultures by *Mycoplasma* species (pleuro-pneumonia-like organisms) is not believed to be a serious hazard, but our appreciation of these organisms is much less than that of ordinary bacteria, and their presence may escape detection. Mycoplasmas grow slowly and generally only on media enriched with blood or serum, and if they are initially present as contaminants they are likely to be outgrown by the more hardy and less fastidious bacteria. However, they should be borne in mind and their presence suspected if bacterial cultures show inconsistencies on repeated testing. Bacterial cultures that have been isolated on media containing antibiotics or from patients treated with antibiotics, may show 'g', 'L' or other aberrant forms, which may be confused with mycoplasmas because they grow slowly and produce very small colonies.

3.3   Screening tests

Screening tests take various forms and, as improvements are constantly being made, only an outline of their development is given here together with a few references for those who propose to use these diagnostic aids. As the main objective of screening tests is economy of time and material, we start with a statement applicable to all, that, for quick results, heavy inoculation is essential.

The tests are of two kinds: (i) *eliminating*, those intended to identify unwanted and (believed to be) unimportant organisms; and (ii) *presumptive*, those tests that, with media containing several substrates (multitest media), will indicate to which major group an organism probably belongs. Both kinds of screening tests rely heavily on the assumption that the test organism is in pure culture, and this assumption must be made at a time in the isolation and identification programme when the odds are against it.

Eliminating tests are usually quite simple as, for example, the inoculation of urea medium when looking for salmonellas or shigellas; if the urea is hydrolysed that particular culture can be discarded, for it would be a most unusual salmonella or shigella that produced urease. Knox (1949) elaborated on this principle by placing coverslips (to detect gas production) and impregnated test papers on the surface of a plate of multitest medium inoculated with a test organism; from the plate, it was possible to detect H_2S production, mannitol, sucrose, and lactose fermentation, and swarming of the organism. In conjunction with a tube of urea medium the tests covered a wide range; some of the tests, when positive, suggested that the organism was unlikely to be a pathogen and that the culture could be discarded. Lányi & Adám (1960) combined the impregnated paper discs of the Knox plate with a selective basal medium so that colonies from the primary plate could be used as inocula; deoxycholate in the medium prevented interference by many organisms likely to be present in cultures of faeces.

The elimination of any culture carries the risk of loss of a rarely encountered organism or one that may be an unrecognized pathogen; this is the penalty for discarding primary plates before investigations are completed. The moral is never to discard a specimen or primary plate until all tests have been completed and the identification made satisfactorily. This may seem a counsel of perfection but most of us learn it by bitter experience; and it did lead to the discovery, among other things, of penicillin by Fleming (1922).

Presumptive identifications can be made by inoculating media containing several substrates and one or more indicator(s). Some of these media contain inhibitory substances so that a colony from a selective medium can be used as inoculum, but most multitest media require the inoculum to be a pure culture. By a judicious choice of indicators and substrates, multitest media may show a sufficient range of colour or other changes to make a preliminary allocation of the test organism to a major group or subdivision. Multitest media and methods only justify themselves when they are both quick and accurate so that effort can be concentrated on cultures showing the reactions of established pathogens; to use multitest media to make the final identification is indefensible. But by eliminating unwanted organisms, workers in busy laboratories should have time to investigate the presumptive pathogens by the more informative and reliable tests described in Chapter 4.

Because lactose fermentation was believed to be of paramount importance, Russell (1911) put ten times more lactose than glucose in his double-sugar medium. Kligler (1917, 1918) introduced lead acetate to the medium, which was blackened when sufficient

H$_2$S was produced. In another variation, substituting mannitol for lactose, Kligler & Defandorf (1918) claimed to be able to distinguish the Shiga from the Flexner dysentery bacillus. To increase the differentiating power still further, Kendal & Ryan (1919) experimented with various combinations of sugars and ended with two double-sugar tubes which included glucose, lactose, sucrose, and mannitol. Other combinations and the addition of other substrates to bring in more characters have followed, and another two-tube test (Kohn, 1954 as modified by Gillies, 1956) became popular for the screening and presumptive identification of intestinal pathogens. Kligler's Iron Agar (1917, 1918) formed the basis of TSI (Triple Sugar Iron Agar) which was apparently developed simultaneously but independently by Sulkin & Willet (1940) and by workers in the Difco Laboratories (*Difco Manual*, 1953). Although TSI was introduced as a multitest medium it has become an unofficial standard for H$_2$S production at the low degree of sensitivity that has differential value among enteric bacteria.

Screw-capped containers, which do not allow volatile products to escape and so may affect the colour of indicators, are not particularly suitable for multitest media (Marcus & Greaves, 1950).

Most multitest sloped media are intended for use in the identification of enterobacteria; others are aimed at detecting pathogenic vibrios (Hsu, Liu & Liao, 1964), and Chapman (1946, 1952) described some for identifying staphylococci. Multitest media have been exploited commercially especially for the identification of enterobacteria, which are not only common and widely distributed but are easily identified and placed in their major groups by simple biochemical tests. Many schemes or systems have been marketed in the USA, Europe and the Far East, though few have had more than a fleeting popularity.

Identification methods that rely heavily on prelimi-nary screening on multitest media should not be used; it is far better to work with pure cultures on agar slopes and use them to inoculate all the media needed to make an identification. There are many disadvantages in multitest media, not least the possible interaction of one chemical reaction with another; acid produced from a fermentable sugar may inhibit the blackening of the iron indicator in TSI medium (Bulmash, Fulton & Jiron, 1965), and ammonia produced from peptone may inhibit urease production (Stewart, 1965). There may also be interference in biochemical reactions, as nitrite interferes with the detection of indole when tested by some of the older methods (Smith, Rogers & Bettge, 1972).

3.4 Rapid tests

In the previous edition of this *Manual*, single substrate and rapid tests which could be used for screening were described. Clarke & Cowan (1952) developed a series of micromethods in which constitutive and induced enzymes in heavy suspensions of bacteria acted on the test substrate in a buffered solution. They believed, together with Manclark & Pickett (1961), that bacterial characterizing tests should be carried out as far as possible in such a way so that the organism acted on only one substrate in each test. This view has since been confirmed by the many different rapid methods which have been marketed commercially since the API system was first described by Buissière & Nardon in 1968. Despite some early discrepancies with conventional test results (Smith, Rogers & Bettge, 1972), these rapid characterization tests have now become an integral part of the routine in many laboratories, either as short sets for screening purposes, as with enterobacteria, or as extensive sets for species identification, as with the genus *Bacillus*. In view of their importance and widespread use, we discuss them more fully in Section 4.6.

4
Bacterial characters and characterization

Features such as brightly coloured pigments may be characteristic of a few species as well as a good pointer to the nature of the organism and its ultimate identification. But pigments may mislead, as in the Biblical case of bleeding polenta which is no longer considered to be a miracle but a phenomenon that can be produced experimentally by a bacterium and in nature is commonly produced by a yeast (Merlino, 1924; Gaughran, 1969; Cowan, 1956a, 1970b). As bacteria present few gross diagnostic features they must be looked at closely; the characters sought and the tests applied will depend on knowledge and expertise as well as experience with similar organisms; the approach to identification will be conditioned by professional training and intuitive skill. The observations made and the tests applied are aimed at characterizing the organism so that it can be described (the technical term for the list of characters is a description) and compared with descriptions of other, previously identified and classified organisms.

4.1   Bacterial characterization

The difference between characterization for classification and for identification lies not so much in the tests themselves as in the emphasis placed on the results of the tests. Although it is not universally accepted, most taxonomists now support the Adansonian concept that, for classification, equal weight should be given to each character or feature. The relationships between strains can be calculated and expressed as similarity either of positive characters (Sneath, 1957b) or by taking account of both positive and negative features (Hill et al., 1961; Floodgate, 1962; Lockhart & Hartman, 1963); the results of such comparisons can be analysed labori-

ously by making a large number of calculations, or more easily by letting a computer do the hard work (Sneath, 1978).

We accept the Adansonian concept for classification, but for identification we attach much weight to some characters, regarding them as having great distinguishing value; we give less weight to others, and no weight at all to some features. Excessive weighting is given to coagulase production by staphylococci; heavy weighting is placed on the urease and phenylalanine deaminase systems in identifying *Proteus* and *Providencia* species, and on urease in distinguishing between *Alcaligenes faecalis* and *Bordetella bronchiseptica*. Little emphasis is placed on gelatin hydrolysis or liquefaction by staphylococci or micrococci but more weight is given to the same test among the enteric bacteria or the pseudomonads. The variable weighting attached to these characters is largely based on experience but it is always hoped that the assimilation of data from a wide range of bacteria will, in the future, enable the value of a feature to be expressed in a quantitative manner; this has already been done for the Enterobacteriaceae by Edwards & Ewing (1962, 1972) and more recently by Farmer et al. (1985).

If everyone had ready access to a computer, an almost unlimited number of characters or features could be used, but with tables we are restricted by memory and limited by our ability to recognize similarities and differences when making multiple mental comparisons simultaneously. Because of these limitations a mechanical aid (named the Determinator) was developed by Cowan & Steel (1960, 1961) and tables suitable for use with it were constructed. The original Determinator was restricted by its size to about twenty-five features, but in the simplified form this limitation was removed and, in theory at least, fifty or more features could be included in the tables. Few ever used this device, but the tables, which can be used by simple inspection, led to the development of this *Manual* and indirectly to a more elaborate mechanical device for the identification of enterobacteria (Olds, 1966, 1970). By selection and weighting the number of features used in the individual tables was restricted, and the identification made in stages. At one time Cowan & Steel intended to make tables with the smallest number of tests essential for identification. In the event each second-stage table includes sufficient detail to provide an adequate, but not exhaustive, characterization.

4.2   Choice of characters

In choosing characters for the tables we prefer those that seem to be most constant and tests that give the most reproducible results. Unfortunately, nearly all tests are influenced by factors that are difficult to control, and it is therefore difficult to specify standard methods. All we can do is to recommend that the materials used (media and reagents) should be controlled as far as possible (see Appendix A) and that environmental factors, such as temperature and the duration of incubation, should be standardized. Various workers have discussed the choice of characterizing tests and methods, and each has their own preference. Sneath & Johnson (1972) suggested statistical methods by which the influence of test error on the correctness of identification could be measured; they estimated that within one laboratory (where the error is likely to be least) test error will be about 5% and they considered that a test with a laboratory error greater than 10% would not be suitable for taxonomic work. We would emphasize the desirability of keeping to the same method of doing a test so that its idiosyncrasies and difficulties become known, and, within the one laboratory, the results become reasonably comparable. We have made innumerable comparative tests but could seldom say unequivocally that one method was better than all the others. To keep the results reasonably comparable we chose certain methods and these became our laboratory standards. Often the choice of method was a compromise between two, sometimes conflicting, demands: firstly to know the truth, and secondly to be able to distinguish between two otherwise similar organisms. It is essentially a compromise to express qualitatively (as positive or negative) what is really a quantitative reaction. An example is the production of hydrogen sulphide; when an organism is grown in a medium with an adequate sulphydryl content, and a sensitive indicator (lead acetate paper) is used, the ability to produce even small amounts of H_2S can be detected, but the method is not discriminatory and the results are useless for distinguishing between those salmonellas that produce much and those that produce only a little H_2S. However, with a medium deficient in −SH compounds and with a poor indicator (ferrous chloride), only an organism with great ability to produce H_2S is positive in the test.

Sometimes a test is carried out by different methods when dealing with different groups of organisms. Again taking H_2S production as the example: in the genus *Brucella* the organisms are grown on a medium rich in −SH compounds and lead acetate papers are changed each day so that the result of the test can be expressed as 'H_2S produced on the first two days' or 'from the 1st to the 5th day'. We do not know of any other group of organisms in which this technique is used, and its application to other groups might give information of value. On occasions it is thus essential to indicate the method to be used to obtain the results given in a table.

4.3   Characters not used in the tables

Before describing the characters chosen for use in the tables, we think we should state our reasons for omitting some time-honoured characters and tests. Certain features are not used in the diagnostic tables because they are subjective; for example, the smell of staphylococci growing on agar media is unmistakable but also indescribable. The recognition of the finer shades of pigments is a subjective observation; we try to keep to the primary colours and avoid such indefinite subdivisions as, for example, coral red and sky blue.

We do not ususally describe colony morphology as this will vary with the medium on which the organism is grown and, except with bacteria such as *Corynebacterium diphtheriae* var. *gravis*, is seldom sufficiently characteristic to have diagnostic value.

22

We do not consider that the descriptions of cultures on agar slopes are worth much, and we rarely pay any attention to the type of growth in broth except to note the presence or absence of a pellicle. In a few cases (e.g. *Bacillus anthracis*) the type of growth in gelatin stab cultures is characteristic, but the inverted fir-tree growth can only be seen when the gelatin columns are deep and the cultures are incubated at about 22 °C. On the whole we pay little attention to the type of liquefaction of gelatin and are content to record the test as 'gelatin liquefied' (positive) or 'not liquefied' (negative).

Thus, in this *Manual* there are no diagrams of the different shapes, edges, surfaces, and elevations of colonies, or of the shape of liquefaction seen in gelatin stab cultures; the elimination of these relics of early bacteriology makes unnecessary a glossary of descriptive terms that now have but limited use. However, lest we should be accused of too biochemical an approach to classification and identification, we must state our belief that cell morphology and thus microscopy does have an important place in characterization.

We do not describe serological techniques since the role of serology in classification and identification lies chiefly in the finer subdivisions used for epidemiological purposes. For those who wish to pursue serological analysis we recommend the monographs by Kauffmann (1954), Edwards & Ewing (1962, 1972), and Ewing (1986). The latter are essentially practical treatises and contain such relevant and important details as the identity of the best strains to use for immunization and absorption. However, as the primary subdivision of the streptococci depends on the serological method of grouping introduced by Lancefield (1933) and as this is used in Table 6.3b, we describe the methods of preparing extracts of streptococci necessary for this test in Appendix C.

We do not describe fluorescence microscopy or fluorescent antibody (FA) methods as they are now subjects in themselves. We suspect however that not all laboratories have the necessary equipment and expertise available to use them. Those who want guidance should consult reviews by Cherry & Moody (1965), Georgala & Boothroyd (1968) and Nairn (1976).

4.3.1 Antibiotic sensitivity. To clinicians, the sensitivity of an infecting organism to antibiotics that can be used therapeutically is clearly important. Hence, antibiotic sensitivity tests have become an important part of the clinical laboratory routine and there is a tendency to regard the results of these tests, expressed in an antibiogram, as valuable characteristics for the identification of an organism. Although it is possible to say in general terms that certain species are sensitive or resistant to a particular antibiotic, sensitivity to antibiotics is not a character that has much diagnostic value among the bacteria of medical interest, and with occasional exceptions (e.g. the resistance of most campylobacters to nalidixic acid), the antibiogram has only a minor part to play in identification work. In the case of obligate anaerobes, however, sensitivity to metronidazole is a valuable diagnostic character which serves to distinguish anaerobes as a group from aerobes and facultative organisms (Tables 6.1 and 7.1). While an unusual antibiogram can point to a misidentification (Abrams, Zierdt & Brown, 1971), the list of sensitivities and resistances of a strain from a treated patient may simply reflect the effectiveness or failure of treatment. And, since strains which become resistant *in vivo* do not usually change their other characters (Brown & Evans, 1963), the deletion of the antibiogram removes only a highly variable character from consideration when the identification is made.

Non-fermenting and non-saccharolytic Gram-negative rods belong to groups of bacteria that have so many negative and so few positive characters that it is tempting to accept the antibiogram as a useful tool, if only as an auxiliary one (Pedersen, Marso & Pickett, 1970; Gilardi, 1971b). We think that this has limitations when trying to identify such strains from patients, for the possibility of resistance developing as a result of treatment, or from the influence of transfer and resistance factors (Garrod, Lambert & O'Grady, 1981) must not be overlooked. So, although the antibiogram is important and should be reported to the clinician, it should play only a small part in the preliminary characterization and description necessary for accurate identification of organisms isolated from man and other animals especially if they have been treated with or fed antibiotics. However, sensitivity or resistance to antibacterial agents or antibiotics, especially if they are not used for treatment or included in animal foods, can be helpful in the preliminary screening and differentiation of certain organisms or groups of organisms: for example the sensitivity of pseudomonads and many vibrios to the pteridine derivative O/129, the sensitivity of most anaerobes to metronidazole and the resistance of most campylobacters to nalidixic acid.

4.4   Primary tests used in the tables

When the tables for this *Manual* were first prepared, the Gram reaction was used as the starting point with morphology, fundamental reactions such as ability to grow in air, catalase and oxidase production, and the method of carbohydrate breakdown, for subsequent subdivisions. One advantage of a table is that several characters of different groups can be seen simultaneously and compared, whereas this is not possible with the genealogical type of chart or dichotomous key. We were surprised to find that most bacteria could be placed in a genus or small group of genera by using the results of a limited number of selected tests.

4.4.1   Gram reaction.
Gram did not describe a stain but a method in which he used stains and solutions devised by others; to this day its mechanism is not fully understood, but we do know that the Gram reaction is a stable characteristic of a bacterium. Gram positivity (the ability to resist decolorization with ethanol or acetone) is a feature of relatively young bacterial cells of some species; as they age, the cells lose this characteristic and apparently become Gram-negative. It is important, therefore, to examine young cultures, preferably before the end of the logarithmic phase of growth. Genuinely Gram-negative bacteria do not retain the first stain which is easily removed by the decolorizing agent. Thus, as in many other tests, a positive finding (in this case retention of the purple stain) has much more significance than a negative result which may, in fact, be false due to (i) the age of the culture, or (ii) excessive decolorization with powerful solvents such as acetone. There are many variations of Gram's staining method (and each works well in the hands of those who practise it); the one we use under the name of Lillie's modification is simple and gives good results but, as acetone is used, the decolorization can be overdone. A modification by Preston & Morrell (1962) is claimed to be foolproof. Recently, a rapid paper-strip method has been marketed for distinguishing between Gram-positive and Gram-negative organisms though it has doubtful practical and no taxonomic value.

4.4.2   Morphology
is affected by the medium on which the organism is grown and by the temperature of incubation. Organisms are typical and in their most natural state in young cultures; in wet, unstained preparations, they are best observed by phase-contrast or dark-ground microscopy. Such examination will show not only the shape(s) of organisms but, when prepared from suitable material (see Section 3.3.5), will show motility if it is present, and whether the cells remain rigid (as in most bacteria), flex (spirochaetes), or glide (cytophagas). The distinction between spheres (cocci) and rods (bacilli) is not always clear-cut, and genera such as *Acinetobacter* and *Moraxella* cannot be placed categorically in one morphological group. Although it is usual to describe organisms of both these genera as either coccobacilli or short rods, electron micrographs clearly show the coccal nature of some acinetobacter strains (Thornley, 1967). Baumann, Doudoroff & Stanier (1968b) found that the differences in morphology of these genera corresponded with the growth phase: plump rods in the logarithmic phase and coccoid forms in the stationary phase. Brzin (1965) described what she called a sphaeroplasting effect, in that prolonged incubation of '*Acinetobacter anitratus*' (*Acinetobacter calcoaceticus*) strains at 37 °C produced polymorphism.

Bizarre-shaped cells may suggest particular genera and the presence of clubs or dumb-bell forms will call for staining by methods such as those of Neisser or Albert or with Loeffler's methylene blue, capable of showing metachromatic granules.

Electron microscopy is still not yet available in all diagnostic laboratories and without it the site of insertion of bacterial flagella cannot be determined accurately. Fortunately such information is not often needed for the identification of motile bacteria, and we use it only for the genus *Campylobacter* for which the simple flagella stain of Kodaka *et al.* (1982) is recommended. Scanning electron microscopy seems to have special advantages in the identification of the actinomycetes (Williams & Davies, 1967).

4.4.3   Acid fastness is shown when an organism resists decolorization by strong acids or mixtures of ethanol and mineral acid; this is characteristic of a few bacteria and when positive is diagnostic of mycobacteria. Nocardias are sometimes acid-fast but seldom resist the vigorous decolorization which mycobacteria successfully endure. The 'hot' staining method of Ziehl–Neelsen (Ziehl, 1882; Neelsen, 1883) is usually used to demonstrate acid fastness but 'cold' staining methods are also used (Aubert, 1950), as well as fluorescent techniques with auramine or rhodamine.

4.4.4   Spores are stained by a modification of Moeller's (1891) method (itself a modified Ziehl–Neelsen method) in which ethanol is used for decolorization. The staining method is simple and seldom causes difficulty but young spores do not resist decolorization and they may or may not take up the counterstain. For clostridial spores, the malachite green method of Schaeffer & Fulton (1933) is preferred. In older cultures some bacilli may shed their spores so that in rod-shaped bacteria unstained areas occur and the stained spores may lie free of the cells from which they developed. As an alternative to staining, phase-contrast microscopy may be used. An indirect method of demonstrating the presence of spores is to show that a culture can survive heating at 80 °C for 10 minutes.

A problem that faces the bacteriologist is the tendency for sporing organisms to lose the ability to produce spores. The asporogenous state may be permanent, or it may be a temporary reaction to a particular environment, when a change of medium or temperature of incubation could suffice to restore the strain's ability (or need) to form spores. Subculture to a starch-containing medium, such as Potato Agar, is often successful in restoring the ability of an aerobe to form spores; in other instances a deficiency of manganese in the medium may be the cause of the asporogenous state and the remedy is a supplement of 'trace elements'. Often the cause is unknown and the best general advice, based on the restoration of many asporogenous strains of *Bacillus* in the National Collection of Type Cultures to the sporing state, is to use a medium containing 'soil extract' (Appendix A2.6.35).

The meaning of the term 'spore' in bacteriology has been the subject of much discussion. As a purist,

R. E. Buchanan (see also Cross, 1970) insisted that bacterial spores were 'endospores' formed actively within the bacterial cell in contrast to the 'fragmentation spores' of *Nocardia* species. But most bacteriologists do not regard the nocardias as a sporing organism, and we think that the simple word spore tells us all we need to know about it. As we understand the bacterial spore, it is a body resistant to heat and disinfectants that is formed by relatively few bacteria; of the animal pathogens the only sporing bacteria are members of the genera *Clostridium* and *Bacillus*. Historically, anaerobic spore-forming bacteria were important in war wounds; their occasional involvement in a wide variety of clinical syndromes is, however, now recognized.

Sterilization techniques are checked by including spore suspensions in drums containing dressings and gloves; some spores are more heat-labile than others, and spores of a resistant species (usually of *Bacillus stearothermophilus*) are used. After sterilizer tests, the spore suspensions returned to the laboratory should be incubated at about 50 °C and the cultures observed for at least a week. It is important to identify any strain that appears to survive sterilization; a mesophilic spore-former would suggest post-sterilization contamination.

In connection with the acid-fast and spore-forming characters of organisms, certain other problems need to be discussed. Should every culture be stained by Ziehl–Neelsen's and Moeller's methods or tested for heat-resistance, or should these tests be restricted to Gram-positive organisms or to those cultures which, from their morphology, colony form, rate of growth, and other characters, we suspect may be acid fast or able to produce spores? We do not know of any Gram-negative bacteria that are genuinely acid fast and it is therefore reasonable to omit the Ziehl–Neelsen stain for Gram-negative organisms. Should we stain all cultures for spores and, failing to find them, try again after further cultures on Soil Extract Agar or other spore-encouraging media? We know that these tests are not done as a routine and, as the majority of cultures will show negative results, we do not suggest that the search for sporing forms need be made in every case. All we would stress is that when spores are not looked for, a mental note should be made that they have not been excluded, and that their possible presence should be borne in mind.

4.4.5 **Motility** may be studied in a hanging-drop or other wet preparation. Some strains are only sluggishly motile when first isolated; motility may be speeded by using Craigie's technique (Craigie, 1931; Tulloch, 1939) in which the organism is inoculated into a central tube of sloppy agar and, after incubation, a subculture is made from those organisms that, by their motility, have migrated outside the central tube. Motility may be inferred by observing the spreading growth in a semisolid agar (Tittsler & Sandholzer, 1936) which may be seen better when a tetrazolium dye is incorporated in the medium; as the organisms grow the dye is reduced, and the medium changes colour (Kelly & Fulton, 1953). The temperature of incubation is important; most motile organisms are motile at lower temperatures (e.g. 15–25 °C) and may not be motile at the temperature (e.g. 37 °C) optimal for growth.

The problem pertaining to motility is: should all strains be tested or only rods? If we only examine the rods we shall overlook the motility of many strains of *Enterococcus (Streptococcus) faecium*, of *Micrococcus agilis*, and other cocci. When these tests become part of the daily routine they do not take up much extra time; they are only time-consuming and upsetting of routine when they are 'special tests'. These remarks refer to the motility shown by aerobic organisms; anaerobes present special problems in that motility will be inhibited by the air present in hanging-drop preparations. Capillary tube preparations, sealed at each end, from cooked meat cultures, are more likely to show motility in clostridia.

Some bacteria (cytophagas) are motile by a gliding movement and special media and techniques are necessary to observe it. This type of movement is affected not only by the concentration of agar in the medium, but also by the concentration of peptone. Such organisms are not likely to be found in pathological specimens because the methods used by medical bacteriologists are not suitable for showing this gliding motility. Lautrop (1961), Halvorsen (1963) and Piéchaud (1963) thought that they had found a similar motion in '*Bacterium anitratum*' (*Acinetobacter calcoaceticus*) and *Moraxella lwoffii* (*Acinetobacter lwoffii*), but this was not true gliding motility and the organism should be regarded as non-motile (Lautrop, 1965).

4.4.6 **The ability to grow in air** is a character shared by all bacteria except anaerobes and strict microaerophiles such as campylobacters; it is a feature needed in Table 6.1 for the identification of certain anaerobes (especially *Clostridium perfringens*) in which spore formation may be difficult to show, and which, without this character, would appear to be placed among the lactobacilli, corynebacteria, or other Gram-positive rods. Failure to grow in air may be due to a deficiency of carbon dioxide, and growth in an atmosphere of air with added CO_2 should be attempted. Three important clostridia, *Cl. histolyticum*, *Cl. tertium* and *Cl. carnis*, grow mod-erately well in air and are regarded as 'facultative aerobes'.

All these difficulties can be largely overcome by relying on the universal sensitivity of anaerobes to metronidazole. Both aerobes and facultative anaerobes (whether CO_2-dependent or not) are uniformly resistant to metronidazole under anaerobic conditions.

4.4.7 **Ability to grow under anaerobic conditions** is fairly widespread among bacteria but as it is not universal the knowledge that an organism cannot grow under these conditions can be diagnostically important. Some of these organisms are strict aerobes, others may need carbon dioxide for growth. In contrast the ability of some *Bacillus* species to grow anaerobically can also be diagnostically useful.

4.4.8 **Carbon dioxide requirement**. An incubator in which the concentration of CO_2 can be regulated or an anaerobic jar from which the appropriate amount of air is evacuated and replaced with CO_2 are necessary for defined conditions; if these are not essential, a candle jar can be used which gives an atmosphere of about 2.5% CO_2 and 17% O_2 (Morton, 1945); for anaerobes, a CO_2 gas-generating kit in an anaerobic jar yields a final atmosphere of CO_2 (10%) and hydrogen in the absence of oxygen.

4.4.9 **The catalase test** is simple and seldom causes difficulty, but because some strains of lactobacilli, pedicococci, and a few strains of *Enterococcus (Streptococcus) faecalis* appear to form catalase, Gutekunst, Delwiche & Seeley (1957) questioned the validity of the test 'as an overriding classification feature'. False catalase reactions by some lactobacilli grown in low (0.05%) concentrations of glucose (Dacre & Sharpe, 1956) are due to an azide-insensitive, non-haem catalase (pseudocatalase) and can be avoided by using media with 1% glucose without added haematin (Whittenbury, 1964).

A few species (e.g. *Aerococcus viridans*) produce a weakly positive reaction which may easily be missed by those looking only for strong reactions. Gagnon, Hunting & Esselen (1959) described a simple method in which some of the growth of the organism under test was spread on discs of filter paper and dropped into 3% H_2O_2; when catalase was present the evolution of gas quickly brought the discs to the surface. Alternatively, a commercial paper-strip method is available for the detection and measurement of hydrogen peroxide production (Appendix C1.17).

Those who work with mycobacteria have different criteria for the catalase test; the methods are semi-quantitative and positive results are graded by the height of the column of bubbles in a standard test (see Appendix C3). Another method, the catalase drop test, can be used for rapid results.

To reduce the danger from aerosols, as with cultures of *Yersinia pestis*, Burrows, Farrell & Gillett (1964) stab-inoculate agar containing 0.5% H_2O_2 and, using low power magnification, look for effervescence; if a disinfectant that lowers surface-tension (e.g. cetrimide, 0.5%) is added to the agar, the oxygen bubbles persist longer and further reduce the danger from aerosols.

4.4.10   The oxidase test was first used to demonstrate colonies of *Neisseria* species in mixed cultures (Gordon & McLeod, 1928; McLeod *et al.*, 1934; McLeod, 1947), but following the test devised by Kovács (1956) it is now used also to distinguish pseudomonads from the enteric bacteria. When precautions are taken to avoid oxidation of the reagent, the test is sensitive and useful in classification and identification (Steel, 1961). Leclerc & Beerens (1962) use a technique similar to Kovács' but substitute the more stable dimethyl for the tetramethyl compound. Brisou *et al.* (1962) suggested a modification of Kovács' method that is said to make the result of the test more clear-cut and easier to read. In the USA the term 'cytochrome oxidase' is used for the reaction, and the methods recommended are those of Gaby & Hadley (1957) and Ewing & Johnson (1960), which are less sensitive than Kovács' method.

Tests for oxidase resemble those for H_2S in that methods differing in sensitivity can be used; as in the H_2S test, greater bacterial differentiation can be obtained by using a method of low sensitivity. Steel (1962b) found Kovács' method too sensitive for staphylococci, some of which gave weak or delayed reactions; he obtained taxonomically more helpful results by using Gaby & Hadley's (1957) method, with which all staphylococci were oxidase negative. However, with the description of many more species of staphylococci (e.g. *S. sciuri*), this is no longer the case.

4.4.11   The Oxidation–Fermentation (OF) test. To find out whether the attack on carbohydrates is by oxidation or by fermentation, the OF test is done by growing the bacterium in two tubes of Hugh & Leifson's (1953) medium; in one tube the medium is covered with a layer of soft paraffin (petrolatum). It is important to use a solid form as liquid paraffins cannot be expected to give comparable results. Oxidizers show acid production in the open tube only; fermenters produce acid in the paraffin-covered tube and, starting from the bottom, in the open tube. The usual sugar included in the Hugh & Leifson medium is glucose but, because of the occurrence of organisms which do not seem to attack glucose but break down other sugars (Hugh & Ryschenkow, 1961; Koontz & Faber, 1963) the need for a test using the basal medium with maltose or pentoses should be considered. Park (1967), who had some indefinite results in a modified Hugh & Leifson medium, developed a simple test to show that the glucose had been utilized and was no longer present in the medium.

The OF basal medium may be used for all the 'sugar reactions' needed to characterize bacteria (Gilardi, 1971a). Various modifications to the medium have been suggested, including a useful peptone-free medium by Board & Holding (1960); to avoid confusion we do not use the term 'Hugh & Leifson test', but prefer the more descriptive term Oxidation–Fermentation (OF) test.

With the OF test three points deserve mention. (i) The organism may not be able to grow in the Hugh & Leifson type medium, in which case the test must be repeated using a basal medium enriched with 2% serum or 0.1% yeast extract. (ii) The organism may grow but not produce acid in either tube. This result should be confirmed by inoculation of Park's (1967) modified Hugh & Leifson medium containing glucose. (iii) Leifson (1963) found that bromothymol blue was toxic to some bacteria, and modified the OF medium for marine organisms.

The OF test is one of the most important tests carried out in the early stages for identification of aerobic bacteria. Most genera are composed of bacteria that either oxidize or ferment glucose; when a genus contains some species that attack glucose by oxidation and other species by fermentation, there would seem to be good reason to reconsider the taxonomy of the genus and the desirability of dividing it.

Some organisms do not appear to be able to attack a sugar readily, and often show acid production only after several days of incubation. Lederberg (1950) found that this delay was due to failure of the sugar to reach the inside of the bacterial cell, and the ONPG test (Section 4.5.35) was devised to reveal quickly the potential fermentative power of these 'late lactose fermenters'.

4.5   Secondary tests used in the tables

These notes give some background information about the secondary tests used. Details of special media used for the biochemical tests are given in Appendix A; the reagents and methods are described in Appendix C.

4.5.1   Acetylmethylcarbinol production. The Voges–Proskaüer or **VP test** can be carried out in many ways and with almost any desired degree of sensitivity. It is now generally thought that the older methods (Harden & Norris, 1912) are too slow and insensitive, but there is less agreement about the method to be recommended or the sensitivity that gives the best differentiation between taxa. Although Clark & Lubs (1915) specified 30 °C for the test, the MR and VP tests were often carried out on cultures that had been incubated at 37 °C. For many years, water bacteriologists recommended 30 °C (Report, 1956b) and we now know that some enterobacteria such as *Hafnia* often give a negative VP result at 37 °C but a positive reaction at 30 °C or lower. In a comparative trial it was found that incubation for 5

days (at 30 °C) was the minimum time needed to detect by Barritt's method (1936) all the positive results among the enterobacteria (Cowan & Steel, 1964); for other organisms (e.g. staphylococci) longer incubation up to 10 days gave a greater number of positive results. Others have reported that acetylmethylcarbinol (acetoin) may be broken down and used as a carbon source by various coliform organisms (Linton, 1925; Paine, 1927; Ruchhoft *et al.*, 1931; Tittsler, 1938), *Bacillus* species (Williams & Morrow, 1928) and staphylococci (Segal, 1940). Taylor (1951) found that O'Meara's (1931) fumarate medium prevented the breakdown of acetylmethyl carbinol by soft-rot bacteria and allowed it to accumulate.

Outside the field of enteric bacteria it has been found that phosphate may interfere with the production of acetoin; Smith, Gordon & Clark (1946) recommended a medium in which the phosphate is replaced by NaCl, and Abd-el-Malek & Gibson (1948b) used a simple glucose peptone broth without added salt or phosphate. Cowan & Steel (1964) compared Glucose Phosphate Broth with the media recommended by Smith, Gordon & Clark and by Abd-el-Malek & Gibson, and they came to the conclusion that Glucose Peptone Broth was the most suitable medium for *Bacillus* and *Staphylococcus* and Glucose Phosphate Broth was best for the enterobacteria and most other organisms.

After comparing different methods for the VP test for many years, Cowan & Steel (1964) chose Barritt's (1936) method as a satisfactory standard; the sensitivity was found to be mid-way between O'Meara's (1931) and Batty-Smith's (1941) methods. For a useful review of the VP test see Eddy (1961). It should be noted, however, that commercial kits usually employ pyruvate as the substrate for the VP test; this is more sensitive and yields more positive reactions than with Glucose Phosphate Broth, especially with streptococci.

4.5.2   Aesculin hydrolysis is a test of value for streptococci, many anaerobic genera and some other organisms. The glycoside aesculin contains molecules of the aglycone 6,7-dihydroxycoumarin and glucose; hydrolysis of aesculin may be demonstrated in one of two ways. The usual method is to incorporate the glycoside in a nutrient base together

with a ferric salt; aesculin hydrolysis is indicated by a brown coloration due to reaction of the released aglycone molecule with the iron. In addition, hydrolysis of aesculin, which is naturally fluorescent in UV light, can be confirmed by the loss of fluorescence, thus obviating possible confusion with pigment-producing organisms. Alternatively, utilization of the related glucose portion of the aesculin molecule by the organism can be detected by acid or acid and gas production.

4.5.3   Bile solubility is used to distinguish pneumococci from the viridans types of streptococci; however, the test is not specific for *Streptococcus pneumoniae*. The pneumococcus differs from other streptococci in having an autolytic enzyme which can be demonstrated by allowing a digest broth culture to age in the incubator; at 24 hours the broth is turbid but after a few days the medium becomes clear owing to lysis of the bacterial cells. Bile and bile salts activate the autolytic enzyme, and thus speed up cell lysis. They will not, however, produce clearing of a heat-killed culture or one that is too acid; the suspension to be tested should therefore be about pH 7.2. At one time crude bile was used for the test but the isolation of various bile salts in a pure state showed that certain of them were more active than others (Downie, Stent & White, 1931). Sodium deoxycholate is satisfactory and can be obtained in a reasonable state of purity.

4.5.4   Buffered single substrate (BSS) tests are, as their name implies, attempts to avoid the usual biochemical tests made in complex media with the concomitant risk that metabolic products may interfere with the specific reactions under test. The risk is real and is most obvious in sugar reactions tested in peptone-containing media on organisms that oxidize carbohydrates; for example, as long ago as 1955 Pickett showed that brucellas were able to produce acid from several sugars in an otherwise inert milieu.

Various methods have been used to exploit the BSS principle; tablets containing substrate and buffer (Hoyt, 1951; Pickett & Scott, 1955; Hoyt & Pickett, 1957) were dissolved in small volumes of water, steamed, and the solutions heavily inoculated with the test organism. As the biochemical tests were carried out within a few hours, the results probably

depended on the presence of preformed enzymes. The micromethods of Clarke & Cowan (1952), which largely depended on preformed enzymes, had the disadvantage that the preparation of the heavy suspensions of test organisms involved too many manipulations for use in a routine laboratory.

Pickett (1970) and Pickett & Pedersen (1970b) have developed a series of tests (or rather of test surroundings) in which the organism can act on one substrate at a time; the principle is applied to sugar reactions, decarboxylases, deamidases, and hydrolases. The tests are particularly useful for characterizing non-saccharolytic bacteria and those that oxidize carbohydrates – the so-called non-fermenters. We should point out that characterizations based on BSS tests will not always be the same as those made by conventional methods, nor will they match the characters shown in most of our tables (cf. Tables 7.6a,b).

4.5.5   A positive CAMP test, described by Christie, Atkins & Munch-Petersen (1944), is the production of a clear zone around a colony in an area of a blood agar plate that has been affected by staphylococcal β-toxin; this bald statement needs amplification, for the clearing takes place only on blood agar made with sheep or ox blood, and not on media made with human, rabbit, horse, or guinea-pig blood. The important point in carrying out this test is that the agent produced by the bacterial cells must come in contact with the sheep (or ox) red cells before the staphylococcal β-haemolysin. The test is almost specific for strains of *Streptococcus agalactiae* from man or animals; Christie, Atkins & Munch-Petersen (1944) failed to find any other streptococcal species that produced the clear zone, but some haemolytic strains of groups E, P, and U give positive CAMP reactions (Shuman *et al.*, 1972). *Pasteurella haemolytica* also gives a positive reaction (Bouley, 1965). A modified CAMP test utilizing a culture of β-haemolytic group B streptococci on horse Blood Agar is of value in the identification of strains of *Cl. perfringens* which produce α-toxin (Gubash, 1978, 1980).

Fraser (1961) described a somewhat similar synergistic haemolytic effect that may occur when *Corynebacterium ovis* and *C. equi* are grown together on Blood Agar made with washed blood cells from sheep but not from the horse. Unlike the CAMP phenomenon this observation does not seem to have led to the development of a useful specific diagnostic test.

4.5.6 Carbohydrate breakdown.

The division of bacteria into fermenters, oxidizers, and non-utilizers by the OF test of Hugh & Leifson (1953) is one of the most heavily weighted of the primary tests used in the progressive system of identification in this *Manual*, and carbohydrate utilization also features in the secondary tests. The latter so-called 'fermentation tests' were used by early bacteriologists to distinguish one organism from another and elaborate diagnostic tables were based on them (see, for example, Castellani & Chalmers, 1919). The introduction of the simple inverted inner tube for gas collection (Durham, 1898) and the use of pH indicators enabled the production of gas and acid to be detected by inspection. Screw-capped bottles and tubes are not satisfactory for sugar tests because the CO_2 evolved by the bacteria during growth is trapped and, by lowering the pH value of the medium, may change the colour of the indicator and suggest a (false) positive result. If screw-capped containers are used, the caps should therefore be loosened about an hour before the indicator colour is observed.

Too much emphasis is possibly placed on bacterial differentiation by the reactions of individual sugars (apart from glucose; Section 4.4.11). In classification by numerical methods the composition of taxa is essentially the same whether or not the sugar reactions are included in the characters analysed (Focht & Lockhart, 1965). In the genus *Acinetobacter* acid production from several sugars is mediated by a non-specific aldolase (Baumann, Doudoroff & Stanier, 1968*b*).

The failure to standardize methods has led to discrepant results in the hands of different workers, and it is only within recent years that taxonomists have given adequate thought to the significance of acid production by a bacterium growing in a medium containing a carbohydrate. Peptones are also present in such a medium and, during growth of the organism, these are broken down to substances that are alkaline in reaction; if, in the medium, there is a carbohydrate, alcohol, or other substance commonly called a 'sugar' that can be broken down by the bacteria either by oxidation or by fermentation, acid will be pro-

duced, but it will be detected by a pH indicator in the medium only when the acid produced from the sugar exceeds the alkali from the peptone. The visibility of the reactions is also influenced by (i) the buffering properties of the medium, and (ii) the indicator used; for example, bromthymol blue shows acid production when the pH value falls to 6.0 or less, whereas bromcresol purple does not change colour until the pH has fallen to about 5. Peptone Water Sugars, which are commonly used in the UK, have less buffering power and yield less alkali than the broth-based sugars used extensively in the USA and elsewhere. With Peptone Water Sugars we prefer Andrade's indicator (which becomes pink at about pH 5.5) or bromcresol purple (yellow at about pH 5), and it is fortunate that in these media the enterobacteria give similar results to those with broth-based sugars containing bromthymol blue (yellow at about pH 6.0).

With apparently non-saccharolytic bacteria the results obtained in peptone-containing sugar media may be misleading in assessing their carbohydrate-attacking ability because a small amount of acid produced will be masked by the breakdown products from peptone. Pickett (1955) and Pickett & Nelson (1955) overcame this difficulty by using buffered peptone-free media; with cresol red as indicator they showed that acid was produced from several sugars by the apparently 'non-fermenting' *Brucella* species. The development of these methods (Pickett, 1970) is outlined in Section 4.5.4. Another method to reveal the acid-producing potential of '*Acinetobacter anitratus*' (*Acinetobacter calcoaceticus*) (Stuart, Formal & McGann, 1949) and of slow lactose-fermenting coliform organisms (Lowe & Evans, 1957) is to increase the carbohydrate concentration to five or even ten per cent. A peptone-free modification of the Hugh & Leifson (1953) OF medium has been suggested (Board & Holding, 1960; Holding & Collee, 1971) in which acid production correlates well with utilization of glucose; it can be used for aerobic, oxidizing bacteria, and also for bacteria that require additional growth factors.

Some bacteria will not grow on simple media and need an enriched sugar medium. Many streptococci and corynebacteria are grown in media containing serum; neisserias in media enriched by serum or ascitic fluid; and haemophilic bacteria in sugar media to which X and V factors have been added.

Organisms that oxidize sugars do not readily show acid production when they are grown in tubes of liquid media, and more reliable results are obtained when they are grown on the surface of solid media, thus exposing the organisms to an adequate supply of air. Oxidizers such as *Pseudomonas* species do not give reliable 'sugar reactions' on peptone-containing media and they should be grown on media with an ammonium salt as the main nitrogen source. Smith, Gordon & Clark (1952) used ammonium salt sugars (ASS) for their work on *Bacillus* species, some of which ferment and others oxidize carbohydrates. Bacteria may be grown on peptone-containing broth and then centrifuged and resuspended in water or saline so that, when added to a buffered solution of carbohydrate, the bacterial enzymes act on a single substrate (see, for example, Davis, 1939; Clarke & Cowan, 1952; Le Minor & Ben Hamida, 1962).

Snell & Lapage (1971) compared four methods of detecting glucose breakdown, one of which was positive only when all the glucose had been utilized. Peptone water sugars gave the fewest positive results and the ammonium salt sugars the most; a modified OF medium (Park, 1967), tested for residual glucose, gave results almost as good as those with ASS. Snell & Lapage (1971) confirmed that *Pseudomonas maltophilia* could attack glucose when methionine, an essential growth factor, was added to the ASS medium, thus showing that it was suitable, when supplemented, for testing fastidious bacteria.

Carbohydrate fermentation by anaerobes can be demonstrated in liquid media incubated under anaerobic conditions although gas production alone is unreliable as an indicator since it is often evolved also from proteins. As anaerobiosis decolorizes pH indicators, it is usual to add them after incubation.

Many anaerobes do not grow satisfactorily in ordinary liquid sugar media, and it is necessary to use an enriched basal medium for fermentation tests. The horse blood agar plate-fermentation method of Phillips (1976) is consistently successful, giving rapid and unambiguous positive or negative results.

4.5.7   Carbon source utilization (CSU) tests are used extensively in classification work; their application to identification is limited mainly to tests for the utilization of citrate. The mineral basal medium used by Owens & Keddie (1969) for studies on nitrogen nutrition can be used for the CSU tests; it may be supplemented when necessary with an amino acid mixture or with yeast extract (0.02%) and vitamin B_{12} (2µg/litre).

Gordon & Mihm (1957) used organic acids as carbon sources in the basal medium described in Section A2.6.8. But relatively few CSU tests are used in routine diagnostic laboratories, although commercial kits are available for non-fermenters and yeasts.

Citrate utilization is tested in Koser's (1923) citrate medium or in a similar medium solidified by agar (Simmons, 1926). Vaughn et al. (1950) believed that the addition of agar invalidated the test. The medium must be in chemically clean tubes (see Appendix A1.1). In tests of this kind the inoculum should be small and free from medium on which the organism has grown. To avoid carry-over, use a straight wire instead of a loop, and inoculate from a dilute suspension in water, saline or buffer. All growth should be confirmed by subculture (again using a straight wire) to another tube of the same citrate medium.

Other citrate media, such as Christensen's, contain additional nutrients and do not test the ability of the organism to use the citrate radical as the sole carbon source. An organism growing in Koser's or Simmons' medium will grow on Christensen's medium, but one growing on Christensen's medium may not grow on the other two media (but see Piéchaud & Szturm-Rubinsten, 1963).

4.5.8   Chitinolytic activity can be shown as a clear halo around growth on Chitin Agar. As chitin is insoluble in water a purified preparation is suspended in Salt (for halophiles) or Water Agar and layered on a base of Nutrient Agar (Appendix C3.11).

4.5.9   The coagulase test was developed from observations that certain staphylococci clotted plasma from the goose (Loeb, 1903), man, horse, and sheep (Much, 1908); Gratia (1920) introduced the name staphylocoagulase for the active agent. At least two substances, bound and free coagulases, are concerned, but the tube methods for carrying out the coagulase test do not distinguish between them; the slide test (Cadness-Graves et al., 1943) detects bound coagulase. A growing number of commercial preparations are available for testing coagulase production, including both bound and free forms.

The type of plasma used in the test may affect the result; the anticoagulant should not be citrate alone for this will be removed by citrate-using bacteria such as 'Klebsiella aerogenes' (K. pneumoniae subsp. aerogenes) (Harper & Conway, 1948) or certain streptococci (Evans, Buettner & Niven, 1952), with the result that a clot will form after prolonged incubation and give the (false) appearance of a delayed positive coagulase test. Harper & Conway (1948) recommended that heparin should be added to citrated plasma to prevent clotting of fibrin when the citrate is withdrawn. A filterable coagulase-like factor produced by some streptococci will not clot heparinized plasma (Wood, 1959). The species of animal from which the plasma is derived is important: for staphylococci of human origin, plasma from man or rabbit should be used; sheep and bovine plasma give fewer positive results and guinea-pig plasma gives even fewer. When strains from animals other than man are under test, it is advisable to use plasmas from several animal species, including the one from which the strains were isolated.

The coagulase test is simple, so simple that there are almost too many ways of doing it. Williams & Harper (1946) compared many of these methods, including that recommended internationally for testing for free-coagulase (Subcommittee, 1965), and those given in Appendix C 3.12 are based on their conclusions as well as our own experience. We draw attention however to a few important points. Occasionally a strain will be isolated that produces so much fibrinolysin early in its growth that a clot from coagulase action never becomes visible. Sometimes a small clot forms early but lyses quickly; for this reason a reading should be made an hour after starting the test. Some strains produce only small amounts of coagulase and the clot may only be seen after overnight incubation. Each batch of plasma should be tested to confirm that it is suitable for the coagulase test; filtered plasma is generally unsuitable. Positive and negative controls should be included in the tests put up each day. The use of fibrinogen was investigated by Cadness-Graves et al. (1943) and was found to be a suitable substitute for plasma. Reconstituted dried plasma can also be used (Colbeck & Proom, 1944).

4.5.10 Decarboxylases for amino acids are characteristic for different bacterial groups among the Enterobacteriaceae (Møller, 1954a, c). Initially the determination of the decarboxylases was a research problem but Møller (1955) developed simpler technical methods so that the decarboxylase pattern became a useful taxonomic tool at a higher level than antigenic structure. The method is not specific for decarboxylation and may indicate other metabolic processes such as deamination, deamidation, and transamination (Cheeseman & Fuller, 1966); however, these distinctions are not made in this *Manual*. Glutamic acid decarboxylase, which is characteristic of *Escherichia*, *Shigella*, *Providencia*, *Morganella* and *Proteus*, cannot yet be determined simply, but arginine dihydrolase, and lysine and ornithine decarboxylases can now be detected readily by observing the colour change of an indicator. Falkow (1958) introduced even simpler tests but they were not satisfactory with klebsiellas; they cannot therefore be used with organisms of unknown identity. Arginine is hydrolysed by some but not all streptococci and corynebacteria (Niven, Smiley & Sherman, 1942); methods of detecting arginine hydrolysis by pseudomonads are described by Sherris et al. (1959) and Thornley (1960). Steel & Midgley (1962) found the decarboxylase patterns of different genera and species taxonomically useful. Møller's methods are not always satisfactory with the non-fermentative bacteria, and BSS decarboxylase tests (Pickett & Pedersen, 1970b) may give a greater number of positive results.

4.5.11 Denitrification. Many bacteria isolated in medical and veterinary laboratories are denitrifiers, that is, they not only reduce nitrate to nitrite but also reduce nitrite to nitrogen gas. This in itself upsets the reading of the nitrate reduction test (see Section 4.5.31 and Table 4.1). The gas may be detected in an inverted inner (Durham) tube in Nitrate Broth or in the butt of slopes of the Fluorescence-denitrification (FN) agar medium of Pickett & Pedersen (1968).

4.5.12 Deoxyribonuclease (DNase) can be shown by growing the test organisms as streaks on or as stab-inocula in a medium (either defined or complex) containing DNA, and after incubation for 36 hours, flooding the plate with 1 N-HCl. A clear zone around the growth indicates DNase production. The temperature of incubation may be important. Jeffries, Holtman & Guse (1957) advise incubating at several temperatures as the enzyme may act at a temperature other than that for optimum growth; with *Bacillus megaterium* they obtained zone sizes of 0.2 cm at 37 °C, 0.5 cm at 30 °C, and 0.9 cm at 25 °C. Alternatively, decolorization of toluidine blue or methyl green by the breakdown products of DNA is a sensitive and suitable method for organisms such as campylobacters and staphylococci (Gilardi, 1978). The presence of DNase is often used in clinical laboratories for the presumptive characterization of *Staphylococcus aureus*, either as well as or instead of coagulase for presumptive pathogenicity.

4.5.13 Digestion of meat, inspissated serum, Dorset Egg medium or casein are used as indicators of proteolytic activity. At one time gelatin liquefaction was used to detect proteolysis, but gelatinase is not a true proteolytic enzyme.

4.5.14 Ethylhydrocuprein or **optochin inhibition** of pneumococcal growth was described by Moore in 1915, but as a diagnostic test it has had a chequered career. Soon after its introduction it fell into disrepute and, as a means of distinguishing pneumococci from viridans streptococci, it was superseded by the bile solubility test, especially when the more highly purified bile salts became available (Downie, Stent & White, 1931). The optochin test has since come into its own again in the form of absorbent paper discs impregnated with ethylhydrocuprein for direct application to inoculated plates (Bowers & Jeffries, 1955; Bowen *et al.*, 1957). In the concentration recommended by Bowers & Jeffries for direct application to inoculated plates, a small zone (1–2 mm beyond the disc) of inhibition may occur with a few viridans streptococci but pneumococci are inhibited more obviously with zones extending to 5 mm or more. The advantage of the optochin test over bile solubility is that the disc can be applied to any plate culture of the organism under test, whereas for bile solubility the suspension or broth culture must be of about neutral pH value. If small zones of inhibition are ignored and 5 mm is the minimum zone recorded as positive, the specificity of the optochin test for the pneumococcus is high. Bowers & Jeffries (1955) found that only one of 243 pneumococci failed to be inhibited; the exception was found to be avirulent for mice and was thought to be in the R form (though R pneumococci are bile-soluble).

4.5.15 Biochemical tests in enriched media. Delicate or fastidious organisms are often grown in media enriched with serum or other supplements which can introduce uncontrolled and uncontrollable side-effects. Whenever such supplements are used the enriched medium (without the test substrate) should be used as a control. For example, Cobb (1966) reported that *Corynebacterium bovis* produced ammonia from Christensen's urea medium supplemented with 3% serum. In a control experiment he found that the organism produced acid from the basal medium without urea (the basal medium contained glucose); when urea was present the test culture produced an alkaline reaction, confirming that alkalinity (the positive urease indicator) of the test was due to urea breakdown.

An alternative method of dealing with fastidious organisms is to culture them on a suitable medium, wash off the growth with water or saline, centrifuge it, resuspend in water and use the suspension in a BSS test (Section 4.5.4). In this way *Haemophilus influenzae* has been shown to produce a powerful urease (Sneath & Johnson, 1973). Similarly, *Helicobacter pylori* was described as urease-negative until Langenberg *et al.* (1984) showed that it gives a rapid reaction in a BSS test with Christensen's urea broth.

4.5.16 Gelatin hydrolysis or **liquefaction** is shown by a test in which the organism grows in a nutrient medium solidified by gelatin; the disadvantages of the liquefaction test are that: (i) different samples of gelatin vary in gelling power; (ii) the cultures are incubated at a temperature (22 °C) below the melting point of the medium (about 25 °C) so that mesophilic organisms may grow very slowly or not at all; (iii) some bacteria will not grow in the medium. To overcome the second of these difficulties the cultures may be incubated at the optimal temperature for growth and later refrigerated to see whether the gelatin has retained its gelling property; uninoculated medium incubated in parallel acts as a control.

Gelatin stab cultures may need weeks of incubation before showing liquefaction. Hucker (1924*a*), working with micrococci, found a curious relationship between the length of incubation and the first appearance of liquefaction; when the number of liquefying strains was plotted against duration of incubation there were two peaks, one after about 1–2 weeks, and the second after about 3 months. The significance of tests of such long duration is doubtful (the gelatin may be denatured) and they are quite useless in identification work. However, the gelatin stab test should not be discarded; some species will liquefy it overnight, others will take longer, and these differences may be helpful in distinguishing between species such as *Enterobacter cloacae*, which takes a week or more, and *Serratia marcescens*, which liquefies gelatin in 1–2 days. For identification work the duration of incubation must be limited to a reasonable period, and one of the rapid methods should be used in parallel. Frazier's (1926) test has the advantage that the gelatin is in agar and the medium does not melt at 37 °C. After growth of the organism, the plate is flooded with an acid mercuric chloride solution which reacts with the gelatin in the medium to produce an opacity; where gelatin has been hydrolysed the medium remains clear. Frazier's (1926) method is preferred for anaerobes though it is now considered safer to use 30% trichloracetic acid instead of the acid solution of mercuric chloride.

A rapid method devised by Kohn (1953) uses gelatin–charcoal discs hardened by formaldehyde; these do not melt at 37 °C and can be added to Peptone Water cultures, which are then returned to the incubator; preformed or induced enzyme will hydrolyse the gelatin and liberate the charcoal particles. Lautrop (1956a) found that the action of gelatinases was influenced by the presence of calcium ions and recommended that test organisms should be suspended in physiological saline with 00.1 M-CaCl$_2$. Greene & Larks (1955) devised an even quicker micromethod in which Kohn's discs were used (Appendix C3.23). Thirst (1957b) and Hoyt & Pickett (1957) developed microscope-slide techniques which were similar to one described by Pickford & Dorris (1934), who found that the gelatin of photographic plates and film could be removed by proteolytic enzymes and bacteria. LeMinor & Piéchaud (1963) describe a method in which the silver sulphide of exposed and developed film can be seen to be released when the gelatin is liquefied.

4.5.17 Gluconate is converted by some bacteria to 2-ketogluconate, which can be detected by the appearance of a reducing substance in the medium.

Haynes (1951) found this test helpful in identifying *Pseudomonas aeruginosa*. Shaw & Clarke (1955) simplified the test and reported that it was useful for klebsiellas. When *Klebsiella* species were compared with *Enterobacter*, Cowan et al. (1960) found that klebsiellas with IMViC reactions − − + + and *Enterobacter* species were gluconate-positive, but klebsiellas with other IMViC reactions were often gluconate-negative.

4.5.18 Growth or failure to grow on specified media can indicate (i) nutritional needs; (ii) sensitivity or insensitivity to substance(s) in the medium; and (iii) ability to use a specified compound as source of a particular nutritional factor. Examples of the characters revealed are: (i) growth on Blood Agar but not on the basal medium indicates a need for enrichment with blood; (ii) (a) failure to grow on MacConkey Agar, accompanied by growth on Nutrient Agar, shows sensitivity to bile salts; (b) growth on media containing 6.5% NaCl shows an unusual degree of salt tolerance; (iii) failure to grow on Koser's Citrate medium shows that the organism cannot use citrate as a carbon source under the test conditions. These utilization tests must be adequately controlled to prevent carry-over from the medium on which the inoculum was grown (see Citrate utilization, Section 4.5.7).

4.5.19 Haemolysin production and **haemolysis** are not always cause and effect; the ability to produce a soluble haemolysin is not necessarily associated with zones of haemolysis on Blood Agar plates (Elek & Levy, 1954). Streptococci produce haemolytic zones on the surface of Blood Agar made from the blood of most animal species and these organisms are rightly named haemolytic streptococci. The haemolysins produced by streptococci may be oxygen-labile (streptolysin O) or oxygen-stable (streptolysin S) and they need different conditions for their production; on Blood Agar plates, however, they produce similar zones of haemolysis. Streptolysin O is an antigenic extracellular protein; streptolysin S is non-antigenic, cell-bound and requires for its release a 'carrier' agent contained in serum or starch. Brown (1919) studied the nature of the haemolytic zones around streptococcus colonies in poured plates and labelled the types of haemolysis α (green zone, cell envelopes intact), β (clear, colourless zone, cell envelopes disrupted) and γ (no action on red cells). The term γ-haemolysis is an anachronism for 'non-haemolytic' and describes a negative result. The application of the terms α and β has been extended to the haemolytic zones seen around bacterial colonies on the surface of Blood Agar, and though not in strict accord with Brown's usage, it is a convention that is well understood and is included in Table 6.3*b*.

The β-haemolysis seen on Blood Agar plates is usually due to streptolysin S: some strains of *S. pyogenes* produce only the O haemolysin and are consequently non-haemolytic on Blood Agar unless incubated anaerobically. Streptococci that produce α-haemolysis or green zones on Blood Agar are often described as 'greening' or 'viridans' streptococci. The species name '*Streptococcus viridans*,' previously attached to several different kinds of greening streptococci never adequately characterized, is not now used. Indeed Sherman (1937) applied the epithet usefully to describe the 'viridans' group of streptococci which are commensal rather than pathogenic. *Streptococcus mitior* is probably most representative of the organisms previously named '*S. viridans*'. Many of the viridans streptococci are unable to break down the hydrogen peroxide which they produce and this may contribute to the 'greening' phenomenon on Blood Agar medium as well as interfering with haemolysin activity and affecting their viability.

Staphylococci behave differently on plates made with the blood of different animal species and it is misleading to speak of haemolytic staphylococci because the haemolysis may be due to a haemolysin or to a lipolytic enzyme (Orcutt & Howe, 1922). The soluble haemolysins can be used to detect the toxins produced by some strains of staphylococci; thus rabbit cell haemolysin is one manifestation of α-toxin, and sheep cell 'hot–cold' lysin is a characteristic of β-toxin. These toxins are not used in characterizing different species of *Staphylococcus* and so do not appear in the diagnostic tables.

As with staphylococci, the haemolytic activity of the different haemolysins produced by strains of *Clostridium* depends partly on the species of red cells used. Thus, the α-toxin of *Cl. perfringens*, which is a 'hot–cold' lysin, is relatively inactive against horse erythrocytes, but is highly lytic for sheep red cells. The θ-toxin (oxygen-labile haemolysin) of *Cl. perfringens*, however, is strongly haemolytic for the erythrocytes of both these animals. Because some of the clostridial haemolysins are species-specific, these toxins could be used to show the finer subdivision of the genus. Synergistic haemolysis on horse blood agar by α-toxin-producing *Cl. perfringens* and β-haemolytic group B streptococci forms the basis of the so-called CAMP test for the confirmation of *Cl. perfringens* (Gubash, 1980). The haemolytic activity of certain vibrios has some distinguishing value when tested with special media containing red blood cells from particular animal species (Sakazaki, Tamura & Murase, 1971; Barrett & Blake, 1981).

4.5.20   Hippurate may be hydrolysed to benzoate by bacterial action, and the ability to do this is limited to certain bacteria, for which it is an important characteristic. The end product is tested for by the addition of ferric chloride, which precipitates both hippurate and benzoate but the hippurate is more readily soluble in excess. The final concentration of iron is critical; to find the optimal amount of $FeCl_3$ required, uninoculated tubes of medium, on which a titration can be made, should be incubated with the test cultures.

The methods of Ayers & Rupp (1922) and Hare & Colebrook (1934) for streptococci use a relatively rich basal medium in which the organism will grow without hippurate. The Hajna & Damon (1934) method for coliform organisms uses Koser's medium (without citrate) as a base and so becomes a test of the organism's ability to use hippurate as a source of carbon as well as its ability to hydrolyse it. Thirst (1957*a*) added an indicator so that the growth may be seen more readily.

The rapid test of Hwang & Ederer (1975) was originally described for group B streptococci, but it is a convenient method for campylobacters.

4.5.21   Hydrogen sulphide production by bacteria is such a common feature that, of itself, it has little differential value. The H_2S test is one that can be made as sensitive as required (for a review see Clarke, 1953*a*); with an adequate sulphur source (cysteine) and a delicate indicator (lead acetate papers) almost all the enteric bacteria can be shown to be able to produce H_2S. Tested in this way an accurate estimate can be obtained of an organism's catabolic power in relation to sulphur compounds, but it is not possible to distinguish readily between those organisms with much and those with little ability to produce H$_2$S. With a poor medium or a less sensitive indicator (ferrous chloride or lead acetate in the medium) only the strong H$_2$S-producers are detected. This kind of test of low sensitivity allows clear distinctions to be made between *Escherichia* and *Salmonella* and even between different salmonellas. Two media yield results of this kind: Ferrous Chloride Gelatin and Triple Sugar Iron Agar (TSI). Both are recommended by the international Enterobacteriaceae Sub-Committee (Report, 1958) and their formulae are given in Appendix A. Lead acetate papers are not only ten times more sensitive than lead acetate in the medium, but they eliminate the toxicity of lead for the growing bacteria (ZoBell & Feltham, 1934). In the *Brucella* group the time of H$_2$S production may be significant; this is found by changing the lead acetate papers each day.

4.5.22 **Indole** is volatile and can be detected either by testing the medium with *p*-dimethylaminobenzaldehyde or by a paper strip impregnated with oxalic acid held near the mouth of the container by the cap or stopper. Both methods are sensitive and usually give the same result; occasionally all the indole volatilizes and only the paper strip is positive. Extraction of the indole from the liquid culture increases the sensitivity of the test; ether, xylol and petroleum have been used, but all are potentially dangerous if, following the usual bacteriological techniques, the mouth of the tube is flamed. Kovács' (1928) reagent has the advantage that the solvent (amyl alcohol) is present in the test solution. Oxalic acid papers (Gnezda, 1899; Holman & Gonzales, 1923) and papers soaked in *p*-dimethylaminobenzaldehyde (Kohn, 1954) are both sensitive indicators for indole.

Temperature of incubation may affect the result; Taylor (1945–6) found three strains of *Escherichia coli* that were indole-negative at 37 °C but positive at 30 °C. Some organisms (e.g. *Clostridium* species) may break down indole; Reed (1942) found that with some species this happened so slowly that indole could always be detected in cultures 1–10 days old, but *Clostridium sporogenes* used it so quickly that it gave negative results when cultures were grown for only one day in a medium containing 1 mg indole per 100 ml broth.

Unless indole has previously been extracted with xylol, sodium nitrite present in broth may interfere with its detection by Ehrlich's or Kovács' reagents (Smith, Rogers & Bettge, 1972).

4.5.23 **Inhibition of bacterial growth** by a defined or a biological agent may be a useful identifying characteristic and is used in several of the tables; it occurs in different forms, ranging from inhibition by chemicals such as KCN or dyes to inhibition by bile salts or antibiotics. Inhibition by KCN (Appendix C3.32), optochin (C3.22) and the pteridine derivative O/129 (C3.41) are described in the sections indicated.

Commercially available antibiotic discs keep pace with prevailing fashion; they are available as single discs containing different amounts of antibiotic and as 'rings' with multiple discs for several antibiotics or different concentrations of them. Antibiotic sensitivity results are clearly important clinically but have only limited potential in helping to identify the organism isolated (see Section 4.3.1).

4.5.24 **The KCN test** distinguishes those bacteria that can grow in the presence of cyanide and those that cannot grow in the stated concentration. When a strain is reported as KCN positive it means that it grows in Møller's (1954b) KCN medium and that it is therefore resistant to the concentration used. KCN-negative strains, i.e. those that do not grow, should be subcultured to the basal medium without KCN; if they cannot grow in the basal medium the test is without significance. Møller (1954b) used waxed corks to prevent loss of cyanide from the tubes; these are unpleasant to handle and the use of small screw-capped bottles is preferable (Rogers & Taylor, 1961).

Those who use the test assume certain responsibilities for safety; KCN and HCN are extremely toxic and the KCN solution should be kept in a locked cupboard. After use, the cyanide in the medium should be destroyed by adding ferrous sulphate and alkali before the tubes or bottles are autoclaved.

4.5.25 **Lecitho-vitellin (LV)** is the lipoprotein component of egg-yolk and it can be obtained as a clear yellow liquid by mixing egg-yolk with saline (Macfarlane, Oakley & Anderson, 1941). This liquid becomes opalescent when mixed with certain bacterial toxins or lecithinases; flocculation and separation of a thick curd of fat may follow. When lecithinase-forming organisms grow on a solid medium containing LV, the lecithinase diffuses into the agar and produces zones of opalescence around individual colonies. This reaction can be inhibited by adding certain antitoxic or antilecithinase sera to the surface of the medium before inoculation. Lipolytic organisms also produce an opalescence on LV Agar and it is often accompanied by a distinctive 'pearly layer' or iridescent film; the presence of free fatty acid can be demonstrated by treating the medium, after incubation, with copper sulphate solution (Willis, 1960). The ability to produce an opacity on LV Agar is useful in the division of the genera *Bacillus* and *Clostridium*, but other organisms, such as *Staphylococcus aureus*, may also give positive reactions. Egg-yolk emulsified in an equal volume of sterile saline is a practical and satisfactory substitute for LV for incorporation in solid media such as Egg-Yolk Agar (McClung & Toabe, 1947).

The LV reaction is not due solely to a lecithinase; Willis & Gowland (1962) consider that separation of insoluble protein, splitting of fats from lipoprotein complexes, and the coalescence of particles of free fat are all involved. In many laboratories media containing human serum (Nagler, 1939) have been replaced by egg-yolk media.

Although *Pseudomonas aeruginosa* is known to produce a lecithinase, the egg-yolk reaction is usually negative; from this Stanier, Palleroni & Doudoroff (1966) argued that the egg-yolk reaction is specific for only one kind of lecithinase and that other types do not produce opacity with egg-yolk. The actions of four types of lecithinase are discussed by Willis (1969); only one (lecithinase C) is usually produced by bacteria.

4.5.26   The malonate test was introduced by Leifson (1933) to help distinguish *Escherichia coli* from '*Klebsiella aerogenes*' (*K. pneumoniae* subsp. *aerogenes*), and with these organisms he found a perfect correlation with the VP test. Shaw (1956) showed that most strains of the Arizona group were malonate positive and most other kinds of salmonella were malonate negative. As both these groups are VP-negative there is thus no correlation between the malonate and VP tests. The test was described as a fermentation by Leifson and as a utilization by Shaw

in spite of the fact that she added yeast extract to stimulate growth.

4.5.27   Metabolic fatty acids. The metabolic products that have received most attention, especially among the anaerobic bacteria, are the volatile fatty acids of the series formic to heptanoic, certain other short-chain carboxylic acids (notably lactic and succinic acids) and the low-molecular-weight alcohols. Minute quantities of these compounds may be analysed by gas–liquid chromatography (Holdeman, Cato & Moore, 1977). Qualitative and quantitative differences in end-products of metabolism are associated with different genera and species, and since these characteristics are stable they are of considerable taxonomic value for certain organisms (e.g. *Fusobacterium*).

4.5.28   The methyl red (MR) test, and the **Voges–Proskaüer (VP)** test for acetylmethylcarbinol or acetoin, may be carried out with the same liquid culture. The tests are mainly used to distinguish various coliform organisms from each other; all these ferment glucose vigorously and the pH value of the glucose medium falls quickly. When methyl red is added after overnight incubation the cultures of all these organisms will give an acid reaction with the dye, i.e. MR-positive. After further incubation *Escherichia coli* cultures produce even more acid and in spite of phosphate buffer in the medium may be self-sterilizing; the MR test remains positive. Cultures of *Klebsiella pneumoniae* subsp. *aerogenes*, on the other hand, decarboxylate and condense the pyruvic acid to form acetylmethylcarbinol, the pH value rises and, when methyl red is added, the colour is yellow, i.e. MR-negative. Nowadays there is a tendency to do biochemical tests earlier but the temptation to speed up the MR test should be resisted; it should never be read until the cultures have been incubated for at least 2 days at 37 °C or 3 days at 30 °C. The reaction cannot be accelerated by increasing the glucose content of the medium; Clark & Lubs (1915) found that, in media with much above 1% glucose, cultures of '*K. aerogenes*' (*K. pneumoniae* subsp. *aerogenes*) did not revert to become MR-negative. Despite its simplicity, we suspect that the MR test is rarely used in clinical laboratories.

37

4.5.29   Milk (usually as Litmus Milk or Bromcresol Purple Milk) is a good nutrient medium in which most organisms will grow and it has a fairly constant composition since man only interferes by removing the cream and adding an indicator. Although highly esteemed elsewhere, in the medical laboratory Litmus (or Bromcresol Purple) Milk occupies a secondary position and most bacteriologists believe that the information it gives can be obtained with more certainty by using other media; for this reason, we do not use it in the tables. An objection to milk is that unless a change takes place in the appearance of the medium (e.g. acid or clot formation) it is difficult to be sure that growth has occurred.

Milk contains lactose, galactose, a trace of glucose, casein, and mineral salts. Acid production from the fermentation of lactose is shown by a change in colour of the indicator, and, when much acid is produced, by the formation of a clot. But another form of clot may be produced by rennet; in this case the clot forms first and later, like the fibrin clot in blood, contracts and expresses a clear whey. In contrast the acid clot does not contract. When the bacterium also produces proteolytic enzymes the clot may be peptonized. Apart from the rennet clot (for which milk is a unique medium) all the other reactions can be detected more easily by using media appropriate for each reaction.

Caseinase activity may be detected in a solid medium by incorporating skimmed milk in a nutrient agar base. Proteolysis is shown by the development of clear zones in the medium around areas of growth. Alternatively, substitution of soluble casein for milk gives a clear medium in which casein hydrolysis is seen as a clear zone around growth after the plate is flooded with 30% trichloracetic acid or with acid mercuric chloride solution (cf. Frazier's gelatinase test, Appendix C3.23).

4.5.30   Niacin (nicotinic acid) production is a feature characteristic of human tubercle bacilli and it distinguishes them from bovine tubercle bacilli and other mycobacteria (Pope & Smith, 1946). Several modifications of the test method have been devised; all are based on the extraction of niacin from the bacterial growth and subsequent detection by a colorimetric reaction. If used, the test must be done with care not only because of infection risks but also because one of the reagents (cyanogen bromide) is lachrymatory and toxic.

4.5.31   Nitrate reduction may be shown either by detecting the presence of one of the breakdown products, or by showing the disappearance of nitrate from the medium. The products of reduction may include nitrite, hyponitrite, hydroxylamine, ammonia, nitrous oxide, or gaseous nitrogen. The first test to be applied aims at showing the presence of nitrite. When this test is negative (i.e. nitrite is not detected) the medium is tested to see whether there is residual nitrate; if this test also is negative it confirms that the first stage of the breakdown has been completed and the nitrite further broken down.

In uninoculated Nitrate Broth and with cultures of organisms that do not reduce nitrate, the test for nitrite is negative until zinc dust (ZoBell, 1932) or other reducing agent is added to the culture medium to reduce the nitrate contained in it. To detect small amounts of residual nitrate the amount of zinc added may be critical (Steel & Fisher, 1961). The tests are very sensitive and it is important to check the uninoculated medium for nitrite, which should not be present.

Some workers prefer to carry out the test in a semisolid medium (ZoBell, 1932); others insist that free access to oxygen is necessary for nitrate reduction by aerobes.

Conn (1936) discussed the difficulty of recording the results of the nitrate reduction test, and advised that the terms positive and negative be avoided. Instead the actual finding(s) should be recorded; the possibilities are shown in Table 4.1.

An entirely different method was described by Cook (1950) who found that when nitrate was included in Blood Agar base, nitrate-reducing bacteria growing on the Blood Agar medium reduced the haemoglobin to methaemoglobin; this method has the advantage that the change seen is apparent even when the organism can also reduce nitrite. A convenient alternative way of performing the test is to apply a blotting paper disc impregnated with potassium nitrate on an inoculated plate of plain Blood Agar.

4.5.32   Nitrite reduction can be brought about by certain bacteria incapable of reducing nitrate (ZoBell, 1932). It can be shown by growing the organism in a

38

Table 4.1 *Interpretation of tests for reduction of nitrate and nitrite*

Culture medium	Test applied	Result	Interpretation
Nitrate Broth	1 For nitrite	Colour not changed (negative)	Nitrite not present (see Test 3)
	2 For nitrite	Red colour (positive)	Nitrate reduced to nitrite
	3 Zinc dust	(A) Colour not changed	Nitrite not present: therefore nitrate in original medium has been reduced completely by the bacteria
		(B) Red colour	Nitrate in medium reduced to nitrite by zinc but not by bacteria
Nitrite Broth	4 For nitrite	(C) Red colour	Nitrite present; not (all) reduced
		(D) Colour not changed	Nitrite reduced by bacteria and has disappeared from the medium

broth containing 0.01% $NaNO_2$ and, after sufficient time for the reduction to take place, testing for residual nitrite (Table 4.1).

4.5.33 The **nitrogen nutrition** of bacteria can be studied in a mineral base with a chelating agent (Owens & Keddie, 1969). The method has considerable interest in classification work but the standards of chemical cleanliness required are higher than some bacteriological laboratories can meet. But this should not deter anyone from trying the method.

4.5.34 O/129 sensitivity. The pteridine derivative O/129 (Appendix C1.18; C3.41) was regarded as almost specific in inhibiting the growth of vibrios, although the number of strains showing resistance to this agent seems to be increasing (Matsushita, Kudoh & Ohashi, 1984; Gerbaud *et al.*, 1985). However, it is still a useful differential test to apply to any non-fluorescent, oxidase-positive, Gram-negative rod. Simple methods, such as drops of a 10% suspension on an inoculated plate of Nutrient Agar containing 0.5–1% NaCl are adequate though dried discs containing 150 μg of this 'vibriostatic agent' may give more reproducible results; discs containing 10 μg have some differential value within the genus. The discs can be prepared in the laboratory or obtained commercially (Lee & Donovan, 1985).

4.5.35 The **ONPG** (*o*-nitrophenyl-ß-D-galactopyranoside) test is used to detect potential lactose fermenters which, in ordinary media, either take several days to produce acid or do not produce any acid.

Lactose fermentation depends on two enzymes, (i) an induced intracellular enzyme, β-galactosidase, which attacks lactose, and (ii) a permease which regulates penetration of the lactose through the cell wall. Kriebel (1934) found that late lactose-fermenters produced acid more quickly when the concentration of lactose was increased to 5%; Chilton & Fulton (1946) recommended 10% lactose in agar. However, the results of the 5 and 10% lactose tests and the ONPG test for β-galactosidase do not always agree (Lapage, Efstratiou & Hill, 1973). Lederberg (1950) used ONPG for the study of β-galactosidase, and Le Minor & Ben Hamida (1962) developed a rapid ONPG test for toluene-treated bacterial cultures. Lowe (1962) found that toluene treatment was not essential to liberate the β-galactosidase and that overnight incubation of cultures in peptone water containing ONPG hydrolysed the colourless substrate to the yellow *o*-nitrophenol.

4.5.36 Phenylalanine can be converted by oxidative deamination to phenylpyruvic acid (PPA) which, like many other keto acids, can be identified by adding ferric chloride (Singer & Volcani, 1955). The phenylalanine test was used by Henriksen & Closs (1938) who found that *Proteus* species gave the strongest reactions but '*Klebsiella aerogenes*' (*K. pneumoniae* subsp. *aerogenes*) also gave some positive results. Since then Henriksen (1950) and others (Buttiaux *et al.*, 1954; Singer & Bar-Chay, 1954; Shaw & Clarke, 1955) have found it to be almost specific for *Proteus*, *Morganella* and *Providencia*. This specificity prompted Singer & Bar-Chay to put the

Providence organisms into the genus *Proteus*; however, the two genera are now recognized as distinct.

The phenylalanine deaminase of *Moraxella phenylpyruvica* seems to be weaker than that of *Proteus* species and the usual methods do not work well with it. Snell & Davey (1971) describe a method in which the tubes are agitated at 37 °C and give positive results in about an hour.

4.5.37 Phosphatase activity was used by Barber & Kuper (1951) to aid the identification of pathogenic staphylococci; they found a high degree of correlation between phosphatase and coagulase production. By prolonging the incubation period, Baird-Parker (1963) demonstrated phosphatase production in 378 of 546 strains of staphylococci and 10 of 677 strains of micrococci. Some workers prefer a liquid medium and Lewis (1961) compared the plate and tube methods; he found that essentially similar results were obtainable in a liquid medium incubated for 6 hours and on a solid medium incubated for 18 hours with coagulase-positive staphylococci, but the tube method showed far fewer phosphatase-positive coagulase-negative strains. Among enteric bacteria, Vörös *et al.* (1961) found that phosphatase was produced only by strains of *Proteus* and *Providencia*; using the same technique Cowan & Steel (1974) were unable to confirm this specificity and found positive reactions also in the *Salmonella*, *Shigella*, *Klebsiella* and *Escherichia* groups; for this reason, we no longer include the phosphatase test in the tables for identification of enterobacteria in this *Manual*.

4.5.38 Pigment formation often has considerable diagnostic value and it is an advantage to know how to encourage it. Although the pigments produced are seldom photosynthetic, most bacteria dealt with in this *Manual* form pigment better in the light; this is most noticeable in the staphylococci and serratias, but also occurs in the pseudomonads and in chromobacteria. The effect of light on pigment production by mycobacteria has become a means of distinguishing species. Temperature and medium also influence the intensity of pigmentation; most bacteria produce pigments better at temperatures below the optimum for growth, such as 22 °C for mesophils.

Medium probably has the biggest effect on the development of pigment. In some cases the simple addition of glucose will enhance pigmentation, in other cases this will inhibit it. The old adage that 'one man's meat is another man's poison' applies also to bacterial pigment production and different formulae are needed for different organisms. The elimination of all meat extracts and the addition of mannitol are beneficial for *Chromobacterium* and *Janthinobacterium* and may improve pigmentation of *Serratia* strains (Goldsworthy & Still, 1936, 1938); quite different media are needed to encourage pigmentation by pseudomonads (see Appendix A2.4). On routine laboratory media, some strains of *Pseudomonas cepacia* produce yellow or brown non-fluorescent pigments which are soluble in water and chloroform. On chemically defined media, the pigments may exhibit a wide variety of colours depending on the carbon source used for growth (Lennette *et al.*, 1982).

The characteristic black pigment produced by some strains of the *melaninogenicus–oralis* group of *Bacteroides* during growth on media containing blood is due to the formation of protohaemin, and the red fluorescence of their colonies in ultraviolet light is due to protoporphoryn, a precursor of protohaemin (Shah *et al.*, 1979). Yellow-green fluorescence in long-wave ultraviolet light is also exhibited by colonies of *Clostridium difficile*.

4.5.39 Poly-β-hydroxybutyric acid (PHB) may accumulate as a cellular reserve material; it was used by Stanier, Palleroni & Doudoroff (1966) in their characterization of *Pseudomonas* species. The chemical method of extracting and identifying this polymer (Williamson & Wilkinson, 1958) is not suitable for routine use, but examination of wet preparations of the organism by phase-contrast microscopy or of films stained by weak carbol fuchsin will reveal the intracellular deposits. PHB is produced most abundantly when the organism is grown in a medium containing D, L-β-hydroxybutyrate; after growth, films are stained with Sudan black and counterstained with safranin to reveal the purple-black deposits of PHBA within cells.

4.5.40 Survival under certain adverse conditions (usually heat) may have diagnostic significance; for example, streptococci that survives heating at 60 °C for 30 minutes (and which form the basis of the recently described genus *Enterococcus*) are likely to belong to Lancefield Group D. The tests themselves are not easy to standardize and the methods used by different authors vary greatly. For example, after the heating test for *Enterococcus* (*Streptococcus*) *faecalis* an immediate subculture may fail to show growth, whereas if the heated broth is incubated overnight, a subculture is more likely to yield growth. Other factors may affect the result, including the nature of the medium or suspending fluid in which the heating is carried out, its pH value, the time allowed for the medium to heat up to the desired temperature, and the type of container, particularly the thickness of the glass, in which the sample is heated. Some authors (Abd-el-Malek & Gibson, 1948*a*) always used milk, which they regarded as a medium of more constant composition than man-made infusions and enzymic digests.

While the testing of vegetative bacteria for survival has its difficulties, the testing of spore suspensions is even more full of pitfalls. The heat stability of spores not only varies from one species to another, but even in the same species will vary from strain to strain, and spores of the same strain grown on different occasions do not necessarily have the same resistance to heat. For a discussion of this subject the reader is referred to papers by Kelsey (1958, 1961). 'Heat-shock' of bacterial spore suspensions is a useful technique employed to initiate germination. The resistance of spores to ethanol is used in the so-called 'alcohol-shock' treatment, which also destroys the accompanying vegetative forms.

4.5.41 Temperature range for growth and the optimal growth temperature are characteristic of different groups of bacteria; of those in the medical and veterinary fields the optimal temperature is usually between 35 and 40 °C but the range for growth varies considerably. Some species (e.g. *Neisseria gonorrhoeae*) have only a narrow range and rapidly die at temperatures outside the range; other organisms have a wide growth and an even wider survival range. In all cases the optimal temperature for growth is near the maximum of the temperature range.

Biochemical tests are usually made on cultures grown at the temperature optimal for growth; however, this may not be optimal for the development of the product to be tested. For example, acetoin production by hafnias occurs at a lower temperature than the growth optimum. Some salmonellas are able to grow on a medium containing an ammonium salt as nitrogen source at 30 °C but will not grow on this medium at 37 °C, the optimal temperature for growth on media providing organic nitrogen.

The ability of an organism to grow at 20–22, 30, and 37 °C are tested in many laboratories and the diagnostic tables show, in general, the more specialized tests used for different groups of bacteria; for these, adjustable water baths or incubators are needed. In the differentiation of species of *Mycobacterium* (Table 6.10*b*) growth or survival is shown at several different temperatures.

4.5.42 Temperature tolerance. Most mesophilic bacteria in the vegetative state are killed at 56 °C for 30 minutes. A few species such as *Staphylococcus aureus, Aerococcus viridans*, and some streptococci (mostly belonging to the genus *Enterococcus*) survive heating at 60 °C for 30 minutes; this degree of heat-tolerance can be used as a screening test for them.

4.5.43 Tween 80 test for lipolytic activity (Sierra, 1957). Tween 80 is the oleic acid ester of a polyoxyalkylene derivative of sorbitan. It can be included in a suitable nutrient medium and the test culture(s) streak-inoculated on the surface; after incubation at the optimal temperature for the organism(s) under test, the plate is examined for opaque haloes around the growth. The opacity, which indicates lipolytic activity, is due to crystal formation.

Tween 80 can also be incorporated in a liquid medium, which is used for the much longer period of incubation (up to 21 days) needed by mycobacteria (Kubica & Dye, 1967).

4.5.44 Urease activity is tested in Christensen's (1946) urea medium which supports the growth of many bacteria. The urease activity of *Proteus, Providencia* and some *Klebsiella* species can be shown in a highly buffered urea medium (Stuart, van Stratum & Rustigian, 1945) in which other enterobacteria appear to be urease negative. *Proteus* species can use urea nitrogen but most other urease-producing organisms need an additional nitrogen source for growth. Urease activity provides a useful test for distinguishing between *Clostridium bifermen-*

41

tans and *Clostridium sordelli*. Urease activity is shown by alkali production from urea solutions, but, in at least two methods (Elek, 1948; Ortali & Samarani, 1955), Nessler's reagent is added to show the presence of ammonia.

4.6   Rapid methods for the screening and identification of bacteria

Rapid, multitest micromethods – manual and mechanized – have now become firmly established in microbiological practice. Many of the early methods relied upon heavy inocula with preformed constitutive enzymes to demonstrate biochemical activity in miniaturized conventional methods (Clarke & Cowan, 1952). The majority of micromethods were developed for the Enterobacteriaceae, but more recently special methods have been introduced for the non-fermenters, anaerobes, streptococci and staphylococci.

The pioneering work of Buissière & Nardon (1968) on single substrate multi-test methods from which the API system evolved has led also to the development of several off-the-shelf kits with special plastic strips for single-step procedures for bacterial identification. The current emphasis is for reproducibility, speed, standardization and ease of use. Other microtest identification systems with 96-well microplates have been developed both commercially and by individual laboratories, as have multiple inoculation procedures for agar plates containing different substrates. Paper discs impregnated with substrates have also been used. All these techniques depend on a definitive result within 48 hours of inoculation and many can now provide presumptive identifications within 4 hours. The standard of quality control by manufacturers is higher than most individual laboratories can provide: we do not think, for example, that many laboratories could carry out melting-point analyses on their test substrates before the medium is prepared.

The use of numerical taxonomic techniques, first described by Sneath (1957*b*) and discussed more fully in Chapter 8, has become so refined that data derived from such studies can now be used for computer-assisted identification of bacterial strains. Many commercial kits utilize such databases and several different procedures are available for interpreting the

patterns of results. Most commercial kit manufacturers provide indices of coded test-result patterns or profiles in numerical order which give a primary level of identification; for further help, many manufacturers operate telephone desks for direct assistance usually with the aid of a computer. The indices are normally prepared by combining test results to form octal sets as described in Chapter 10.

4.6.1   Manual biochemical systems.
We do not intend in this section to review all the commercially available identification and screening kits, but rather to illustrate the methodology used with examples of kits currently available in the United Kingdom. We will describe the overall principles but not the specific methods as these may be found in the product literature issued with each kit; new commercial kits are launched frequently and clinical evaluations of them are usually published in scientific journals such as the *Journal of Clinical Microbiology*.

There are two varieties of manual micromethods: (i) dehydrated substrates contained in plastic wells or compartments or on absorbent paper discs or strips, and (ii) multiple conventional substrates incorporated in agar for inoculation with one or more organisms.

4.6.1.1   Dehydrated substrates.
The combination of several dehydrated substrates in one package or kit allows for 'unitary' identification, where all the tests are inoculated or the results interpreted in one step. Certain impregnated paper discs, such as those for indole or oxidase, are also available as individual conventional tests. For use, all kits with dehydrated substrates are inoculated with suspensions of the test organisms; as the required density of organisms may vary according to the kit, the suspensions should be prepared as described by each manufacturer. We make no apology for reminding users of this *Manual* that the bacterial cultures for identification must be pure.

In the Minitek system individual impregnated paper discs from a wide range can be combined in a plastic tray. Some of the tests need a layer of sterile mineral oil or paraffin to ensure an adequate microaerophilic reaction; and after incubation for 18–24 hours, some tests require the addition of reagents. To use the manufacturer's Index of the most likely sets of results for the Enterobacteriaceae, 14 specified tests must be used. This system has not proved popular in the United Kingdom for several reasons, including: the freedom of test choice; the fact that a set of 14 tests is insufficient for a reasonable identification level for the Enterobacteriaceae; and the plethora of other kits available at similar cost. A 4 hour test version is now available but requires heavier inocula. The system can be used for the identification of anaerobes by choosing an appropriate set of substrate discs and incubation conditions appropriate for anaerobic identification.

The Micro–ID system depends on the presence of preformed constitutive enzymes in the bacterial suspensions and so allows identification of the Enterobacteriaceae in only 4 hours. Each kit consists of 15 substrates dehydrated on paper discs in compartments in one plastic tray; the compartments hold both substrate and reagent discs. The test reactions are recorded after 4 hours (in one test after the addition of KOH) as a 5-digit octal profile. This can be interpreted by reference to the manufacturer's Profile Index. The system does permit some flexibility in recording the test results as the kits may be refrigerated overnight before final interpretation: trays inoculated later in the day can thus be placed in the refrigerator for reading the following morning.

API have a wide range of kits available for many groups of medical bacteria. The API20E kit was designed for identifying enterobacteria, and consists of 20 special compartments ('Ivan Hall tubes') in a plastic strip. After incubation for 18–24 hours and the addition of appropriate reagents for the tryptophan deaminase, indole, and VP tests, it provides a 7-digit octal set of results or profile which can be looked-up in the Profile Index or referred to the manufacturer for computer-assisted identification. Since its introduction in the 1970s it has become one of the most popular identification kits with a good reputation for reproducibility and reliability as well as a worldwide database. Indeed the API50 test kits are currently regarded as one of the most convenient means for the identification of *Bacillus* species (Berkeley *et al.*, 1984).

The advent of plastic 96-well microtitre trays for serological analysis provided scope for other kits with potential for some degree of automated reading. Manufacturers have opted in most instances for a combination approach either by making part of the tray available for antibiotic sensitivity tests or by subdividing the tray to allow several organisms to be examined simultaneously, e.g. 4 sets of 24 or 3 sets of 32 tests. For these kits, further manufacturing technology was required to ensure not only that the media remained at the bottoms of the wells when dehydrated but, more importantly, that they rehydrated uniformly when the bacterial suspension was added.

4.6.1.2 Agar-based identification systems. These identification systems fall into two groups: those in which one inoculation serves for all the tests for one organism, and those which require multiple inoculations of several media with several organisms. The principal drawback with these systems is the limited shelf-life of the media as, with prolonged storage and evaporation, some concentration of the constituent materials inevitably occurs.

The Enterotube (Roche) is useful in circumstances where the full paraphernalia of a laboratory is not always available. A single plastic compartmentalized tube is divided into 11 chambers each containing media with single or multiple substrates. A thin metal rod runs through the base of each chamber; inoculation is achieved by touching a single colony on a solid medium with one end of the rod and pulling it through the whole tube, thus inoculating the medium in each chamber. The rod is then re-inserted to block the passage between the chambers and so ensure that no cross-contamination occurs between them. Reagents are added after overnight incubation and colour changes observed and recorded. Kits are available for both the fermenting and non-fermenting Gram-negative rods although only the former are currently regarded as satisfactory.

A variety of multiple agar media in differing commercial formats have been marketed with varying success. One system used a multitest medium in a single tube followed later by a circular plastic mould with several compartments, each of which had to be stab-inoculated. These all required considerable manipulation at the inoculation stage and because of this drawback have not proved widely acceptable.

Multi-point inoculation techniques for identifying bacteria have been available for many years. A commercial version (Cathra Replireader), marketed in the later 1970s, consisted of several agar plates with different substrates together with a replicate-inoculation device for suspensions of multiple organisms for identification. A maximum of 36 isolates could be inoculated onto each of the 17 test plates for identification; extra plates containing antibiotics for sensitivity testing were also available. The method proved efficient and economic (Baer & Washington, 1972; Waterworth, 1980) but has failed to gain widespread acceptance principally because of quality control and supply problems with the commercially prepared agar plates incorporating the identification substrates. However, this kind of rapid methodology has re-emerged commercially following the recent availability of accurate automated volume-control systems for the manufacture of packaged substrates for bacterial identification and antibiotic sensitivity purposes. An increasingly wide range of agar-based substrates has become available in tablet form (Mast) and this methodology, in association with multipoint agar-based antibiotic sensitivity testing, has proved convenient, flexible, efficient and economical. Various schemes to provide computerized databases have been proposed but because of the variety of different media and suppliers we think it unlikely that any single method will take precedence. Rather, we suspect that the trend will be towards laboratories creating and supporting their own databases (Clayton et al., 1986). The principal advantage of this approach lies in effective and ongoing in-house quality control and assessment both of laboratory procedures and in the identification of organisms. Provided that the test reactions are monitored carefully in comparison with selected control organisms (see Appendix D) this approach will provide most of the advantages described by Clarke & Cowan in 1952.

4.6.2 Other rapid methods

4.6.2.1 Monoclonal antibodies.
The recent introduction of monoclonal antibodies, produced from single cloned hybridoma B cells, has considerable potential for bacterial identification purposes. As each B cell line produces a single immunoglobulin the antibodies have become known popularly as monoclonals. More details about the production and diagnostic use of monoclonal antibodies can be obtained from the publications of Kohler & Milstein (1975), Nowinski et al. (1983) and McLauchlin et al. (1988).

Direct tests are becoming increasingly available for many bacterial antigens and they have an enormous potential in rapid, definitive microbiology not only in the diagnostic laboratory but also at the bedside or in the surgery. Indeed commercially available kits to detect Group A streptococci in throat swabs within minutes are already available and we think that this area of rapid methodology is likely to develop considerably.

4.6.2.2 DNA probes.
This recently developed technique depends on the natural process whereby single-stranded DNA is attracted to complementary strands to form double-stranded hybrids. Single-stranded, radiolabelled bacterial DNA (the probe) can thus be used to seek out complementary DNA strands in material such as culture preparations, bacterial colonies and even clinical specimens directly. The procedure is usually carried out on a solid phase such as a nitrocellulase filter; double-stranded DNA hybrids or duplexes remain bound to the filter while the single-stranded, unbound DNA is washed off. The technique has numerous potential applications and could be used, for example, to rapidly screen large numbers of samples effectively and economically. The following references will provide the reader who wishes to explore this technique with a few leads: Escherichia coli (Moseley et al., 1982; Romick, Lindsay & Busta, 1987), Neisseria (Totten et al., 1983) and Mycobacterium (Cooper et al., 1989).

4.6.3 Mechanized or automated methods.
In this section we first discuss screening methods which help with the handling of clinical specimens, and then methods that assist with the identification of bacteria isolated from them. As before, we intend this as an introduction to the principles and the technology rather than as a review of every method. Evaluations and descriptions of the latest methods are usually published in scientific journals such as the Journal of Clinical Microbiology.

Mechanized methods have been used in many clinical laboratories particularly outside the UK. The majority of these systems utilize micromethods with in addition automated interpretation of test reactions. The principal drawbacks are the high capital and revenue costs, especially for the examination of relatively few specimens.

4.6.3.1   Screening methods. The ability to detect the presence of potential pathogens in a clinical sample with a semi-automated method would be a boon to all laboratories: the advantages of processing more than 1 000 specimens per day are obvious. Several methods are commercially available though only for a limited range of specimens, notably urine, CSF, sputum and blood cultures.

Several mechanized screening methods for urine have been described. They include the measurement of optical densities after incubation of small samples in suitable growth media; the quantitative measurement of the luminescence of bacterial ATP; measurement of the relative uptake of certain dyes or of comparative fluorescence; and enumeration and measurement of the size of the particles in urine samples with modified blood cell counters. Each method has its devotees (and sceptics) and we make no judgement on their relative merits although we are sure that these procedures will develop and become more widespread in the future.

The screening of blood cultures has proved a larger problem. The incorporation of special substrates into blood culture media has allowed the application of radioisotope and infrared methodology as well as uncomplicated, visual gas production methods. Much effort has been directed towards measuring the minute changes in electrical conductivity across defined media in the presence of rapidly growing bacteria, though effective control of the inherent variables has proved expensive to implement successfully.

4.6.3.2   Identification methods. Apart from manual methods which lend themselves to mechanized or automated interpretation, an array of specialized systems have been developed for the identification of pure cultures. Once again the enterobacteria have been the prime area of interest, although the Gram-negative non-fermenters have an appreciable following.

The instruments available are based on manual methods and many still use the same test reactions but with specially developed substrates in plastic cartridges or cuvettes suitable for automated reading in photometers. The more expensive instruments incorporate microcomputers which analyse the reaction patterns and provide a computer-assisted identification of each test isolate.

The majority of the instruments are capable of providing accurate levels of comparative identification. However, published evaluations often fail to stress the basic microbiological concepts discussed in Section 5.2, and we cannot stress too strongly again that pure cultures are imperative.

4.6.4   General aspects. Although microbiological mechanization and rapid methodology have relatively high capital costs and revenue consequences, other factors should also be considered. The shorter time from isolation to identification is an obvious advantage provided it can be completed within a normal working day. The increased sensitivity and specificity derived from automation and strictly controlled manufacturing conditions should provide microbiologists with firmer information upon which to base clinical judgement.

We do not think, however, that the basic principles of microbiology will be understood so easily by the next generations of microbiologists if in future the materials and methods are simply to be taken from the refrigerator or shelf as kits. We believe strongly that time-honoured media and methods have an important part to play in training microbiologists. We wonder also, when instruments break down (as they will inevitably), whether the expertise of traditional procedures will be available? It seems to us that diagnostic microbiology is at a turning point and the new technology route should be followed with some caution.

5
Theory and practice of bacterial identification

It goes without saying that adequate clinical information is essential to enable appropriate culture media to be chosen for primary isolation. We believe that the subsequent investigation of the organism(s) thus isolated should be approached with an open mind; the organism(s) should be regarded as unknown and the process of identification started from the basic (primary) characters.

5.1   Theory of identification

In theory the identification of a bacterium consists of a comparison of the unknown with the known, the object being the ability to say that the unknown is like A (one of the known bacteria) and unlike B–Z (all other known bacteria); another and arguably equally important objective is to be able to say that the unknown organism is the same as A and thus to give it a name or identification tag. When we say that it is A we imply that it is different from all the other known bacteria, B–Z. All identification schemes depend on knowing a great deal about the already identified (or known) units, but the human memory can cope with only a small proportion of this knowledge, so memory aids are essential. In practice there are at present two distinct methods of making the identification; but the feasibility of a third method using a computer, first suggested by Payne (1963), was demonstrated by Dybowski & Franklin (1968) and is discussed in Chapter 10.

The first method is familiar to all biologists and uses the dichotomous key. Characters are taken in turn and the keys are most successful when the features can be expressed unequivocally as either positive or negative. Although *Streptomyces* species are not described in this *Manual*, Küster's (1972) claim that dichotomous keys are the most workable for the

classification and identification of that genus deserves notice. In choosing the sequence of characters he tried to take first those that were easiest to determine, and he followed the same sequence for all subdivisions of the genus. Küster's scheme used seven characters which he was able to determine from observations made of cultures grown on only two media. With this economy of effort he (i) made primary groupings from the colour of the aerial mycelium, and (ii) subdivided these groups by the presence or absence of a distinctive pigment on the reverse side of the vegetative mycelium. The other characters used were, in order (iii) melanin reaction, (iv) formation of soluble pigment, (v) morphology of the spore-producing/bearing structures (sporophores), (vi) morphology of spores, and (vii) further subdivisions made on the utilization of one or more carbohydrates. The only dichotomous key to deal comprehensively with bacteria is that developed by Skerman (1949, 1959–67) and the successive versions have been increasingly useful.

Another form of dichotomous key, the flow chart, can make allowance for the variable reactions given by strains of some bacterial species as in that prepared by Manclark & Pickett (1961). Thus, in this *Manual* what we call a 'd' character (different reactions in different strains, positive in some, negative in others) is treated in the flow chart as both positive and negative, and the species appears in at least two places.

Tables make up the second memory aid, and these are widely used in all laboratories. It is easier to see the essential characters in a table than in pages of descriptive matter, which is seldom precise and often made unnecessarily vague by phrases such as 'most strains are...', 'some strains do not...', 'not infrequently strains...', and the impossible 'strains showing no...'.

Table 5.1. *Symbols used in Chapters 6 and 7 and equivalent descriptive terms*

Symbol	Meaning and descriptive equivalent
+	85-100% strains are positive (all, most, many, usually)
d	16-84% strains positive (many, several, some)
-	0-15% strains positive (none, one, few, some)
( )	Delayed reaction in test or delayed growth
(d)	Different reactions given by different strains; positive reactions often delayed
w	Weak reaction or growth
(w)	Reaction or growth delayed and weak
w/-	Weak reaction or no reaction with different strains; positive reactions are weak or growth is feeble
D	Different reactions given by lower taxa (genera, species, varieties)
?	Not known or insufficient information
.	Not applicable

Table 5.2. *Additional symbols used in some tables in Chapters 6 and 7*

Symbol	Meaning
A	Aerobic atmosphere preferred
C	Curved in shape
F	Fermentative; fermentation
G	Gas produced
H	Helical or spiral in shape
J	Generally positive in young cultures; inconstant in older cultures
M	Microaerophilic conditions preferred
NT	Not testable
O	Oxidative; oxidation
[O]	Under aerobic conditions
[Ø]	Under anaerobic conditions
R	Rod-shaped (bacillus)
r	Resistant (to antibiotic, etc)
S	Sphere; coccus
s	Susceptible; sensitive (to antibiotic, etc)
T	Spores terminal
U	Spores central
V	Spores subterminal or central; variable in position
X	Spores oval; ellipsoidal
Y	Spores round
VP	Voges–Proskaüer test

Letters in bold type in tables are serological designations. Superior italic letters are explained in footnotes to the individual tables.

The construction of diagnostic tables would be simplified if all strains of one species behaved alike, and if the results of all tests could be expressed unambiguously as either positive or negative. Unfortunately as neither of these is ever likely to happen, we are forced to use various symbols to indicate the constancy or inconstancy of bacterial characters.

The symbols now in use were developed from those applied by Kauffmann, Edwards & Ewing, (1956) and later adopted in reports of the Enterobacteriaceae Subcommittee of what has become the International Committee on Systematic Bacteriology of the International Union (formerly Association) of Microbiological Societies (ICSB of IUMS). Neither Kauffmann nor the Subcommittee fixed any numerical values to the symbols and in the first edition of this *Manual* a small table was given showing the values used in preparing the diagnostic tables for that edition. In Table 5.1 we show the assessment of these values and the gradings used in Chapters 6 and 7 of this third edition; we also show the approximate equivalents of descriptive terms used for reactions or expressing the results of tests; these equivalents (which are subjective) are necessary because so few characterizations are expressed quantitatively. Few laboratories other than those with reference functions have examined a sufficient number of strains of the less common bacteria to make test results expressed as percentages meaningful; exceptions to this statement are the Centers for Disease Control, Atlanta, Georgia, USA and the National Collection of Type Cultures, London, UK which, over a period of years, have handled large numbers of cultures and contributed many publications in which the results were expressed quantitatively. The tables of Lennette *et al.* (1985) for a large range of bacteria, and those of Edwards & Ewing (1962, 1972) and Ewing (1986) for a more limited range, are particularly valuable.

Some characters are almost invariably positive or negative; unfortunately characters of such constancy are usually shared by similar organisms, and although they are important for characterization (and may appear in the miniature definitions given in Chapters 6 and 7), they have little value in distinguishing an organism from its neighbours, and thus seldom appear in the second-stage tables.

The tables can form the basis of a set of diagnostic punched cards to be used with similar cards on which the characters of the unknown organisms are punched. Sorting the cards of the unknowns with those of the knowns can be one of the quickest, most accurate and least burdensome ways of arriving at the identification of an organism (cf. Riddle *et al.* 1956). We describe the use of the diagnostic tables in such a punched card system of identification in Chapter 9. The diagnostic tables can also form the basis for computer-assisted identification, which we discuss in Chapter 10.

5.2   Practice of identification

So far in this *Manual* we have discussed principles and indicated how all identification is based on a comparison of the organism we wish to identify with organisms of known identity. The accuracy of the identification depends on the thoroughness of the preparatory work such as media making, preparing stains and reagents, and the degree of care taken in carrying out, observing and recording the results of the various tests.

In Chapter 3 we drew attention to the fact that bacteria isolated on inhibitory and selective media were likely to be mixed cultures, and we indicated some of the steps to be taken to purify a culture. It is not easy to be sure that such a 'purified' culture is incontrovertibly pure, and when there is any doubt whatever, it is safer and saves time to repeat the purification process. To identify a culture takes a great deal of effort and to suspect at the end that the culture may be impure is not only aggravating to the laboratory worker and the delay in receiving the report frustrating to the clinician, but it also indicates that the bacteriologist has wasted much time and material. Common organisms really are the commonest; and when an organism cannot be identified or seems to be an exotic species, we should consider the possibility that either our culture material is impure, or we have made some error in observation or recording. This happens to all of us and it reflects adversely on our ability and integrity when we fail to repeat observations, and go ahead believing that our results are infallible.

There are various routes by which an identification can be arrived at; medical bacteriologists often have the advantage that they know what they are looking for, and at an early stage direct their investigation into certain special channels. This may sometimes turn out to be a disadvantage; for example, the

selective media used may inhibit the growth of a pathogen whose presence is unsuspected. Steel (1962a) discussed the different techniques used for identification of pure cultures. Basically there are three approaches to the problem; in the first, which we call the *blunderbuss* method, every conceivable test is done, and when all the results are available, the characters of the organism are compared with those listed in standard texts including *Bergey's* manuals of determinative and of systematic bacteriology. If all tests appropriate to the organism have been included, it should be possible to make the identification, but quite often other (possibly unheard of) characters are mentioned so that additional tests are needed; this is such a common experience that few bacteriologists follow the blunderbuss method. However, such a comprehensive investigation is necessary when the organism has to be characterized for its description as a new species.

The second approach is based on *probabilities* and a judicious assessment of what kind of organism is causing the particular infective process. Thus, from a boil one would expect to isolate *Staphylococcus aureus*, or from the stools of a patient with an intestinal upset, one of the enterobacteria, and it would be reasonable to do tests that are likely to lead to as rapid an identification as is consistent with accuracy. When the most probable causal organism seem to be excluded, the investigator should continue with an open mind and follow the third approach.

The third approach is the step-by-step or *progressive* method as used in this *Manual*, in which the first step aims at determining a few fundamental characters such as those used in Tables 6.1 and 7.1. When these characters are known (usually in 24 hours but occasionally needing 48 hours) another set of media can be inoculated to enable appropriate tests (given in second-stage tables) to be made; the number of these tests will always be less than that needed when the blunderbuss method is followed. Sometimes additional tests are needed for the better identification of a species, and these are shown in third-stage tables.

In deciding what media to inoculate we are guided by the tests to be carried out, and we must decide for or against classical methods that are slow, as for example gelatin stab-cultures to show liquefaction or hydrolysis. Time can be saved by using multitest media in which several reactions can be observed at one time; such methods are used mainly in the pre-liminary screening of large numbers of cultures, and they are useful in that 'non-pathogens' or organisms thought to be of low-grade pathogenicity can be detected and discarded without more ado, thus restricting further tests to those organisms that appear to fit into groups that contain potential pathogens.

Other rapid methods may be considered: not only are they quicker than standard procedures but some, at least, give more clear-cut results; that of Clarke (1953a) for H$_2$S production is, however, very sensi-tive and yields more positive results than are shown in the diagnostic tables. The range and use of rapid methods is discussed in Section 4.6.

When all the tests have been completed the results are compared with the appropriate table(s); in this edition some species can be identified at the second stage, in others both the second- and third-stage tables should be consulted. For various reasons a species (or genus) may be shown in more than one table; we hope that these double entries will make identification easier for users of this *Manual*.

In using the progressive tables in Chapters 6 and 7 it is important to remember that occasionally an organism of undoubted identity will have an anoma-lous character (such as a positive oxidase reaction in a strain of *Salmonella typhi*) so misleading that it will be impossible to make the identification from the tables. We have not made provision for exceptions such as this; neither have we made double entries for motile and non-motile variants of the same species. We would also remind those using Table 6.1 that asporogenous strains of *Bacillus* species can and do occur. Not all *Bacillus* species are Gram-positive but most of those likely to be isolated in medical labora-tories are, and the genus is therefore described only in Chapter 6. However, *Gemella*, because its staining character (usually Gram-negative) can be misleading, is shown in tables in both Chapters 6 and 7.

6
Characters of Gram-positive bacteria

In characterization by stages, the first-stage table is combined with a figure and shows how, with a small number of selected characters, Gram-positive bacteria can be divided into groups that correspond to those used in orthodox classifications. Not all of the theoretically possible combinations of characters are shown in Table 6.1 because many of them do not seem to occur in nature. Each shaded square indicates the genus or genera that have the characters shown in the same column in the table above it. Equivocal characters, those difficult to determine, and characters markedly influenced by culture medium or test method can make a genus span more than one column; we have therefore tried to concentrate on the reactions given by most strains of a species in the kind of media likely to be used in routine diagnostic laboratories (majority reactions or characters) though in doing this we may perhaps have introduced a tidiness that is not warranted by the biological nature of the scheme. An example of generic spread is seen with *Aerococcus*, which appears in the third and fourth columns of Table 6.1; in this case, the reason for the spread is that the catalase reaction is not always easy to read and may be interpreted in different ways by different workers. Those who expect a large volume of gas to be produced may record the feeble reaction of *A. viridans* as negative whereas others, who habitually work with streptococci and are conversant with truly negative results in this test, will take more notice of the small bubble of gas that may be produced and record it as positive. Conflicting readings of this kind occurred when two laboratories co-operated in the work which led to the description of the new species *Aerococcus viridans* (Williams, Hirch & Cowan, 1953).

6.1 Division into major groups

As in previous editions of this *Manual*, the Gram-positive bacteria are divided into several major groups, using the characters shown in the upper part of Table 6.1; they are shown as rectangles with broken lines and are numbered to correspond with the diagnostic tables in which further characterizing details are given. These major groups of bacteria are not accretions of related genera but are groups of convenience, groups of similarly shaped organisms, or groups of organisms that give similar results in the limited number of tests applied in the first stage of our identification scheme. Indeed, we emphasize that the groupings of the Gram-positive non-spore-forming rods encompassing diphtheroids (Section 6.5), actinomycetes (Section 6.7) and organisms intermediate between them (Section 6.6) are highly artificial. The classification of the bacteria in these groups has undergone marked changes in the past decade and is still not fully resolved (see Kandler & Weiss, 1986; Jones & Collins, 1986). The genus *Corynebacterium*, for example, is taxonomically close to *Mycobacterium* and *Nocardia* but, unlike them, corynebacteria are not acid-fast; since acid-fastness is an important identifying character in routine diagnostic laboratories, the corynebacteria are therefore grouped together with morphologically similar organisms as 'diphtheroids' in Section 6.5. The same considerations apply also to the Gram-negative bacteria which we deal with in Chapter 7 though they do include a 'group of difficult organisms' comprising miscellaneous bacteria that cannot reasonably be attached to other groups. Our intention in using major groups is to be strictly practical and accordingly the size of certain bacterial groups is determined to

Table 6.1. *First-stage table for Gram-positive bacteria*

	1	2	3	4	5	6	7	8	9	10	11	12	13	14	15	16	17	18	19	20	21
Shape	S	S	S	S	S	S	S	R	R	R	R	R	R	R	R	R	R	R	R	R	R
Acid fast	–	–	–	–	–	–	–	–	–	–	–	–	–	–	–	–	–	–	w	+	+
Spores	–	–	–	–	–	–	–	–	–	–	–	–	–	–	–	–	+	+	–	–	–
Motility	–	–	–	–	–	–	–	–	–	–	–	–	–	–	–	–	D	D	–	–	–
Growth in air	+	+	+	+	+	+	–	+	+	+	+	+	+	–	–	–	d	+	+	+	+
Growth anaerobically†	–	+	w	w	+	+	+	–	+	+	+	+	–	+	+	+	+	D	–	–	?
Catalase	+	+	w	–	–	–	–	+	+	+	+	–	+	+	–	–	–	+	+	+	+
Oxidase	+	–	–	–	–	–	–	–	–	–	–	–	?	?	?	?	?	d	–	–	–
Glucose (acid)	D	+	+	+	+	+	+/–	–	–	+	+	+	+	+	+	–	D	d	+	+	+
Carbohydrates [F/O/–]	O/–	F	F	F	F	F	F/–	–	–	F	F	F	F	F	F	–	F/–	F/O/–	O	O	O/NT

Organism	1	2	3	4	5	6	7	8	9	10	11	12	13	14	15	16	17	18	19	20	21
Micrococcus [a]	+	6.2																			
Staphylococcus		+																			
Aerococcus			+	+																	
Streptococcus					+	+															
Enterococcus					+	+															
Lactococcus					+	+															
Pediococcus [b]						+															
Gemella				6.3		+	+														
Anaerobic cocci *								+													
Kurthia									+	+											
Corynebacterium												+									
Listeria												+									
Brochothrix												+									
Erysipelothrix												+									
Lactobacillus												+									
Arcanobacterium												+									
Arachnia [c]												+									
Rothia													+								
Propionibacterium														+							
Actinomyces														+							
Bifidobacterium														+	+						
Eubacterium																+					
Clostridium [d]																	+				
Bacillus								◇	◇	◇		◇						+			
Nocardia [e]																			+	+	
Mycobacterium																					+

Cultural characters references within the matrix: 6.4, 6.5, 6.6, 6.7, 6.8, 6.9, 6.10.

*	*Peptococcus* and *Peptostreptococcus*.
a	Also *Stomatococcus*.
b	Also *Leuconostoc*.
c	Also *Actinomyces odontolyticus*.
d	Exceptions: *C. histolyticum*; *C. tertium*; *C. carnis*.
e	Also *Actinomadura*.
†	Anaerobic growth of anaerobes inhibited by metronidazole.
D	Different reactions in different species of the genus.
d	Different reactions in different strains.
F	Fermentation.
O	Oxidation.
w	Weak reaction.
?	Not known.
◇	Asporogenous variants.
+	Typical form.

Cultural characters of these organisms can be found in tables with the number indicated.
S Sphere (coccus).
R Rod-shaped (bacillus).
NT Not testable.

Other symbols used in the table are explained in Tables 5.1 and 5.2 on p. 47.

some extent by the size of tables that will fit into the page. We think that embracing the major groups in this way will help in identifying bacteria logically in stages or by steps. The consequences of the groupings can be seen in Chapter 9, which uses information from Tables 6.1 and 7.1 in a scheme of identification to the level of genus utilizing punched cards. The same information is used for the computer-assisted bacterial identification programs described in Chapter 10. The bacterial groups are not named but colloquial or descriptive tags, such as anaerobic cocci and enterobacteria have been applicable to some of them. Some of the groups overlap, thus showing that they are not conventional taxa.

Some characters that depend on biochemical and molecular biological techniques are very useful in bacterial classification but are not appropriate for day-to-day diagnostic work. Such characters include, for example, the chemical composition of the cell wall (of distinctive and particular value in the classification of Gram-positive bacteria), the lipid composition (including fatty acid profiles), isoprenoid quinone structural types, whole cell protein patterns and metabolic product profiles. These, together with the information derived from DNA–base ratios, DNA restriction patterns, DNA–DNA and DNA–rRNA homology values and rRNA oligonucleotide sequence cataloguing (see Goodfellow & Minnikin, 1985; Gottschalk, 1985) can be of great importance in classification but they are not characters that can be determined by simple tests. They do, however, play an important part in bacterial identification at the reference laboratory level.

6.2   The staphylococci and micrococci
(Staphylococcus, Micrococcus, Stomatococcus, Aerococcus)

Characters common to members of the group: Gram-positive cocci: aerobic. Catalase-positive; oxidase-negative (some exceptions). Indole and H$_2$S not produced.

Grouping these genera of Gram-positive cocci together has been traditional though controversial for many years. At one time there were seemingly interminable arguments about *Staphylococcus* and *Micrococcus,* whether they should be separate or combined, and if combined what they should be

named. Later, it was generally thought that only one group of catalase-positive Gram-positive cocci was justified, for which the name *Staphylococcus* was preferred by medical and *Micrococcus* by non-medical bacteriologists. By the time Cowan (1962*b*) reviewed the situation, a distinction was made between those cocci that fermented glucose anaerobically (the staphylococci) and those that oxidized the sugar or did not produce acid from it (the micrococci). Other test results, including those for acetyl methylcarbinol (acetoin) and oxidase as well as sensitivity to lytic substances and serology, also favoured their separation. This has been strongly supported by numerical taxonomy (Hill, 1959; Feltham, 1979) and DNA studies (Silvestri & Hill, 1965; Kocur, Bergan and Mortensen, 1971) which clearly demonstrated significant differences in the GC base ratios between *Staphylococcus* (31–33%) and *Micrococcus* (69–75%); the recently created genus *Stomatococcus* (56–64%) is also clearly separate. Further confirmation of their validity as separate genera has come from studies of the structure of the cell wall (Schleifer & Kandler, 1972), and of components such as menaquinones (Jefferies *et al.*, 1968), fatty acids (Jantzen *et al.*, 1974) and fructose aldolases (Fischer *et al.*, 1983). More recently, sequencing of 16S ribosomal RNA has permitted the phylogeny of the genera to be determined (Schleifer and Stackebrandt, 1983). Indeed, Stackebrandt and Woese (1979) suggest that *Staphylococcus* is related to *Bacillus* but is a valid genus; *Micrococcus,* on the other hand, appears to be mixed with *Arthrobacter* in the coryneform group. In their view, *Planococcus,* a marine, single-species genus which is usually considered with staphylococci and micrococci, should be placed in the genus *Bacillus* together with *Sporosarcina,* but as these organisms are not pathogenic for man we mention them here only to dismiss them. Recent reviews on these topics include those of Goodfellow (1985, 1987), Alderson (1985) and Schleifer (1986).

Table 6.2*a* shows the main distinguishing features between staphylococci and the micrococci. The genus *Stomatococcus,* described by Bergan & Kocur (1982) with a single species *S. mucilaginosus,* was previously included within *Micrococcus.* We show it separately in Table 6.2*a* but for convenience include it with the micrococci in Table 6.2*c*. We also include *Aerococcus,* the α group of Shaw, Stitt & Cowan

(1951) in these tables because it can cause confusion. This genus resembles more closely the streptococci (see Section 6.3) and can be distinguished readily from staphylococci by its failure to hydrolyse arginine and to reduce nitrate; we discuss it more fully in Section 6.3.2.

The aerobic, packet-forming cocci previously referred to as the 'sarcinas' are now included in *Micrococcus* (Hubálek, 1969) thus limiting the genus *Sarcina* to anaerobic packet-forming cocci only (Shaw, Stitt & Cowan, 1951). The latter have been associated occasionally with postoperative complications of the genito-urinary tract.

With such wide differences between *Staphylococcus* and *Micrococcus* it is surprising that it has proved so difficult to develop reliable differential characterization tests for strains of these genera. Several tests have been proposed though most of them are known to have exceptions (Baker, 1986). We list some of the differential tests in Table 6.2a and consider them here. The concept that staphylococci fermented glucose whereas micrococci oxidized it (or at least produced no acid from it) formed the basis for several variations of the Oxidation–Fermentation (O–F) test of Hugh & Leifson. However, as the results varied so much, a standardized test with a modified Baird-Parker (1963) medium was recommended for staphylococci (Subcommittee, 1965, 1976). Later, a thioglycollate broth test which obviated the need for a pH indicator and an oil seal was introduced (Kloos & Schleifer, 1975b); this test depends on the extent of growth in relation to the air/medium interface. Most staphylococci grow well throughout the broth medium though *S. saprophyticus* and similar strains appear to be oxidizing because they grow poorly in the anaerobic part of the tube; in contrast micrococci, except for *M. kristinae* which ferments glucose, grow only near the surface of the medium. Despite these exceptions, the ability to grow under anaerobic conditions is an important characteristic of *Staphylococcus* strains.

The detection of cytochrome *c* in the oxidase test with 6% tetramethylphenylenediamine in dimethyl sulphoxide as the reagent (Faller & Schleifer, 1981) is characteristic of *Micrococcus* strains, although *S. sciuri* and *S. caseolyticus* are also positive. The more usual oxidase reagent is significantly less sensitive but still gives a positive reaction for most strains of

Table 6.2a. *Second-stage table for* Staphylococcus, Micrococcus, Stomatococcus *and* Aerococcus

	1	2	3	4
Growth under anaerobic conditions	+	–	+	w
Catalase	+	+	w	w
Oxidase	–	d	–	–
Carbohydrate attack	F	O/–	F	F
VP	+	–	+	–
Arginine hydrolysis	+	–	–	–
Nitrate reduced	+	–	+	–
Lysozyme	r	s	?	?
Lysostaphin	s	r	r	?

1 **Staphylococcus** s = sensitive
2 **Micrococcus** r = resistant
3 **Stomatococcus**
4 **Aerococcus**

Other symbols used in the tables are explained in Tables 5.1 and 5.2 on p. 47.

Micrococcus (Boswell, Batstone & Mitchell, 1972). A positive result thus indicates that the organism is probably not a staphylococcus.

The production of acetylmethyl carbinol (acetoin) from glucose in the Voges–Proskaüer (VP) test has been used as a valuable character for separating the two genera (Kocur & Martinec, 1962). As the presence of phosphate can interfere with acetoin production (though not among enterobacteria; see Section 4.5.1) Baird-Parker (1963) emphasized the need to use a phosphate-free medium and to incubate for up to 14 days at 30 °C for staphylococci and micrococci. Under these conditions, all staphylococci except *S. intermedius, S. hyicus*, and *S. simulans* give a positive VP reaction whereas most micrococci are negative except for *M. kristinae*. It should be noted, however, that some commercial strip methods use pyruvate as the substrate and can therefore give results which differ from those with the Baird-Parker method (Marples & Richardson, 1982).

The hydrolysis of arginine is also a useful test for separating staphylococci from micrococci (Peny & Buissiere, 1970; Feltham, 1979). Methodology is important but perhaps of more importance is the occurrence of arginine-negative strains of *S. epidermidis* (Marples & Richardson, 1981) and of arginine-positive strains of *Micrococcus* (Marples & Richardson, 1980).

53

The susceptibility of some *Micrococcus* species to lysozyme (Fleming, 1922) and of some *Staphylococcus* species to lysostaphin (Schindler & Schuhardt, 1964) as well as the greater resistance of staphylococci to erythromycin (Schleifer & Kloos, 1975b) and bacitracin (Falk & Guering, 1983) and the resistance of micrococci to the nitrofurans (Curry & Borovian, 1976) have all been proposed as simple methods for separating strains of the two genera. These approaches may have some differential value but they are not definitive. Serology (slide agglutination) has also been used successfully for distinguishing between micrococci and coagulase-negative staphylococci (Nakhla, 1973).

Although staphylococci are usually smaller than micrococci, neither this nor their Gram reaction are reliable criteria for their differentiation. Equally, pigmentation, though previously much stressed, is one of the least important characteristics of staphylococci; indeed non-pigmented (white) colony variants occur frequently. The pigmented 'violagabriellae' variant of *S. epidermidis* was regarded by Steel (1964) as an aberrant strain but Marples (1969) found that it occurred not uncommonly on human skin. Its reddish-purple pigmentation shows up well on simple media such as CYLG (Casein–yeast–lactate–glucose) or Potato Agar but is easily missed on media containing blood. Most staphylococcal pigments tend towards orange in colour whereas micrococcal pigments are typically greenish-yellow; but exceptions abound. Contrary to the usual belief, O'Connor, Willis & Smith (1966) did not find that exposure to daylight impaired pigmentation; Willis, O'Connor & Smith (1966) regarded fatty acids as more important and recommended a milk-cream agar.

Despite the absence of a single wholly reliable routine laboratory test, we do not think that microbiologists experience much difficulty in correctly identifying a strain as a *Staphylococcus* or as a *Micrococcus*.

For the selective isolation of staphylococci, particularly in food-poisoning investigations, Mannitol Salt Agar (Chapman, 1946), the egg-yolk tellurite medium of Baird-Parker (1962) and the potassium thiocyanate medium (SK) of Schleifer & Krämer (1980) are useful for inhibiting the growth of Gram-negative and other organisms; and Phenolphthalein-phosphate Agar may be used for the rapid detection of *S. aureus* colonies in mixed cultures (Barber & Kuper, 1951).

6.2.1   Staphylococcus (Tables 6.2a,b). For years, the genus *Staphylococcus* was regarded as virtually equivalent to *Staphylococcus aureus*, the main species pathogenic for man. The ability to coagulate citrated plasma virtually defined this potential pathogen and coagulase-negative staphylococci were disregarded. However, the taxonomy of this genus has undergone considerable revision, firstly in the recognition of phenotypes (Baird-Parker, 1963, 1965a,b) within the genus and, more recently, of species among the coagulase-negative human staphylococci (Schleifer & Kloos, 1975a; Kloos & Schleifer, 1975a,b) and secondly in the extension of taxonomic interest to animal and environmental staphylococci (Kloos, Schleifer & Smith, 1975a,b, 1976; Devriese *et al.*, 1983). The potential pathogenicity of coagulase-negative staphylococci, particularly in urinary tract and foreign body infections, has also become accepted (Parker, 1981; Sewell *et al.*, 1982).

Some 26 species of staphylococci have now been validly described and we list these with their identifying characters in Table 6.2b. Species 1–14 are associated with man; the remainder are essentially animal strains though they may sometimes occur in opportunist infections in man. In man, *S. aureus* remains the predominant pathogen though *S. saprophyticus* can cause primary infections of the urinary tract (Hovelius, 1986). In addition, *S. epidermidis*, *S. haemolyticus* and *S. capitis* together with biotypes within *S. hominis* – such as the recently described *S. lugdunensis* (Freney *et al.*, 1988) – are all able to act as opportunist pathogens (Parker, 1981). The few tests needed to differentiate all these species are marked with an asterisk (*) in Table 6.2b.

Staphylococcal strains, particularly those of *S. aureus*, can produce a number of extracellular proteins which may have enzymic activities and may be toxic to tissues; although these products can have some differential value, they are not used in species identification and are not shown in the diagnostic tables. Some are recognized as haemolysins, as for example the α toxin, which is also the dermonecrotic toxin; this protein is antigenic and forms the basis for a clinical antibody test. The β-haemolysin is characteristic of animal strains of *S. aureus* though its production can be inhibited by the acquisition of temperate phages. Many enzymes have toxic effects on tis-

Table 6.2b. *Third-stage table for* Staphylococcus

	1	2	3	4	5	6	7	8	9	10	11	12	13	14	15	16	17	18	19	20	21	22	23	24	25	26
Growth anaerobically	+	+	+	+	+	w	w	+[a]	+	w	+	+	w	w	w	+	+	w	–	–	w	–	–	w	+	+
Oxidase	–	–	–	–	–	–	–	–	–	+	+	–	–	+	–	+	–	+	–	–	–	–	w	+	–	–
*VP	+	–	–	–	+	+	–	?	+	+	+	–	+	+	–	+	+	–	–[?]	–	–	d	–	–	+	+
*Coagulase	+	+	d	–	–	–	d	?	–	–	–	–	–	–	–	–	–	–	–	–	–	–	–	–	–	–
Acid from																										
Lactose	+	+	+	+	D	–	–	–	D	+	+	+	+	–	+	+	d	+	+	+	d	d	+	–	–	–
*Maltose	+	–	–	d	+	–	d	–	+	+	d	–	+	+	+	d	–	+	+	+	+	+	d	+	+	–
Mannitol	+	+	+	d	+	+	–	–	+[b]	d	d	+	–	–	–	–	+	–	+	+	+	+	+	+	–	–
Fructose	+	+	+	+	+	+	+	+	d	+	+	+	+	+	+	+	+	+	+	+	+	+	+	+	+	–
Sucrose	+	+	+	+	+	+	+	–	+	+	+	+	+	+	+	+	+	d	+	+	+	+	+	+	+	–
*Trehalose	+	+	+	+	–	+	+	–	+	+	+	+	+	+	+	+	d	d	–	+	+	–	+	+	+	d
Xylose	–	–	–	–	–	–	–	?	–	–	–	–	–	+	+	–	?	?	d	+	+	d	–	–	–	–
Cellobiose	–	–	–	–	–	–	–	–	–	–	–	–	–	–	–	–	?	?	+	–	+	+	+	+	–	–
Raffinose	–	–	–	–	–	–	–	?	–	–	–	–	–	–	–	–	–	–	+	–	+	–	+	+	–	–
Mannose	+	+	+	+	+	+	+	?	–	–	–	d	–	–	+	+	+	–	d	+	+	+	+	d	+	+
*Phosphatase	+	+	+	+	+	+	d	?	d	d	–	w	–	+	+	+	?	?	+	–	+	+	+	+	+	+
Nitrate	+	+	+	+	+	+	+	+	+	+[d]	+	+	+	+	+	+	–	–	–	+	+	+	+	+	+	+
*Arginine	+	+	+	+	+	+	–	+	+	+[d]	+[d]	+	d	–	–	+	–	–	–	–	?	–	+	?	–[c]	+
Urea	d	+	+	+	+	–	–	+	–	–	+	–	–	d	–	–	–	+	–	+	+	–	d	–	+	?
Protease	+	D	+	+	w	w	–	?	–	–	–	–	–	–	+	–	–	+	–	–	+	–	w	+	?	?
*Novobiocin	s	s	s	s	s	s	s	s	s	s	s	s	r	r	r	s	s	s	r	r	r	r	r	r	s	s

1 **Staphylococcus aureus;**
 S. pyogenes; Micrococcus
 pyogenes var. aureus
2 **Staphylococcus intermedius**
3 **Staphylococcus hyicus**
4 **Staphylococcus chromogenes**
5 **Staphylococcus epidermidis;**
 Staphylococcus saprophyticus; S. albus;
 Micrococcus pyogenes var. albus

6 **Staphylococcus capitis**
7 **Staphylococcus auricularis**
8 **Staphylococcus saccharolyticus**
9 **Staphylococcus haemolyticus**
10 **Staphylococcus hominis**
11 **Staphylococcus warneri**

12 **Staphylococcus simulans**
13 **Staphylococcus saprophyticus**
14 **Staphylococcus cohnii**
15 **Staphylococcus xylosus**
16 **Staphylococcus caprae**
17 **Staphylococcus carnosus**

18 **Staphylococcus caseolyticus**
19 **Staphylococcus arlettae**
20 **Staphylococcus equorum**
21 **Staphylococcus gallinarum**
22 **Staphylococcus kloosii**
23 **Staphylococcus lentus**

24 **Staphylococcus sciuri**
25 **Staphylococcus lugdunensis**
26 **Staphylococcus schleiferi**

s = sensitive
r = resistant

a No growth anaerobically
b Usual reaction
c Ornithine decarboxylated
d Inferred reaction
* These tests are usually sufficient to identify the species that may infect man

Other symbols used in the table are explained in Tables 5.1 and 5.2 on p. 47.

sues, including the PV leucocidin of Panton & Valentine (1932); fibrinolysin (Hájek & Maršálek, (1971); deoxyribonuclease (Elston & Fitch, 1964); phosphatase (Pennock & Huddy, 1967); coagulases (Cruickshank, 1937; Cadness-Graves *et al.*, 1943); and the so-called α, β and δ toxins or haemolysins. Some strains can also produce enterotoxins (A–E) with a powerful emetic effect in man and certain animals. Some strains of *S. aureus* (of phage group I) produce toxins which cause the 'toxic shock syndrome'; enterotoxin B has also been implicated in toxic shock (Schlievert, 1986). Many laboratories now screen isolates for DNase activity to identify them as presumptive pathogenic staphylococci. Of all these factors, however, the production of coagulases which can clot plasma is still a reliable and widely used test for the recognition of potentially pathogenic staphylococci, particularly those associated with acute infections.

Two different coagulase methods can be used for presumptive pathogenic staphylococci: the tube test which detects 'free' coagulase and the slide test for 'bound' coagulase (also called the clumping factor). In tube tests, human strains produce coagulases which clot human and rabbit plasma but not always bovine plasma; conversely, bovine strains give a positive coagulase reaction more frequently with bovine than with human plasma. This test as well as the slide test for clumping factor ('pseudoagglutination' of staphylococci) are therefore best performed with rabbit plasma, which is commercially available; human plasma should be avoided unless it has been strictly controlled for clotting capability and absence of inhibitors. A variety of commercial slide agglutination screening tests are also available; some detect only the clumping factor but others also detect the staphylococcal cell-wall component 'protein A' which binds non-specifically to γ globulins (Grov, Myklestad & Oeding, 1964). None of these slide tests is as reliable as a strictly controlled tube coagulase test (Dickson & Marples, 1986) but because of their ease of use and rapidity they are widely used as a good indicator of pathogenic potential.

Taxonomically four main clusters or groups of species can be recognized respectively around *S. aureus*, *S. epidermidis*, *S. saprophyticus* and *S. sciuri* though the validity of all the 26 species is undeniable.

The '**aureus**' group of species includes *S. aureus*,

S. intermedius, *S. hyicus*, *S. chromogenes* and, more distantly, *S. simulans*. Although these species share several phenotypic characteristics (Feltham, 1979; Goodfellow *et al.*, 1983), DNA hybridization clearly separates them (Schleifer, 1986). Although *S. intermedius* and *S. hyicus* cause infections in certain animals they have not been implicated yet in human disease.

Strains of *S. aureus* can also be subdivided into a number of biotypes which reflect different sources. Meyer (1966) distinguished the 'hominis' from the bovis variety and Háyek & Maršálek (1971) further elaborated the differences, calling the hominis strains biotype A, some strains B, bovine strains C and other animal strains D, E & F. The E & F biotypes are now recognized as *S. intermedius*. Biotype A strains are associated with man; they usually produce fibrinolysin and the α haemolysin, and are susceptible to an internationally accepted set of phages for typing isolates from human infections (Asheshov & Rountree, 1975). Strains of bovine origin, biotype C, produce β haemolysin but not fibrinolysin and, except for phage 42D, they are susceptible only to special sets of phages developed for typing isolates from animals.

Strains of *S. intermedius* and *S. hyicus* do not possess clumping factor for slide tests and they take longer to produce a clot in the tube test than human *S. aureus* isolates (Devriese *et al.*, 1978). *S. chromogenes* and *S. simulans* are coagulase-negative.

Acetoin production (VP test) is useful for differentiating *S. aureus* (positive) from the other coagulase-positive staphylococcal strains (negative).

The '**epidermidis**' group of species includes three subgroups: (i) *S. epidermidis*, *S. capitis* and some strains of *S. warneri*; (ii) *S. hominis* and the rest of *S. warneri*; (iii) *S. haemolyticus*, *S. caprae* and *S. saccharolyticus*. A distinguishing feature of the '*epidermidis*' group is that almost all strains are sensitive to novobiocin in concentrations up to 1.6 μg/ml in agar media (Schleifer & Kloos, 1975*a*).

S. epidermidis, followed by *S. haemolyticus*, are the commonest coagulase-negative species associated with human infections other than those of the urinary tract (Nord *et al.*, 1976; Marples & Richardson, 1981). *S. epidermidis* is relatively active biochemically but does not acidify mannitol or trehalose; *S. haemolyticus* usually acidifies both these sugars. The other species in the 'epidermidis' group are less active biochemically, less well defined and less likely to be associated with disease or to exhibit multiple resistance to antibiotics. Any of the species could be encountered as contaminants and occasional opportunist infections have been reported (Fleurette et al., 1987). Taxonomic developments in this group should be expected. For S. epidermidis useful serological and phage typing schemes have been developed (Pillet & Orta, 1977; de Saxe et al., 1981).

The 'saprophyticus' group of species includes S. saprophyticus, S. cohnii and S. xylosus. They are all resistant to novobiocin and exhibit anomalous resistance to penicillins and fusidic acid (Richardson & Marples, 1980). S. saprophyticus appears to act as a primary pathogen causing urinary tract infections in young women (Maskell, 1974) and possibly prostatitis and urethritis in men (Hovelius, 1986). The skin is probably the main source of these infections though the less pathogenic S. cohnii is the usual novobiocin-resistant commensal species present in adult skin (Namavar et al., 1978). S. xylosus is an uncommon cause of human infection and most isolates are of animal origin (Marples & Richardson, 1981). The 'saprophyticus' taxon is frequently used as a collective 'dump' in medical microbiology laboratories.

The 'sciuri' group of species comprises S. sciuri and S. lentus, both of which are also novobiocin-resistant. These species are of animal origin and differ from other staphylococci in giving a positive oxidase reaction and in their ability to ferment cellobiose. Numerical taxonomy (Feltham, 1979) and DNA hybridization (Schleifer, 1986) indicate that they are only distantly related to other species of Staphylococcus. However, some strains resembling S. sciuri and S. gallinarum have been isolated from human infections; such strains may give anomalous reactions in clumping factor tests.

In summary, the staphylococci include the primary pathogens S. aureus and S. saprophyticus as well as the opportunist pathogens S. epidermidis and S. haemolyticus. The other species appear to be of lesser clinical significance though they may be involved, for example, in implant surgery and immunosuppressive therapy. In spite of the extended discussion about the genus Staphylococcus and its species, they are relatively easy to isolate and identify.

Minidefinition: *Staphylococcus. Gram-positive cocci in clusters. Non-motile; nonsporing. Aerobic and facultatively anaerobic. Catalase-positive; usually oxidase-negative. Hydrolyse arginine; produce acetoin. Attack sugars by fermentation. Type species: S. aureus; NCTC strain 8532.*

6.2.2 Micrococcus (Tables 6.2a,c). Hucker (1924b) originally included both staphylococci and micrococci in the genus *Micrococcus* but, as described in Section 6.2, opinions have since changed. Whether or not this varied and somewhat rambling genus should be absorbed into or linked with *Arthrobacter* we leave for taxonomists to sort out (Alderson, 1985; Goodfellow, 1987). It is, however, undoubtedly separate from *Staphylococcus* and is currently a valid genus. Organisms that fit the current description of micrococci are commonly encountered in routine laboratories either as environmental contaminants or as commensals from normal skin and only occasionally from infections. The difficulty is to recognize when these colonially distinct 'non-pathogens' do cause infection and, for this, simple reliable tests are required. Unfortunately, the characters that can be readily detected (Table 6.2c) are less convincing than those obtained by more complex methods such as DNA hybridization, cell-wall component analysis and the like though not all the species listed should be regarded as wholly secure.

The characters shown in Table 6.2c are based on descriptions by Kloos, Tornabene & Schleifer (1974). Many of the criteria are negative yet these species can actively metabolize a wide variety of substrates; presumably the test systems are at fault in failing to detect such activity.

In contrast to the staphylococci, pigment production among micrococci is a stable and important differential character; although its taxonomic significance is uncertain, we do, however, use it in Table 6.2c. The differences between *M. luteus*, the classical micrococcus, and *M. varians* are not great; they both form easily recognizable lemon-yellow, mounded colonies of varied texture. The yellow–orange colonies of *M. kristinae* (which behaves biochemically like a staphylococcus) and the bright orange colonies of *M. nishinomiyaensis* together with the pink and red colours of *M. roseus* and the motile *M.*

Table 6.2c. *Third-stage table for* Micrococcus *and* Stomatococcus

	1	2	3	4	5	6	7	8	9
Motility	−	−	−	−	−	−	+	−	−
Oxidase	+	+	+	+	+	+	+	+	−
VP	−	−	−	+	−	−	−	−	+
Pigmentation	Y	Y	C	Y	O	C	R	R	−
Carbohydrates, acid from									
Glucose	−	+	−	+	d	−	−	d	+
Fructose	−	+	−	+	−	−	−	d	+
Sucrose	−	d	−	+	−	−	−	−	+
Arginine	−	−	−	−	−	+	−	−	−
Nitrate reduced	−	+	−	−	+	−	−	+	+
Lysozyme	s	r	d	r	r	s	s	s	?
Methicillin	s	s	s	s	s	r	s	s	s

1 **Micrococcus luteus**; *Micrococcus afermentans; Micrococcus lysodeikticus; Staphylococcus afermentans*
2 **Micrococcus varians**; *Micrococcus lactis; Staphylococcus lactis*
3 **Micrococcus lylae**
4 **Micrococcus kristinae**
5 **Micrococcus nishinomiyaensis**
6 **Micrococcus sedentarius**
7 **Micrococcus agilis**
8 **Micrococcus roseus**; *Staphylococcus roseus*
9 **Stomatococcus mucilaginosus**

Y = yellow   s = sensitive
C = cream   r = resistant
O = orange
R = red

Other symbols used in the table are explained in Tables 5.1 and 5.2 on p. 47.

agilis differ from any staphylococcal pigmentation and are usually obvious though a few isolates, particularly when young, may cause some confusion.

None of the species are regarded as clinically significant though there are occasional reports of infections with strains similar to *M. lylae* and the marine species, *M. sedentarius* (Old & McNeill, 1979; Marples & Richardson, 1980; Fleurette *et al.*, 1987). These strains, which are of uncertain taxonomic status, are described as non-pigmented, able to hydrolyse arginine and resistant to methicillin.

Stomatococcus mucilaginosus, an oral commensal organism in man, may be associated with occasional opportunist infections. It can be recognized by the sticky adherent nature of colonies on solid media and by a positive aesculin reaction together with the test characters shown in Table 6.2c.

In summary, the micrococci comprise mostly environmental and saprophytic strains. The main question is one of recognition and exclusion except for the occasional strain possibly associated with disease. Certainly it is essential before discarding any isolate that might be a *Micrococcus* to make sure it is not a *Staphylococcus*. And that, fortunately, is not too difficult.

Minidefinition: *Micrococcus. Gram-positive cocci in small or large clusters. Non-motile; non-sporing. Aerobic. Catalase-positive; usually oxidase-positive. Do not usually produce acetoin. Attack sugars oxidatively or not at all. Type species: M. luteus; NCTC strain 2665.*

6.2.3 Aerococcus (Tables 6.2a; 6.3a,b). This genus was described and named by Williams, Hirch & Cowan (1953). The cocci, which formed the α-group of Shaw, Stitt & Cowan (1951), were isolated from environmental samples such as air, dust, and dairy utensils, and were regarded as intermediate between staphylococci and streptococci though nearer to the latter. The catalase reaction is feeble and may be described in different ways by different observers; to some it will be regarded as negative, to others it will be weakly positive. Since the catalase reaction is important for distinguishing between staphylococci and streptococci, we include the characters of *Aerococcus viridans* in Table 6.2*a* among the Gram-positive, catalase-positive cocci (*Staphylococcus, Micrococcus*) as well as in Tables 6.3*a* and *c* with the catalase-negative streptococci. Like streptococci, the aerococci do not reduce nitrate to nitrite; however, production of the enzyme leucine aminopeptidase by all streptococci (Table 6.3*b*) but not by staphylococci, micrococci or aerococci provides a basis for their separation.

Minidefinition: *Aerococcus. Gram-positive cocci in pairs, fours, and small clusters. Non-motile; non-sporing. Aerobic and microaerophilic; facultatively anaerobic. Catalase feebly positive or negative; oxidase-negative. Attack sugars fermentatively without gas production. Type species: A. viridans; NCTC strain 8251.*

6.3 The streptococci

(*Streptococcus, Lactococcus, Enterococcus, Aerococcus, Leuconostoc, Pediococcus* and *Gemella*)

Characters common to members of the group: **Gram-positive cocci; non-motile (rare exceptions). Aerobic, facultatively anaerobic. Catalase-negative; oxidase-negative. Carbohydrates fermented; gas not produced. Nitrates not reduced. Indole and H$_2$S not produced.**

With so many shared characteristics, this group of genera is fairly homogeneous and does not include any unexpected members except *Gemella*, which is somewhat different; we give the reasons for including it here in Section 6.3.6. We have also included the strictly anaerobic peptococci and peptostreptococci (see Section 6.4) in Table 6.3*a* because there can be difficulties in distinguishing them from streptococci and other members of this group.

In addition to its inclusion in the staphylococcus–micrococcus group (Section 6.2.3), *Aerococcus viridans* appears here because it is an organism inter-

Table 6.3*a*. *Second-stage table for* Streptococcus, Enterococcus, Aerococcus, Gemella, Pediococcus, Leuconostoc, Peptococcus *and* Peptostreptococcus

	1	2	3	4	5	6	7	8
Growth in air + 10% CO$_2$	+	+	+	+	+	+	−	−
Gas from glucose	−	−	−	−	−	+	−	d
Growth in 6.5% NaCl broth	−	+	+	−	d	−	−	−
Growth on Acetate Agar at pH 5.4	−	−	−	−	+	d	−	−
Growth in 40% bile	D	+	+	−	−	−	−	−
Sensitive to metronidazole	−	−	−	−	−	−	+	+

1 Streptococcus (pyogenic, viridans and lactic divisions): see Table 6.3*b*.
2 Enterococcus (*Streptococcus*: enterococcus division): see Table 6.3*b*.
3 Aerococcus: see Tables 6.2*a*; 6.3*b*.
4 Gemella: see Table 6.3*b*.
5 Pediococcus: see Table 6.3*b*.
6 Leuconostoc: see Table 6.3*b*.
7 Peptococcus: see Table 6.4.
8 Peptostreptococcus: see Table 6.4. *P. putridus; Streptococcus putridus*

Symbols used in the table are explained in Tables 5.1 and 5.2 on p. 47.

Table 6.3b. *Third-stage table for* Streptococcus, Enterococcus, Lactococcus, Pediococcus, Aerococcus *and* Gemella

	1	2	3	4	5	6	7	8	9	10	11	12	13	14	15	16	17
Haemolysis	β	β/–	β	α	β	β	β	β/–	β	α/–	β/–	β	α	α/β	α/β	–	–
Requires CO_2 for growth	–	–	–	–	–	–	–	d	–	–	–	–	d	–	–	–	+
Growth at 45 °C	–	–	–	–	–	–	–	–	–	–	–	–	–	–	–	–	–
Growth in 6.5% NaCl broth	–	d[a]	–	–	–	–	–[a]	–[a]	–	–	–[a]	–	–	–	–	–	–
Growth on 40% Bile Agar	–	+	–	–	–	–	–	d	–	–	d	d	–	d	–	–	–
Leucine aminopeptidase	+	+	+	+	+	+	+	+	+	+	+	+	+	+	+	+	+
Bile–aesculin test	–	–	–	–	–	–	–	–	–	–	d	–	–	–	–	–	–
Voges–Proskaüer test[b]	–	+	–	–	–	–	–	+	+	+	–	–	–	–	–	–	–
Pyrrolydonylarylamidase	+	–	–	–	–	–	–	–	–	d	d	–	d	–	–	+	+
Phosphatase	+	+	+	+	+	+	+	+	+	d	–	+	–	D	d	–	–
Pyridoxal or cysteine dependence	–	–	–	–	–	–	–	–	–	–	–	–	–	–	–	+	–
Hydrolysis of																	
hippurate	–	+	–	–	–	–	–	–	–	+	–	d	–	–	–	–	–
aesculin	d	–	–	d	d	d	d	+	+	+	+	–	d	+	d	–	–
arginine	+	+	+	+	+	+	+	+	+	+	+	+	d	+	–	–	–
starch[c]	–	–	–	–	–	–	–	–	–	–	–	–	–	–	–	–	–
Sensitive to																	
bacitracin (0.1 unit)	+	d	d	d	–	–	–	–	–	d	d	d	+	d	d	–	–
optochin	–	–	–	–	–	–	–	–	–	–	–	–	+	–	–	–	–
H_2O_2 production	–	–	–	–	–	–	–	–	–	–	–	–	+	+	+	–	–
Fermentation of																	
pyruvate	–	–	–	–	–	–	–	–	–	–	–	–	–	–	–	–	–
ribose	–	+	–	+	d	+	+	–	+	+	–	+	–	–	–	–	–
arabinose	–	–	–	–	–	–	–	–	–	–	–	–	–	–	–	–	–
mannitol	D[d]	–	–	–	–	–	–	d	+	+	–	–	–	–	–	–	–
sorbitol	–	–	–	d	+	–	–	–	+	+	–	–	–	–	–	–	–
adonitol	–	–	–	–	–	–	–	–	–	–	–	–	–	–	–	–	–
sucrose	+	+	+	+	+	+	+	+	+	+	+	+	+	+	+	d	(w)
lactose	+	d	–	+	+	d	d	d	d	+	+	+	+	+	+	d	–
trehalose	+	+	–	+	–	+	+	+	+	+	+	+	+	+	d	d	(w)
raffinose	–	–	–	–	–	–	–	d	–	d	D[e]	–	d	d	d	d	–
inulin	–	–	–	–	–	–	–	–	–	+	d	–	d	d	–	–	–
starch	+	d	+	+	+	+	+	d	d	d	+	+	d	d	d	d	(w)
Polysaccharide from sucrose	–	–	–	–	–	–	–	–	–	–	–	–	–	Dx/–	–/Dx	–	–
Motility	–	–	–	–	–	–	–	–	–	–	–	–	–	–	–	–	–
Yellow pigment	–	–	–	–	–	–	–	–	–	–	–	–	–	–	–	–	–
Lancefield antigen	A	B	C	C	C	C	G	–/F/ G/C/A	E/P/ U/V/–	–/E	R/S/ T/–	L	–	–/H	–/O/K–	–	

1 **Streptococcus pyogenes**; *S. haemolyticus*
2 **Streptococcus agalactiae**
3 **Streptococcus equi**
4 **Streptococcus dysgalactiae**
5 **Streptococcus zooepidemicus**
6 **Streptococcus equisimilis**
   Streptococcus spp. group C
7 **Streptococcus** spp. group G (large colony variety); *Streptococcus canis*
8 **Streptococcus anginosus**; *'S. milleri'*; minute colony haemolytic streptococci; *S. intermedius*–MG; *S.constellatus*
9 **Streptococcus porcinus**; *S. lentus*
10 **Streptococcus uberis**
11 **Streptococcus suis**
12 **Streptococcus** spp. group L
13 **Streptococcus pneumoniae**; pneumococci
14 **Streptococcus sanguis**
15 **Streptococcus oralis**; *'S. mitior'*
16 **Streptococcus** spp. pyridoxal or cysteine dependent
17 **Streptococcus morbillorum**

α Green zone around colonies on Blood Agar
β Clear, colourless zone around colonies on Blood Agar
a Some strains will grow in 4% NaCl broth
b More strains positive in a medium containing pyruvate than in Glucose Phosphate Broth
c Zone of clearing greater than 2 mm diameter around growth on Starch Agar stained with Lugol's iodine
d Strains of M-type 6 and M-type 55 ferment mannitol

e Strains of Lancefield serological Group R ferment raffinose
f May be opposite reaction with strains of serotypes d or g
g Positive reactions with strains of serotypes b, d and g
h Usually positive with human isolates
j Both antigens may be present in a single strain
Dx = Dextran (glucan)
Lv = Levan (fructan)

Other symbols used in the table are explained in Tables 5.1 and 5.2 on p. 47.

Table 6.3b. (contd).

	18	19	20	21	22	23	24	25	26	27	28	29	30	31	32	33	34
Haemolysis	–/β	α/–	–	α/–	β	α	–/α/β	–/α	α/–	α	–/α/β	–	–/α	–/α	–/α	α	β/α/–
Requires CO_2 for growth	–	–	–	–	–	–	–	–	–	–	+	–	–	–	–	–	–
Growth at 45 °C	+	+	+	+	+	+	+	d	d	d	–	–	–	–	+	–	–
Growth in 6.5% NaCl broth	+	+	+	+	+	+	+	–[a]	–[a]	–[a]	–[a]	–[a]	–[a]	–	+	+	–
Growth on 40% Bile agar	+	+	+	+	+	+	+	+	+	+	d	d	+	d	+	+	–
Leucine aminopeptidase	+	+	+	+	+	+	+	+	+	+	+	+	+	d	+	–	+
Bile–aesculin test	+	+	+	+	+	+	+	+	+	+	d	d	d	d	+	d	–
Voges–Proskaüer test [b]	+	+	+	+	+	+	+	+	+	+	+	+	+	+	+	d	w
Pyrrolydonylarylamidase	+	+	+	+	+	+	+	–	–	–	–	–	d	d	–	d	+
Phosphatase	–	–	–	–	–	–	–	–	–	–	–	d	–	–	–	–	+
Pyridoxal or cysteine dependence	–	–	–	–	–	–	–	–	–	–	–	–	–	–	–	–	–
Hydrolysis of																	
hippurate	d	d	–	–	+	d	d	–	–	–	–	–	d	–	d	d	–
aesculin	+	+	+	+	+	+	+	+	+	+	+[f]	+	+	+	+	d	–
arginine	+	+	+	+	+	–	+	–	–	–	–[g]	–	+	–	+	–	–
starch [c]	–	–	–	–	–	–	–	+	–	–	–	–	–	–	–	–	–
Sensitive to																	
bacitracin (0.1 unit)	–	–	–	–	–	–	–	–	–	–	–	d	d	–	d	d	d
optochin	–	–	–	–	–	–	–	–	–	–	–	–	–	–	–	–	–
H_2O_2 production	–	d	–	+	–	d	–	–	–	–	–[f]	–	–	d	+	+	–
Fermentation of																	
pyruvate	+	–	–	–	–	(w)	–										
ribose	+	+	+	+	+	+	+	–	–	–	–	–	+	d	+	d	–
arabinose	–	+	+	+	+	d	–	d	–	–	–	–	d	d	d	–	–
mannitol	+	+	+	+	+	+	–	d[h]	–	–	+	–	d	d	–	d	–
sorbitol	+	d	d	–	–	+	–	–	–	–	+[f]	–	–	–	–	d	–
adonitol	–	–	–	–	–	+	–	–	–	–	–	–	–	–	–	–	–
sucrose	+	+	+	+	+	+	+	–	+	+	+	+	d	d	d	d	+
lactose	+	+	+	+	+	+	+	+	+	+	+	+	d	d	d	–	+
trehalose	+	+	+	+	+	+	d	+	d	–	+	d	d	+	+	+	d
raffinose	–	d	d	+	+	–	–	+	+	d	+	+	–	d	–	d	–
inulin	–	d	–	+	+	d	–	d	d	d	+	d	–	–	–	d	–
starch	+	d	–	–/w	+	–	–	+	–	–	–	d	+	–	–	–	d
Polysaccharide from sucrose	–	–	–	–	–	–		Dx/–	–	–	Dx	Lv/Dx	–	Dx/–	–	–	–
Motility	–	–	–	+	+	–	–	–	–	–	–	–	–	–	–	–	–
Yellow pigment	–	–	+	+	–	–	–	–	–	–	–	–	–	–	–	–	–
Lancefield antigen	D	D	D	D	D	Q/D[j]	D	D	D	D	–/E	–/K	N	–	D/–	–	–

18 **Enterococcus faecalis**; *S. faecalis*
19 **Enterococcus faecium**
20 **Enterococcus mundtii**
21 **Enterococcus casseliflavus**
22 **Enterococcus gallinarum**
23 **Enterococcus avium**
24 **Enterococcus durans**; *S. faecium* var *durans*; *S. durans*
25 **Streptococcus bovis** biotype I
26 **Streptococcus bovis** biotype II
27 **Streptococcus equinus**
28 **Streptococcus mutans**, serotypes c, e and f
29 **Streptococcus salivarius**
30 **Lactococcus lactis**
31 **Leuconostoc** spp.
32 **Pediococcus** spp.
33 **Aerococcus** spp.; *Pediococcus*; *Gaffkya* spp.
34 **Gemella haemolysans**; *Neisseria haemolysans*

α Green zone around colonies on Blood Agar
β Clear, colourless zone around colonies on Blood Agar
a Some strains will grow in 4% NaCl broth
b More strains positive in a medium containing pyruvate than in Glucose Phosphate Broth
c Zone of clearing greater than 2 mm diameter around growth on Starch Agar stained with Lugol's iodine
d Strains of M-type 6 and M-type 55 ferment mannitol

e Strains of Lancefield serological Group R ferment raffinose
f May be opposite reaction with strains of serotypes d or g
g Positive reactions with strains of serotype b
h Usually positive with human isolates
j Both antigens may be present in a single strain
Dx =Dextran (glucan)
Lv = Levan (fructan)

Other symbols used in the table are explained in Tables 5.1 and 5.2 on p. 47.

mediate between the catalase-positive and catalase-negative Gram-positive cocci with characteristics of both groups; within that spectrum it is nearer to the streptococci than to the staphylococci.

6.3.1   Streptococcus (Tables 6.3a,b). Rational classification of the streptococci remained problematical until the demonstration of serologically identifiable polysaccharide group antigens by Lancefield (1933, 1940) and the definition by Sherman (1937) of four major divisions which are still in current use: the pyogenic streptococci, the viridans streptococci, the enterococci and the smallest group, the lactic (milk) streptococci. Subsequent efforts to correlate Lancefield's serological groups with divisions based on cultural and biochemical characteristics were bedevilled by a host of exceptions as well as by aberrant strains. Isolates that do not match any well-defined streptococcal species continue to occur; some, such as pyridoxal-dependent strains (Bouvet *et al.*, 1985) might form a useful species or taxon, but others differ only slightly from species currently recognized. The application of newer taxonomic techniques, especially DNA hybridization, cell-wall analysis, and fatty acid and enzyme profiles, have certainly revealed natural relationships among, for example, the pyogenic streptococci (Kilpper-Bälz & Schleifer, 1984); in contrast, the results of such tests alone would suggest that organisms as different as the oropharyngeal commensal *Streptococcus salivarius* and the lactic organism *Streptococcus* (now *Lactococcus*) *thermophilus* should form a single species (Farrow & Collins, 1984a) though the former is of no use as a starter culture for the production of yoghurt (Marshall, Cole & Phillips, 1985). The possible return of the pneumococcus to the former genus *Diplococcus* now seems unlikely but the idea that enterococci should form a separate genus, *Enterococcus*, has been revived (Schleifer & Kilpper-Bälz, 1984; Collins *et al.*, 1984) is now widely recognized.

Despite the mass of information currently available on the characterization of streptococci, haemolysis is still of considerable differential as well as predictive pathogenic use even if limited in taxonomic value; this is reminiscent of the 1920s (Brown, 1919) when streptococci were divided into the haemolytic (those producing β haemolysis), the viridans (those producing green or α haemolysis) and the non-haemolytic (unfortunately mislabelled γ haemolytic) on Blood Agar plates. Although the kind of haemolysis on this medium is not always clear-cut, especially as the hydrogen peroxide produced by some streptococci can interfere with haemolysin activity and contribute to 'greening' by its action on haemoglobin, it is nevertheless a useful starting point when present. In the present divisions, the pyogenic streptococci include many of the common pathogens of man and domestic animals: most but not all of them are β haemolytic and serological methods are particularly useful for their identification (Table 6.3b). Among the viridans streptococci (which include the pneumococci) and the enterococci (the latter belonging to Lancefield serological group D but having differing haemolytic properties), biochemical and physiological tests are more satisfactory than serology for species identification; the enterococci are generally more salt-tolerant, and also more heat-resistant than other streptococci. These traditional characterization procedures, despite their limitations, are usually adequate if time-consuming but they do not constitute a single comprehensive identification scheme for all the streptococci isolated in diagnostic laboratories. As a step towards such an objective, Colman & Ball (1984) suggested that miniaturized identification systems supplemented with a few other tests (including Lancefield grouping, bacitracin and optochin sensitivity and pyridoxal dependence) might suffice for the majority of strains. Outside the medical, dental and veterinary fields, the lactic streptococci, now transferred to the new genus *Lactococcus* (Schleifer *et al.*, 1985), are important to the milk, dairy and cheese industries; as they are rarely if ever pathogenic, we show *L. lactis* only in Table 6.3b.

The concept of 'species' as defined for streptococci is in general lower and less firm than for most other genera, it is therefore important to appreciate that 'aberrant' strains do occur and that in practice exceptions to the characters shown in Table 6.3b are likely to be encountered from time to time. Moreover, the precipitin reactions for the Lancefield antigens are not always straightforward; difficulties can occur, particularly with Group D strains, some extracts of which will not react with otherwise satisfactory antisera unless the antigen is precipitated with ethanol (Smith & Shattock, 1962). Some strains of *S.*

sanguis and *S. salivarius* do not react with any of the grouping antisera and their identification depends on other characters. Many streptococci seem to be sensitive to oxygen on first isolation so that their detection in clinical material may be more successful under anaerobic conditions. Added CO_2 is often advantageous for growth and some strains of pneumococci will not grow without it initially (Austrian & Collins, 1966) though the requirement is usually lost rapidly on subculture.

Among the pyogenic streptococci, *S. pyogenes* (Lancefield Group A) remains the major pathogen of man. Usually the first step in its recognition is the presence of β haemolytic colonies on Blood Agar plates due to the oxygen-stable 'S' lysin; many isolates, however, are only weakly haemolytic and slashing the agar during inoculation of plates or anaerobic incubation often increases the extent of haemolysis with such strains. Some isolates lack the 'S' lysin completely and are therefore non-haemolytic; the need for investigation of such strains, including determination of their Lancefield group antigen, may become apparent only because they are bacitracin-sensitive (Maxted, 1953) or because of their biochemical reactions. All Group A streptococci produce pyrrolydonylarylamidase (PYRA) but fail to ferment ribose; this combination of characteristics distinguishes them from strains of Groups B, C and G (Table 6.3b); it can, however, occur among other streptococci including strains of enterococci, pneumococci and aerococci as well as *S. suis* though not among those of *S. anginosus* (often called '*S. milleri*' by clinical microbiologists) that cross-react with group A antiserum. We suspect that in the future such biochemical tests may well replace some of the present conventional methods for the identification of the pyogenic streptococci. Strains of *S. pyogenes* can be typed serologically by determination of the M and T protein antigens; the latter is stable but, unlike the former, is not related to virulence. Recent changes in the pattern and severity of infections with *S. pyogenes* as well as the association of particular M/T types with certain clinical syndromes (Gaworzewska & Colman, 1988) suggest that this reference laboratory procedure could usefully be applied more often for epidemiological purposes.

The streptococci of Lancefield Group B (*S. agalactiae*) isolated from human infections are often not only haemolytic but may also produce pigmented colonies (Tapsall, 1987). These linked characters occur much less often in strains isolated from bovine infections (Butter & de Moor, 1967). Anaerobic incubation on media containing starch is the best method of detecting the tan-coloured pigment produced by these strains (Islam, 1977). Irrespective of their haemolytic reactions on Blood Agar plates, Group B streptococci of both human and animal origin produce, with rare exceptions, a substance that will lyse sheep or ox but not human, horse, rabbit or guinea-pig red cells which have been exposed to a sphingomyelinase C such as the β-lysin of staphylococci or the α-toxin of *Clostridium perfringens* (Sterzik & Fehrenbach, 1985). This phenomenon, known as the CAMP reaction (Christie, Atkins and Munch-Petersen, 1944) can occur also with some strains of *S. uberis* (Roguinsky, 1969) and of *Listeria monocytogenes*.

Several different species of streptococci possess the Lancefield Group C antigen (Table 6.3b); in addition, some strains of *S. anginosus* ('*S. milleri*') cross-react with this Group antiserum. A positive Voges–Proskaüer reaction and failure to ferment ribose will distinguish the latter. Subdivision of Lancefield Group C strains is based traditionally on tests for the fermentation of lactose, trehalose and sorbitol and on the presence or absence as well as the nature of haemolysis on Blood Agar media; there is, however, a need for new and more specific tests probably based on their enzyme activities. *S. zooepidemicus*, an animal pathogen, occasionally causes serious infections in man (Michalcu *et al.*, 1982; Barnham *et al.*, 1987) but the suggestion that it should be transferred to *S. equi* (Farrow & Collins, 1984b) because of homology in DNA hybridization results fails to take account of differences in their pathogenicity and host-specificity: *S. equi* causes strangles in horses whereas *S. zooepidemicus* causes pyogenic infections in many different animals. This objection applies also to their suggestion that the human commensals and opportunist pathogens (Efstratiou, 1983) at present called *S. equisimilis* and the 'pyogenes-like' strains of Lancefield Group G, should be transferred to the species *S. dysgalactiae*.

Strains of Lancefield Group G that are pathogenic for animals have been brought together as *S. canis* (Clark *et al.*, 1984; Devriese *et al.*, 1986); these animal isolates all form β-galactosidase and chymotrypsin. The 'human' strains of Group G can be distinguished from *S. canis* because they are more 'pyogenes-like' in fermenting trehalose and in producing β-glucuronidase, streptokinase and hyaluronidase. Some strains of *S. anginosus* ('*S. milleri*') cross-react with Group C antiserum and these have the same pattern of reactions as other members of Group C except that they ferment raffinose more often (Smith & Sherman, 1938).

The minute-colony-producing organisms assembled together as '*S. milleri*' are serologically heterogeneous and taxonomic agreement has yet to be reached; however, as the name *S. milleri* is still in widespread clinical use, we continue to give it alongside the present correct name *S. anginosus*. They are, however, biochemically homogeneous (Table 6.3*b*) and all give a positive VP reaction, form phosphatase and hydrolyse arginine but fail to ferment either ribose or sorbitol and do not produce β-glucuronidase (Ruoff & Ferraro, 1986). They can be regarded as forming one aggregated species ('*S. milleri*') irrespective of their haemolysis (Colman & Williams, 1972) or, alternatively, they may be subdivided into haemolytic strains called *S. anginosus*, and non-haemolytic organisms labelled *S. intermedius* if they ferment lactose and *S. constellatis* if they do not (Facklam, 1984). Another approach, suggested by Coykendall, Wesbecker & Gustafson (1987), is to apply the name *S. anginosus* rather than '*S. milleri*' to the single species but accept three biotypes: biotype 1 strains are mostly haemolytic and do not ferment lactose or hydrolyse aesculin; biotype 2 strains, which may or may not be haemolytic, split aesculin and ferment lactose and sometimes starch; biotype 3 strains are like those of biotype 2 but additionally ferment either raffinose or mannitol, or both of them. We think, however, that the use of a single name for all these organisms is useful meanwhile because clinically they all produce similar suppurative diseases (Van der Auwera, 1985) although strains of biotype 3 occur also as commensals in the vagina (Ball & Parker, 1979; Poole & Wilson, 1979).

The species *S. porcinus*, also known under differing names '*S. infrequens*' and '*S. lentus*', is serologically heterogeneous and includes those streptococci, pathogenic for pigs, that belong to Lancefield serological Groups E, P, U and V. These β-haemolytic streptococci possess a distinctive set of physiological and biochemical characters (Wessman, 1986) by which they can be identified, though full characterization would also require demonstration of their actual Group antigen (Table 6.3*b*).

Some strains of *S. uberis* cross-react with Group E and others with Groups G, P or U antisera (Roguinsky, 1969, 1971). Useful reactions for the differentiation of these viridans streptococci from *S. agalactiae* include the fermentation of mannitol and sorbitol, hydrolysis of aesculin and hippurate (Cullen, 1969) and a positive VP reaction; the absence of heat, salt and bile tolerance distinguishes them from the enterococci.

S. suis, another serologically heterogeneous species which is pathogenic for pigs, includes more than eight distinct serotypes. Of these, serotype 1 is known also as Group S and serotype 2 as Group R streptococci. Again, confirmation of the serotype is an aid to identification of this species, particularly in occupation-related cases of meningitis caused by Group R strains. Early descriptions of these strains suggested a greater physiological homogeneity than has been found subsequently (Hommez *et al.*, 1986).

Streptococci of Group L have been isolated from a variety of animal sources and occasionally from man. They can be mistaken for *S. pyogenes* (Group A streptococci) because they not only produce β-haemolysis but are often sensitive to bacitracin and may even cross-react with the 'A' reagent in some commercial grouping kits. Tests for the fermentation of ribose and the production of pyrrolydonylarylamidase (PYRA) distinguish them from *S. pyogenes*; and cross-reactions with group A sera do not occur with less sensitive precipitin tests.

Despite all the characters shown in Table 6.3*b*, pneumococci are usually identified by their sensitivity to optochin, bile solubility or by agglutination with a polyvalent serum (OMNI-serum) though as always occasional exceptions occur. Some strains of *S. oralis* (also known as '*S. mitior*') are sensitive to optochin and bile-soluble strains of *Enterococcus* (*Streptococcus*) *faecalis* also occur; moreover, rough strains of pneumococci may not be lysed by bile (Lund, 1959). OMNI-serum contains antibodies to the choline-containing 'C-substance' present in the cell-walls of pneumococci as well as in some strains of *S. oralis* ('*S. mitior*') and some batches of the

Lancefield Group C reagent in grouping kits may agglutinate them (Lee & Wetherall, 1987). Other test characters are therefore necessary for correct identification. Non-capsulated strains of pneumococci isolated from outbreaks of conjunctivitis are more difficult; if they are both bile-soluble and optochin-sensitive there is little doubt about their identification (Shayegani et al., 1982), but if they are not soluble in bile and not capsulated, procedures such as polyacrylamide gel electrophoresis of intracellular proteins may be needed for species identification (Pease, Douglas & Spencer, 1986).

The aggregated 'species' S. sanguis is serologically heterogeneous and includes Groups H and W (Ball, 1985). Several subdivisions of this species have been proposed, including one with two subspecies corresponding to Groups 1 and 3 of Coykendall & Specht (1975). The presence of alkaline phosphatase distinguishes Coykendall & Specht's Group 1, which has this property, from Group 3, which does not. Strains that lack the glucosyltransferase enzymes responsible for the formation of glucan (dextran) from sucrose are now included with S. sanguis. A key characteristic of S. sanguis is its ability to hydrolyse arginine (Table 6.3b) as this character correlates with others including cell-wall composition (Price et al., 1986).

Cell-wall analysis provided the clue that led eventually to the precise definition of the organism formerly called 'S. mitior' by Colman & Williams (1972) but now accepted as S. oralis (Kilpper-Bälz, Wenzeg & Schleifer, 1985); since the name 'S. mitior' is still used widely we continue to give it alongside S. oralis. Facklam (1977) would allot the same organism either to the species S. mitis or to S. sanguis II, the latter containing the raffinose-fermenting strains. The presence in the cell wall of ribitol and the absence of large amounts of rhamnose were first noted by Colman & Williams (1965); subsequently, the presence of choline and an unusual mucopeptide structure called 'Lys-direct' (Kilpper-Bälz, Wenzeg & Schleifer, 1985) confirmed that the cell-wall composition was unusual. Some of these strains form dextran from sucrose and for this reason were once classed with S. sanguis. The dextran-positive strains are generally more active biochemically and nearly all of them produce α-galactosidase, β-galactosidase and phosphatase as well as fermenting raffinose, lactose and starch (Colman & Ball, 1984). Neither the dextran-formers nor the other members of the species S. oralis hydrolyse arginine or give a positive VP reaction.

Some organisms that are similar in cell-wall composition to S. oralis (Roberts et al., 1979) require supplements of pyridoxal hydrochloride (10 µg/ml) for growth in many culture media. They can be recognized most conveniently by satellitism around disks containing 20 µg of this substance. The production of pyrrolydonylarylamidase (PYRA) is a key character of these organisms. Bouvet and her colleagues (1985) describe three biotypes: one produces α- and β-galactosidase and ferments trehalose, the second does not produce any of these enzymes but forms glucuronidase, and the third produces none of them.

S. morbillorum grows better anaerobically than in air even with added CO_2. Like one of the pyridoxal-dependent biotypes, the only positive test characters may be the production of leucine aminopeptidase and pyrrolydonylarylamidase. Unlike Gemella species, phosphatase is not formed and the VP reaction is negative (Berger & Pervanidis, 1986).

Among the streptococci that carry the Lancefield Group D antigen there are two disparate clusters of species (Table 6.3b). All the species will grow on Bile–aesculin Agar but, as this property occurs also in other species, a negative test result is more significant. One cluster fulfils Sherman's criteria for enterococci and will grow in 6.5% Salt Broth, survive heating at 60 °C for 30 minutes and will grow at 45 °C. These organisms have now been transferred to the genus Enterococcus, and we deal with them in Section 6.3.2.

The other cluster of Lancefield Group D species – namely S. bovis with its two biotypes and S. equinus – are less tolerant of salt. S. bovis biotype I can be distinguished from S. mutans by the presence of the D antigen and by the active hydrolysis of starch. When cultured in sucrose-containing media, S. bovis biotype I usually produces a water-soluble glucan (dextran), and on Sucrose Agar it forms watery spreading colonies. The glucan formed by S. mutans is less soluble and adherent hard colonies, not unlike those of S. sanguis, develop on Sucrose Agar. Facklam (1972) observed variants, now called S. bovis biotype II, which are less active than biotype I;

they can be distinguished from *S. salivarius* by the presence of the D antigen and the failure to form levan from sucrose.

What were at first regarded as biotypes and serotypes (a–f) of *S. mutans* are now accepted by dental microbiologists as separate species. In medical laboratories, isolates of one or other of the serotypes c, e and f (not to be confused with Lancefield groups A–F) predominate (Perch, Kjems & Ravn, 1974) and for these the epithet *mutans* is retained (Table 6.3*b*). Strains of serotype 'a' are inhibited by bacitracin discs containing 0.1 unit and these are known as *S. cricetus* (Coykendall, 1977). *S. rattus* was formed for strains of serotype b; they hydrolyse arginine. Strains of serotypes d and g, collectively termed *S. sobrinus*, usually form peroxide and fail to ferment sorbitol. When cultured on Sucrose Agar, a white halo develops around the colonies (Beighton, 1985) presumably due to the production of a highly branched glucan (mutan).

It is not difficult to identify typical strains of *S. salivarius* as they form soft, domed colonies on Sucrose Agar owing to the production of a fructan (levan) from sucrose. Some strains produce a glucan as well as a fructan and they form craggy colonies on Sucrose Agar. Clinical material occasionally contains streptococci whose classification is uncertain because they appear to share some properties of *S. salivarius* and *S. bovis* biotype II though they can be distinguished from both of those species. All three taxa give a positive Voges–Proskaüer reaction and hydrolyse aesculin but not arginine. The atypical strains can be distinguished from *S. salivarius* by their failure to form an extracellular polysaccharide from sucrose, and from *S. bovis* biotype II because they do not carry the Lancefield D antigen or give a positive result in the bile–aesculin test. *S. salivarius* will grow in media made selective by the addition of sodium azide (0.02%) and sucrose (5%); with such media it can be isolated from faeces.

The transfer of *S. lactis* and its subspecies to a new genus, *Lactococcus*, was proposed by Schleifer *et al.* (1985) and this has now been accepted. These organisms are already regarded by dairy microbiologists as more like lactobacilli than streptococci. In medical laboratories strains are occasionally isolated, but the name *L. lactis* should not be applied, unless the Lancefield N antigen has been identified in the culture and other characters demonstrated, including the hydrolysis of arginine, growth in 4% but not in 6.5% Salt Broth and growth at 10 °C and 40 °C but not at 45 °C. Similarly *S. equinus* is a precisely defined species and we do not think that failure of a viridans streptococcus to ferment lactose should be given over-riding importance. The presence of D antigen, a positive bile–aesculin test and the failure to hydrolyse arginine or to grow in 6.5% Salt Broth are additional minimal requirements for the identification of an isolate as *S. equinus*.

> **Minidefinition:** *Streptococcus. Gram-positive cocci in pairs or chains. Non-motile. Non-sporing. Aerobic, facultatively anaerobic. Catalase- and oxidase-negative. Attack carbohydrates fermentatively. Type species: S. pyogenes; NCTC strain 8198.*

6.3.2 Enterococcus (Tables 6.3*a*,*b*). This genus was originally proposed by Kalina (1970) for a group of streptococci first described by Thiércelin & Jouhard (1903) and known collectively as 'faecal streptococci'. Recent nucleic acid and taxonomic studies support the separation of these organisms from other Group D streptococci (Bridge & Sneath, 1982, 1983; Farrow *et al.*, 1983; Kilpper-Bälz *et al.*, 1982; Schleifer & Kilpper-Bälz, 1984). With increasing recognition of the generic name *Enterococcus* in clinical and other laboratories, its taxonomic position is now secure and we accord with this view. The genus currently contains several species listed in Table 6.3*b*. However, an alternative view which we prefer is to regard *Enterococcus* as comprising only two species: *E. faecalis*, and *E. faecium* with its five varieties. This situation has still to be resolved.

Growth in 6.5% Salt Broth, survival after heating at 60 °C for 30 minutes and growth at both 10 °C and 45 °C are all satisfactory characterization tests for differentiating *Enterococcus* from *Streptococcus* species (Table 6.3*a*). Growth at pH 9.6, often used previously for this purpose is not recommended as media at this pH are usually unstable. With the exception of *E. faecalis*, Collins, Farrow & Jones (1986) offer a concise review of the properties of this genus. Unlike the other species, *E. faecalis* ferments pyruvate (Gross, Houghton & Senterfit, 1975). The yellow pigment produced by *E. casseliflavus* may be demonstrated either by transferring some of the growth from a Nutrient Agar culture to a filter paper or, alternatively, by inspection of the packed cells after centrifugation of a broth culture. Two species, *E. gallinarum* and *E. casseliflavus*, are motile.

Minidefinition: *Enterococcus. Gram-positive cocci in pairs or short chains. Non-motile (except two species). Non-sporing. Aerobic, facultatively anaerobic. Catalase- and oxidase-negative. Attack carbohydrates fermentatively. Type species: E. faecalis; NCTC strain 775.*

6.3.3   Aerococcus (Tables 6.2a; 6.3a,b). The name *Aerococcus viridans* was introduced for Gram-positive cocci that did not form chains, were either catalase-negative or only feebly positive and which were present in the air of occupied rooms (Williams, Hirch & Cowan, 1953). If the catalase reaction is recorded as negative then *Aerococcus* must be distinguished from the streptococci; and if positive, from staphylococci and micrococci (Section 6.2). Although aerococci closely resemble pediococci, *Aerococcus* is now accepted as a separate genus; however, the organism isolated from lobsters, previously called *Gaffkya* and subsequently *Pediococcus homari* (Deibel & Niven, 1960) as well as '*P. urinae-equi*' (Whittenbury, 1965b; Sakaguchi & Mori, 1969) from horses are now regarded as aerococci (Kelly & Evans, 1974).

Like the staphylococci and micrococci, aerococci lack leucine aminopeptidase and this differentiates them from the streptococci which possess this enzyme. In agar shake cultures, growth with nearly all strains of aerococci is maximal just below the surface and they are thus microaerophilic. Glucose is fermented with the formation of $L(+)$ lactic acid but without gas production (Deibel & Niven, 1960).

Unlike the pediococci, aerococci do not grow on Acetate Agar at pH 5.4 but they share with the enterococci (with which they may be confused) the ability to grow on 40% Bile Agar and in 6.5% NaCl Broth. On Blood Agar, colonies (<1 mm) produce zones of α haemolysis.

Aerococci have been isolated occasionally from the skin of infants, from patients with endocarditis, and from urines and wound swabs. That they can be isolated from repeated specimens taken from patients with infection suggests that they are capable of mis-

chief, if only as opportunist pathogens (Colman, 1967; Parker & Ball, 1976).

Minidefinition: *Aerococcus. Gram-positive spheres in pairs, fours and small clusters. Non-motile; non-sporing. Aerobic and microaerophilic. Catalase-negative or only feebly positive; oxidase-negative. Attack sugars fermentatively without gas production. Type species: A. viridans; NCTC strain 8251.*

6.3.4   Pediococcus (Tables 6.3a,b). A genus of Gram-positive, catalase-negative, lactic-acid-producing cocci which form pairs and tetrads and which occur in beer, meat-curing brines and fermenting vegetable juices. In the clinical laboratory, the species that cause spoilage of beer are unlikely to be encountered as they do not grow at temperatures above 30 °C. Some of the diversity in this genus has been reduced by transferring '*Pediococcus urinae-equi*' and *P. homari* (from lobsters) to *Aerococcus* (Kelly & Evans, 1974). Strains of pediococci similar to those present in silage, cheese and fermented sausages have been isolated from the human mouth (Sims, 1966), and occasional strains resistant to vancomycin (30 μg disc) from blood cultures (Colman & Efstratiou, 1987).

Unlike streptococci and aerococci, pediococci grow on Acetic Acid or Acetate Agar at pH 5.4 (Whittenbury, 1965b). They grow on Blood Agar incubated in air; and in Glucose Broth they produce sufficient DL or $L(+)$ lactic acid (Garvie, 1984) to give a final pH or 4 or less. Gas is not produced from glucose, nor are extracellular polysaccharides such as dextran or levan formed from sucrose. A few strains give a pseudo-catalase reaction on media containing haem compounds but not on Nutrient Agar containing glucose (0.05% w/v). Pediococci are distinguished from *Leuconostoc* species by their inability to produce slimy colonies on carbohydrate-containing media or to produce CO_2 from glucose (Gibson & Abd-el-Malek, 1945).

The characteristics of some species have been reviewed by Garvie (1984) and the properties of most strains isolated from clinical specimens are like those of *P. pentosaceus*. Some strains of this species carry the Lancefield group D antigen (Colman 1967) and also share some biochemical properties with these streptococci (Table 6.3b).

Minidefinition: *Pediococcus. Gram-positive cocci forming tetrads or pairs. Catalase-negative; oxidase-negative. Attack sugars fermentatively without gas production. Microaerophilic. Acid-tolerant. Type species: P. damnosus; NCTC strain 1832.*

6.3.5   Leuconostoc (Tables 6.3a,b). Species of this genus are normally present in plant materials, dairy products and other fermented foodstuffs as well as in spoiled foods so that they are likely to be encountered in public health laboratories; such isolates are usually vancomycin-resistant (Orberg & Sandine, 1984). They have also been isolated occasionally from blood cultures (Colman & Ball, 1984) and, as with pediococci, some were resistant to vancomycin (Buu-Hoï, Branger & Acar, 1985). In the clinical laboratory, dextran-forming cultures of *Leuconostoc mesenteroides* may be confused initially with *Streptococcus bovis* biotype I because both yield watery colonies on Sucrose Agar and share other biochemical characteristics (Table 6.3b). The leuconostocs differ from other Gram-positive 'catalase negative' cocci in that they grow in air with or without added CO_2. They form a natural group with the heterofermentative lactobacilli, especially *Lactobacillus confusus* and *L. viridescens* (Garvie, 1984), producing CO_2 from glucose; this property can be demonstrated in shake cultures in an enriched medium such as the MRS Agar of de Man, Rogosa & Sharpe (1960) but not in inverted inner (Durham) tubes in liquid medium.

Minidefinition: *Leuconostoc. Gram-positive cocci in pairs or short chains. Microaerophilic. Catalase-negative. Attack sugars fermentatively and produce gas. May form dextran from sucrose. Type species: L. mesenteroides; ATCC strain 8293.*

6.3.6   Gemella   (Tables   6.3a,b). *Gemella haemolysans* was first described as a species of *Neisseria* by Thjøtta & Bøe (1938) but it was later transferred to a new genus, *Gemella*, by Berger (1961) who also described it as Gram-negative. It is easily decolorized in Gram-stained smears but belongs with the Gram-positive bacteria close to the streptococci because of its cell-wall composition and DNA G+C ratio among other things (Reyn 1970;

Stackebrandt *et al.*, 1982). It has been suggested that *G. haemolysans* is synonymous with *Streptococcus morbillorum* (Facklam & Wilkinson, 1981) but, although the final classification of *Gemella* species is not yet settled, the balance of evidence favours its separation from *S. morbillorum* (Berger & Pervandis, 1986) and we follow this here by showing it separately in Table 6.3b; because it is so readily decolorized (or over-decolorized) we also show *Gemella* in Table 7.3 with *Neisseria* and *Branhamella* species because of the characteristics usually sought for those genera. It can be separated from them by its failure to form catalase or oxidase. The apparent similarity to *S. morbillorum* is probably due to the lack of reactivity of both organisms in the tests conventionally used for streptococci (Table 6.3b). There are, however, several distinguishing properties. Although CO_2 stimulates the growth of both on agar media, *G. haemolysans* prefers aerobic and *S. morbillorum* anaerobic conditions. *G. haemolysans* gives a positive reaction in the Voges–Proskäuer test and reduces nitrite but not nitrate (Berger & Pervanidis, 1986) whereas *S. morbillorum* gives none of these reactions. The haemolysis (α or β) from which the specific epithet is derived occurs slowly on rabbit Blood Agar and on horse Blood Agar prepared with a Columbia base; it does not occur with sheep blood.

Minidefinition; *Gemella. Gram-positive (but easily decolorized) cocci. Aerobic, facultatively anaerobic. Catalase-negative, oxidase-negative. Attacks sugars by fermentation, producing little acid and no gas. Type species: G. haemolysans; ATCC strain 10379.*

6.4   The anaerobic Gram-positive cocci
(*Peptococcus, Peptostreptococcus*)

***Characters common to members of the group*: Gram-positive cocci. Strictly anaerobic. Sensitive to metronidazole. Catalase-negative (except the type species *Peptococcus niger*).**

Peptococcus and **Peptostreptococcus** (Tables **6.3a, 6.4**) are genera of Gram-positive anaerobic cocci that can use peptones or amino acids as primary sources of energy. They are part of the normal flora of man and animals, especially of the oropharynx,

Table 6.4. *Second-stage table for* Peptococcus *and* Peptostreptococcus

	1	2	3
Sensitive to discs containing			
Metronidazole (5 µg)	+	+	–
Vancomycin (5 µg)	+	+	+
Liquoid (1000 µg)	–	+	–
Carbohydrates, acid from			
Glucose	–	+	+
Fructose	–	+	+
Indole	+	–	–
*Propionate from threonine	–	+	–
*Iso-caproic acid from			
glucose	–	+	–

*For laboratories with gas chromatography facilities.

1 **Peptococcus asaccharolyticus**
2 **Peptostreptococcus anaerobius**
3 *streptococci*

Symbols used in the table are explained in Tables 5.1 and 5.2 (p. 47).

colon and vagina; as opportunist pathogens they are often isolated, usually in mixed culture, from clinical material. Blood Agar containing neomycin and other antibiotics is selective for them (Watt & Brown, 1983); growth is usually slow (2–4 days) and haemolysis does not occur (Watt & Jack, 1977). The identification of isolates is not easy, partly because the definitions of individual species are in a state of flux but mostly because it depends greatly on their enzyme activities and on analysis of the metabolic end-products by gas–liquid chromatography (Ezaki & Yabuchi, 1985). Recent taxonomic changes in the Gram-positive anaerobic cocci have left *Peptococcus niger* (a rare clinical isolate) as the sole species in the genus *Peptococcus*. All other species formerly in this genus have been transferred to *Peptostreptococcus* (Ezaki *et al.*, 1983; Holdeman-Moore, Johnson & Moore, 1986). In practice, all metronidazole-sensitive Gram-positive cocci may be confidently regarded as peptostreptococci. The arrangement of cells in Gram-stained smears is not reliable for distinguishing peptostreptococci, which are supposed to form chains, from the peptococci, which should not. Confusion may sometimes occur with microaerophilic streptococci but, unlike the streptococci, peptococci and peptostreptococci are sensitive to metronidazole; they are also sensitive to vancomycin (5 µg disc) in con-

trast to the Gram-negative anaerobic cocci (Section 7.2.3) which are resistant (Rogosa *et al.*, 1958; Watt, Bushell & Wallace, 1984; Holdeman *et al.*, 1986). Hofstad (1985) claims that sensitivity to novobiocin is a reliable characteristic of peptostreptococci but Watt, Wallace & Bushell (1986) dispute this. However, among strains of anaerobic cocci, *Peptostreptococcus anaerobius* can be distinguished readily by its sensitivity to Liquoid (polyanethol sulphonate) as shown by wide zones of inhibition (Wideman *et al.*, 1976). We show this and other features which differentiate peptococci from peptostreptococci in Table 6.4, which includes also streptococci for comparison. Those who wish to study these genera and their species further should consult Holdeman, Cato & Moore, 1977; Holdeman-Moore, Johnson & Moore, 1986.

> **Minidefinitions**: *Peptococcus. Gram-positive cocci, often in clusters. Strict anaerobes. Sensitive to metronidazole. Feeble fermentative powers: clinical isolates do not ferment glucose. Type species: P. niger; NCTC strain 11805.*
> *Peptostreptococcus. Gram-positive cocci, often in chains. Strict anaerobes. Sensitive to metronidazole. Sugars attacked fermentatively and gas may be produced. Type species: P. anaerobius; NCTC strain 11460.*

6.5   The diphtheroids
(Corynebacterium, Listeria, Brochothrix, Kurthia)

***Characters common to members of the group*: Gram-positive rods, not spore-forming. Aerobic, facultatively anaerobic. Catalase positive, oxidase negative.**

There is some similarity in morphology between all the members of this group for which the descriptive label 'diphtheroid' (derived from the specific epithet of *Corynebacterium diphtheriae*) is traditionally used in clinical laboratories although it has no taxonomic meaning. The grouping is convenient but artificial as *Corynebacterium* belongs to the high G+C mole % branch of the Gram-positive bacteria whereas the other genera have a low G+C mole % DNA content (Stackebrandt & Woese, 1981).

Most members of the group grow better on media

enriched with blood or serum though none require X or V factors. Haemin stimulates the growth of *Corynebacterium matruchotii* under anaerobic conditions but can be inhibitory with aerobic incubation. The classification of the vaginal organism first called '*Haemophilus vaginalis*' and later '*Corynebacterium vaginale*' has been resolved by the creation of a new genus *Gardnerella* though its actual taxonomic position is still uncertain; we deal with it in Section 7.10.2 but include it for comparison in Table 6.5*b*. Some notes on the current species of *Corynebacterium* are given in Section 6.5.1. It should be noted that *C. bovis* is atypical in that it is oxidase-positive and that the newly described skin commensal organism *C. amycolatum* does not contain detectable mycolic acids.

6.5.1 Corynebacterium (Tables 6.5*a*, 6.5*b*) cur-
rently comprises animal pathogens and commensals together with some saprophytic organisms; the plant pathogens previously included in the genus have all been reclassified in the genera *Arthrobacter*, *Clavibacter*, *Curtobacterium*, or *Rhodococcus* (see Davis *et al.*, 1984; Collins & Cummins, 1986).

In the medical field some organisms previously placed in the genus are now excluded. '*Corynebacterium acnes*' is now classified in the genus *Propionibacterium* and we deal with it in Section 6.7. '*Corynebacterium haemolyticum*' and '*C. pyogenes*' have been transferred to the genera *Arcanobacterium* and *Actinomyces* respectively and they are dealt with in Sections 6.6 and 6.7. '*Corynebacterium equi*' and '*C. hoagii*' represent a single species and are now classified as *Rhodococcus equi*. On the other hand, the organisms previously forming the monospecific genus '*Bacterionema*' and those of the species '*Brevibacterium ammoniagenes*' (associated with nappy rash in infants) have been reclassified in the genus *Corynebacterium* as *C. matruchotii* and *C. ammoniagenes* (Collins, 1982*a*, 1987).

The organisms previously regarded as *C. renale* have been shown to represent three distinct species, *C. renale*, *C. cystitidis* and *C. pilosum* (Yanagawa & Honda, 1978). The organisms *C. minutissimum*, associated with erythrasma of the skin, and *C. mycetoides*, reported to cause tropical ulcers in man, have been reinstated in the genus *Corynebacterium*

Table 6.5*a*. *Second-stage table for* Corynebacterium, Listeria, Brochothrix *and* Kurthia

	1	2	3	4
Growth at 37 °C	+	+	−	d
Motility	−	+	−	+
Catalase	+	+	+ [c]	+
Carbohydrate attack	F/−	F	F	−
VP	− [a]	+	+	−
H$_2$S	−	− [b]	−	d

1 **Corynebacterium**
2 **Listeria;** *Listerella*
3 **Brochothrix**
4 **Kurthia**
a One species positive. *C. cystitidis.*
b Some strains of *L. grayi* and *L. murrayi* produce small amounts of H$_2$S (lead acetate paper method)
c Catalase-positive at 20–25 °C; negative at 30 °C; also media-dependent

Other symbols used in the table are explained in Tables 5.1 and 5.2 on p. 47.

(Collins, 1982*b*; Collins & Jones, 1983). In addition, new species have been described: *C. jeikeium* (Jackman *et al.*, 1987) for the multi-antibiotic resistant diphtheroids previously designated 'Group JK corynebacteria' (Riley *et al.*, 1979; Ersgaard & Justensen, 1984) and *C. amycolatum* for some recent isolates from skin (Collins, Burton & Jones, 1988).

The description of the genus is now based largely on chemical characters not easily determined in routine laboratories (Collins & Cummins, 1986). Consequently, it is sometimes difficult to distinguish corynebacteria from members of other coryneform genera such as *Microbacterium*, *Dermobacter* and *Brevibacterium*. Similarly, although more than 20 species in the genus represent distinct taxa, it is not easy to choose phenotypic characters that allow their differentiation. We show the characters likely to be of most value in identifying corynebacteria of medical importance in Table 6.5*b*.

The work of Barksdale (1981) and Maximescu *et al.* (1974) among others has shown that a group of related species or varieties are able to produce diphtheria toxin when lysogenized by a suitable bacteriophage. The group includes the three cultural varieties of *C. diphtheriae*; *C. pseudotuberculosis*, which is traditionally accorded species status; and the strains previously designated '*C. ulcerans*', a taxon which

Table 6.5b. *Third-stage table for* Corynebacterium *and* Gardnerella

	1	2	3	4	5	6	7	8	9	10	11	12	13	14	15	16	17	18
Motility	–	–	–	–	–	–	–	–	–	–	–	–	–	–	–	–	–	–
Catalase	+	+	+	+	+	+	+	+	+	+	+	+	+	+	+	+	+	–
Metachromatic granules	D	–	+	+^{b}	+	+	+	+	+	+^{a}	+	+	+	–	+	+	+	d
Haemolysis	D	+	d	–	–	–	–	–	–	–	–	–	–	–	–	–	–	+
Growth improved by blood/serum	+	+	+	+	+	+	+	+	+	+	+	?	+	+	+	+	+	+
Carbohydrate breakdown – [F/O/–]	F	F	F	F	F	F	F	F	F	F	F	F?	F	?^{c}	–	?^{c}	F	F
Carbohydrates, acid from:																		
glucose	+	+	+	+	+	+	+	+	+	+	+	+	+^{c}	–	+^{c}	+	+	+
lactose	–	–	d	–	–	–	–	–	–	–	–	d	–	–	d^c	–	–	d
maltose	+	+	+	+	+	d	+	+	+	+	–	+	d^c	–	+^{c}	+	+	+
mannitol	–	–	–	–	–	–	–	–	?	–	–	?	?	–	?	–	–	–
salicin	–	–	–	–	–	–	–	–	?	–	+	–	–	–	–	–	–	+
starch	D	+	+	–	+	–	+	+	–	–	–	+	–	–	–	–	d	d
sucrose	–^{d}	–	d	+	+	–	–	–	+^{e}	+	–	–	–	–	–	–	d	d
trehalose	–	+	–	–	+	d	+	+	–	–	–	d	–	–	d^c	d	d	–
xylose	–	–	–	–	–	–	+	–	–	–	–	–	?	–	?	–	–	d
VP	–	–	–	–	–	–	–	–	?	?	–	–	?	–	–	–	+	–
Aesculin hydrolysis	–	–	–	–	–	–	–	–	?	+	?	–	?	–	–	–	–	–
Nitrate reduced	+	–	d	+	+	–	+	–	–	+	+	–	d	–	+	–	?	–
Gelatin liquefaction	–	+	d	–	–	–	–	–	–	–	–	d	–	–	–	–	–	–
Urease	–	+	+	–	d	+	+	+	–	d	+	–	–	+	–	–	d	–
Arginine hydrolysis	–	–	+	–	–	?	?	?	?	?	?	?	?	?	–	?	–	–
Pyrazinamidase	–	–	–	+	+	+	+	+	+	+	?	?	?	+	+	?	?	?
Casein digestion	–	+	–	–	–	+	–	–	–	–	–	–	–	–	–	–	–	d
Phosphatase	–	–	–	–	–	–	–	–	+	–	?	+	?	–	+	+	?	?

1 **Corynebacterium diphtheriae**
2 **'Corynebacterium ulcerans'**
3 **'Corynebacterium pseudotuberculosis;**
  'C. ovis'; 'C. pseudotuberculosis-ovis';
  Preisz-Nocard bacillus
4 **Corynebacterium xerosis**
5 **Corynebacterium kutscheri;** *'C. murium';*
  'C. pseudotuberculosis-murium'
6 **Corynebacterium renale;** *'C. renale' type I*

7 **Corynebacterium pilosum;**
  'C. renale' type II
8 **Corynebacterium cystitidis;**
  'C. renale' type III
9 **Corynebacterium minutissimum**
10 **Corynebacterium matruchotii;**
  'Bacterionema matruchotii'
11 **Corynebacterium ammoniagenes;**
  Brevibacterium ammoniagenes'
12 **Corynebacterium striatum;**
  'C. flavidum'

13 **Corynebacterium jeikeium;**
  Group JK corynebacteria
14 **Corynebacterium pseudodiphtheriticum;**
  'C. hofmannii' (and variant
  spellings of both epithets)
15 **Corynebacterium bovis**
16 **Corynebacterium mycetoides**
17 **Corynebacterium amycolatum**
18 **Gardnerella vaginalis;** *'C. vaginale'.*

a Characteristic morphology – rods attached to filaments (whip-handles)
b Scanty granules
c Positive when Tween 80 added to medium
d Occasional strains positive
e Occasional strains negative
D different results in the varieties (*gravis, mitis* and *intermedius*) of *C. diphtheriae*

Other symbols used in the table are explained in Tables 5.1 and 5.2 on p. 47.

for practical reasons is treated separately in Table 6.5b. This group of toxigenic organisms appears to differ from other members of the genus in being pyrazinamidase-negative and neuraminidase-positive (Barksdale, 1981).

When diphtheria was common, smears prepared from the growth on Loeffler's serum slopes (or directly from throat swabs) and stained with methylene blue were often sufficiently characteristic for experienced workers to report not only the presence of *C. diphtheriae* but also the identity of the variety. Typically, the *gravis* variety exhibits club-shaped and dumb-bell forms with scanty metachromatic granules though in the cells there are always areas stained in different shades of blue. The *mitis* type accords with the textbook picture of *C. diphtheriae*: pleomorphic rods with numerous metachromic granules and cells arranged in 'V' and 'W' shapes. The *intermedius* variety, inappropriately named not from the characteristics of the organism but from the severity of disease in Leeds in the early 1930s (Anderson *et al.*, 1933), is least like the textbook description, consisting of short rods with alternating bands of light and dark blue stain without any metachromatic granules: the so-called 'barred' appearance. Of the diphtheroid organisms found in the human throat, *C. xerosis* may mimic the *gravis* type of *C. diphtheriae* but after subculture it becomes more uniform in shape and, like other diphtheroids, tends to form bundles of cells: the so-called palisade arrangement. Of the animal pathogens, *C. pseudotuberculosis* ('*C. ovis*') and *C. kutscheri* ('*C. murium*') are similar in morphology to the *mitis* variety of *C. diphtheriae*. The morphology of *C. matruchotii* – rods attached to filaments (whip handles) – is characteristic; and branching can also occur in aerobic or acidic conditions.

The typical colony forms of *C. diphtheriae* are best seen on Chocolate–Tellurite Agar (Appendix A2.2.2). Most *gravis* strains produce 'daisy head' colonies; *mitis* strains yield colonies with a smooth surface, black in the centre but surrounded by a clear grey zone – the so-called 'poached egg' appearance; and *intermedius* strains produce the smallest colonies, grey in colour, with a smooth glistening surface. '*C. ulcerans*' resembles *C. diphtheriae* var. *gravis* in some respects but can be differentiated by biochemical tests (Table 6.5*b*).

Clinically, it is important not only to identify diphtheria bacilli by their cultural and morphological characters but also to establish whether or not they are toxigenic. This is usually performed with cultures *in vitro* by a modified Elek double diffusion precipitin method (see, for example, Jameson, 1965) instead of by animal inoculation.

Corynebacteria may not grow well enough in Peptone Water sugars to show their fermentative abilities. It is preferable to use Serum sugars or a medium such as that of Hugh & Leifson (1953) with the appropriate carbohydrate substituted for glucose. Tween 80, and aeration, improve the growth of *C. bovis* so that it may produce acid from carbohydrates and give a positive VP reaction (Jayne-Williams & Skerman, 1966). Tween 80 also improves the growth of *C. jeikeium*.

Minidefinition: *Corynebacterium. Gram-positive rods which under most conditions of growth do not branch. Non-motile; non-sporing; not acid-fast. Aerobic and facultatively anaerobic. Catalase-positive; usually oxidase-negative. Attack sugars fermentatively or do not attack them. Type species: C. diphtheriae; NCTC strain 11397.*

6.5.2   Listeria (Tables 6.5*a, c*). This organism, isolated from epidemic infection among laboratory animals, was first described by Murray, Webb & Swann, (1926) as *Bacterium monocytogenes* because among other characters it induced a monocyte response in their blood. The generic name, *Listerella* was chosen to honour Lord Lister, the surgeon, but as this had already been used in zoology and botany the genus was later renamed *Listeria* (Pirie, 1940). At one time it was thought to be closely related to *Erysipelothrix* although it differed from this genus in several respects and subsequent taxonomic studies have supported their separation (Davis *et al.*, 1969; Stuart & Pease, 1972). *Listeria monocytogenes* is now known to be a fairly hardy non-sporing organism, widespread in soil and vegetation, which can cause a variety of infections referred to as listeriosis in a number of different animals, including man. In recent years there has been a marked increase in the reported incidence of listeriosis (Seeliger, 1961; Gitter, Bradley & Blampied, 1980) which it is difficult to ascribe wholly to better methods of isolation and identification. In farm animals infection is associated with poor-quality silage; in man, food, including pre-cooked and chilled meals, has also been implicated in its transmission (McLauchlin, 1987). Faecal carriage of *Listeria* is not uncommon, particularly among abbattoir workers and those involved in the meat trade.

Following the recent transfer of the non-pathogenic species *L. denitrificans* to a new genus, *Jonesia* (Rocourt, Wehmeyer & Stackenbrandt, 1987*a*), *Listeria* now contains six species in addition to *L. monocytogenes*. The taxonomic position of two of them, *L. grayi* and *L. murrayi*, has been controversial (Seeliger & Jones, 1986) but recent genomic evidence confirms their place in *Listeria* (Rocourt, Wehmeyer & Stackebrandt, 1987*b*); neither of them is pathogenic for man. The remaining species,

L. innocua, L. seeligeri, L. welshimeri and *L. ivanovii*, are essentially genomic in derivation from *L. monocytogenes* (Rocourt, Schrettenbrunnner & Seeliger, 1983) and they are thus not easy to distinguish in routine laboratories.

Like *Brochothrix*, which they closely resemble, all *Listeria* species survive and grow slowly at low temperatures (1–5 °C); this unusual ability is used to advantage for their selective isolation by 'incubation' in the refrigerator. This procedure is, however, slow so that selective and enrichment media such as Thallous Acetate–Nalidixic Acid Agar and Thiocyanate– or Thallous Acetate–Nalidixic Acid Broths (Kramer & Jones, 1969) should also be used. We can recommend a recently described selective medium that contains an aesculin–ferric ammonium citrate indicator system (Curtis *et al.*, 1989) on which *Listeria* produces blackening; the best results are obtained by incubation at 30 °C. On solid blood-free media, *Listeria* colonies have such a characteristic clear, bright blue-green iridescent colour and appearance when viewed by obliquely transmitted white light that they can be recognized readily even on heavily contaminated plates. Equally characteristic is the 'tumbling' or 'head-over-heels' motility in broth cultures 'incubated' at room temperature. Another characteristic of the genus is the production of acetoin. We list these and other differential test characters for the identification of *Listeria* species in Table 6.5*c*. Most but not all strains of *L. monocytogenes* show β haemolysis on Blood Agar plates though the zones can be narrow and care must be taken not to mistake them for streptococci; unfortunately the type strain is non-haemolytic, atypical in the CAMP test and phenotypically identifies with *L. innocua*. *Listeria* species can easily be confused with corynebacteria, especially as they can grow on tellurite-containing media; they can also tolerate high concentrations of bile salts and grow well on MacConkey Agar. *L. ivanovii*, which gives wide zones of β-haemolysis, is important as a cause of abortion in sheep; it corresponds almost entirely with serovar 5 of the O and H antigenic typing scheme for *L. monocytogenes* of Seeliger & Hohne (1979). For epidemiological purposes, however, phage typing (Audurier *et al.*, 1979; Rocourt *et al.*, 1985) is preferable as it is reproducible and highly discriminatory.

Minidefinition: *Listeria. Gram-positive rods; motile, non-sporing; not acid-fast. Aerobic and facultatively anaerobic. Catalase-positive; oxidase-negative; produce acetoin. Attack sugars by fermentation. Type species: L. monocytogenes; NCTC strain 10357. (Recommended typical strain, NCTC 11994).*

6.5.3 Brochothrix (Tables 6.5a,c) is a genus consisting currently of two species, *B. thermosphacta* and *B. campestris*. The former is an important spoilage organism of film-wrapped, refrigerated meat; it has also been isolated from fish and other products such as milk and cottage cheese. The latter, isolated recently from soil and grass (Talon *et al.*, 1988), is phenotypically similar to *B. thermosphacta* (Table 6.5c). There is no evidence that either of them are pathogenic for man but we include them because they may need to be differentiated from similar organisms, including *Listeria*, which occur in food products.

Both species grow well between 4 and 25 °C with limited growth at 30 °C and none at 37 °C (Gardner, 1981; Talon *et al.*, 1988). They are non-haemolytic and in young cultures (< 24h) two colony types frequently occur with such different morphology that the plates may be regarded mistakenly as contaminated. They do not show the blue-green iridescence exhibited by *Listeria* colonies under obliquely transmitted white light. Glucose added to the growth medium greatly increases colony size and the growth has a distinctly sour smell. They do not grow on media selective for lactobacilli such as the Acetate Agar of Rogosa, Mitchell & Wiseman (1951) and poorly, if at all, on the MRS medium of de Man, Rogosa & Sharpe (1960). They may be isolated on the selective streptomycin-thallous acetate-cyclohexamide agar (STAA) medium of Gardner (1966) on which *Listeria* and lactobacilli fail to grow. The organisms are catalase-positive but production of the enzyme is dependent on both the growth medium and the temperature of incubation (Davidson, Mobbs & Stubbs, 1968); Blood Agar base is usually suitable and incubation should be at 20–25 °C and not at 30 °C.

Minidefinition: *Brochothrix. Gram-positive rods; occur singly or in chains; non-motile; non-sporing; not acid-fast. Aerobic and facultatively anaerobic. Catalase-positive; oxi-*

Table 6.5c. *Third-stage table for* Listeria, Brochothrix *and* Kurthia

	1	2	3	4	5	6	7	8	9	10	11
Anaerobic growth	+	+	+	+	+	+	+	+	+	−	−
Motility	+[a]	+[a]	+[a]	+[a]	+[a]	+[a]	+[a]	−	−	+	+
β-haemolysis (horse Blood Agar)	+[b]	−	w	−	+[c]	−	−	−	−	−	−
CAMP test with											
Staphylococcus aureus	+	−	+	−	−	−	−	−	−	−	−
Rhodococcus equi	−	−	−	−	+	−	−	−	−	−	−
Blue-green colony colour:											
oblique illumination (24 h)	+	+	+	+	+	+	+	−	−	−	−
Bird's feather growth:											
Nutrient Gelatin slant	−	−	−	−	−	−	−	−	−	+	+
Catalase	+	+	+	+	+	+	+	+[d]	+[d]	+	+
Growth at:											
4 °C	+	+	+	+	+	+	+	+	+	+	+
37 °C	+	+	+	+	+	+	+	−	−	d	+
45 °C	w[g]	w[g]	w[g]	w[g]	w[g]	w[g]	w[g]	−	−	−	+
Growth with											
8% NaCl (2 days)	+	+	+	+	+	+	+	+	−	d	d
10% NaCl (2 days)	+	+	+	+	d	+	+	d	−	−[e]	−[e]
Carbohydrate breakdown [F/O/−]	F	F	F	F	F	F	F	F	F	−	−
Carbohydrates, acid from:											
glucose	+	+	+	+	+	+	+	+	+	−	−
mannitol	−	−	−	−	−	+	+	+	d	−	−
α-methyl-D-mannoside	+	+	d	+	−	+	+	?	?	−	−
L-rhamnose	+	d	−	d	−	−	d	−	+	−	−
sucrose	−	d	?	?	d	−	−	+	d	−	−
D-xylose	−	−	+	+	+	−	−	+	+	−	−
VP	+	+	+	+	+	+	+	+	+	−	−
Hydrolysis of:											
Aesculin	+	+	+	+	+	+	+	+	+	−	−
Hippurate	+	+	+	+	+	−	−	−	+	+	+
Phosphatase	+	+	+	+	+	+[f]	+[f]	+	+	−	+
Nitrate reduced	−	−	−	−	−	−	+	−	−	−	−
H₂S produced	−	−	−	−	−	d	d	−	−	d	−

  1 Listeria monocytogenes; *Listerella monocytogenes*
  2 Listeria innocua
  3 Listeria seeligeri
  4 Listeria welshimeri
  5 Listeria ivanovii
  6 Listeria grayi
  7 Listeria murrayi
  8 Brochothrix thermosphacta
  9 Brochothrix campestris
  10 Kurthia zopfii
  11 Kurthia gibsonii

a Motility must be tested at 20–25 °C
b Not all strains of *L. monocytogenes* are β haemolytic – the type strain (ATCC 15313) is non-haemolytic
c A very wide zone of β-haemolysis (or multiple zones) exhibited by *L. ivanovii*
d Catalase positive at 20–25 °C; negative at 30 °C; also media dependent
e A few strains grow with 10% (w/v) NaCl
f Weak phosphatase production with some strains
g About the upper limit for growth of *Listeria* – some strains may give poor growth at 45°C

Other symbols used in the table are explained in Tables 5.1 and 5.2 on p. 47.

dase negative. Produce acetoin. Acid produced from a wide variety of sugars by fermentation. Type species: B. thermosphacta; NCTC strain 10822.

6.5.4   Kurthia (Tables 6.5a,c) is not usually regarded as a pathogen, but we include it as strains have been isolated from meat and dairy products and occasionally from clinical material (Keddie, 1981).

Surface colonies are rhizoid but unlikely to be confused with *Bacillus* species; they are not haemolytic. Two species, *K. zopfii* and *K. gibsonii*, are recognized though other psychrophilic strains occur with many *Kurthia*-like characters (Shaw & Keddie, 1983; Keddie & Shaw, 1986). Growth occurs in the range –5 ° to 35 °C for *K. zopfii* and –5 ° to 45 °C or more for *K. gibsonii*. They give negative reactions in most of the usual biochemical tests. The 'bird's feather' growth on Nutrient Gelatin slopes (Keddie & Shaw, 1986) is highly distinctive for both species.

> **Minidefinition:** *Kurthia. Gram-positive rods in chains; motile but non-motile variants occur; not acid-fast. Strictly aerobic. Acid not produced from sugars in peptone media. Acetoin not produced. Nitrate not reduced. Type species: K. zopfii; NCTC strain 10597.*

6.6   The coryneform–actinomycete intermediate group

(Lactobacillus, Listeria, Erysipelothrix, Arachnia, Actinomyces, Arcanobacterium)

***Characters common to members of the group:* Gram-positive rods, usually diphtheroid in morphology but may show rudimentary branching; non-sporing; not acid-fast. Attack sugars fermentatively. Mostly facultative anaerobes.**

Despite pressure to be more definitive, we have retained the descriptive term 'coryneform–actinomycete intermediate' as used previously in this *Manual* for this large group of organisms because they have relatively few common characters other than 'coryneform' cell morphology. The organisms can be divided broadly into two subgroups: (i) the lactic-acid producing 'bacilli' and (ii) the branching rods (actinomycetes); between these two subgroups are organisms with intermediate characters. We deal with the actinomycetes in Section 6.7 but for comparison include the genus *Actinomyces* in Tables 6.6a,b; we describe it in Section 6.7.1 but for completeness include the minidefinition in Section 6.6.6.

Orla-Jensen (1919) divided the lactobacilli into three subgenera, '*Thermobacterium*', '*Streptobacterium*' and '*Betabacterium*', on the basis of fermentative activity and temperature of growth. These names have no standing in nomenclature now but it is a tribute to Orla-Jensen's work that the species of the genus *Lactobacillus* can still be divided into three similar groups of thermobacteria, streptobacteria and betabacteria broadly equivalent to those of Kandler & Weiss (1986); these groups are shown in Table 6.6a. Two of the groups are homofermentative (sugars fermented mostly to lactic acid) and the third (betabacteria) are heterofermentative (sugars fermented partly to lactic acid and partly to volatile acids including CO_2). The species characteristics of some of the lactobacilli are given in Table 6.6b.

Though normally regarded as catalase-negative, some strains of lactobacilli (also some leuconostocs and pediococci) produce a catalase in media containing only low concentrations of glucose. These 'pseudocatalases' are insensitive to sodium azide (Johnston & Delwiche, 1962) and are not produced when the organisms are grown on media containing 1% glucose (Whittenbury, 1964).

The genus *Erysipelothrix* has some resemblance to *Lactobacillus*; it has also often been compared to and combined with *Listeria* (see Section 6.5) and we therefore show these organisms in Table 6.6a for comparison together with *Brochothrix* and *Kurthia*. We also show *Erysipelothrix rhusiopathiae* in Table 6.7 for comparison with the propionibacteria of medical significance.

The monospecific genus *Arachnia* resembles the genus *Propionibacterium* in producing propionic acid as the major-end product of carbohydrate metabolism. *Arcanobacterium haemolyticum* (formerly *Corynebacterium haemolyticum*) closely resembles the genus *Actinomyces*.

Some genera and species in this large group are shown in more than one of the Sections and Tables. This arrangement is deliberate so that additional characters can be introduced and direct comparisons thus

Table 6.6a. *Second-stage table for* Lactobacillus, Listeria, Brochothrix, Kurthia, Erysipelothrix, Arachnia, Arcanobacterium *and* Actinomyces

	1	2	3	4	5	6	7	8	9	10	11
Oxygen requirements:											
Strictly aerobic	+	–	–	–	–	–	–	–	–	–	–
Strictly anaerobic	–	–	–	–	–	–	–	–	–	–	+
Facultatively anaerobic/microaerophilic	–	+	+	+	+	+	+	+	+	+	–
Motility	+	–	+^{a}	–	–	–^{b}	–	–	–	–	–
Catalase	+	+^{c}	+	–	–	–^{d}	–	–	w/–	–^{k}	–
Growth at 5 °C	+	+	+	+	–	–^{e}	–^{e}	–	–	–	–
Growth at 15 °C	+	+	+	+	–^{f}	D	D	?	?	?	–
Gas from glucose	–	–	–	–	–	–	+	–	–	–	+
Carbohydrates, acid from:											
arabinose	–	+	–	–	–	D	D	–^{g}	–	D	
maltose	–	+	+	+	+	+	+	+	d	d	+
melezitose	–	+	+^{h}	–	–	D	–	–	–	D	–
salicin	–	+	+	–	+	+	–	d	?	D	–
VP	–	+	+	–	–	–	–	–	–	–	+
Nitrate reduced	–	–	–^{i}	–	–	–	–	+	d	D	+
H$_2$S production^j	D	–	–	+	–	–	–	d	–	D	+

1 **Kurthia** spp.
2 **Brochothrix** spp.
3 **Listeria** spp.; *Listerella*
4 **Erysipelothrix** spp.
5 **Lactobacillus**; group I, thermobacteria
6 **Lactobacillus**; group II, streptobacteria
7 **Lactobacillus**; group III, betabacteria
8 **Arachnia propionica**
9 **Arcanobacterium haemolyticum**; *'Corynebacterium haemolyticum'*
10 **Actinomyces** spp.
11 **Clostridium perfringens** *(asporogenous variants); C. welchii*

a Motility must be tested at 20–25 °C
b Motility (by peritrichous flagella) occurs in a few species but is usually lost on sub-culture
c Catalase produced when incubated at 20–25 °C; also media dependent
d A few species may produce 'pseudocatalases' on low-glucose containing media
e Occasional species show some growth at 5 °C
f A few species grow at 15 °C
g Strains of serovar 1 may produce acid
h *L. grayi* and *L. murrayi* do not produce acid
i *L. murrayi* reduces nitrates
j H$_2$S production in Triple Sugar Iron Agar
k *A. viscosus* is catalase positive

Other symbols used in the table are explained in Tables 5.1 and 5.2 on p. 47.

made between a greater number of similar or possibly similar organisms. For these reasons we show as stated the characters of *Actinomyces* in Table 6.6 but deal with the genus in Section 6.7.1.

We would remind readers that the minidefinitions of genera, especially of those seldom seen in clinical laboratories, do not necessarily apply to all species in them as they have been drawn up essentially with those species of medical concern in mind.

6.6.1 Lactobacillus (Tables 6.6a,b) is a large genus with some 50 species. They occur in vegetation and dairy products and in man where they form part of the normal flora of the gut and vagina. Apart from their association with dental caries (Rogosa *et al.*, 1953) lactobacilli are generally regarded as non-

pathogenic, but there are reports of their involvement in human disease; *L. casei* subsp. *rhamnosus* as well as *L. acidophilus*, *L. gasseri*, *L. plantarum* and occasionally *L. salivarius* have been associated with bacterial endocarditis, septicaemia and other infections (Sharpe, Hill & Lapage, 1973; Berger, 1974; Bayer *et al.*, 1978; Bourne *et al.*, 1978; Lorenz *et al.*, 1982; Dickgiesser, Weiss & Fritsche, 1984). Döderlein's bacillus is not a bacteriological entity; most lactobacilli from the human vagina seem to be *L. acidophilus* (Rogosa & Sharpe, 1960).

Some organisms isolated from meat and fish, notably *L. piscicola* (shown to be synonymous with *L. carnis*) and *L. divergens*, have been reclassified recently in a new genus *Carnobacterium* (Collins *et al.*, 1987) as *C. piscicola* and *C. divergens* respec-

Table 6.6b. *Third-stage table for* Lactobacillus, Listeria, Erysipelothrix, Arachnia, Arcanobacterium *and* Actinomyces

	1	2	3	4	5	6	7	8	9	10	11	12	13	14
Growth at 15 °C	−	−	−	−	−	+	+	+	−	+	+	?	?	?
Growth at 45 °C	+	+	+	+	+	−[a]	−	−	d	w[e]	−	d	?	−
Gas from glucose	−	−	−	−	−	−	−	+	+	−	−	−	−	−
Carbohydrates, acid from:														
arabinose	−	−	−	−	−	−	d	+	d	−	−	d[f]	−	D
galactose	+	+	d	+	+	+	+	d	+	d	+	+	+	D
lactose	+	−	d	+	d	d	+	d	+	d	+	+	+	+
maltose	+	d	d	+	d	+[b]	+	+	+	+	+	+	d	d
mannitol	−	d	−	+	−	+[b]	+	−	−	−	−	+	−	D
melezitose	−	−	−	−	−	+[b]	d	−	−	+	−	−	−	D
melibiose	d	−	−	+	d	−	+	+	+	−	−	d	−	D
raffinose	d	−	−	+	d	−	+	d	+	−	−	+	−	D
salicin	+	+	d	d	+	+[b]	+	−	−	+	−	d	?	D
sorbitol	−	−	−	+	−	+[b]	+	−	−	−	−	d	−	−[g]
trehalose	d	+	d	+	d	+[b]	+	−	d	+	−	d	d	D
Aesculin hydrolysis	+	+	−[c]	d	+	+	+	d	d	+	−	−	−	D
Nitrate reduction	−	−	−	−	−	−	−[d]	−	−	−	−	+	d	D
Arginine hydrolysis	−	+	d	−	−	−	−	+	+	−	+	−	−	−

1 **Lactobacillus acidophilus**
2 **Lactobacillus jensenii**
3 **Lactobacillus delbrueckii**
4 **Lactobacillus salivarius**
5 **Lactobacillus gasseri**
6 **Lactobacillus casei**
7 **Lactobacillus plantarum**
8 **Lactobacillus brevis**
9 **Lactobacillus fermentum** (not 'L. fermenti'; now also includes L. cellobiosus)
10 **Listeria monocytogenes;** Listerella monocytogenes
11 **Erysipelothrix rhusiopathiae;** E. insidiosa
12 **Arachnia propionica;** Actinomyees propionicus
13 **Arcanobacterium haemolyticum;** Corynebacterium haemolyticum
14 **Actinomyces** spp.

a Only *L. casei* subsp. *rhamnosus* grows at 45 °C
b *L. casei* subsp. *tolerans* does not produce acid from these carbohydrates
c Only those strains previously named 'L. leichmanni' hydrolyse aesculin
d Some strains reduce nitrate but only if glucose limited to keep pH above 6
e 45 °C about upper limit of growth for *Listeria*
f Strains of serovar 1 may produce acid
g Some strains of *A. israelii* and *A. pyogenes* may produce acid

Other symbols used in the table are explained in Tables 5.1 and 5.2 on p. 47.

tively; sporing forms of lactobacilli have been classified in the genus *Sporolactobacillus* (Kitahara & Suzuki, 1963). None of these genera is regarded as pathogenic and they are not considered in this *Manual*.

The species composition of *Lactobacillus* has changed considerably in the last decade; many new species have been described, but others have been reduced in rank. For example, *L. bulgaricus* and *L. lactis* are now regarded as subspecies of *L. delbrueckii*; and *L. cellobiosus* as a biovar of *L. fermentum*.

Of the three groupings of lactobacilli (thermobacteria, streptobacteria and betabacteria) the heterofermentative betabacteria can produce gas from glucose under certain conditions. Such gas production is not likely to be confused with that from clostridia (and

their non-sporing variants) which is vigorous and occurs in a variety of media incubated anaerobically. In contrast, heterofermentative lactobacilli (and *L. delbrueckii*) produce ammonia from arginine (Kandler & Weiss, 1986). For the sugar reactions of lactobacilli, the MRS medium (Appendix A2.6.25) of de Man, Rogosa & Sharpe (1960) is usually used; Whittenbury (1963) showed that a soft agar medium was advantageous.

The characters of lactobacilli likely to be isolated in medical laboratories are shown in Table 6.6b but we do not show the subspecies of *L. delbrueckii*, *L. casei* and *L. plantarum*. The specialized methods used in the detailed characterization of lactobacilli are outside the scope of this *Manual*; we refer readers for information to papers by Sharpe (1979, 1981) and Kandler & Weiss (1986).

Minidefinition: *Lactobacillus. Gram-positive rods often coryneform; chain formation common; typically non-motile and non-sporing. Not acid-fast. Microaerophilic or facultatively anaerobic. Catalase-negative. Complex growth requirements; grow best about pH 6.0. Attack sugars fermentatively. Type species: L. delbrueckii; ATCC strain 9649.*

6.6.2 Listeria (Tables 6.5a,c; 6.6a,b) was at one time regarded as closely related to *Erysipelothrix* and placed in that genus. However, Barber (1939), supported later by numerical taxonomic work (Davis & Newton, 1969; Davis *et al.*, 1969) always maintained the separation of the two genera. Stuart & Pease (1972) thought that *Listeria* resembled the enterococci and *Erysipelothrix* the other streptococci. The catalase test and motility do, however, distinguish between them. We describe *Listeria* more fully in Section 6.5.2 but repeat the minidefinition here.

Minidefinition: *Listeria. Gram-positive rods; motile; non-sporing; not acid-fast. Aerobic and facultatively anaerobic. Catalase-positive; oxidase-negative; produce acetoin. Attack sugars by fermentation. Type species: L. monocytogenes; NCTC strain 10357. (Recommended typical strain NCTC 11994).*

6.6.3 Erysipelothrix (Tables 6.6a,b). Until recently this genus contained only one species, *E. rhusiopathiae*, the causative organism of swine erysipelas and human erysipeloid. Despite agreement about its pathogenicity it has a chequered history, having been placed at various times in no less than eleven different genera with fourteen different epithets (Shuman & Wellmann, 1966). This nomenclatural difficulty was finally resolved with the issue of Opinion 32 (1970) conserving the name *Erisipelothrix* which is now included in the *Approved Lists of Bacterial Names* (1980). A second species *E. tonsillarum* (not 'E. tonsillae'), has been described recently on the basis of DNA hybridization but as it cannot yet be distinguished from *E. rhusiopathiae* by morphology or biochemical tests (Takahashi *et al.*, 1987) we mention it only for completeness. Both species are microaerophilic and grow well on Nutrient Agar

especially with the addition of serum (5–10%); crude, but not purified, bile salts (Hutner, 1942) and Tween 80 (Ando, Moriya & Kuwahara, 1959) seem to act well as substitutes for serum. The optimum temperature for growth is 30–37 °C within the range 5–42 °C. White & Shuman (1971) showed that the fermentation reactions of *Erysipelothrix* strains varied with the medium and the indicator used, but most of them show a consistent pattern under the same conditions of growth. They recommended a basal medium with peptone, meat extract and 10% horse serum. We have obtained reliable results with Nutrient Broth sugars containing phenol red as the indicator, but known strains should always be included as controls (Jones, 1986). Tests for the production of H_2S should be done preferably in Triple Sugar Iron Agar (Wood, 1970).

Twenty-two serovars of *E. rhusiopathiae* have been distinguished on the basis of heat-stable somatic antigens. Serovars 1 and 2 are common; the others are rare (Kucsera, 1973; Wood, Haubrich & Harrington, 1978; Nørrung, 1979). All the strains of *E. tonsillarum* examined so far belong to serovar 7 (Takahashi *et al.*, 1987).

Minidefinition: *Erysipelothrix. Gram-positive rods, often in filaments; not branching; non-motile; non-sporing; not acid-fast. Microaerophilic and facultatively anaerobic. Catalase negative; oxidase-negative; H_2S-positive. Acid produced from a wide variety of sugars by fermentation. Type species: E. rhusiopathiae; NCTC strain 8163.*

6.6.4 Arachnia (Tables 6.6a,b; 6.7), a diphtheroid rod that may show filaments with branching, which can grow aerobically but prefers anaerobic conditions; CO_2 is not required for either aerobic or anaerobic growth. As it is catalase-negative, *Arachnia* appears in the first-stage table (6.1) in the same major grouping as *Lactobacillus* and *Erysipelothrix* and hence we include it in Tables 6.6a and b. Morphologically, *Arachnia* resembles the actinomycetes and physiologically the propionibacteria; we therefore show its characters also in Table 6.7 and give additional information about it in Section 6.7.3.

Minidefinition: *Arachnia. Gram-positive diphtheroid or branched rods and filaments. Non-motile; not acid-fast. Facultatively aer-*

obic but grows best anaerobically. Catalase-negative. Attack sugars by fermentation with propionic and acetic acid as the main end-products.

6.6.5   Arcanobacterium (Tables 6.6a,b; 6.7). A genus of microaerophilic, Gram-positive, irregular rods containing the single species *A. haemolyticum*, formerly called *Corynebacterium haemolyticum* (Collins, Jones & Schofield, 1982). The species was previously closely associated with *Corynebacterium pyogenes* (now *Actinomyces pyogenes*) but it has since been shown to be distinct by numerical taxonomic, chemotaxonomic and genomic techniques (Schofield & Schaal, 1981; Collins *et al.*, 1982). The organisms were first isolated from nasopharyngeal and other infections among American soldiers in the Pacific and, as the name implies, the colonies are β-haemolytic on Blood Agar (Hermann, 1961).

In young (18 h) Blood Agar cultures, Gram-positive slender rods predominate which become granular, segmented and in older cultures may appear as cocci. They grow poorly on media without the addition of blood or serum and prefer anaerobic conditions. An atmosphere with added CO_2 considerably enhances growth. Serum should not be used for fermentation tests as false positive reactions may occur. The tests important for characterization are shown in Tables 6.6*a* and *b*.

> **Minidefinition:** *Arcanobacterium. Gram-positive, irregular rods, may appear coccoid; non-motile, non-sporing. Microaerophilic. Typically catalase-negative. Attack sugars by fermentation. Type species: A. haemolyticum; NCTC strain 8452.*

6.6.6   Actinomyces (Tables 6.6a,b; 6.7). This genus is discussed in Section 6.7.1 but for comparative purposes we show the generic characters in Tables 6.6*a,b* and repeat the minidefinition here.

> **Minidefinition**: *Actinomyces. Gram-positive rods which may show rudimentary branching. Non-motile; non-sporing; not acid-fast. Microaerophilic and anaerobic. Catalase-negative (two exceptions). Attack sugars fermentatively. Type species: A. bovis; NCTC strain 11535.*

6.7   The actinomycetes

(Actinomyces, Propionibacterium, Arachnia, Rothia and Bifidobacterium)

***Characters common to members of the group*: Gram-positive, short to filamentous rods with branching, even if rudimentary. Non-motile; not acid-fast. Aerial mycelium not produced. Attack sugars fermentatively.**

The term 'actinomycetes' is not easy to define. Some taxonomists use it to refer to *Mycobacterium, Nocardia, Streptomyces* and related groups; others use it to encompass all Gram-positive bacteria with a high DNA G+C content (> 55 mol %). We use it as in the previous edition of this *Manual* for a diverse group of organisms which show true branching but which have wide variations in atmospheric requirements between the genera and species. Moreover, they all belong to the 'actinomycete' branch of the Gram-positive bacteria as defined by Stackebrandt & Woese (1981). With the exception of *Rothia*, which grows best in air (Gerencser & Bowden, 1986), the organisms in this group are anaerobic or microaerophilic; with some, notably *Actinomyces*, added CO_2 improves growth and others may also benefit. The colonial morphology of the organisms varies from smooth to rough 'breadcrumb-like' formations, both of which can be displayed by the same strain thus suggesting that the culture may be mixed; some are filamentous or spider-like. The test characters, including pigmentation, can also vary considerably with the composition of the medium and the pH as well as with the concentration of oxygen so that for species identification particular attention to media and cultural conditions is essential. Further information, with illustrations, is given in the reviews by Slack & Gerencser (1975), Schaal & Pulverer (1981), Gerencser & Bowden (1986), Cummins & Johnson (1986), Schaal (1986*a,b*) and Scardovi (1986).

All the members of this diverse group ferment glucose and are sensitive to penicillin and the β-lactam antibiotics. Their cultural characters, which are shown in Table 6.7, are not always stable and we warn against placing too much reliance on them individually; identification of this group of organisms more than most should be based on a summation of characters. As a rule of thumb, the more pigmented an isolate, the less likely it is to be pathogenic.

6.7.1   Actinomyces (Table 6.7). There is a wide range of morphological types amongst this genus. Most strains of *Actinomyces israelii* are filamentous with a rough colonial morphology, while many strains of *A. naeslundii*, *A. viscosus* and *A. odontolyticus* are more diphtheroidal in cell morphology with smooth colony forms. Growth of all strains is enhanced with added CO_2, though *Actinomyces meyeri* (formerly *Actinobacterium meyeri*) grows best and should be cultured under anaerobic conditions (Cato *et al.*, 1984). For growth *Actinomyces* require a rich medium, such as that provided by a meat infusion broth or a medium with added serum.

Differentiation between species based solely on either cell or colonial morphology is not feasible. Table 6.7 shows the tests most useful for characterization; these have been chosen as reasonably reproducible, taking into account the variation likely to occur with different media. We do not include two recently described species, *A. denticolans* and *A. howellii* (the latter catalase-positive), isolated from dental plaque in cattle (Dent & Williams, 1984a,b).

The common cause of actinomycosis in man is *A. israelii*, the pus from lesions usually containing yellowish to brown particles, the so-called 'sulphur granules'. Until recently the cervicofacial region was the site most frequently affected but during the last decade there has been a marked increase in isolations of *A. israelii* from women using intrauterine contraceptive devices (IUDs) or vaginal pessaries. *Actinomyces* species isolated from other clinical infections include: *A. meyeri* from brain abscesses; *A. eriksonii*, now regarded as a *Bifidobacterium* (Scardovi, 1986), from throat and abdominal lesions; and *A. naeslundii* and *A. viscosus* from the tonsils and mouth where they occur normally as commensals but may be associated together with *A. odontolyticus* in dental decay and with carious teeth.

The classical animal infection is 'lumpy jaw' in cattle caused by the type species, *A. bovis*. Other species associated with animal infections of veterinary concern include *A. pyogenes* (formerly *Corynebacterium pyogenes*) causing mastitis in cattle (Reddy, Cornell & Fraga, 1982); *A. israelii*, causing infections similar to *A. bovis*; *A. suis*, which affects the soft tissues of cattle; *A. viscosus* from the teeth of hamsters; and the recently isolated *A. hordeovulneris*, a cause of canine actinomycosis (Buchanan *et al.*, 1984).

The increasing incidence of *A. israelii* infections as well as recent research into dental decay have led to improvements in the isolation and characterization of these microorganisms which were previously regarded as 'unusual'. The most reliable identification techniques are those based on classical tests (Slack & Gerencser, 1975; Schofield & Schaal, 1981) rather than on commercial rapid test kits, which have not yet proved reliable for these organisms. Although characters are given in Table 6.7 for differentiation of the more common species, the classification of the genus is still far from satisfactory. However, there appear to be three distinct groupings consisting of: (1) *A. israelii;* (2) *A. naeslundii*, *A, viscosus* and *A. odontolyticus;* and (3) *A. bovis* and *A. pyogenes.*

A. israelii is a well-defined species which can be readily distinguished from others (Holmberg & Nord, 1975; Pine, 1970; Schofield & Schaal, 1981; Schaal, 1986a); it possibly deserves recognition as a separate genus within the *Actinomycetaceae*. *A. bovis*, although the type species of the genus, differs from all the other species in its cell-wall composition (Schleifer & Kandler, 1972; Schaal, 1986a) and in its biochemical characteristics (Schofield & Schaal, 1981). The only species with which it can be associated is the recently described *A. pyogenes*, previously classified as *Corynebacterium pyogenes* (Collins & Jones, 1982; Reddy, Cornell & Jones, 1982; Reddy, Cornell & Fraga, 1982). There may thus be some justification for removing *A. bovis* from the genus though this would create nomenclatural difficulties and we would prefer the *status quo* to be maintained meanwhile. *A. viscosus* produces catalase, will grow aerobically and does not hydrolyse aesculin or reduce nitrite.

Minidefinition: *Actinomyces. Non-motile Gram-positive rods which may show true though rudimentary branching. Non-sporing; not acid-fast. Microaerophilic and anaerobic. Catalase-negative (two exceptions). Attack sugars fermentatively. Type species: A. bovis; NCTC strain 11535.*

6.7.2   Propionibacterium (Table 6.7). A genus of heterogeneous Gram-positive bacteria that produce

Table 6.7. *Second-stage table for* Propionibacterium, Arachnia, Actinomyces, Rothia, Bifidobacterium *and* Erysipelothrix

	1	2	3	4	5	6	7	8	9	10	11	12	13	14	15
Growth in air	–	–	w/–	+	w/–[c]	+	w/–[c]	d[c]	d[c]	+	w/–[c]	–	+	–	+
Growth anaerobically	+	+	+	+[b]	+	+	+	+	+	+	+	+	–[d]	+	+
CO$_2$ required for growth	–	–	–	–	+	+	+	+	+	+	+	?	–[d]	–	?
CO$_2$ improves growth	+	+	+	+	+	+	+	+	+	+	+	?	–[d]	–	?
Catalase	+[a]	+[a]	+[a]	–	–	–	–	–	–	+	–	–	+	–	–
Carbohydrates, acid from:															
glycerol	–	–	+	d	+	–	–	d	–	d	d	–	(w)	?	–
lactose	–	–	d	+	+	+	+	d	d	d	d	+	d	+	+
maltose	–	+	+	+	d	d	+	+	d	+	+	+	+	+[e]	+
mannitol	d	–	–	+	–	–	d	–	–	–	–	+	–	D	–
raffinose	–	+	–	+	–	–	+	+	–	+	–	+	–	+	–
salicin	–	–	+	d	–	–	+	d	d	d	–	+	+	D	–
sorbitol	d	–	–	d	–	–	d	–	–	–	–	+	–	D	–
sucrose	–	+	+	+	+	–	+	+	d	+	+	+	+	+	(w)
trehalose	–	+	+	d	–	d	d	+	d	d	–	+	+	D	–
xylose	–	–	–	–	–	d	+	d	d	–	+	+	–	D	–
melezitose	–	d	–	–	–	d	d	d	–	d	–	?	d	D	–
melibiose	–	d	–	d	d	–	+	+	–	d	–	?	–	+	–
VP	–	–	–	–	–	–	–	–	–	–	–	–	(d)	?	–
Aesculin hydrolysis	–	–	+	–	–	–	+	+	d	–	–	d	+	?	–
Starch hydrolysis	–	–	–	–	+	d	–	d	d	d	–	–	–	?	–
Nitrate reduced	–	–	–	+	–	d	d	+	+	d	–	–	+	–	?
Indole	+	–	–	–	–	–	–	–	–	–	–	d	–	?	–
Gelatin liquefaction	+	–	+	–	–	d	–	–	–	–	–	?	d	?	–
Growth in 10% bile	+	+	+	+	d	d	–	d	–	d	–	?	+	?	?

1 **Propionibacterium acnes**; *Corynebacterium acnes*; Voss' *C. acnes*; group I; *C. parvum* (Cummins & Johnson, 1974).
2 **Propionibacterium granulosum**; Voss' *C. acnes* group II
3 **Propionibacterium avidum**
4 **Arachnia propionica**; *Actinomyces propionicus*
5 **Actinomyces bovis**
6 **Actinomyces pyogenes**; *Corynebacterium pyogenes*
7 **Actinomyces israelii**
8 **Actinomyces naeslundii**
9 **Actinomyces odontolyticus**
10 **Actinomyces viscosus**; *Odontomyces viscosus*; the hamster organism
11 **Actinomyces meyeri**
12 **'Actinomyces eriksonii'**; probably *Bifidobacterium* spp. (Scardovi, 1986))
13 **Rothia dentocariosa**; *Nocardia dentocariosa*
14 **Bifidobacterium** spp. *Lactobacillus bifidus*
15 **Erysipelothrix rhusiopathiae**; *E. insidiosa*

a Catalase reaction improved if culture exposed to air before testing
b Better growth anaerobically
c Poor growth may occur in air; growth improved with CO$_2$ but best anaerobically
d Some growth anaerobically with added CO$_2$; Schofield & Schaal (1981) report stimulation of growth by CO$_2$
e Some strains of *Bifidobacterium bifidus* are negative

Other symbols used in the table are explained in Tables 5.1 and 5.2 on p. 47.

propionic acid as one of the end-products of their fermentative metabolism. It contains two main groups of organisms with different habitats: those from cheese and dairy products; and those which occur as commensals in the skin and the respiratory and intestinal tracts of man and animals. The former, which represent the original members of the genus and are thus often referred to as 'classical' propionibacteria (see Cummins & Johnson, 1986), are not considered here. The latter, exemplified by the anaerobic acne bacillus, occur frequently as contaminants of clinical material and as part of a mixed microbial flora in opportunist infections. The acne bacillus, originally ill-placed in the genus *Corynebacterium*, was eventually transferred to *Propionibacterium* as proposed by Douglas & Gunter (1946) but only after a protracted debate, until agreement early in the 1970s, about whether or not '*C. acnes*' was representative of all the anaerobic diphtheroids. Clinically, *P. acnes* and *P. granulosum* are the two species most frequently isolated from purulent infections, though previously there was some doubt about the separate identity of the latter species (Voss, 1970; Johnson & Cummins, 1972); unlike the other representatives of the genus neither of them will grow in air. With freshly isolated strains, variation in characterization test results does occur, particularly with aesculin and casein hydrolysis and in the carbohydrate fermentation patterns; however, some reports of such variation in results between different laboratories may have been due to mixed cultures (Cummins & Johnson, 1986). The taxonomic status of the anaerobic species *P. lymphophylum*, which has been isolated from urinary tract infections, is doubtful; it may well not be a member of the genus (Cummins & Johnson, 1986).

> **Minidefinition:** *Propionibacterium. Gram-positive diphtheroidal rods; may be coccoid, bifid or even branched. Non-motile; non-sporing. Anaerobic to aerotolerant. Catalase-positive. Attack sugars by fermentation with propionic acid as the main end product. Type species: P. freudenreichii; NCTC strain 10470.*

6.7.3 Arachnia (Table 6.7).

As its name implies, one important character differentiating this single species genus, *Arachnia propionica*, from *Actinomyces* is the production of propionic acid from the fermentative breakdown of glucose, now usually detected by gas chromatography. Diaminopimelic acid is also present in the cell wall (Johnson & Cummins, 1972). Originally described as an actinomycete (Buchanan & Pine, 1984), this organism is facultatively aerobic but grows best under anaerobic conditions; CO_2 is not required (Schaal, 1986b) and the finding of Schofield & Schaal (1981) that it may be stimulatory under certain cultural conditions remains to be clarified.

Arachnia propionica can cause clinically typical actinomycosis, and it may be difficult to distinguish from cultures of *Actinomyces israelii* contaminated with *Propionibacterium acnes*. Isolation techniques to ensure purity are thus, as always, of paramount importance. The colonies of *A. propionica* are rough and the cells are usually filamentous and may be branched. It can be distinguished from *Actinomyces israelii* not only by analysis of the end-products of fermentation but also by its inability to ferment melibiose, melezitose and xylose or to hydrolyse aesculin (Table 6.7). The two serovars recognized within the species differ from each other in some of their physiological characteristics (Schaal, 1986b).

> **Minidefinition:** *Arachnia. Gram-positive diphtheroidal or branched rods and filaments. Non-motile; not acid-fast. Facultatively aerobic but grows best anaerobically. Catalase-negative. Attack sugars by fermentation with propionic and acetic acids as the main end-products. Type species: A. propionica; ATCC strain 14157.*

6.7.4 Rothia (Table 6.7).

This group of catalase-positive Gram-positive rods, represented by the single species *R. dentocariosa*, was previously contained within *Nocardia* until Georg & Brown (1967) created a new genus for it. Unlike *Nocardia*, it ferments carbohydrates and never produces conidia or a mycelium. *R. dentocariosa* has been isolated from carious teeth but its role in infection remains unclear. The organism usually grows best under microaerophilic conditions and not at all under anaerobic conditions. It produces rough, wrinkled colonies on solid media; microscopically it shows branching filaments which fragment easily and appear diphtheroidal or even coccoid as the culture ages; fresh isolates fragment less easily. Strains grow in the presence of 10% bile and produce ammonia from serine. For further information, see Gerencser & Bowden (1986).

> **Minidefinition:** *Rothia. Gram-positive diphtheroidal or filamentous rods; pleomorphic but do not form a mycelium or produce aerial hyphae. Non-motile; not acid-fast. Microaerophilic and aerobic. Catalase-positive. Attack sugars by fermentation. Reduce nitrite to ammonia. Type species: R. dentocariosa; NCTC strain 10917.*

6.7.5 Bifidobacterium (Table 6.7)

species are mainly diphtheroidal in morphology but are characterized by crudely branching forms, often T or Y shaped. The majority of strains require anaerobic growth conditions. Bifidobacteria occur in the human oral cavity, intestinal tract and vagina and in the faeces and rumen contents of animals and birds (Reuter, 1971; Scardovi *et al.*, 1971; Slack & Gerencser, 1975; Scardovi, 1981).

The taxonomic status of the genus is uncertain, as are several of the 20 species given in the *Approved Lists of Bacterial Names* (1980). A variety of fermentation patterns have been described and this is the usual method for speciation. We make no attempt at species characterization and show in Table 6.7 only their collective characteristics. *Bifidobacterium bifidum*, previously known as *Lactobacillus bifidus*, is probably the best known species and, because of its limited ability to attack sugars, is the easiest to identify (Scardovi *et al.*, 1971; Scardovi, 1981, 1986). They resemble lactobacilli in cell-wall structure and carbohydrate metabolism (Kandler, 1970) but we believe current taxonomic work is likely to show that *Bifidobacterium* is separate from both the lactobacilli and the actinomycetes.

> **Minidefinition:** *Bifidobacterium. Gram-positive rods with a tendency to form rudimentary branches. Non-motile; non-sporing; not acid-fast. Anaerobic. Catalase-negative. Attack sugars by fermentation. Type species: B. bifidum; ATCC strain 29521.*

6.8   The anaerobic bacilli
(*Clostridium, Eubacterium*)

***Characters common to members of the group*: Gram-positive rods; spore-forming (except *Eubacterium*); not acid-fast. Anaerobic. Sensitive to metronidazole.**

The degree of anaerobiosis required by members of this group ranges from the strict (*Clostridium tetani, C. chauvoei, Eubacterium* species) through the less exacting species (*C. perfringens*) to the facultative aerobe *C. histolyticum*. The techniques for the culture of anaerobes have become more sophisticated and greater use is now made of commercially available anaerobic cabinets for all manipulative procedures, although anaerobic jars still play a major and satisfactory role in most general laboratories.

In the past, many species were undoubtedly created too readily among anaerobic organisms, sometimes on the basis of a single isolate or character. However, following promulgation of the *Bacteriological Code* and the *Approved Lists of Bacterial Names*, several

species with previously well-known names (e.g. '*C. tetanomorphum*' and '*C. subterminale*') have been discarded either because viable cultures with the characters listed were not found *extant* or because they were shown to be identical with other approved species. The species of current medical interest, which now include for example *C. barati* and *C. ramosum* are shown in Table 6.8. *C. putrefaciens*, despite its name, is not strongly proteolytic and is unlikely to be isolated often as it grows best at room temperature but not at 37 °C; we include it for comparison as it is fairly salt-tolerant and is associated with the spoilage of brine-cured ham and other foods. We also continue to include *Eubacterium*, a genus of Gram-positive bacilli which do not produce spores, in Table 6.8 to obviate the remote possibility of confusion with non-sporing variants of clostridia.

6.8.1   Clostridium (Tables 6.6*a*, 6.8). In this genus, species characterization in the diagnostic laboratory depends partly on spore morphology as well as on tests for particular enzyme activities. For those with gas–liquid chromatography facilities, identification can be assisted by the detection of other metabolic products. Many species of clostridia can be further subdivided into varieties or types by the different toxins (enzymes) they produce (Sterne & Warrack, 1964). However, as few bacteriologists have the specific antitoxins available or the expertise to carry out the tests, we do not give third-stage tables to show these toxin types; such isolates should be referred if necessary to a reference laboratory. Those interested in the finer subdivisions are referred to publications by Brooks, Sterne & Warrack (1957) for *Clostridium perfringens*; Oakley, Warrack & Clarke (1947) and Oakley & Warrack (1959) for *C. novyi*; and Smith (1977) for *C. botulinum*. It should be noted that *C. sporogenes* and proteolytic strains of *C. botulinum* are closely similar genetically and in their general cultural characters, the only significant difference between them being the production of a neurotoxin by *C. botulinum* although the former is usually haemolytic. The clostridia of wound infections are dealt with extensively by Willis (1969, 1977, 1988). Infections caused by clostridia, including sporadic cases of enteritis, are not generally transmissible from person to person, so that in outbreaks of food-poisoning due to certain toxin types of

Table 6.8. *Second-stage table for* Clostridium

	1	2	3	4	5	6	7	8	9	10	11	12	13	14	15	16	17	18	19	20	21	22	23
Motility	+	−	−	+	+	+	+	−	+	+	+	+	+	+	+	+	+	+	+	+	+	−	D
Spore position and shape	UX	UX	UX	TX	VX	VX	TXY	TX	VX	VX	VY	UX	UX	VX	VX	VX	VX	VX	VX	TY	VX	VX	−
Growth at 37 °C	+	+	+	+	+	+	+	+	+	+	+	+	+	+	+	+	+	+	+	+	+	−	+
Carbohydrates, acid from:																							
glucose	+	+	+	+	+	+	+	+	+	+	+	+	+	+	+	+	+	+	−	−	−	−	D
lactose	+	+	+	+	+	+	+	+	+	+	+	−	−	−	−	−	−	−	−	−	−	−	D
sucrose	+	+	+	+	−	+	+	+	+	−	+	d[a]	d[a]	−	−	−	−	−	−	−	−	−	D
salicin	+	−	+	+	−	+	+	+	−	d[a]	d[a]	−	−	−	−	−	−	−	−	−	−	−	D
Nitrates reduced	−	d[a]	+	+	−	−	−	−	d[a]	d[a]	+	−	−	−	−	−	−	−	−	−	−	−	D
Indole	−	−	−	−	−	−	−	−	−	+	−	−	−	+	+	−	−	−	+	−	−	−	D
Gelatinase	−	+	−	−	−	−	−	−	+	+	−	+	+	+	+	+	+	d[a]	+	+	+	−	D
Caseinase	−	−	−	−	−	−	−	−	−	−	−	+	−	+	+	+	−	+	−	+	−	−	−
Urease	−	−	−	−	−	−	−	−	−	−	−	d	−	−	+	d	−	−	−	+	−	−	?
Egg yolk:																							
lecithinase C	−	+	+	−	−	−	−	−	−	−	−	−	−	−	+	+	+	−	−	−	−	−	D
lipase	−	−	−	−	−	−	−	−	−	−	−	+	+	+	−	−	+	−	−	−	−	−	−

1 **Clostridium butyricum**	9 **Clostridium chauvoei**; *C. fesseri*	18 **Clostridium difficile**
2 **Clostridium perfringens;**	10 **Clostridium septicum**	19 **Clostridium subterminale**
Welchia perfringens 'C. welchii'	11 **Clostridium sphenoides**	20 **Clostridium tetani**; *Plectridium tetani*
3 **Clostridium barati**; *C. paraperfringens*	12 **Clostridium botulinum** (A,B,F)*	21 **Clostridium histolyticum**
4 **Clostridium tertium**	13 **Clostridium botulinum** (C,D,E)†	22 **Clostridium putrefaciens**
5 **Clostridium fallax**	14 **Clostridium novyi**; *C. oedematiens*	23 **Eubacterium** spp.
6 **Clostridium carnis**	15 **Clostridium bifermentans**	
7 **Clostridium ramosum**	16 **Clostridium sordelli**; *C. bifermentans*	
8 **Clostridium innocuum**	17 **Clostridium sporogenes**	

* Mainly proteolytic	T spores terminal
† Mainly non-proteolytic	U spores central
a More strains positive than negative	V spores subterminal/central; variable in position
	X spores oval (ellipsoidal)
	Y spores round

Other symbols used in the table are explained in Tables 5.1 and 5.2 on p. 47.

C. perfringens, and of botulism, secondary cases do not occur. In the more recently recognized association of *C. difficile* with pseudomembranous colitis and antibiotic-associated diarrhoea there is some evidence that hospital cross-infection may occur (Mulligan, 1988); however, epizootics due to a variety of clostridial infections can cause considerable losses among flocks and herds of animals.

The isolation of clostridia is not usually difficult but their purification requires patience and skill, and may take several weeks. Isolation techniques usually involve enrichment culture of material heated at 80 °C for 10 minutes to destroy vegetative organisms; treatment with ethanol ('alcohol shock') prior to enrichment serves the same purpose. However, it is prudent to culture unheated material as well in case there are insufficient spores present in the heated material to yield any subsequent growth. After incubation for 24–48 hours, subcultures are made to other media (e.g. Blood Agar plates). For *C. tetani*, we recommend the use of a modified Fildes' method in which the material is inoculated onto a small area of a Blood Agar plate. After incubation for about 10 hours, subcultures are made from the advancing edge of the fine growth swarming across the plate; *C. tetani* swarms more rapidly than other bacteria so that the edge of growth often yields the organism in pure culture. Infections and cultures may, however, be mixed with more than one clostridial (or other anaerobic) species present; their separation and identification, which may need the use of specific antisera and sometimes animal inoculation, is one of the more satisfying achievements in clinical bacteriology.

Some comments on the tests for the characters

shown in Table 6.8 are needed. In Gram-stained films of the clostridia, some species, especially the strict anaerobes such as *C. tetani* and *C. novyi*, sometimes stain Gram-negatively, particularly in old cultures. The spores show as circular or oval unstained areas within the cells but they can be stained by the malachite green method. Clostridial spores may be situated centrally, terminally or in between, and they usually distend the bacillary body. Since their position is often variable (and the judgement subjective), the spore data in Table 6.8 should be used cautiously and 'flexibly'. Terminal spherical (drumstick) spores are characteristic of *C. tetani*, while the virtual absence of spores is characteristic of many strains of *C. perfringens* and of *C. fallax*, which is now accepted as a species of *Clostridium* (Willis, 1960). Because *C. perfringens* does not produce spores readily detectable in cultures (including paradoxically strains isolated from material heated to destroy all vegetative organisms) and because it does not need strict anaerobic conditions for growth, we have included it also in Table 6.6*a* for other Gram-positive bacteria which grow better anaerobically than they do aerobically. The non-sporing eubacteria might possibly be confused with 'asporogenous' variants of clostridia though only if microscopy alone is considered. Among the common clostridia only *C. perfringens* and *C. butyricum* form capsules; all are motile except *C. perfringens*, *C. barati* and *C. innocuum*. The clostridia typically produce colonies of irregular shape. Some species such as *C. sporogenes* form frankly rhizoidal colonies; others, such as *C. tetani*, rarely produce discrete colonies except in young cultures, their growth characteristically appearing as a thin transparent 'swarming' film. *C. perfringens* is one of the few commonly encountered clostridia which forms a circular, entire colony.

Haemolysis, considered alone, is not a definitive feature of clostridia. Though many species are haemolytic on Blood Agar plates, different strains of a single species may vary considerably. Some species produce more than one haemolysin, and different haemolysins vary in their activity with the nature of the red cells used.

Gelatinase activity is common among clostridia. All strongly proteolytic clostridia digest gelatin, but there are many gelatinolytic species that do not attack complex proteins such as casein. For the detection of gelatinase activity we prefer Frazier's (1926) acid mercuric chloride method (Appendix C3.23) though it is safer to use 30% trichloracetic acid instead of the mercuric chloride solution. For proteinase activity Milk or Casein Agar is usually used; the strongly proteolytic clostridia, such as *C. histolyticum* and *C. bifermentans*, can hydrolyse a variety of complex proteins. As a useful rule, strongly proteolytic species rarely ferment lactose.

The fermentation reactions of most clostridia may be determined in Peptone Water sugar media; for exacting species we recommend the plate method of Phillips (1976) (Appendix C3.8.1) The usual fermentable sugars are glucose, lactose and sucrose, with salicin as a useful addition. Strongly saccharolytic species such as *C. perfringens* and *C. butyricum* ferment all the three basic sugars; weakly saccharolytic organisms ferment only glucose. Species that do not ferment glucose do not attack any of the basic sugars and they constitute the group of 'non-saccharolytic clostridia'. Indole production is a feature only of *C. bifermentans*, *C. sordelli*, *C. sphenoides* and *C. tetani* among the species under consideration.

Egg-yolk reactions, of great importance for the identification of clostridial species, depend on lecithinase C and lipase activity, both types of enzyme producing quite distinct opacity changes in Egg-Yolk Agar (Willis, 1962). Lecithinase C hydrolyses lecithin into phosphorylcholine and an insoluble diglyceride, the reaction resulting in intense diffuse opaque haloes in the medium around colonies and zones of growth; these reactions are inhibited by appropriate antitoxic sera. The lecithinase C-producing species comprise *C. perfringens*, *C. bifermentans*, *C. sordelli*, *C. novyi* and *C. barati*. It should be noted, however, that occasional strains of *C. perfringens* may fail to produce lecithinase.

The lipase hydrolyses free fats into glycerol and free fatty acids, and the reactions in Egg-Yolk Agar appear as zones of intense opacity usually limited in extent to that part of the medium immediately beneath colonies or zones of growth; in addition there is a 'pearly' surface layer overlying the growth. *C. sporogenes*, *C. botulinum* and *C. novyi* are the lipolytic species. It is worth noting that *C. novyi* is the only species that produces both a lecithinase and a lipase.

Urease activity serves to distinguish *C. sordelli* from *C. bifermentans*; indeed it is a sound practice to check the urease activity of all lecithinase C-positive isolates.

The soluble 'exotoxins' produced during growth and acting on specific substrates such as erythrocytes, proteins, lecithin and lipids are responsible for many of the differential cultural characters of clostridia. Other important clostridial toxins do not have recognizable *in vitro* activity, and require demonstration of their characteristic pharmacological effects *in vivo* in animals; such toxins include tetanospasmin and botulinum neurotoxin. The enterotoxin of *C. difficile* also falls into this category, but is exceptional in having useful identifiable cytopathic effects on cultures of tissue cell monolayers (Donta, 1988; Levett, 1988). These effects and their inhibition by antitoxin are also used to identify the presence of the enterotoxin in faecal preparations from cases of pseudomembranous colitis.

> **Minidefinition**: *Clostridium. Rods, Gram-positive in young cultures; typically motile (non-motile forms occur). Not acid-fast. Produce spores that are usually heat-resistant. Anaerobic; some species facultatively aerobic. Metronidazole-sensitive. Catalase-negative. Some species attack sugars fermentatively, others not at all. Type species: C. butyricum; NCTC strain 7423.*

6.8.2 Eubacterium (Tables 6.7; 6.8). These non-sporing anaerobic rods are probably quite unimportant in clinical bacteriology; they are part of the normal intestinal flora and have not been convincingly incriminated as pathogens. Holdeman, Cato & Moore, (1977) characterized 19 species, but we include only one, *E. lentum*, in Table 6.8 for the inexperienced in case of confusion with non-sporing variants of clostridia.

> **Minidefinition**: *Eubacterium. Gram-positive rods; do not branch. Non-sporing; not acid-fast. Anaerobic. Metronidazole-sensitive. Attack sugars fermentatively or not at all. Type species: E. limosum; ATCC strain 8486.*

6.9 The aerobic spore-formers
(*Bacillus*)
***Characters common to members of the group:* Gram-positive rods. Not acid-fast.**

Grow under aerobic conditions and produce heat-resistant spores.

The genus *Bacillus* embraces a large number of rod-shaped spore-forming species with a great diversity of properties. Neither the genus nor many of the species contained within it are taxonomically homogeneous and this is reflected in the variability of many of the characters listed in the first-stage (primary) identification table for Gram-positive bacteria (Table 6.1). Apart from non-sporing variants, the variable characters include (i) the Gram-reaction, (ii) motility, (iii) ability to grow under anaerobic conditions, (iv) the oxidase reaction, and (v) the method by which carbohydrates are broken down. Of these, the variability of the Gram-reaction is the most disturbing to the neatness of the identification scheme used in this *Manual* because it is based on the primary division of bacteria into Gram-positive and Gram-negative organisms. *Bacillus* is generally regarded as a genus of Gram-positive organisms but we must emphasize that strains of some species are Gram-positive only in the early stages of growth, and others may actually be Gram-negative (Gordon, Haynes & Pang, 1973; Claus & Berkeley, 1986) even though they all have cell walls which are structurally Gram-positive in type. We continue, however, to justify the more rigid but less scientific treatment of *Bacillus* as a genus of mostly Gram-positive bacilli on the grounds that the important species of medical interest, particularly *B. anthracis* and *B. cereus*, are clearly Gram-positive. We would remind readers, however, that the minidefinitions in this *Manual* do not necessarily apply to every species in a genus.

The laboratory identification of *B. anthracis* is a matter of some clinical urgency; the identification of other species is rarely so pressing. It should be noted, however, that *B. anthracis* is not the only species of medical and veterinary interest. *B. cereus* is now well recognized as a cause of food-poisoning (Kramer *et al.*, 1982) and of occasional tissue infections in man and other animals (Gilbert *et al.*, 1981; Norris *et al.*, 1981). Several other species including *B. macerans*, *B. sphaericus*, and *B. subtilis*, have also been implicated in various infections, mostly in immunodeficient or severely compromised patients (Logan, 1988). It is therefore important to recognize their potential pathogenicity and to examine further specimens rather than just dismiss *Bacillus* isolates from clinical material as contaminants.

In spite of the different reactions of *Bacillus* species (and of strains) shown in Table 6.1 for first-stage separation, these tests do not provide an adequate basis for subdividing the genus into species. Several unsuccessful attempts have been made to subdivide it with characters such as motility, optimal temperature for growth, nutritional requirements (Proom & Knight, 1955) and chromatographic techniques (Jayne-Williams & Cheeseman, 1960) but none have given a better arrangement than that described in the monograph of Smith, Gordon & Clark (1952) based on traditional biochemical tests, spore position and morphology. This classification, which was revised by Gordon, Haynes & Pang (1973) and divides the genus into species in three groups, has been adhered to substantially ever since. In such a heterogeneous and complex genus, this is marked tribute to the excellence of their work.

6.9.1   Bacillus (Tables 6.9a,b,c). Primary allocation to this genus is made on the basis of aerobic growth of spore-forming rods. As there are now more than 60 valid species, we include in Table 6.9a only those species recognized by Smith, Gordon & Clark (1952) as well as others which can grow on ordinary media under the conditions normally used in medical laboratories. We have omitted numerous species which would not normally be isolated in a medical laboratory either because they require special medium supplements for growth or because the physical conditions such as temperature needed for growth are quite different from those of medically important bacteria.

Recently, the identification of *Bacillus* species has been approached by methods such as pyrolysis mass spectrometry (Shute *et al.*, 1984), pyrolysis gas chromatography (O'Donnell *et al.*, 1980), DNA homology (Seki *et al.*, 1978; Krych, Johnson & Yousten, 1980; Priest, 1981) and enzyme electrophoresis (Baptist, Mandel & Gherna, 1978) though few of them have been adopted in routine diagnostic laboratories. In general the *Bacillus* species identified by these methods accord with those of Gordon, Haynes & Pang (1973) based on spore morphology and biochemical reactions. The latter tests are described in detail by Claus & Berkeley (1986). They are carried out at 30 °C except for the thermophile, *B. stearothermophilus*, which is used for checking the

efficiency of hospital sterilizers. It will not grow at this low temperature and should be incubated at 45–60 °C. Wolf & Barker (1968) and Walker & Wolf (1971) recognized three major varieties (or groups of organisms) within *B. stearothermophilus* which we show in Table 6.9a. Of these, Group I includes for example '*B. thermodenitrificans*', Group II *B. pallidus* and Group III resembles most closely *B. stearothermophilus sensu stricto*; they recommended incubation at 55 °C for characterization tests with tese organisms. We have excluded the psychrotrophic species (Larkin of Stokes, 1967) which occur commonly in frozen and refrigerated foods but which grow poorly, if at all, at or above 30 °C.

The shape, position and size of spores can be determined by phase-contrast microscopy, or alternatively with a spore stain such as that described by Schaeffer & Fulton (1933) (Appendix B2.3.1).

Acid production within 7 days should be examined in an agar medium with an ammonium salt as the primary nitrogen source and supplemented with a little yeast extract (Appendix A2.5.5). The ability to grow anaerobically can be a useful diagnostic feature but it may be difficult to determine. Indeed several species, notably *B. subtilis*, described as strict aerobes can grow, albeit weakly, under anaerobic conditions; in addition, other species, such as *B. licheniformis* (which was originally described as an anaerobe) may lose their capacity for fermentation. Several media, broth or agar-based, have been used for this test. They include Glucose Broth and the 'anaerobic agar' of Gordon, Haynes & Pang (1973) as well as the latter medium with the additoin of 1% glucose (Claus & Berkeley, 1986). We prefer to use agar media, incubated anaerobically, as the results are usually clearer than with liquid media. Nutrient (tryptose) Agar (or even Blood Agar) may also be used in deep tubes (or plates) with or without a pH indicator provided the medium is thoroughly pre-reduced preferably for 2–3 days before inoculation. Visible growth or colour change within 7 days confirms the ability to grow anaerobically. Whatever medium is used, it is important to ensure anaerobiosis, to use appropriate control cultures and to interpret the results carefully.

With the recent description of numerous new members, the genus *Bacillus* has become unwieldy though many of the species can still be identified by conventional tests. It can, however, be laborious

Table 6.9a. *Second-stage table for* Bacillus *species*

	1	2	3	4	5	6	7	8	9	10	11	12	13	14	15	16	17	18	19	20	21	22	23	24
Gram reaction	+	+	+	+	d	+	+	+	+	+	+	+	d	d	−	d	+	−	−	+	+	d	d	d
Chains of cells	+	+	+	+	d	d	+	+	+	+	+	d	d	d	−	d	+	+	+	d	+	+	−	d
Motility*	−	+	−	+	+	+	+	+	+	+	+	+	−	+	+	+	+	+	+	+	+	+	+	+
Cell length > 3μm	+	+	+	+	−	−	d	−	−	−	−	−	−	+	−	d	d	d	d	−	+	−	−	−
Spore position and shape	VX	VX	VX	VX	VX	VX	VX	VX	VX	VX	VTX	VTX	TYX	VX	VX	VTX	VX	VX	VX	TY	VTX	VX	VX	VTX
Swelling of cell body by spore	−	−	−	−	−	−	−	−	−	−	−	d	+	+	+	+	+	+	+	+	−	d	+	+
Growth at 50 °C	−	d	d	d	d	−	−	d	+	+	d	+	+	−	+	d	d	+	−	−	d	+	+	+
Growth in 10% NaCl	+	d	d	d	+	−	−	+	+	+	+	−	+	−	−	−	−	−	−	−	−	−	−	−
Anaerobic growth	+	+	+	+	d	d	−	−	d	+	−	+	+	+	−	+	+	+	+	−	−	d	−	−
Carbohydrates, acid from ASS:																								
glucose	+	+	+	+	+	+	+	+	+	+	+	+	+	+	−	+	+	+	+	−	−	+	+	+
cellobiose	−	d	d	d	d	d	+	+	+	+	+	+	−	+	−	+	d	+	+	−	−	+	+	d
galactose	−	−	−	−	−	d	+	d	+	+	d	d	−	d	−	+	−	+	+	−	−	−	d	−
mannose	−	d	d	d	d	+	+	d	+	+	+	d	d	d	−	+	d	+	+	−	−	+	d	+
melibiose	−	−	−	−	−	−	d	−	+	d	d	−	−	−	−	+	−	+	+	−	−	−	−	+
raffinose	−	−	−	−	−	d	d	d	d	+	+	d	−	+	−	+	−	+	+	−	−	d	d	+
salicin	−	d	d	d	d	d	+	+	+	+	+	+	d	+	−	d	d	+	+	−	−	d	+	d
xylose	−	−	−	−	−	−	d	−	+	+	+	d	+	d	−	d	−	+	+	−	−	−	−	−
ONPG	−	−	−	−	d	−	−	−	−	−	−	d	d	d	d	+	−	+	+	−	−	+	+	−
Utilization of citrate	−	d	d	d	d	−	+	+	+	+	+	d	d	−	d	−	−	d	d	d	−	d	d	d
Urease	−	d	d	−	−	−	d	d	−	−	−	−	−	−	d	−	−	d	−	d	−	−	−	−
Indole	−	−	−	−	−	−	−	−	−	−	−	−	+	+	−	−	−	−	−	−	−	−	−	−
VP	+	+	+	+	−	−	−	+	+	+	+	+	d	+	−	−	+	+	+	−	−	+	+	+
Nitrate reduction	+	+	+	+	+	d	d	−	+	+	+	d	d	−	−	d	d	+	+	d	−	+	+	d
Casein hydrolysis	+	+	+	+	+	−	+	+	+	+	+	d	d	+	+	d	d	−	+	d	d	+	+	d
Hippurate hydrolysis	−	−	−	−	−	−	d	−	d	+	−	−	−	−	+	d	−	−	−	d	−	−	−	−
Starch hydrolysis	+	+	+	+	+	+	+	+	+	+	+	+	+	+	−	+	+	+	+	−	d	+	+	+
Oxidase	d	d	d	d	+	+	−	−	−	−	−	d	+	+	+	−	−	+	−	+	+	−	−	−

1 **Bacillus anthracis**
2 **Bacillus cereus; *B. anthracoides***
3 **Bacillus mycoides**
4 **Bacillus thuringiensis**
5 **Bacillus firmus**
6 **Bacillus lentus**
7 **Bacillus megaterium**
8 **Bacillus pumilus**

9 **Bacillus subtilis**
10 **Bacillus licheniformis**
11 **Bacillus amyloliquefaciens**
12 **Bacillus coagulans**
13 **Bacillus pantothenticus**
14 **Bacillus alvei**
15 **Bacillus brevis**
16 **Bacillus circulans**

17 Bacillus laterosporus
18 Bacillus macerans
19 Bacillus polymyxa
20 Bacillus sphaericus
21 Bacillus badius
22 Bacillus stearothermophilus (Group I: Wolf & Barker, 1968; Walker & Wolf, 1971).
23 Bacillus stearothermophilus (Group II: Wolf & Barker, 1968; Walker & Wolf, 1971).
24 Bacillus stearothermophilus (Group III: Wolf & Barker, 1968; Walker & Wolf, 1971).

* All motile species may produce non-motile variants

T spore terminal
V spore central/subterminal
X spore oval (ellipsoidal)
Y spore round

Other symbols used in the table are explained in Tables 5.1 and 5.2 on p. 47.

Table 6.9b. *Supplementary tests for the identification of* B. anthracis *and closely related species*

	1	2	3	4
Motility	−	+	−	+
Rhizoid colony formation	−	−	+	−
Crystalline inclusions	−	−	−	+
Capsule formation [a]	+	−	−	−
'String of pearls' test [b]	+	−	−	−
Lysis by Y phage [c]	+	−	−	−
Haemolysis on 5% Blood Agar	−	+	+	+

1 **Bacillus anthracis**
2 **Bacillus cereus**; *B. anthracoides*
3 **Bacillus mycoides**
4 **Bacillus thuringiensis**

a Capsule formation after growth on Bicarbonate Agar with Serum plates incubated with 5–10% carbon dioxide, or in an anaerobic jar without catalyst, containing a carbon dioxide generator, at 37 °C overnight. Use Giemsa stain and examine microscopically for capsule formation. (Appendix A2.6.5).
b 'String of pearls' formation after growth in medium containing 10u/ml Penicillin G. (Appendix C3.57). Data from Parry, Turnbull & Gibson (1983).
c Data from Brown *et al* (1958).

Symbols used in the table are explained in Tables 5.1 and 5.2 on p. 47.

Table 6.9c. *Supplementary tests for the identification of* B. subtilis *and closely related species*

	1	2	3
Acid from inulin	+	d	−
Arginine dihydrolase	−	+	−
α-D-Arabinosidase production	d	+	−
α-D-Glucosidase production	+	+	−
β-D-Glucosidase production	+	d	−
L-Tryptophan-aminopeptidase production	−	+	+
Anaerobic growth	−	+	−
Propionate utilization	−	+	−
Chain formation	d	d	+
DNA hydrolysis	+	+	−
CMC hydrolysis [a]	+	+	−

1 **Bacillus subtilis**
2 **Bacillus licheniformis**
3 **Bacillus amyloliquefaciens**

a Carboxymethylcellulose hydrolysis. Culture on Nutrient Agar with 0.5% CMC for 48 h at 30–37 °C. Flood plate with 2M HCl for 10 min, then Ethanol until a white precipitate is formed (about 8 h).

Symbols used in the table are explained in Tables 5.1 and 5.2 on p. 47.

and computer-assisted schemes have been developed to aid identification. One scheme, claimed to give rapid and reproducible results (Logan & Berkeley, 1981, 1984; Berkeley, 1984), utilizes the API miniaturized biochemical system with 12 tests from the API20E and all of those in the API50CHB kit, together with supplementary morphological tests. An alternative probablistic scheme, described by Priest & Alexander (1988), is based on traditional tests for 30 morphological and physiological characters. It permits identification of 44 common *Bacillus* species, including many environmental isolates, within a few days. In the second-stage identification table (6.9a), we have used data from both of these studies.

There are a few areas where species differentiation is complicated or unclear which need comment. *B. cereus*, *B. anthracis*, *B. mycoides* and *B. thuringiensis* are all closely related species which have been the subject of much controversy. *B. anthracis* was regarded by Gordon, Haynes & Pang (1973) as a pathogenic variety of *B. cereus*; they suggested also that *B. mycoides* and the insect pathogen, *B. thuringiensis*, should be regarded as sub-species of *B. cereus*. This is because they differ from *B. cereus* in only a few characteristics which are virtually all plasmid-associated and can be lost, whereupon they become indistinguishable from *B. cereus* by the usual characterization tests. Had Smith, Gordon & Clark (1952) followed the principles of the *Bacteriological Code* at that time, *B. anthracis* would have been the species and *B. cereus* the variety as the epithet '*anthracis*' antedated that of '*cereus*'. However, they gave good reasons for regarding *B. cereus* as the parent form and thus for disregarding the less scientific requirements of the *Bacteriological Code*. In contrast, Leise *et al.* (1959) and Burdon & Wende (1960), citing several distinguishing features, argued that *B. anthracis* should remain as a separate species with its medically meaningful name. Currently, each of the four similar organisms in this group still retain species status and can be differentiated by the tests listed in Table 6.9b. It should be noted, however, that Logan *et al.* (1985) were able to distinguish virulent, avirulent and intermediate strains of *B. anthracis* from strains of each of the other species in the group.

Differentiation between *B. subtilis* and *B. licheniformis* is normally achieved by virtue of the ability of the latter to grow anaerobically but it should be remembered that *B. subtilis* has a limited capacity to grow in the absence of air and this can be confusing. The industrially important, amylase-producing species, *B. amyloliquefaciens*, described by Priest *et al.* (1987) is easily confused with *B. subtilis* but can be distinguished by the tests shown in Table 6.9c.

Although the species *B. firmus* and *B. lentus* are readily distinguished (Table 6.9a), several other poorly described taxa have properties similar to them (Gordon, Hyde & Moore, 1977) and are difficult to identify. Such taxa, however, are usually associated with saline or slightly alkaline environments and are less likely to be encountered in the clinical laboratory. Nevertheless, should difficulty be experienced in identifying these or other *Bacillus* isolates, the detailed and more extensive computer-based systems of Logan & Berkeley (1984) or Priest & Alexander (1988) should be consulted.

> **Minidefinition:** *Bacillus. Rods, mainly Gram-positive in young cultures. Motile (some non-motile forms occur). Not acid-fast; produce heat-resistant spores under aerobic conditions. Aerobic; some species facultatively anaerobic. Oxidase-variable; catalase-positive. Species differ in the manner in which they attack sugars; some do not attack them. Type species: B. subtilis; NCTC strain 3610.*

6.10 The acid-fast rods

(Mycobacterium, Nocardia)

> ***Characters common to members of the group:*** **Gram-positive rods, occasionally coccoid; non-motile. Acid-fast. Aerobic to microaerophilic. Attack sugars oxidatively.**

The characteristic acid-fastness varies in general from weak to strong from *Nocardia* to *Mycobacterium*, although this also depends to some extent on the age of the culture. Rapidly growing mycobacteria, such as *M. fortuitum*, certainly lose their acid-fastness in older cultures, but in practice there is rarely any difficulty in deciding whether or not a strain is acid-fast. If such a problem should arise, then smears of the strain should be decolorized, one with 25% and another with 5% sulphuric acid for 1 minute. This will help to distinguish between the genuine acid-fast strains, which are resistant to the 5% acid, and other strains which are decolorized by it.

Table 6.10a. *Second-stage table for* Nocardia *and* Actinomadura madurae

	1	2	3	4
Acid fast	d	d	d	–
Aerial hyphae	+	+	+	+
Carbohydrates, acid from:				
adonitol	–	–	–	+
arabinose	–	–	–	+
inositol	–	+	+	d
maltose	–	d	–	d
mannitol	–	+	+	+
rhamnose	d	–	–	+
xylose	–	–	–	+
Decomposition of:				
casein	–	–	+	+
hypoxanthine	–	+	+	–
tyrosine	–	–	+	+
urea	+	+	+	–
xanthine	–	+	–	–

1 *Nocardia asteroides*
2 *Nocardia otitidis–caviarum; N. caviae*
3 *Nocardia brasiliensis; N. mexicana; N. pretoriana*
4 *Actinomadura madurae; N. madurae*

Symbols used in the table are explained in Tables 5.1 and 5.2 on p. 47.

6.10.1 Nocardia (Table 6.10a).

Although mainly soil organisms, nocardias are capable of causing infections and are isolated occasionally in medical laboratories. Since the previous edition of this *Manual*, opinion has consolidated and several species that were once regarded as nocardias have now been assigned to other genera. Thus *Nocardia madurae*, the cause of 'Madura foot', is now classified in a new genus as *Actinomadura madurae* (Goodfellow & Lechevalier, 1986); however, as we do not refer to this species elsewhere in this *Manual*, we have included it in Table 6.10a. Similarly, '*Mycobacterium rhodocrous*' is now assigned to the 'plant' genus *Rhodococcus* (Goodfellow, 1986) but as it has no medical significance we do not include it.

The definition of the genus *Nocardia* now rests largely on the presence, within the cells, of characteristic lipids such as mycolic acids with 46 to 60 carbon atoms in the chains (Minnikin & O'Donnell, 1983) and of large amounts of meso-diaminopimelic acid in the cell wall (Goodfellow & Cross, 1983). Tests for these acids are not, however, suitable for routine diagnostic laboratories so that, if necessary, strains should be referred to a reference laboratory.

The species pathogenic for man are *N. asteroides*, *N. brasiliensis* and '*N. caviae*', now renamed *N. otitidis-caviarum*. They can be isolated from clinical specimens by the use of Sabouraud's Dextrose Agar, Beef-heart-infusion Blood Agar, or Lowenstein–Jensen medium (Schaal, 1984). Their colonies vary in both morphology and colour depending on the composition and consistency of the medium. They usually have an aerial mycelium which makes them look 'velvety' but if this is absent the colonies are matt in appearance. The pigmentation may diffuse into the medium and often ranges from creamy-white and salmon-pink to an orange-tan colour. There are several other species of *Nocardia* which can be differentiated by means of some 150 characters (Orchard & Goodfellow, 1980) but as they are not clinically significant we have excluded them. In general, the nocardias are rather slow-growing organisms and precise identification can take months rather than days but as the infections with which they may be associated are usually chronic, this delay is not of much consequence.

Minidefinition: *Nocardia. Gram-positive or Gram-variable rods and filaments which sometimes show branching. Some strains weakly or partly acid-fast. Non-motile. Produce aerial hyphae. Aerobic. Catalase-positive. Attack sugars by oxidation. Type species: N. asteroides; NCTC strain 11293.*

Table 6.10b. *Second-stage table for* Mycobacterium

	1	2	3	4	5	6	7	8	9	10	11	12	13	14
Growth at 25 °C	−	−	+/G	+/G	+/G	+/g	+/g	+/g	+/g	+/g	+/g	+/g	+/G	−
37 °C	+	+	+/g	+/g	+/g	−	+/G	+/G	+/G	+/G	+/g	+/g	+/G	+/g
45 °C	−	−	−	−	−	−	−	−	−	−	−	V	+	+
Growth in presence of:														
PNBA	−	−	−	+	+	+	+	+	+	+	+	+	+	+
thiacetazone	−	−	−	+	+	+	−	+	+	+	+	+	+	+
Atmospheric preference	A	M	?	?	A	M	?	A	M	A	M	M	A	?
Pigment in light	−	−	+	+	−	−	+	+	+	−	−	d	−	V
Pigment in dark	−	−	−	+	−	−	−	+	+	−	−	d	d	V
Tween hydrolysed	d	−	+	?	−	−	+	?	+	d	+	−	+	?

1 **Mycobacterium tuberculosis***; human type of tubercle bacillus
2 **Mycobacterium bovis***; bovine type of tubercle bacillus
3 **Mycobacterium marinum***; *M. balnei*
4 **Scotochromogenic psychrophils**
5 **Mycobacterium chelonei**; *M. borstelense; M chelonei*
6 **Mycobacterium ulcerans***
7 **Mycobacterium kansasii****

8 **Flavescens group**
9 **Gordonae group**; *M. aquae*
10 **Fortuitum group**; *M. minettii; M. perigrinum*
11 **Terrae group**
12 **Avium–intracellulare – scrofulaceum group****; *M. avium; M. intracellulare; M. marianum*
13 **Smegmatis–phlei group**
14 **Mycobacterium xenopi****

* Always clinically significant
** Frequently clinically significant
A Aerobic
M Microaerophilic
V Variable in different growth conditions
G Good growth
g Growth but not vigorous

Other symbols used in the table are explained in Tables 5.1 and 5.2 on p. 47.

6.10.2 Mycobacterium (Table 6.10b). The taxonomy of mycobacteria has benefited greatly from the studies of the International Working Group on Mycobacterial Taxonomy, an *ad hoc* group of bacteriologists who have examined a large number of strains by a variety of methods or by clearly defined techniques. As a result some 41 valid species of *Mycobacterium* were described by Kubica (1978), of which *M. tuberculosis* and *M. bovis* are well known as human and animal pathogens. Although the latter is naturally resistant to pyrazinamide, these two pathogens are probably variants of one species, *Mycobacterium tuberculosis*, and should therefore be termed *M. tuberculosis* subsp. *hominis* and *M. tuberculosis* subsp. *bovis*. However, as there are differences in both epidemiology and treatment, it is important to distringuish between them. For this reason they are usually regarded as separate 'species' and we accord with this traditional usage.

In previous editions of this *Manual*, we relied on several biochemical and cultural tests for the identification of strains. In this edition, we use the scheme devised by Marks (1976) as it relies on a small number of simple tests to assign mycobacteria to species or to groups without the need to use laboratory animals. The quantitative catalase test described in the previous edition of this *Manual* is difficult to perform accurately and is best done in reference laboratories where numerous strains are examined as a routine. Oxidative attack on sugars also has a degree of variability when used by routine laboratories because of the long-term incubation period needed and the greater likelihood of contamination. The essential point of the scheme is that strains should be identified only as far as is clinically necessary. Further identification is possible, for example, by phage typing, agglutination tests or by thin-layer chromatography of the cell-surface lipids, but as these tests are the province of reference laboratories, they are outside the scope of this *Manual*.

In tissues, mycobacteria often occur alone at first though secondary infection with organisms of lesser pathogenicity is liable to occur subsequently. The isolation of slowly growing mycobacteria from sputum and other material containing organisms able to grow rapidly therefore requires measures to kill or at least inhibit the multiplication of such flora. We therefore utilize the greater resistance of mycobacte-

ria to chemical agents and treat the material with either acid or alkali for 10 to 30 minutes. After neutralization, this material is inoculated on media suitable for the growth of mycobacteria and incubated for up to 8 weeks before being discarded as negative. For primary isolation, egg-based Lowenstein–Jensen medium containing malachite green is usually used; the same medium with the addition of pyruvate instead of glycerol is also used routinely for the isolation of *M. bovis* as well as for some drug-resistant strains of *M. tuberculosis*. As the medium must not be allowed to dry out during this prolonged period of incubation, the use of screw-capped containers is recommended.

As this *Manual* is concerned primarily with bacteria of medical importance, the species *M. paratuberculosis* (Johne's bacillus), *M. microti* (the vole bacillus) and *M. lepraemurium* (the marine leprosy bacillus) have been excluded. *M. leprae*, the human leprosy organism, has still not been grown on artificial media and can be detected only by Ziehl–Neelsen staining of specimens or by inoculation and propagation in the nine-banded armadillo (Kirchheimer & Storrs, 1971) or the footpad of the mouse (Shepard, 1960). Growth in both of these animals is very slow and their use is for research rather than diagnosis. For growth of *M. paratuberculosis*, special media supplemented with mycobactin, a mycobacterial extract with an iron-chelating ability, or with killed acid-fast bacteria, are needed. Many of the slow-growing species are causally associated with chronic infections but the faster-growing mycobacteria are rarely significant. Some species such as *M. tuberculosis* are always clinically significant whereas others such as *M. kansasii* may be present as incidental contaminants. Multiple isolation of such strains from a patient, especially in large numbers, indicates clinical significance as does isolation from an aspirate or from tissues.

For the identification of mycobacteria, the acid-fast nature of strains must first be demonstrated; in tissues, the organisms usually stain well but care must be taken, especially when the numbers are small, to ensure that false positive results are not reported because of the presence of contaminating acid-fast organisms in the reagents (see, for example, Carson *et al.*, 1964). Technically, a distinction used to be made between organisms which were both acid- and alcohol-fast and those that were only acid-fast, but this distinction was difficult to substantiate in practice and is impracticable. Most laboratories now use a mixture of acid and alcohol for decolorization so that the organisms should strictly be described as 'acid- and alcohol-fast', though the term 'AFB' for acid-fast bacilli is universally recognized and accepted.

For differentiation of mycobacteria, the simple scheme shown in Table 6.10*b* relies initially on the ability of strains to grow at one or more of the temperatures 25 °C, 37 °C and 45 °C. Those which grow only at 37 °C are strict mesophiles; those which grow better at 25 °C than at 37 °C are psychrophiles; those which grow better at 37 °C than at 25 °C are mesophiles; those which grow at all three temperatures are wide-range mycobacteria; and those that grow at 45 °C but not at 25 °C are thermophiles. With strict mesophiles, absence of growth in the presence of *p*-nitrobenzoic acid (PNBA) and thiacetazone indicates that the strains are tubercle bacilli. Further differentiation of strains depends on oxygen preference, pigment production and the ability of strains to hydrolyse Tween 80. Where a particular test is not necessary for the identification of a species or group of mycobacteria, the result has been omitted from Table 6.10*b*. *M. marinum* has a narrower temperature range for growth when first isolated but after subculture it may grow at 37 °C.

M. tuberculosis may be differentiated from *M. bovis* by its sensitivity to pyrazinamide, niacin production, nitrate reduction and resistance to thiophene carboxylic acid hydrazide (TCH), but these tests are usually best carried out in reference laboratories. They are also used to identify the BCG (Bacillus Calmette–Guerin) vaccine strain derived from *M.*

bovis (Jenkins *et al.*, 1985).

For epidemiological purposes, *M. tuberculosis* may be subdivided into a number of geographical variants such as the 'Asian' and the 'African I and II' strains (Collins, Yates & Grange, 1982); the latter, isolated respectively in West and East Africa, are also called (illegitimately) '*M. africanum*'. All these variants differ in minor respects from classical *M. tuberculosis* in the tests mentioned above though defining such strains is primarily of epidemiological interest. Two geographical variants of *M. chelonae* also occur which differ in their ability to grow in the presence of 5% NaCl and to utilize citrate for growth (Stanford *et al.*, 1972).

Some strains of *Mycobacterium* produce pigment both in light and in the dark and are termed scotochromogenic, as opposed to strains which produce pigment only in the light and which are designated photochromogenic. Scotochromogenic psychrophils and the Flavescens, Gordonae, Terrae, Fortuitum and Smegmatis–phlei groups are so rarely significant in clinical practice that they do not require further speciation though *M. phlei* is unusual in its ability to grow at 52 °C. If clinical significance is suspected, the strain should be submitted to a reference laboratory with as much information as possible, including the number of isolations, the site and nature of the lesion and medical history.

Minidefinition: *Mycobacterium. Gram-positive rods that do not show branching. Typically acid-fast. Non-motile. Non-sporing and do not produce aerial hyphae. Aerobic or microaerophilic. Attack sugars by oxidation. Type species: M. tuberculosis; NCTC strain 27294.*

7

Characters of Gram-negative bacteria

Although not ideal for making a major subdivision of bacteria, Gram's method of staining is convenient because everyone uses it (in one of its many modifications) when characterizing a bacterium. There is an unfortunate tendency to omit this step, especially when dealing with cultures isolated on selective media which, by virtue of the inhibitory agents they contain, may in theory affect the bacterial staining reactions; it is simply assumed that colonies on selective media have the appropriate (or expected) tinctorial and shapely qualities. This may often be tolerated (and sometimes acceptable) in busy routine laboratories where, in the words of W.S. Gilbert, it may be regarded as 'merely corroborative detail, intended to give artistic verisimilitude to an otherwise bald and unconvincing narrative'. However, our objectives are neither speed nor artistry; we want to know the identity of the organisms and for this we need accurate characterizations. We cannot afford therefore to omit making smears and staining them by Gram's method, even if we do not pursue microscopy any further.

7.1   Division into major groups

Before dealing with the Gram-negative bacteria proper, we would remind readers that there are a few organisms that seem to be on the borderline between the Gram-positive and the Gram-negative, for example *Gemella*, a genus which until recently was thought to consist of Gram-negative cocci. Other bacteria show an unusual phenomenon in that they develop some Gram-positivity as cultures age, in contrast to the Gram-positive bacteria, which usually become Gram-negative as the cells age and degenerate. *Mobiluncus* is a recently recognized genus (Spiegel & Roberts, 1984) in the former category and we suspect it will find a larger place in this *Manual* in

the future; organisms of this group, whose association with the female genital tract is well recognized, are the subject of current taxonomic interest.

There is also a small number of miscellaneous Gram-negative bacteria which cannot reasonably be allocated to any of the other groupings of organisms we recognize in Table 7.1; these we have collected together in Section 7.10 as a 'Group of Difficult Organisms'.

7.2   The Gram-negative anaerobes
(*Bacteroides, Fusobacterium, Veillonella, Acidaminococcus, Megasphaera*)

***Characters common to members of the group*: Gram-negative bacteria; do not form spores. Strictly anaerobic. Sensitive to metronidazole.**

In contrast to the previous edition of this *Manual*, the Gram-negative and strictly anaerobic cocci now include three genera, *Veillonella, Acidaminococcus* and *Megasphaera*, though for practical purposes the last two can be ignored; and the Gram-negative anaerobic non-spore-forming rods are represented by two genera, *Bacteroides* and *Fusobacterium*. Previously, the classification of these anaerobic rods was based mainly though not exclusively on two main criteria (1) morphological: in *Fusobacterium* (formerly called *Fusiformis*) the ends of the rods were pointed or fusiform whereas if rounded they were classified as *Bacteroides*; and (2) fermentation products: *Fusobacterium* produced butyric acid but *Bacteroides* did not do so. As may be imagined, the use of such weak characters for differentiation caused much confusion as well as nomenclatural difficulties (see Holdeman & Moore, 1972; Willis, 1964). In addition to poor and/or conflicting descriptions of

Table 7.1. *First-stage table for Gram-negative bacteria*

	1	2	3	4	5	6	7	8	9	10	11	12	13	14	15	16	17	18	19	20	21	22	23
Shape	R	S	S	S	S/R	R	R	R	R	R	R	R	R	R	R	R/S	R	H/C	H/C	H	R	R	NT
Motility	–	–	–	–	–	–	–	–	+	+	–	–	–	+	D	–	–	+	+	+	–	+	NT
Growth in air	–	–	+	+	+	+	+	+	+	+	+	+	+	+	+	+	–*	–†	–	–	+	+	+
Growth anaerobically	+	+	–	–	–	+	–	–	–	–	–	+	+	+	+	+	+	D	+	+	+	–	+
Catalase	d	D	+	+	+	–	+	+	+	+	+	+	–	+	+	D	–	D	–	–	–	+	?
Oxidase	–	?	+	+	–	+	+	–	+	+	+	+	+	+	–	D	+	+/w	+	–	–	+	?
Glucose (acid)	D	–	+	–	+	–	–	–	–	+	+	+	+	+	+	NT	–	–	–	+	+	–	?
Carbohydrates [F/O/–]	F/–	–	O	–	O/–	F	–	–	–	O	O	F	F	F	F	NT	–	–	–	F	F	–	?

	1	2	3	4	5	6	7	8	9	10	11	12	13	14	15	16	17	18	19	20	21	22	23	
Bacteroides	+																							7.2
Fusobacterium [a]	+																							
Veillonella [b]		+																						7.3
Neisseria			+																					
Branhamella				+																				
Acinetobacter					+																			7.4
Kingella						+																		
Moraxella							+																	
Brucella							+																	
Bordetella pertussis							+																	
Bordetella parapertussis								+																
Bordetella bronchiseptica									+															7.5
Alcaligenes									+															
Shewanella									+															
Pseudomonas (alkali-producers)									+															
Achromobacter										+														
Agrobacterium [c]										+														7.6
Janthinobacterium										+														
Pseudomonas (oxidizers) [d]										+														
Flavobacterium [e]											+													
Actinobacillus												+												
Pasteurella												+												7.7
Aeromonas salmonicida												+												
Cardiobacterium													+											
Chromobacterium														+										
Vibrio														+										7.8
Plesiomonas														+										
Aeromonas														+										7.9
Enterobacteria [f]															+									
Haemophilus																+								
Gardnerella																+								7.10
Eikenella [*]																	+							
Campylobacter																		+						
Helicobacter																		+						
Arcobacter																			+					
Anaerobiospirillum																				+				
Streptobacillus [g]																					+			
Legionella																						+		
Mycoplasma																							+	

* Generally poor growth in air; better growth in air + CO_2.

† No growth in air or anaerobically; growth in 3–10% O_2.

[a] Also *Leptotrichia buccalis*

[b] Also *Acidaminococcus* and *Megasphaera*

[c] Also *Ochrobactrum*

[d] Also *Weeksella*; do not attack carbohydrates

[e] Also *Chryseomonas* and *Flavimonas*

[f] Enterobacteria: *Buttiauxella, Cedecea, Citrobacter, Edwardsiella, Enterobacter, Erwinia, Escherichia, Hafnia, Klebsiella, Kluyvera, Morganella, Proteus, Providencia, Salmonella, Serratia, Shigella, Tatumella, Yersinia* and others.

[g] Also *Shigella dysenteriae* 1: (Shiga's bacillus).

Cultural characters of these organisms can be found in tables with the number indicated.

NT　Not testable by usual methods. Fermentative (Sneath & Johnson, 1973).

+　Typical form

?　Not known

Other symbols used in the table are explained in Tables 5.1 and 5.2 on p.47.

Table 7.2a. *Second-stage table for* Bacteroides

	1	2	3	4	5	6	7	8	9	10	11	12	13	14	15	16	17	18
Growth in air + CO_2	−	−	−	−	−	−	−	−	−	−	−	−	−	−	−	−	+	−
Growth in 20% bile	+	+	+	+	+	+	+	−	−	−	−	−	−	−	−	−	?	−
Aesculin hydrolysis	+	+	+	+	+	+	+	+	+	d^b	−	−	−	+	−	−	−	−
Indole	−	−	+	+	+	−	+	−	−	−	−	−	−	+	−	+	−	−
Gelatinase	−	−	d^b	−	−	+	d^b	+	−	+	+	+	+	+	+	+	−	−
Carbohydrates, acid from:																		
arabinose	−	−	+	+	+	+	+	+	−	−	−	−	−	−	−	−	?	−
glucose	+	+	+	+	+	+	+	+	+	+	+	+	+	+	−	−	−	$−^d$
lactose	+	+	+	+	+	+	+	+	−	+	−	+	−	+	−	−	−	−
rhamnose	d^b	−	+	+	d^c	+	−	−	−	−	−	−	−	d^c	−	−	?	−
salicin	+	−	+	d^c	d^b	−	−	+	−	−	−	−	−	+	−	−	?	−
sucrose	+	+	+	+	+	+	−	+	−	+	−	−	+	+	−	−	−	−
trehalose	+	−	+	+	−	−	−	−	−	−	−	−	−	−	−	−	?	−

1 **Bacteroides distasonis**
2 **Bacteroides fragilis**
3 **Bacteroides ovatus**
4 **Bacteroides thetaiotaomicron**
5 **Bacteroides uniformis**
6 **Bacteroides vulgatus**
7 **Bacteroides splanchnicus**
8 **Bacteroides ruminicola**[a]
9 **Bacteroides capillosus**

10 **Bacteroides melaninogenicus**
11 **Bacteroides disiens**
12 **Bacteroides bivius**
13 **Bacteroides intermedius**[**]
14 **Bacteroides oralis**
15 **Bacteroides asaccharolyticus**
16 **Bacteroides ureolyticus**[*]; *Bacteroides corrodens*
17 **Eikenella corrodens**
18 **Veillonella** spp.

Species 1-6 = *Bacteroides fragilis* 'group'
Species 10-14 = *Bacteroides melaninogenicus - Bacteroides oralis* 'group'
[*]   Urease +ve, nitrate +ve
[**] Some strains are lipolytic
[a]   Two subspecies recognized
[b]   More strains positive than negative
[c]   More strains negative than positive
[d]   May be positive on some media

Other symbols used in the Table are explained in Tables 5.1 and 5.2 on p.47.

these organisms, their apparent sensitivity to aerobic conditions during manipulative procedures also caused considerable problems. All these difficulties led to the development of anaerobic cabinets, especially for reference work. However, *Bacteroides* and *Fusobacterium* will usually tolerate the transient aerobic conditions during routine work at the bench especially if added CO_2 is used for culture (Watt & Jack, 1977). For these reasons Cowan, in the previous edition of this *Manual*, pragmatically refused to distinguish between these genera, recognizing only *Bacteroides*. Since then the separation of *Bacteroides* and *Fusobacterium*, based largely on gas-liquid chromatography of metabolic end-products, has been accepted as have several species which are now included in the *Approved Lists of Bacterial Names* (1980) for each genus. We show these species with

their differential characters in Tables 7.2a and b, though precise identification may take some time and their differentiation in routine diagnostic laboratories is still difficult. For practical purposes, allocation to the overall group 'Gram-negative anaerobic bacteria' is usually adequate as all of them, including *Veillonella* and the related genera *Acidaminococcus* and *Megasphaera*, are sensitive to metronidazole and most are catalase-negative.

7.2.1 Bacteroides (Table 7.2a). We show in Table 7.2a the characters of the species currently recognized in this heterogeneous group as well as those of *Eikenella corrodens* (previously included in *Bacteroides*) which may seem to be anaerobic on first isolation (Eiken, 1958) though it will grow in air with added CO_2 on subculture (Jackson & Goodman,

1972). For comparison we also show *Veillonella* and related species of anaerobic Gram-negative cocci collectively in this Table. The catalase test (which we do not show) ought ideally to be negative for *Bacteroides* species but *B. fragilis* strains usually give positive reactions and other strains vary. The genus contains four clusters of species: the saccharolytic, non-pigment-forming *B. fragilis* group; the saccharolytic pigment-producing *B. melaninogenicus–B. oralis* group; the saccharolytic rumen group; and *B. asaccharolyticus* and related organisms, some of which also produce pigment. Most clinical isolates belong either to the *B. fragilis* group (species 1–7) or to the *B. melaninogenicus–B. oralis* group (species 10–14), together with *B. asaccharolyticus*. Shah & Collins (1989, 1990) have proposed that the genus *Bacteroides* should be restricted to the *B. fragilis* group, and that the *B. melaninogenicus–B. oralis* group should be transferred to a new genus, *Prevotella*. The taxonomic position of many of the other species currently placed in *Bacteroides* is doubtful.

Of the *B. fragilis* group, two species, *B. fragilis* and *B. thetaiotaomicron*, are commonly found as pathogens. As a rule, members of this group are resistant to aminoglycosides, penicillin, colistin and vancomycin. Surface colonies on horse Blood Agar are circular, entire, convex and smooth; haemolysis is usually absent. Microscopically, the cells are short Gram-negative rods with rounded ends; vacuoles may be present when cultured in media containing a fermentable carbohydrate.

The *B. melaninogenicus – B. oralis* group as well as *B. asaccharolyticus* comprise the black pigment-producing species, the pigment becoming evident after prolonged incubation (3–5 days) on Blood Agar plates. In young cultures (1–2 days) the species in this group produce a brick-red fluorescent pigment (protoporphyrin) visible under long-wave ultraviolet light (Wood's lamp, 365 nm); fluorescence disappears as colonies develop their brown-black pigmentation (protohaemin). Microscopically, the cells are usually coccobacillary in morphology.

B. ureolyticus (formerly *B. corrodens*) has a distinctive 'pitting' colonial morphology on solid media owing to 'corrosion' of the agar surface. Pitting colonies may only become apparent after incubation for several days, particularly when isolated in mixed culture, as is usual with this species. Colonially, *B. ureolyticus* may be confused with the capnophilic facultative anaerobe *Eikenella corrodens* (Section 7.10.3). The former is readily distinguished by urease production, metronidazole sensitivity and gelatinase production. Moreover, the growth of *B. ureolyticus* is enhanced by supplementing media with sodium formate and fumaric acid.

B. splanchnicus, an uncommon clinical isolate, may be confused initially with members of the *B. fragilis* group since it is resistant to aminoglycosides and grows well on bile-containing media. This species is distinguished by non-fermentation of sucrose although gas chromatography provides better differentiation.

B. disiens, *B. bivius* and *B. oralis* are easily confused with *B. fragilis* but growth in the presence of 20% bile effectively separates them. Moreover, *B. disiens* and *B. brevis* do not ferment sucrose.

Minidefinition: *Bacteroides. Gram-negative rods (may be coccobacillary); non-sporing; usually non-motile. Anaerobic; sensitive to metronidazole. Fermentative or non-fermentative. Type species: B. fragilis; NCTC strain 9343.*

7.2.2 Fusobacterium (Table 7.2b). Many of the species currently included in this genus are insecure, and only *Fusobacterium nucleatum* (the type species) is consistently fusiform (spindle-shaped) in cellular morphology. Other species may be pleomorphic, or difficult to distinguish microscopically from *Bacteroides*. Colonies of many strains on Blood Agar fluoresce yellow-green in long-wave ultraviolet light (365 nm). The species commonly encountered in clinical material are sensitive to kanamycin (1000 μg disc) and colistin (10 μg disc), but resistant to vancomycin (5 μg disc). Strains of *F. necrophorum* are usually haemolytic on horse Blood Agar, and many strains are lipase-positive, showing restricted opalescence and a pearly layer on Egg-yolk Agar (Holdeman & Moore, 1972). We show other differential reactions for the few strains encountered most frequently in clinical material in Table 7.2b. We do not, however, include the morphologically large organism of Vincent's angina, previously classified as *'Fusiformis fusiforme'* and now transferred to the genus *Leptotrichia* as the only species, *L. buccalis*,

Table 7.2b. *Second-stage table for* Fusobacterium

	1	2	3	4
Indole	+	+	–	d
Aesculin	–	–	+	–
Growth in 20% bile	–	–	+	+
Carbohydrates, acid from:				
glucose	–	–	+	+
fructose	–	–	+	+
lactose	–	–	+	–
mannose	–	–	+	+
Lipase	d	–	–	–
Propionate from lactate*	+	–	–	–
Propionate from threonine*	+	+	+	+

1 **Fusobacterium necrophorum**
2 **Fusobacterium nucleatum**
3 **Fusobacterium mortiferum**
4 **Fusobacterium varium**

*For laboratories with gas chromatography facilities

Symbols used in the Table are explained in Tables 5.1 and 5.2 on p.47.

which has similar growth requirements. The identification of fusobacteria in routine laboratories is described by Bennet & Duerden (1985).

> **Minidefinition:** *Fusobacterium. Gram-negative rods (may or may not show typical fusiform morphology); non-sporing; non-motile. Anaerobic; sensitive to metronidazole. Non-fermentative or weakly fermentative. Type species: F. nucleatum; ATCC strain 2556.*

7.2.3   Veillonella, Acidaminococcus, Megasphaera (Table 7.3). As with *Bacteroides* and *Fusobacterium*, the identification and classification of *Veillonella* and the two related genera of Gram-negative anaerobic cocci, *Acidaminococcus* and *Megasphaera*, were beset with difficulties (Rogosa, 1971). Technically, there was considerable doubt previously about their purity as many cultures were mixed and probably growing synergistically; and they were extremely intolerant of oxygen, dying out rapidly on minimal exposure to air at the bench. Poor and/or conflicting descriptions occurred frequently but, by using anaerobic cabinets and other procedures to maintain strict anaerobiosis and by means of gas-liquid chromatography, a number of different genera and species were defined and are currently accepted as valid (Rogosa, 1984). The three genera recognized

are all members of the normal flora of the oropharynx and gastrointestinal tract of man. They are rarely encountered in clinical material and their pathogenic significance, if any, is low; we do not therefore give a second-stage table for species identification but we show the generic characters in Table 7.3 for comparison with those of other Gram-negative cocci. Like fusobacteria, they are resistant to vancomycin (5 μg).

Veillonella parvula is the commonest isolate from human material; other species include *V. atypica* and *V. dispar*. Definitive identification of the genus and species requires gas-liquid chromatography of metabolic end products, and a range of biochemical tests. However, *Megasphaera* is distinguished from the other two genera by its large cell size (>2 μm) and ability to ferment glucose, fructose and maltose.

> **Minidefinition:** *Veillonella. Gram-negative cocci: non-motile; non-sporing. Anaerobic; sensitive to metronidazole. Non-fermentative. Type species: V. parvula; NCTC strain 11810.*

7.3   The Gram-negative aerobic cocci
(*Branhamella, Neisseria,*)

***Characters common to members of the group*:** **Gram-negative cocci or coccobacilli. Non-motile. Aerobic.**

Apart from one species, *Neisseria elongata*, which forms long filaments under the influence of penicillin, all other members of the genus *Neisseria* and those of *Branhamella* (which were originally placed in *Neisseria*) as well as those of the anaerobic genus *Veillonella* are all Gram-negative cocci – a morphological characteristic which they share with the coccal forms of *Acinetobacter*. To American bacteriologists, acinetobacters were originally regarded as 'mimeas', a group of poorly-described Gram-negative cocci that could be confused with gonococci. The morphological resemblance is real, especially in direct smears from clinical specimens, but in culture the acinetobacters soon become slightly elongated, coccobacillary and finally assume a true rod-like form. As clinical bacteriologists can encounter the coccal form of acinetobacters we include them in Table 7.3 for comparison with branhamellas and neisserias. The characters of acinetobacters are

Table 7.3. *Second-stage table for* Acinetobacter, Branhamella, Gemella, Neisseria *and* Veillonella

	1	2	3	4	5	6	7	8	9	10	11	12	13
Gram reaction	−	−	−	$+^d$	−	−	−	−	−	−	−	−	−
Aerobic Growth	+	+	+	+	+	+	+	+	+	+	+	+	−
Catalase	+	+	+	−	+	d^e	+	+	+	+	+	+	D
Oxidase	−	−	+	−	+	+	+	+	+	+	+	+	?
Carbohydrate breakdown [F/O/-]	O	O^b	−	F	−	−	O^b	O^b	O^b	O^b	O^b	O^b	−
Pigment production	−	−	−	−	−	−	+	−	d	−	−	+	−
Haemolysis	−/β	−/β	−	β	−	−	−	−	−	−	−	−	−
Growth at 22 °C	+	+	w	+	−	+	+	−	−	−	+	+	w
Growth on Nutrient Agar	+	+	+	w	+	+	+	−	+	$-^g$	+	+	+
Requirement for blood or serum	−	−	−	−	−	−	−	+	−	$+^g$	−	−	−
Carbohydrates, acid from:													
glucose	$+^a$	d^c	−	+	−	d^e	$-^f$	+	+	+	+	+	$-^h$
lactose	d^a	$-^c$	−	−	−	−	−	−	+	−	−	−	−
maltose	−	−	−	+	−	−	$-^f$	−	+	+	+	+	−
sucrose	−	−	−	+	−	−	$-^f$	−	−	−	+	d	−
Nitrates reduced	−	−	d	−	−	−	−	−	−	−	+	−	+

1 **Acinetobacter calcoaceticus;** *'Acinetobacter anitratus';*
  'Moraxella lwoffii var. *glucidolytica'; M. glucidolytica';*
  'Herellea vaginicola'
2 **Acinetobacter lwoffii;** *'Moraxella lwoffii';*
  'Mima polymopha'
3 **Branhamella catarrhalis;**
  'Neisseria catarrhalis'
4 **Gemella haemolysans;**
  'Neisseria haemolysans'
5 **Neisseria cinerea**
6 **Neisseria elongata**
7 **Neisseria flavescens**
8 **Neisseria gonorrhoeae;**
  gonococcus
9 **Neisseria lactamica**
10 **Neisseria meningitidis;**
  'N. intracellularis'; meningococcus
11 **Neisseria mucosa;**
  'Diplococcus mucosus'
12 **Neisseria subflava;**
  N. flava; N. perflava; N. sicca
13 **Veillonella** spp.

a Positive also in glucose Peptone Water and lactose (10%) in Nutrient Agar.
b No change, or alkali produced, in the open tube of Hugh & Leifson's medium.
c Negative in glucose Peptone Water and lactose (10%) in Nutrient Agar.
d Gram-positive but easily decolorised.
e Strains showing no catalase activity and no production of acid from glucose correspond to
  N. elongata subsp. *elongata*; strains producing catalase and weak acidity from glucose correspond to
  N. elongata subsp. *glycolytica*.
f Negative on isolation; subcultures may give positive reactions.
g On first isolation; many strains will grow on Nutrient Agar on sub-culture.
h May be positive in some media.

Other symbols used in the table are explained in Tables 5.1 and 5.2 on p.47.

shown again in Table 7.4*a* with the kingellas and moraxellas and also some other phenotypically similar Gram-negative rods.

At the generic level, veillonellas do not cause problems in identification as their strictly anaerobic habit readily distinguishes them from acinetobacters, branhamellas and neisserias, all of which fail to grow anaerobically; we deal with *Veillonella* in Section 7.2.3 but include it also in Table 7.3 to show some characters of all the Gram-negative cocci together. Although not really a member of this group, *Gemella*

haemolysans was first described as a neisseria and as it usually appears to be Gram-negative, we include it in Table 7.3 for comparison with *Neisseria* species. It is, however, a weakly Gram-positive organism and its rightful place is in Chapter 6 (Section 6.3.4).

7.3.1   Neisseria (Table 7.3). In this genus, many species have been described and, when the lack of reactivity in biochemical tests is taken into account, this at first seems unwarranted. Molecular biological and genetic techniques, however, have confirmed the heterogeneous nature of the constituent species of *Neisseria* and indicated that the genus as circumscribed in the late 1960s needed revision (Kingsbury, 1967; Henriksen & Bøvre, 1968b; Baumann, Doudoroff & Stainer, 1968a; Kingsbury et al., 1969; Bøvre, Fiandt & Szybalski, 1969). Subsequently Catlin (1970) proposed that '*Neisseria catarrhalis*' should form the type species of a new genus, *Branhamella*, and she thought that other species might follow because *N. caviae* and *N. ovis*, by gas-liquid chromatography, form a homogeneous group with *Branhamella catarrhalis* (Lambert et al., 1971). Genetic studies have confirmed the close relationship of these two species to each other and to a third species, *N. cuniculi* (Bøvre, 1980; Bøvre & Hagen, 1981). Though not all taxonomists would include these three species of so-called 'false neisseriae' in the same taxon as the catarrhalis organism, it is nevertheless convenient to consider them together as a single taxon. Bøvre (1979) proposed that this taxon should be regarded not as a genus but as the subgenus *Branhamella* of the genus *Moraxella* in order to reflect the closer relationship of these organisms to each other than to the 'true neisserias'. The close relationship of *Branhamella* to *Moraxella* (and to *Acinetobacter*) and their lack of relatedness to the 'true neisserias' have now been confirmed by rRNA–DNA studies (Rossau et al., 1986). Of the species placed in the sub-genus *Branhamella*, only the catarrhalis organisms is likely to occur in clinical specimens and it is therefore the only organism in this group that we show in Table 7.3. We continue to refer to it by the approved name *Branhamella catarrhalis* rather than *Moraxella (Branhamella) catarrhalis* as proposed by Bøvre (1979).

Neisseria flavescens, a species thought to have caused a limited epidemic of meningitis in Chicago (Branham, 1930), has rarely been isolated since. Prentice (1957) thought that the organism he isolated from a patient with meningitis might be *N. flavescens* and Wertlake & Williams (1968) described the organism from a case of septicaemia. At first none of the Chicago isolates attacked any sugars but after many years of laboratory propagation, the strains originally received from Branham and deposited in the National Collection of Type Cultures, London, as well as those she kept herself, all developed the ability to produce acid from glucose, maltose, and

sucrose. We accordingly include *N. flavescens* in Table 7.3 but show its original characters in the (faint) hope that it may be isolated again and recognized. The exclusion of '*N. catarrhalis*', *N. caviae*, *N. cuniculi* and *N. ovis* from *Neisseria* leaves a genus (excluding *N. cinerea* and *N. elongata* subsp. *elongata*) composed of bacteria that can attack carbohydrates in suitable media; as usually described, *N. flavescens* is said not to attack carbohydrates but the truth of this statement seems doubtful, though the ability may be masked on first isolation. In the minidefinition we therefore exclude species that do not attack any sugars.

Neisserias grow better on the surface of solid media than in equivalent liquid media; most strains grow better in an atmosphere with increased CO_2 and it is doubtful if any will grow under strictly anaerobic conditions. They are not easily characterized as freshly isolated strains grow feebly in artificial culture. Some species are described as Gram-variable or are said to resist decolorization; this may seem to be a difference due to technical variation in different laboratories, but it is reported so frequently that notice should be taken of it. Henriksen & Bøvre (1968b) described the tendency to resist decolorization as a characteristic of the family Neisseriaceae which, in their view at that time, comprised only the genera *Moraxella* and *Neisseria* though it now also includes *Acinetobacter*, *Branhamella* and *Kingella* (but see Rossau et al., 1986). Bacillary forms may occur in *N. elongata* (Bøvre & Holten, 1970) and, judged by the G+C content of DNA and other genetic information, the generic allocation is correct. The pathogenic neisserias grow feebly or not at all in media prepared for the usual biochemical characterization tests, and are thus worthy candidates for the rapid single-substrate tests in which multiplication of the organism is not essential, the reaction occurring between preformed enzymes and the substrate without interference from metabolic by-products. The substrate N-γ-glutamyl-β-naphthylamide has been used for distinguishing gonococci from meningococci (D'Amato et al., 1978; Hoke & Vedros, 1982) and commercial rapid test kits based on this principle are now available for identification of neisserias.

It is often impossible to decide, on purely laboratory information, whether an isolate is a gonococcus or a meningococcus; the sugar reactions of these organisms may be unreliable due to poor growth and, although most meningococci will produce acid from both glucose and maltose, some undoubted meningococci may attack glucose only and, occasionally, neither sugar. More reliable results may be obtained with the rapid sugar fermentation test described by Vedros (1978) which also obviates the need for growth by relying on preformed enzymes. Most neisserias do not produce acid from lactose, but Mitchell, Roden & King, (1965) collected thirty-five lactose-positive strains of meningococcus-like bacteria over a period of fifteen years. Hollis, Wiggins & Weaver, (1969) named these organisms 'Neisseria lactamicus', since corrected to *N. lactamica*.

The species *Neisseria animalis* (Berger, 1960*b*), *N. canis* and *N. denitrificans* (Berger, 1962) as well as those now included in *Branhamella* – *N. caviae* (Pelczar, 1953), *N. cuniculi* (Berger, 1962) and *N. ovis* (Lindqvist, 1960) – are excluded from Table 7.3 as they have not been reported from clinical specimens. In Table 7.3 we show the classical nasopharyngeal commensals, *N. flava*, *N. perflava* and *N. sicca* under the umbrella species *Neisseria subflava* (previously collected together as '*N. pharyngis*') as there seems little to be gained from maintaining their independent status.

> **Minidefinition**: *Neisseria. Gram-negative cocci. Aerobic; catalase-positive; oxidase-positive. Attack sugars by oxidation. Type species: N. gonnorrhoeae; NCTC strain 8375.*

7.3.2 Branhamella (Table 7.3).

This genus was created by removing from *Neisseria* those species which differed significantly in the base composition of their DNA: in *Branhamella* the G+C mol % value varies between 40 and 44, and in *Neisseria* it is about 50. The two genera also differ in the fatty acid composition of the bacterial cells (Catlin, 1970). The lack of a close relationship between these two genera is further confirmed by rRNA–DNA hybridization studies (Rossau *et al.*, 1986). Unfortunately these characteristics are not among those on which generic differentiation depends in diagnostic laboratories but, as shown in Table 7.3, the distinction can be made with tests that are part of the normal routine. We show only *B. catarrhalis* in Table 7.3 as the other three species have not been reported from man.

Like neisserias, but possibly even more so, the bacterial cells of the branhamellas tend to resist decolorization when stained by Gram's method. In contrast, *Gemella*, a Gram-positive coccus with the opposite characteristic (a Gram-positive organism that is easily over-decolorized), is shown in Table 7.3 so that its characters can be compared with those of *Branhamella catarrhalis* and *Neisseria* species.

Of the usual characterizing tests, those for the reduction of nitrate and the production of acid from carbohydrates are among the most useful. With *Branhamella catarrhalis*, the former test is often positive and the latter negative; the other species left in *Neisseria* (excluding *N. cinerea*, *N. elongata* subsp. *elongata*, *N. flavescens* and *N. mucosa*) fail to reduce nitrate and all attack carbohydrate(s) (but see Section 7.3.1).

> **Minidefintion**: *Branhamella. Gram-negative cocci which may resist decolorization. Aerobic. Catalase-positive; oxidase-positive. Do not produce acid from carbohydrates. Generally reduce nitrate to nitrite. Type species; B. catarrhalis; NCTC strain 11020.*

7.3.3 Acinetobacter (Tables 7.3; 7.4*a*)

is a genus in which two species are now recognized (but see Section 7.4.2) in contrast to the 17 listed by Prévot (1961). These two species have a coccal or coccobacillary morphology, and in smears may show a superficial resemblance to the gonococcus or meningococcus. In a series of papers, de Bord (1939, 1942, 1943, 1948) rightly emphasized this morphological similarity but confused the picture by describing briefly (and inadequately) several different organisms, including two new species of *Neisseria*; and, except for the two new neisserias, he placed them all in a new tribe which he named Mimeae. One of the species that mimicked the gonococcus morphologically is now known as *Acinetobacter calcoaceticus* (formerly '*A. anitratus*') and this species (together with *Acinetobacter lwoffii*) is shown in Table 7.3 for comparison with *Neisseria gonorrhoeae* and *N. meningitidis*.

The acinetobacters have much in common with the moraxellas and recent rRNA–DNA hybridization results (Rossau *et al.*, 1986) lend further support to previous suggestions that the two genera should be united; both genera are shown in greater detail in Table 7.4*a*.

Minidefinition: *Acinetobacter. Non-motile, Gram-negative coccobacilli or short rods. Aerobic. Catalase-positive; oxidase-negative. Attack sugars by oxidation or not at all. Do not produce pigment. Arginine test negative. Type species: A. calcoaceticus; ATCC strain 23055.*

7.3.4   Gemella (Tables 6.3 *a*, *c*; 7.3), an organism that is easily decolorized and usually appears to be Gram-negative (as it was first described). In cell structure and mode of division it resembles the Gram-positive bacteria (Reyn, 1970) and in its cultural characters it seems to be close to the streptococci. We describe this organism with the Gram-positive cocci in Table 6.3*a*, *c* and Section 6.3.4, but because of the ease with which it is decolorized, we also show it with the Gram-negative cocci in Table 7.3.

Minidefintion: *Gemella. Gram-positive cocci (but easily decolorized). Aerobic; facultatively anaerobic. Catalase-negative; oxidase-negative. Attack sugars by fermentation; do not produce gas. Type species: G. haemolysans; ATCC strain 10379.*

7.4   The Moraxella–Acinetobacter group: the non- (or weakly) saccharolytic non-motile rods
(*Moraxella, Acinetobacter, Kingella, Brucella, Bordetella*)

***Characters common to members of the group*: Gram-negative coccobacilli or short rods, non-motile (with the exception of *Bordetella bronchiseptica*). Strictly aerobic. Catalase-positive. Do not oxidize many carbohydrates.**

There have been suggestions that the genera *Moraxella* and *Acinetobacter* should be combined, and it is true that they have much in common, hence the inclusion of both in the family Neisseriaceae (together with *Branhamella*, *Kingella* and *Neisseria*). Indeed, species have been transferred from one genus to the other (for example '*Moraxella lwoffii*' to *Acinetobacter lwoffii*) and confusion has arisen because a species and its 'variety' were equated with species in different genera ('*Mima polymorpha*' = *Acinetobacter lwoffii* and '*Mima polymorpha* var.

oxydans' = *Moraxella nonliquefaciens* or *Moraxella osloensis*). Both *Moraxella* and *Acinetobacter* were created for species discarded from other genera. Organisms wrongly placed in the genus *Haemophilus* (because they were not haemophilic) were transferred to *Moraxella*; and the non-motile members of *Achromobacter*, itself formerly an unsatisfactory collection of non-pigmented Gram-negative rods, were transferred to *Acinetobacter*. *Achromobacter* is dealt with in Section 7.6.1.

7.4.1   Moraxella (Table 7.4*a*) was created by Lwoff (1939) for non-haemophilic bacteria that had previously been placed in *Haemophilus*; these bacteria did not need X and/or V factor(s), and did not attack carbohydrates. Most of the organisms placed by Lwoff in this genus had been isolated from the conjunctiva, but other workers added strains from other sources ('*M. lwoffii*' from soil) and also strains that attacked carbohydrates ('*M. lwoffii*' var. *glucidolytica*'); the latter organism was subsequently shown to be '*Bacterium anitratum*' (Brisou & Morichau-Beauchant, 1952), later known as '*Acinetobacter anitratus*' and currently as *Acinetobacter calcoaceticus*. Brisou (1953), Floch (1953) and others excluded '*M. lwoffii*' and the sugar-attacking species from *Moraxella*; Henriksen (1960) also excluded '*M. lwoffii*' and restricted the genus to oxidase-positive organisms. The debate about what should be included and what excluded from the genus was prolonged (it may not have ended yet) and complicated, but most workers (see Baumann, Doudoroff & Stanier, 1968*a*; Henriksen & Bøvre, 1968*b*; Samuels *et al.*, 1972; Lautrop in *Bergey's Manual* (1974) agree that only oxidase-positive, non-saccharolytic organisms should go into *Moraxella*.

An organism resembling *Moraxella lacunata* was isolated from the conjunctiva of guinea-pigs (Ryan, 1964), and *Moraxella bovis* causes conjunctivitis in cattle and horses (strains from horses, formerly regarded as a separate species, *M. equi*, are now included in *M. bovis* (Bøvre, 1984)). Although *Moraxella bovis* has not been reported from human clinical material, it is retained in Table 7.4*a* for completeness. Scandinavian workers report that it is unable to reduce nitrates and that the catalase test is positive; however, in the USA, Pugh, Hughes &

Table 7.4a. *Second-stage table for* Acinetobacter, Bordetella, Brucella, Kingella *and* Moraxella

	1	2	3	4	5	6^a	7	8	9	10	11	12
Catalase	+	+	+	+	+	–	+	+	+	+	+	+
Oxidase	–	–	–	?	+	+	+	+	+	+	+	+
Carbohydrate breakdown [F/O/–]	O	O^b	–	–	O^b	F^b	–	–	–	–	–	–
PHBA* accumulation in cells	–	–	–	?	–	–	–	–	–	+	–	+
Haemolysis on Blood Agar	–/β	–/β	–	?	–	–/β	β	–	–	–	–	–
Growth at 42 °C	d	d	–	?	d	–	–	–	–	–	–	+
Growth on Nutrient Broth/Agar	+	+	+	–	+	+	+	d	d	+	+	+
Growth on MacConkey	+	+	d	–	d	–	–	d	–	d	+	+
Citrate as C source	+	d	–	–	–	–	–	–	–	–	–	d
Carbohydrates, acid from:												
glucose	+^{c}	d^d	–	?	–	–^{e}	–	–	–	–	–	–
ethanol	+	d	–	?	–	–	–	–	–	d	–	–
maltose	–	–	–	?	–	(+)	–	–	–	–	–	–
xylose	+	d	–	?	–	–	–	–	–^{g}	–^{g}	–	–
Nitrate reduced to nitrite	–	–	–	–	+	–^{f}	d	+	+	d	+	–
Nitrite reduced	–	–	–	–	d	–	–	–	–	–	–	+
Gelatin liquefaction	d	d	–	?	–	–	+	+	–	–	–	–
Urease	d	–	+	–	+	–	–	–	–	d^h	d	–
Tween 20 hydrolysis	+	+	–	?	d	d	+	+	d	d	+	–
Tween 80 hydrolysis	+	+	–	?	–	–	d	d	–	d	–	–
Brown pigment on Tyrosine Agar	–	–	+	–	–	–	–	–	–	–	–	–
Growth on 40% bile	+	+	?	–	d	–	–	d	–	d	+	+
Growth stimulation by bile	–	d	?	?	–	–	–	–	–	–	+	–
Growth on 4% NaCl	–	d	–	?	–	–	+	d	d	–	+	+

1 **Acinetobacter calcoaceticus;** *'A. anitratus';* 'B5W'; *'Moraxella lwoffii* var. *glucidolytica';* '*M. glucidolytica';* *'Herellea vaginicola'*

2 **Acinetobacter lwoffii;** *'Moraxella lwoffii';* *'Mima polymorpha'*

3 **Bordetella parapertussis;** *'Haemophilus parapertussis';* *'Alcaligenes parapertussis'*

4 **Bordetella pertussis;** *'Haemophilus pertussis'*

5 **Brucella spp;** *B. melitensis*'(*'Alcaligenes melitensis';* *'Brucella brucei'); B. abortus*'(Bang's bacillus); *B. suis*

6 **Kingella kingae;** *'Moraxella kingii'*

7 **Moraxella bovis;** *'M. equi'*

8 **Moraxella lacunata;** *'M. duplex';* *'M. liquefaciens'*

9 **Moraxella nonliquefaciens;** *'Mima polymorpha* var. *oxidans'*

10 **Moraxella osloensis**

11 **Moraxella phenylpyruvica**

12 **Moraxella urethralis**

* PHBA: Poly–β–hydroxybutyrate
a Biochemically similar strains producing indole correspond to *K. indologenes.*
b No change, or alkali produced, in the open tube of Hugh & Leifson's medium.
c Positive in glucose Peptone Water.
d Negative in glucose Peptone Water.
e Positive on Ascitic Agar + glucose.
f Biochemically similar strains reducing nitrate correspond to *K. denitrificans.*
g May be positive when carried out as a buffered single substrate test.
h Some strains positive on first isolation; the property is soon lost.
β Clear zone of haemolysis around colonies.

Other symbols used in the table are explained in Tables 5.1 and 5.2 on p.47.

McDonald, (1966) found that all their strains reduced nitrates and were catalase-negative. This perhaps represents an example of 'geographical races' of species.

Moraxella phenylpyruvica (Bøvre & Henriksen, 1967) deaminates phenylalanine and tryptophan when suitable methods are used, as do several other *Moraxella* species; the test of Shaw & Clarke (Appendix C3.45) is not sufficiently sensitive and Snell & Davey (1971) recommend the method of Goldin & Glenn (1962).

Of two organisms provisionally placed in the genus *Moraxella*, one, '*M. urethralis* (Lautrop, Bøvre & Frederiksen, 1970), was said to resemble *M. osloensis*. However, more recent DNA data (Bøvre, 1984; Rossau *et al.*, 1986) place *M. urethralis* well apart from the other major taxa and suggest that it is a candidate for a new genus within the family Neisseriaceae. It has since been proposed that a new genus, *Oligella*, should be created for this organism as well as for an *Alcaligenes*-like organism formerly known as Group IVe (Rossau *et al.*, 1987). The other organism, '*M. kingii*' (Henriksen & Bøvre, 1968a), is saccharolytic on media enriched with ascitic fluid, and is now placed in the genus *Kingella* (Section 7.4.3).

The proposal by Henriksen & Bøvre (1968b) to include the so-called 'false neisserias ' ('*Neisseria catarrhalis*', *N. caviae*, *N. cuniculi* and *N. ovis*) in the genus *Moraxella* has not been followed in this *Manual*; '*N. catarrhalis*' will be found in *Branhamella* (Section 7.3.2).

Cultures of *Moraxella* species are sensitive to drying and some strains will not grow at 37 °C unless they are in a moist atmosphere; they grow best when incubated in a closed jar (Henriksen, 1952).

> **Minidefinition**: *Moraxella. Gram-negative rods; non-motile. Aerobic. Catalase-positive; oxidase-positive. Sugars not attacked. Growth improved by the addition of blood or serum but specific growth factors are not known. Type species: M. lacunata; NCTC strain 11011.*

7.4.2   Acinetobacter (Tables 7.3; 7.4a).

A genus proposed by Brisou & Prévot (1954) for non-motile species that, apart from their lack of motility, would have fitted into *Achromobacter* as defined at that time; they included in it, as '*Acinetobacter anitratum*' (*sic*), two species, '*Bacterium anitratum*' (Schaub & Hauber, 1948) and '*Moraxella lwoffii* var. *glucidolytica*,' which had previously been shown to be identical (Brisou & Morichau-Beauchant, 1952). In 1961, Prévot listed 17 species in the genus, but as a taxonomic entity *Acinetobacter* has had a chequered career, with much debate about the species to be included, and whether it should be a separate genus or included in *Moraxella*. The first good descriptions of organisms in the taxon were published by Schaub & Hauber (1948) for '*Bacterium anitratum*' and by Stuart *et al.* (1949) for the 'B5W group'. Ewing (1949a) recognized that these organisms bore some resemblance to the poorly described tribe Mimeae with genera '*Mima*', '*Herellea*', and '*Colloides*' (De Bord, 1939, 1942, 1943, 1948), some strains of which simulated gonococci. Henriksen (1963) and Pickett & Manclark (1965) showed that these names were being misapplied and that because the original descriptions had been vague and ambiguous, considerable confusion had resulted; these names are now no longer in use.

Steel & Cowan (1964) modified the definition of the genus *Acinetobacter* to allow inclusion of bacteria that did not produce acid from carbohydrates; this was an improvement and allowed the inclusion of '*Moraxella lwoffii*', an organism that was misplaced in *Moraxella*. But they were imprudent in suggesting also the transfer to *Acinetobacter* of the glanders bacillus, which has since found a better resting place in the genus *Pseudomonas*.

After considerable bibliographical research, Baumann, Doudoroff & Stanier, (1968b) found a reference to an organism labelled '*Micrococcus calcoaceticus*' which had the characteristics of '*Acinetobacter anitratus*', and thus added yet another name. Because it is the oldest, *calcoaceticus* becomes the nomenclaturally correct specific epithet thus producing the awkward but currently approved combination *Acinetobacter calcoaceticus*. Juni (1984) included both *A. calcoaceticus* and *A. lwoffii* in the same species under the former name; however, we prefer to distinguish the two species as it is not difficult to do so and it may also be helpful clinically. Indeed it was known for some time that *Acinetobacter* was heterogeneous both nutritionally (Baumann, Doudoroff & Stanier, 1968b, see below) and genetically (Johnson, Anderson & Ordal, 1970). The genus is now known to comprise more than 12 genetically distinct species, including *A. calcoaceticus* and *A. lwoffii*; four of the remaining species have been named *A. baumannii*, *A. haemolyticus*, *A. johnsonii* and *A. junii* (Bouvet & Grimont, 1986). However, as the phenotypic distinction between these species depends almost entirely on nutritional characters, we have not tried to include them in the Tables.

One of the characteristics of *Acinetobacter calcoaceticus* is its ability to attack monosaccharides but not higher saccharides in Peptone Water sugars. When the sugar concentration is raised to 5 or 10%, the organism can attack lactose. A non-specific aldose dehydrogenase (Baumann, Doudoroff & Stanier, 1968*b*) is responsible for the oxidative production of acid from several carbohydrates in complex media. As only one enzyme is involved, the pattern of carbohydrates oxidised is of no value for classification though it is still useful for identification.

Biotypes of *Acinetobacter calcoaceticus* occur and these may vary in soap tolerance (Billing, 1955), gelatin liquefaction, and ability to grow at 44 °C (Ashley & Kwantes, 1961). Several biotypes were described by Baumann, Doudoroff & Stanier, (1968*b*); some of these may perhaps correspond to distinct genospecies The nutritional tests necessary for recognition of 12 of the genospecies can be used also for biotyping purposes (Bouvet & Grimont, 1987). In the characterization of *Acinetobacter* species there is general agreement on the main points but some disagreement on detail; urease, for example, has been reported as negative, variable, and positive for the two species we recognize here. The differences may be explained by Henderson's (1967) finding that urease production by members of this genus is suppressed by ammonia produced from peptone and other nitrogenous constituents of the media.

Minidefinition: *Acinetobacter. Non-motile, Gram-negative coccobacilli or short rods. Strictly aerobic. Catalase-positive; oxidase-negative. Attack sugars by oxidation or not at all. Do not produce pigment. Arginine test negative. Type species: A. calcoaceticus; ATCC strain 23055.*

7.4.3 **Kingella (Table 7.4***a***)** is a genus originally proposed to accommodate the catalase-negative '*Moraxella*' species, '*M. kingii*'. On transfer

Table 7.4*b***.** *Third-stage table to distinguish the classical 'species' of* Brucella

	1	2	3
CO_2 requirement	+	–	–
H_2S produced	+ (early)	–	D[a]
Growth in:			
thionin[b] 1/25 000	–	–	+
thionin[b] 1/50 000	–	+	+
basic fuchsin 1/50 000	+	+	–
safranin O 1/5000	d	+	–

1 **Brucella abortus;** Bang's bacillus
2 **Brucella melitensis;** *B. brucei; Alcaligenes melitensis*
3 **Brucella suis**

a American strains positive; produce H_2S over several days. Danish strains do not produce H_2S. See note in text on geographical races.
b Dyes obtained from the National Biological Stains Department, Allied Chemical Corporation, New York, USA.

Other symbols used in the table are explained in Tables 5.1 and 5.2 on p.47.

(Henriksen & Bøvre, 1976) the name was corrected to *Kingella kingae*. Soon afterwards two other species were added to the genus (Snell & Lapage, 1976); one reduces nitrate and generally nitrite (*K. denitrificans*); the other produces indole (*K. indologenes*). Genetic studies demonstrate a close relationship between the 'true neisserias', *K. kingae* and *K. denitrificans*, whereas *K. indologenes* is not closely related to them (Rossau *et al.*, 1986).

Minidefinition: *Kingella. Non-motile, Gram-negative short rods. Aerobic or facultatively anaerobic. Catalase-negative; oxidase-positive. Attack sugars by fermentation in suitable media. Do not produce pigment. Arginine test negative. Type species: K. kingae; NCTC strain 10529.*

7.4.4 **Brucella (Tables 7.4***a***, *b*)** comprises a group of bacteria whose cultural and serological characters blend into each other so that some workers regarded the whole as one species, while others saw them as three not-too-well-defined species; others accepted the three species without question and were willing to consider other candidates for inclusion in the genus. In 1963 the international Brucella Subcommittee (Stableforth & Jones) decided in favour of three species, each divided into biotypes, and then accepted a new species, *Brucella neotomae*, only seven strains of which had then been isolated. Other species were later proposed and *B. ovis* and *B. canis* were provisionally accepted by the Subcommittee (Jones & Wundt, 1971). More recent DNA studies (Verger *et al.*, 1985) show that the genus does, in fact, comprise a single genospecies, *B. melitensis*. We continue, however, to use the 'old' specific epithets although strictly they should be used in a vernacular form for biovar designation (e.g. *Brucella melitensis* biovar Abortus 1). The generic characters are shown in Table 7.4*a*, and some distinguishing features of the three classical species *Brucella abortus*, *B. melitensis*, and *B. suis* are shown in Table 7.4*b*; details of the various biotypes are given in the report of the Brucella Subcommittee (Jones & Wundt, 1971), and the technical methods are described by Morgan & Gower (1966). The tests used to separate the biotypes include investigation of the oxidative metabolism of isolates (Meyer & Cameron, 1961*a*, *b*), the sensitivity to Tbilisi bacteriophage (which is not specific for any 'species') (Parnas, 1961), and serological tests with monospecific antisera (which are not available commercially and are not easy to prepare).

Differentiation kits and the fluorescent antibody reagents available commercially are not adequate for distinguishing between the various biotypes, and their use does not give better results than the tests shown in Table 7.4*b*. The performance of the latter tests must be well controlled at all stages and, since their interpretation is subjective, they can be relied upon only when strains are examined routinely as in a reference laboratory.

In Table 7.4*b* we show H_2S production by *Brucella suis* as 'D', indicating differences between the main biotypes; American strains produce H_2S and Danish strains do not. These may be more examples of 'geographical races' of species.

Brucella neotomae differs from the classical brucellas in that acid production from various sugars can easily be shown in peptone-containing media and it is oxidase negative. *Brucella ovis* is also oxidase negative; it needs CO_2 for isolation and does not produce H_2S or reduce nitrates. We do not show these two 'species' in the tables.

Except for *Brucella neotomae*, brucellas do not produce acid from carbohydrate in media containing peptone, but by avoiding the peptone, acid production from carbohydrate can be shown in the classical *Brucella* 'species' (Pickett & Nelson, 1955).

Minidefinition: *Brucella. Short Gram-negative rods; non-motile. Aerobic or carboxyphilic. Catalase-positive; usually oxidase-positive. Do not show acid production from sugars in peptone-containing media (except for one 'species'). Urease-positive. Type species: B. melitensis; NCTC strain 10094.*

7.4.5 Bordetella (Tables 7.4*a*; 7.5). Apart from clinical association, the species within this genus appear to have few characters in common. The whooping cough organism, *Bordetella pertussis*, does not grow on ordinary media until it has been in laboratory culture for some time, and a medium rich in blood has usually been considered essential for its isolation. Bordet-Gengou is probably the medium most often chosen, and many attempts have been made to improve its selectivity (see, for example, Lacey, 1951). Its nutritional requirements and metabolism were reviewed by Rowatt (1957), and its isolation and identification by Lautrop (1960). Though the whooping cough organism is nutritionally exacting, Turner (1961) showed that it does not require a rich medium; peptones, however, contain substances that are inhibitory to *B. pertussis*, though a meat extract agar without peptone is suitable for isolation of the organism. The other two species in the genus, *B. parapertussis* and *B. bronchiseptica*, though also associated with infections of the respiratory tract, are much less exacting in their nutritional requirements. *B. pertussis* is non-motile and oxidase-positive, *B. parapertussis* non-motile and oxidase-negative, and *B. bronchiseptica* is motile and oxidase-positive. This diversity of primary characters makes it difficult to define the genus and it is small wonder than *B. parapertussis* and *B. bronchiseptica* have each resided in various other genera in the past. In conventional biochemical tests *B. bronchiseptica* is more similar to *Alcaligenes faecalis* than to the other two *Bordetella* species. However, despite the heterogeneity of these characters in the genus, other considerations such as DNA homology confirm that phylogenetically the three species should be included in the same genus.

Minidefinition: *Bordetella. Gram-negative rods; may be motile by peritrichous flagella or non-motile. Aerobic. Catalase-positive; oxidase may be positive or negative. One species (B. pertussis) does not grow in simple media containing peptone. Do not attack sugars. Type species: B. pertussis; NCTC strain 10739.*

7.5 The non-(or weakly) saccharolytic motile rods

(Alcaligenes, Shewanellas, alkali-producing pseudomonads)

***Characters common to members of the group*: Gram-negative rods; motile. Strict aerobes. Catalase-positive; oxidase-positive. Produce acid from only a few carbohydrates.**

The group is heterogeneous but all species come within the descriptive term motile and non-(or weakly) saccharolytic; they do not usually show acid production from glucose in ammonium salt medium. Most of the 'non-fermenters' by definition also fail to produce acid from carbohydrate in media containing peptone, though without it some of them are actively saccharolytic.

It is essential to check the nitrate medium for residual nitrate after a negative nitrite test as the test for nitrite can be negative when nitrate has been reduced, and the test for residual nitrate is an essential part of the nitrate reduction test (see Table 4.1). A feature of the group is its lack of positive characters; rarely, there is an absence of information, shown by question marks in the tables. This absence is understandable for organisms such as *Bordetella pertussis* which are unable to grow in or on the media used for so many tests, but is is surprising for those organisms in this group which grow readily. Johnson & Sneath (1973) described a wide range of tests useful for characterizing these bacteria.

7.5.1 Alcaligenes (Table 7.5). Although ten species of *Alcaligenes* appeared in the *Approved Lists of Bacterial Names* (1980), previous studies have shown that the five marine species and three hydrogen-utilizing species are not closely related to the type species *Alcaligenes faecalis*. All the marine species except *A. aquamarinus* have now been transferred to a new genus, *Deleya* (Baumann, Bowditch & Baumann, 1983).

'*Alcaligenes odorans*' (Málek, Radochová & Lysenko, 1963) was first isolated from stools and urine and named '*Pseudomonas odorans*'; descriptions of the odour have been typically subjective – from valerian to jasmine – and from strawberry-like in young to ammoniacal in old cultures. A variant, '*Alcaligenes odorans* var. *viridans*', has a fruity smell and produces a bright green zone around colonies on Blood Agar (Mitchell & Clarke, 1965; Gilardi & Hirschl, 1969). However, the name '*A. odorans*' no longer has any standing in nomenclature and it is now regarded as a synonym of *A. faecalis* (Kiredjian *et al.*, 1981; Rüger & Tan, 1983; Holmes & Dawson, 1983). *A. ruhlandii* is an earlier, but less well-known synonym of *Achromobacter xylosoxidans* (Kiredjian *et al.*, 1981; Holmes & Dawson, 1983). The latter organism and *Alcaligenes denitrificans* were not in the *Approved Lists of Bacterial Names* but both names have since been revived (Yabuuchi & Yano, 1981; Rüger & Tan, 1983) and these were the only two taxa retained with *Alcaligenes faecalis* in the genus *Alcaligenes* (Kersters & DeLey, 1984*b*). Although *Achromobacter xylosoxidans* is easily separated from *Alcaligenes denitrificans* (the former produces acid in ammonium salt medium from glucose and xylose whilst the latter fails to do so) other considerations show that they are closely related (Kersters & DeLey, 1984*b*). On the other hand, although *A. faecalis* and *A. denitrificans* are almost indistinguishable phenotypically (Table 7.5) they are not closely related genetically. It has been proposed that *Achromobacter xylosoxidans* should be transferred to the genus *Alcaligenes* as *Alcaligenes xylosoxidans* and that *Alcaligenes denitrificans* be made a subspecies, *Alcaligenes xylosoxidans* subsp. *denitrificans* (Kiredjian *et al.*, 1986). Meanwhile, for practical identification purposes, we prefer to retain *Achromobacter xylosoxidans* in *Achromobacter* and *Alcaligenes denitrificans* in *Alcaligenes* together with *Alcaligenes faecalis*. A further species has been proposed: *Alcaligenes piechaudii* (Kiredjian *et al.*, 1986) but it is not easily distinguishable from *A. denitrificans* by conventional biochemical tests and we do not include it in Table 7.5.

Minidefinition: *Alcaligenes. Gram-negative*

rods; motile (by peritrichous flagella). Aerobic. Catalase-positive; oxidase-positive. Do not produce acid from sugars even in suitable media (some strains produce acid from ethanol). Type species: A. faecalis; NCTC strain 11953.

7.5.2   Shewanella (Table 7.5). The only species of this genus known to occur in clinical material (Holmes, Lapage & Malnick, 1975) is *Shewanella putrefaciens*. This organism was once included in *Pseudomonas* but was transferred because of its low DNA G+C content, which is characteristic of

Table 7.5. *Second-stage table for* Achromobacter, Alcaligenes, Bordetella, Shewanella *and the alkali-producing pseudomonads*

	1	2	3	4	5	6	7	8	9	10	11
Brown pigment	−	−	−	−	−	d	−	−	−	−	−
Orange pigment	−	−	−	+	−	−	−	−	−	−	−
Oxidase	+	+	+	+	+	−	+	+	+	+	+
Nitrate reduced	+	+^{a}	−	+	+	−	+	+	−	+	d
Simmons' citrate	+	d	d	−	+	−	+	+	−	d	+
Christensen's citrate	+	+	+	d	+	d	+	+	−	d	+
Urease	−	−	−	d	+	+	d	−	−	d	d
Gelatinase production	−	−	−	+	−	−	−	−	+	−	−
Growth in KCN medium	d	+	d	−	+	−	−	−	d	−	d
H$_2$S from TSI	−	−	−	+	−	−	−	−	−	−	−
Ornithine decarboxylase	−	−	−	d	−	−	−	−	−	−	−
Casein hydrolysis	−	−	−	+	−	−	−	−	−	−	−
Deoxyribonuclease production	−	−	−	+	−	−	−	−	−	−	−
Carbohydrates [in ammonium salt medium], acid from:											
glucose	+	−	−	d	−	−	−	−	−	d	−
arabinose	−	−	−	d	−	−	−	−	−	−	−
ethanol	d	d	+	−	−	−	−	−	d	+	−
fructose	d	−	−	−	−	+	−	−	−	d	−
glycerol	−	−	−	−	−	−	+	−	−	d	d
maltose	−	−	−	d	−	−	−	−	−	−	−
mannitol	−	−	−	−	−	−	+	−	−	−	−
sucrose	−	−	−	d	−	−	−	−	−	−	−
xylose	+	−	−	−	−	−	−	−	−	−	−
Tween 20 hydrolysis	−	−	−	+	−	−	+	+	+	d	+
Tween 80 hydrolysis	−	−	−	+	−	−	+	+	−	−	+
Tyrosine hydrolysis	+	+	+	d	+	−	+	+	d	+	+
Tyrosine, brown pigment production from	−	−	−	d	−	+	−	d	+	d	−
Growth on b-hydroxybutyrate	+	+	+	+	+	−	+	d	+	+	+
PHBA* accumulation in cells	+	d	d	−	d	−	+	−	+	d	+
Growth on Cetrimide Agar	+	+	+	−	−	−	d	d	−	d	−
Growth at 42 °C	d	d	d	d	d	−	−	+	−	+	−
Lecithinase production	−	−	−	+	−	−	−	d	−	−	−

1 Achromobacter xylosoxidans;
  Alcaligenes xylosoxidans subsp. *xylosoxidans*
2 Alcaligenes denitrificans;
  Alcaligenes xylosoxidans subsp. *denitrificans*
3 Alcaligenes faecalis; '*A. odorans*'
4 Shewanella putrefaciens;
  Alteromonas putrefaciens; '*Pseudomonas putrefaciens*'
5 Bordetella bronchiseptica;
  '*Alcaligenes bronchisepticus*'

6 Bordetella parapertussis;
  '*Haemophilus parapertussis*'; '*Alcaligenes parapertussis*'
7 Pseudomonas acidovorans
8 Pseudomonas alcaligenes
9 Pseudomonas diminuta
10 Pseudomonas pseudoalcaligenes
11 Pseudomonas testosteroni

* PHBA: Poly–β–hydroxybutyrate
a Strains also reduce nitrite; strains failing to reduce nitrite correspond to *Alcaligenes piechaudii*.

Other symbols used in the Table are explained in Tables 5.1 and 5.2 on p.47.

Alteromonas (Lee, Gibson & Shewan, 1977). A more recent proposal is to transfer the organism once again, but to the new genus *Shewanella* (MacDonell & Colwell, 1985*b*). The species is somewhat heterogeneous and has been subdivided in various ways by different workers (Holmes, Lapage & Malnick, 1975; Owen, Legros & Lapage, 1978). We retain the organism as a single species which is easily recognisable by its salmon pink pigment, copious H_2S production (positive even on Triple Sugar Iron agar – the only Gram-negative non-fermenter to do so) and decarboxylation of ornithine.

> **Minidefinition**: *Shewanella. Gram-negative rods; motile. Aerobic. Catalase-positive; oxidase-positive. Some strains oxidize a few sugars. Type species: S. putrefaciens; ATCC strain 8071.*

7.5.3 Pseudomonas: the alkali producers (Table 7.5).

Although most pseudomonads produce acid from glucose in the open tube (only) of Hugh & Leifson's oxidation fermentation (O–F) medium (oxidative reaction) and from several carbohydrates in ammonium salt medium (Appendix A2.5.5), a few produce alkali in the open tube of glucose O–F medium and produce acid from only a few (or no) carbohydrates in ammonium salt medium. Such organisms, motile by polar flagella, may easily be confused with *Bordetella bronchiseptica* or *Alcaligenes* species unless flagellar staining is performed.

The members of the group comprise *P. acidovorans, P. alcaligenes, P. diminuta, P. pseudoalcaligenes* and *P. testosteroni*. Their occurrence in clinical material is largely unknown as such strains are not easy to identify because of their non-reactive nature in conventional tests and they have probably often been misidentified in the past as *Alcaligenes* species. In the range of tests given in Table 7.5 the unnamed peritrichously flagellated organism 'Group IVc-2' (Clark *et al.*, 1984) would be easily misidentified as *P. testosteroni* without flagella staining. However, the strains of Group IVc-2 we have examined differed from *P. testosteroni* in that none reduced nitrate, all produced urease, none produced acid from glycerol, all grew at 42 °C and many (78%) produced lecithinase. The revival of *Comamonas terrigena* proposed by De Vos *et al.* (1985) also presents problems

as the only characteristics presented by these authors to differentiate *C. terrigena* from *P. testosteroni* are utilization of carbon sources. It has since been proposed that *P. acidovorans* and *P. testosteroni* should be transferred to the genus *Comamonas* (Tamaoka, Ha & Komagata, 1987) but we disregard this as it is difficult to distinguish the two genera with conventional tests.

> **Minidefinition**: *Pseudomonas (alkali-producers): Gram-negative rods; motile by polar flagella. Aerobic. Catalase-positive; oxidase-positive. Produce alkali in the open tube of O-F medium; attack few or no carbohydrates.*

7.6 The actively saccharolytic motile rods
(*Achromobacter, Agrobacterium, Janthinobacterium*, oxidizing pseudomonads, *Flavobacterium, Weeksella*).

Characters common to members of the group: **Gram-negative rods. Strict aerobes. Catalase-positive; oxidase-positive. Produce acid from many sugars in ammonium salt medium. Motile (except *Pseudomonas mallei*).**

Bacteria that produce pigmented colonies are easy to recognize but they can cause difficulties in biochemical tests (e. g. oxidase) that involve a colour reaction. In such instances, non-pigmented variants, if produced, can be used instead. For other organisms, media have been devised to encourage pigment production and Mannitol Yeast-extract Agar (Appendix A2.4.2) is especially useful for *Janthinobacterium* and *Chromobacterium* species. The temperature of incubation is at least as important as the medium and stronger pigments are usually produced at the lower end of the growth range; 20–25 °C is satisfactory for pigment production by most mesophilic organisms.

The group is heterogeneous but all species come within the descriptive term 'actively saccharolytic'; they invariably show acid production from glucose in suitable media. All the species oxidize carbohydrates and this is best seen in basal media with a low peptone content such as Ammonium Salt (Appendix A2.5.5) and O–F sugars or in buffered single substrate (BSS) tests (Pickett & Pedersen, 1970*b*).

Table 7.6a. *Second stage table for* Ochrobactrum, Achromobacter, Agrobacterium, Chryseomonas, Flavimonas, Janthinobacterium *and* Pseudomonas

	1	2	3	4	5	6	7	8	9	10	11	12	13	14	15	16	17	18	19
Motility	+	+	+	+	d	+	+	+	+	+	+	−	+	d	d	+	+	+	d
Growth at 37 °C	+	+	+	d	−	+	+	+	+	+	+	+	+	+	+	+	+	+	+
Growth at 20–22 °C	+	+	+	+	+	+	+	+	+	+	+	+	+	+	+	+	+	+	+
Brown pigment	−	−	−	−	−	−	−	−	d	−	−	−	−	−	−	−	−	−	−
Violet pigment	−	−	−	−	−	−	−	d	−	−	−	−	−	−	−	−	−	−	−
Green pigment	−	−	−	−	−	−	−	−	d	−	−	−	−	−	−	−	−	−	−
Yellow pigment	−	−	−	−	+	+	+	−	d	−	−	−	−	+	−	−	−	d	−
Orange pigment	−	−	−	−	−	+	−	−	−	−	−	−	−	−	−	−	−	+	+
Growth on MacConkey Agar	+	+	+	+	d	d	+	+	+	+	+	+	+	−	+	+	+	+	d
Oxidase	+	+	+	d	+	+	+	+	+	+	d	+	d	+	+	+	+	+	+
Oxidative in O–F medium	+	+	+	d	d	+	+	+	+	+	d	+	d	d	+	+	+	+	−
Alkaline in O–F medium	−	−	d	−	+	−	−	−	−	−	−	+	−	−	−	−	−	−	−
Nitrate reduced to nitrite	+	+	+	d	d	d	+	+	d	d	d	+	d^{b}	−	d	+	+	+	−
Simmons' citrate medium	+	d	+	d	d	+	−	d	d	d	d	d	+	+	d	+	+	+	+
Christensen's citrate medium	+	+	+	+	d	+	+	+	d	d	d	d	+	d	+	+	+	+	+
Urease	+	+	+	+	d	d	+	−	d	d	d	d	+	−	−	−	−	−	d
Gelatinase production	d	−	−	−	−	+	d	d	d	d	−	+	d	+	−	d	d	d	d
Growth in KCN medium	d	−	d	−	−	−	d	−	d	d	−	−	d	−	+	+	−	−	−
H₂S (PbAc paper)	d	−	−	+	−	−	d	−	d	−	−	−	−	−	−	−	−	−	−
Gluconate	−	−	−	−	−	−	−	d	d	−	−	−	d	−	−	−	−	−	−
Malonate	−	−	−	−	−	+	d	d	d	d	d	−	d	−	+	+	d	d	−
ONPG	−	+	−	d	d	+	+	d	−	d	d	−	+	+	−	+	−	−	−
Carbohydrates acid from:																			
10% glucose	d	d	d	−	−	+	+	+	+	+	+	+	d	−	+	+	+	+	+
10% lactose	−	−	−	−	−	+	+	−	−	+	−	d	−	−	−	−	−	−	−
[in Peptone Water Medium], acid from: glucose	−	−	−	−	d	−	−	−	−	d	d	d	−	−	−	+	d	−	−
[in ammonium salt media], acid from:																			
glucose	+	+	+	+	+	+	+	+	+	+	+	+	d	+	+	+	+	+	+
adonitol	+	−	−	+	−	−	−	d	−	+	d	−	−	−	−	d	−	−	−
arabinose	+	+	−	+	−	−	−	d	−	d	d	−	+	+	+	+	+	+	d
cellobiose	+	−	−	+	−	−	+	−	−	+	d	d	+	+	d	+	−	+	d
dulcitol	+	−	−	−	−	−	+	d	−	−	−	−	−	−	−	−	−	−	+
ethanol	+	+	d	+	d	+	+	d	+	+	+	−	d	d	−	d	d	d	−
fructose	+	+	d	+	d	+	+	d	+	+	+	d	d	+	+	d	d	+	−
glycerol	+	+	+	+	d	+	+	+	+	+	+	+	d	+	+	+	d	d	+
inositol	+	+	+	+	−	+	+	+	+	+	d	−	d	+	+	+	d	d	−
lactose	+	+	+	+	+	+	+	+	+	+	−	d	+	+	+	+	d	−	+
maltose	+	+	+	−	+	+	+	d	+	+	d	d	+	d	+	+	−	d	+
mannitol	+	+	−	+	d	+	+	+	+	+	−	d	d	d	+	+	−	d	+
raffinose	−	−	+	−	+	−	−	−	−	−	−	−	+	+	−	−	−	−	d
rhamnose	+	+	−	−	−	+	+	d	+	−	d	d	+	d	+	+	−	d	−
salicin	d	d	−	d	+	d	−	−	−	d	d	d	d	d	−	d	d	−	−
sorbitol	d	−	−	−	d	−	d	−	−	d	d	−	−	d	−	d	−	−	−
sucrose	d	−	−	d	−	d	d	−	d	d	d	+	+	+	d	d	−	d	−
trehalose	d	+	+	+	+	+	+	d	+	+	d	−	+	+	d	+	−	d	−
xylose	+	+	+	+	+	+	+	+	+	+	+	−	+	+	+	+	+	d	−

Table 7.6a – *continued*

	1	2	3	4	5	6	7	8	9	10	11	12	13	14	15	16	17	18	19
Phenylalanine	d	–	–	–	–	–	–	–	+	–	+	+	–	–	–	–	+	+	–
Arginine dihydrolase	–	–	d	d	–	+	–	–	+	d^a	+	+	d	–	–	–	+	d	–
Lysine decarboxylase	–	–	–	–	–	–	–	–	–	d^a	–	–	–	–	–	–	–	–	–
Ornithine decarboxylase	–	–	–	–	–	–	–	–	–	–	–	–	–	–	–	–	–	–	–
Selenite reduction	–	–	–	–	–	–	–	d	d	+	d	+	+	–	+	+	–	–	–
Casein hydrolysis	–	–	–	–	d	d	d	d	+	+	+	+	+	d	+	+	d	+	+
Deoxyribonuclease production	–	–	–	–	d	+	d	–	d	–	–	+	+	d	–	+	–	–	–
Thornley's arginine	–	d	–	–	–	–	+	–	+	+	d	+	+	+	+	+	+	d	+
Tween 20 hydrolysis	–	–	–	+	+	+	+	+	+	+	d	+	+	+	+	+	+	+	+
Tween 80 hydrolysis	d	–	–	+	+	d	+	d	+	+	d	+	+	+	+	–	+	+	d
Tyrosine hydrolysis	–	d	+	+	+	+	d	–	+	+	d	+	+	+	+	+	+	d	d
Tyrosine, brown pigment from	–	+	+	–	d	d	d	–	d	+	+	+	+	+	–	d	–	d	+
Nitrite reduced	+	+	d	d	–	+	+	+	+	+	–	–	–	–	–	+	–	+	–
PHBA* growth	+	+	+	d	+	+	+	+	+	+	+	+	d	+	+	+	+	+	+
PHBA* accumulation in cells	–	d	d	–	+	–	–	–	+	+	d	+	d	+	+	+	d	d	+
Aesculin hydrolysis	+	+	–	+	+	d	+	+	+	d	d	+	d	–	–	d	–	d	–
Growth in presence of cetrimide	–	d	+	d	–	d	+	–	+	+	+	+	d	–	–	–	+	d	–
Fluorescence – King's medium B	–	–	–	–	–	–	–	–	–	+	+	–	–	–	–	–	+	–	–
Growth at 5 °C	–	–	–	–	–	–	+	+	d	–	–	–	–	–	–	–	–	d	–
Growth at 42 °C	d	d	d	–	–	+	–	–	+	+	d	d	d	d	–	+	+	+	–
3-ketolactose production	–	–	d	+	–	+	–	–	+	–	–	–	–	–	d	–	–	–	–
Lecithinase production	–	–	–	–	–	–	–	–	–	+	d	d	–	d	d	–	d	d	d
Starch hydrolysis	–	–	–	–	–	–	–	d	–	–	–	d	–	d	–	–	–	d	–

1 Ochrobactrum anthropi; *Achromobacter* Group A; *Achromobacter* species biotypes 1 and 2; Groups Vd-1 and Vd-2

2 Achromobacter Group B

3 Achromobacter xylosoxidans; *Alcaligenes xylosoxidans* subspecies *xylosoxidans*

4 Agrobacterium tumefaciens; *Agrobacterium radiobacter*

5 Agrobacterium Yellow Group

6 Chryseomonas luteola; Group Ve, type 1

7 Flavimonas oryzihabitans; Group Ve, type 2

8 Janthinobacterium lividum; 'Chromobacterium lividum'

9 Pseudomonas aeruginosa; 'P. pyocyanea'

10 Pseudomonas cepacia; 'P. multivorans'; 'P. kingii'

11 Pseudomonas fluorescens

12 Pseudomonas mallei; 'Loefflerella mallei'; 'Pfeifferella mallei'; 'Malleomyces mallei'

13 Pseudomonas maltophilia; Xanthomonas maltophilia

14 Pseudomonas paucimobilis; 'Sphingomonas paucimobilis'

15 Pseudomonas pickettii

16 Pseudomonas pseudomallei; 'Loefflerella pseudomallei'; 'L whitmor(e)i'; 'Pfeifferella whitmori'; 'Malleomyces pseudomallei'

17 Pseudomonas putida

18 Pseudomonas stutzeri

19 Pseudomonas vesicularis

*PHBA: Poly-β-hydroxybutyrate.
a More strains positive by Richard's (1968) method.
b Cannot use nitrate as N source.

Other symbols used in the table are explained in Tables 5.1 and 5.2 on p.47.

7.6.1   Achromobacter (Tables 7.5; 7.6a). This was for many years an ill-defined genus of motile Gram-negative rods whose main distinguishing feature was the negative one of not producing pigmented colonies. The genus was never adequately defined and *Achromobacter* became the name of the dump-heap of organisms left unnamed by the rejection of the generic name *'Bacterium'* by the Judicial Commission (Opinion 4 (revised), 1954). Accord-ingly, it was omitted from the *Approved Lists of Bacterial Names* (1980) but was later revived by Yabuuchi & Yano (1981) for the single species *Achromobacter xylosoxidans*, which is of clinical interest (Holmes, Snell & Lapage, 1977). Since this organism is closely related to *Alcaligenes denitrificans*, Kiredjian *et al.* (1986) proposed that *Achromobacter xylosoxidans* should be transferred to the genus *Alcaligenes* with two subspecies, *Alcaligenes xylosoxidans* subsp. *xylosoxidans* and *Alcaligenes xylosoxidans* subsp. *denitrificans*. Despite good scientific evidence for this proposal we prefer to keep *Achromobacter xylosoxidans* and *Alcaligenes denitrificans* as separate taxa (see Section 7.5.1). The characteristics of *Achromobacter xylosoxidans* are compared with *Alcaligenes* in Table 7.5 and with the actively saccharolytic non-fermenters in Table 7.6a.

In a numerical taxonomic analysis of *Achromobacter*-like strains from clinical material Holmes & Dawson (1983) recognized six groups, A to F, of which A and B were by far the largest. Recent taxonomic work shows that groups A, C and D are biotypes of a single species which is not phylogenetically closely related to *Achromobacter xylosoxidans*; the name *Ochrobactrum anthropi* has been proposed for this species. Groups B, E and F still require further taxonomic investigation but we suspect that group B will also ultimately reside in a new genus created to accommodate it. We show *Achromobacter* group B in Table 7.6a together with *Ochrobactrum anthropi* biotype A (= *Achromobacter* group A, which also includes organisms formerly described either as *Achromobacter* biotypes 1 and 2 or as Groups Vd-1 and Vd-2 of Clark *et al.*, 1984).

> **Minidefinition**: *Achromobacter. Gram-negative rods; motile (by peritrichous flagella). Aerobic. Catalase-positive; oxidase-positive. Attack sugars by oxidation. Type species: A. xylosoxidans; NCTC strain 10807.*

7.6.2   Agrobacterium (Table 7.6a). This genus comprises primarily pathogens of plants; indeed, the many species within it have been defined by plant pathologists largely according to their pathogenic effects on plants. Several studies show that a different classification can be achieved when the phytopathogenic effect of strains is not given undue weight. Kersters & DeLey (1984a) recognized three species: *A. tumefaciens* (synonym of *A. radiobacter*), *A. rhizogenes* and *A. rubi*. In addition Holmes & Roberts (1981) described a fourth taxon, the '*Agrobacterium* yellow group', which produced yellow-pigmented colonies and were included in *Agrobacterium* because they formed 3-ketolactose, a test considered specific for agrobacteria (Bernaerts & DeLey, 1963). The '*Agrobacterium* yellow group' is, however, probably much more closely related to *Pseudomonas paucimobilis* as the two differ little in conventional biochemical characters (Table 7.6a). Strains of the group have been isolated from dialysis fluid (Swann *et al.*, 1985) and *A. tumefaciens* and other agrobacteria occasionally from other clinical specimens (Lautrop, 1967; Riley & Weaver, 1977; Kiredjian, 1979; Plotkin, 1980; Freney *et al.*, 1985).

> **Minidefinition**: *Agrobacterium. Gram-negative rods; motile. Aerobic. Catalase-positive; oxidase-positive. Wide range of sugars attacked by oxidation. Type species: A. tumefaciens; ATCC strain 23308.*

7.6.3   Janthinobacterium (Tables 7.6a; 7.8a). *Janthinobacterium lividum* formerly resided in the genus *Chromobacterium* together with *C. violaceum* (DeLey, Seagers & Gillis, 1978). Both these organisms are characterized by the production of violet pigments, which make determination of the oxidase reaction difficult with methods that depend on the production of a purple colour in the test. Snell (1973) was able to find non-pigmented variants suitable for the oxidase test; in their absence, very young cultures are less pigmented and should be used. To encourage pigment production we recommend the use of Mannitol Yeast-extract Agar incubated at 20–25 $^{\circ}$C (20 $^{\circ}$C for *Janthinobacterium lividum* and at 25 $^{\circ}$C for *C. violaceum*). We deal with *Chromobacterium violaceum* in Section 7.8.4.

Chromobacterium was a genus created around a colour and it seems to be as unsuccessful as other genera confined to a particular colour. *J. lividum* and *C. violaceum* are both Gram-negative rods but there are several important differences between them: *J. lividum* grows between 4° and 30 °C, *C. violaceum* between 10° and 37 °C. *J. lividum* oxidizes carbohydrates and its characters are shown in Table 7.6*a*; most strains of *C. violaceum* ferment sugars (a few do so oxidatively) and it is shown with the fermenting Gram-negative rods in Table 7.8*a* together with the characters of *J. lividum* beside it for comparison. At one time or another both species have been labelled *Chromobacterium violaceum*, and in literature before 1958 the names should be viewed with caution.

Chromobacteriosis is a rare disease of man caused by the mesophilic species *Chromobacterium violaceum* (Sneath, 1960); the psychrophile is unlikely to be isolated from clinical material but may arise as an infrequent contaminant of stored refrigerated products such as blood.

> **Minidefinition**: *Janthinobacterium. Gram-negative rods; motile. Produce a violet pigment. Aerobic; psychrophilic. Catalase-positive; oxidase-positive. Sugars attacked by oxidation. Type species: J. lividum; NCTC strain 9796.*

7.6.4 Pseudomonas: the oxidizers (Table 7.6*a*).

This large group of organisms includes pathogens for both animals and plants, but because specimens from animal and plant tissues are studied in different laboratories different tests and techniques are often used; this has resulted, in the past, in a separation into animal and plant species which is quite unjustified, for strains pathogenic for plants may also be pathogenic for animals and *vice versa*. Indeed, different names may be proposed for the same organism by the different groups of workers. For example, *P. cepacia* was proposed for an organism isolated from onions, and later '*P. multivorans*' was suggested for the same organism isolated from soil and clinical material from man (see Holmes, 1986*b*). Until recently, *Pseudomonas aeruginosa* (previously referred to as '*Pseudomonas pyocyanea*' in medical laboratories) and *P. fluorescens* were virtually the only species studied extensively by both groups of workers, but the common ground has now been much extended.

Pseudomonas aeruginosa produces two water-soluble pigments: pyocyanin which gives the green-blue appearance to the areas surrounding colonies or confluent growth on plates; and fluorescin, yellow in colour but which, as its name implies, exhibits characteristic fluorescence in ultra-violet light. While pyocyanin is formed only by *P. aeruginosa*, another green pigment, chlororaphin, is produced by some plant pseudomonads; this pigment is not water-soluble and is seen as crystals in agar media. Other pseudomonads, such as *P. putida*, may produce a fluorescent pigment similar to fluorescin.

Although not closely related phylogenetically, *P. pseudomallei*, originally known as Whitmore's bacillus, has much in common with the fluorescent pseudomonads. Wetmore & Gochenour (1956) found that growth of this organism was generally inhibited on media such as Salmonella–Shigella (SS) Agar, Deoxycholate Citrate Agar, and Cetrimide Agar, on which the fluorescent species would grow. The flagella of *P. pseudomallei* were first described as peritrichate by Legroux & Genevray (1933), but later as polar by Brindle & Cowan (1951) and by Wetmore & Gochenour (1956); all these workers showed that the organism had much in common with the pseudomonads but none suggested transferring it to that genus and it was not included in *Pseudomonas* until the seventh edition of *Bergey's Manual* (Haynes, 1957). Redfearn, Palleroni & Stanier (1966) included *P. mallei* (the glanders bacillus) in their survey of *Pseudomonas* species, and regarded it as a typical but permanently non-motile member of that genus. This organism is closely related phylogenetically to *P. pseudomallei*.

Fortunately, glanders is almost a disease of the past and few now have the opportunity (or the risks) of working with recently isolated cultures. Melioidosis (of which *P. pseudomallei* is the causative organism) is a disease of tropical countries but occasionally occurs in temperate climates in people who were probably infected abroad (Peck, 1986). *Pseudomonas pseudomallei* may be confused with other pseudomonads and although its wrinkled colonial appearance may be characteristic, it is not diagnostic as it can be simulated by *P. aeruginosa* and by *P. stutzeri* (Lapage, Hill & Reeve, 1968). Zierdt & Marsh (1971) state that after incubation for three or four days, colonies of *P. pseudomallei* have an aromatic odour that is distinctive; but without experience of it we do not think that this subjective characteristic can be of much help for identification. Other diagnostic features are the development of bright red colonies on MacConkey agar (and on the basal medium without lactose) and the ability to grow on Deoxycholate Citrate Agar. For most laboratories the isolation of *Pseudomonas pseudomallei* is a rare event and confirmation of isolates should always be obtained from a reference laboratory with access to specific antiserum tested against *Pseudomonas aeruginosa* and other pseudomonads to exclude cross-reactions. *P. mallei* is one of the most dangerous organisms to work with in a laboratory, and *P. pseudomallei*, though probably less dangerous, should be treated with the same respect; both are listed in Hazard Group 3 by the Advisory Committee on Dangerous Pathogens (1984).

Many other pseudomonads have been isolated from clinical material and the hospital environment (see, for example, Gilardi, 1978, 1985a,b) and there has been much effort to find distinguishing features to assess the potential pathogenicity of the different species. Undoubtedly some strains are 'opportunist pathogens' and, as many of them are resistant to disinfectant solutions, they may cause low-grade infections from contaminated catheters, wash-out fluids, and drip lines. Media for the selective isolation of pseudomonads have been reviewed by Park & Billing (1965). Thom *et al.* (1971) found that the addition of nitrofurantoin to King's B medium (Appendix A2.4.3) was easier to prepare than cetrimide media and was equally good for the selective isolation of *Pseudomonas aeruginosa*. On this medium most strains of *Proteus* species, *Escherichia coli*, *Enterococcus faecalis*, and staphylococci were either inhibited completely or grew only feebly after overnight incubation at 37 °C.

Tests to identify the many species are becoming more complex; for example, one of the distinguishing characters is to show by phase-contrast microscopy the presence or absence of poly-β-hydroxybutyrate (PHB) in the cells of cultures grown preferably in a medium with DL-β-hydroxybutyrate as the carbon source, with subsequent confirmation by staining with Sudan Black B. Apart from the accumulation of PHB in the bacterial cells, the tests for characters shown in Table 7.6a do not call for exceptional knowledge or skill and can be performed in most laboratories. The growth of *P. aeruginosa* is often accompanied by iridescence; the mechanism of this phenomenon is still unknown, but it is independent of phage sensitivity (Zierdt, 1971).

Four methods are available for typing strains of *P. aeruginosa* for epidemiological purposes: bacteriocin typing, serotyping by somatic and by flagellar antigens, and bacteriophage typing (Pitt, 1988).

Bacteriocin typing is probably the most popular and since the original description of Gillies & Govan (1966) the technique has been modified to increase its sensitivity and specificity (Fyfe, Harris & Govan, 1984). The discrimination achieved by pyocin typing between clinical isolates of *P. aeruginosa* is adequate for most investigations but the test reproducibility is influenced by media composition, bacterial inoculum and storage of the reference indicator strains.

Pseudomonas aeruginosa is heterogeneous in O-somatic antigen structure and 17 heat-stable (lipopolysaccharide) antigens form the basis of the International Antigenic Typing Scheme (IATS) described by Liu *et al.* (1983). O-typing by slide agglutination is reproducible and the number of clinical strains typable is high (90–95%); few strains give unstable suspensions in saline but about 5% of isolates are polyagglutinable. The frequency of serologically atypical isolates increases greatly in chronic infections, especially cystic fibrosis (Pitt *et al.*, 1986). The discriminatory power of O-typing is fair but certain groups such as O6, O10, and O11 predominate and together account for over 40% of all strains. Subtyping by minor antigens is useful in dividing strains of serogroup O6 (Pitt, 1980a).

About 90% of clinical strains are typable with flagella (H) antisera. In combination with O-typing, H antigens increase discrimination between strains as many combinations of H factors occur (Lányi & Bergan, 1978). Some H antigens undergo diphasic variation and this property adversely affects the reproducibility of H-typing (Pitt, 1980b).

Bacteriophage typing has been used extensively by various workers and a standard set of phages is recommended (Bergan, 1978). Some laboratories favour the coding of lytic results by designating distinct patterns with numbers but others prefer to compare the patterns after taking account of the known variability of the method. Phage-typing cannot be used alone for precise type-identification despite the

Table 7.6b. *Buffered single substrate (BSS) tests for* Pseudomonas(*Pickett &*
Pedersen, 1970b,c)

	1	2	3	4	5	6	7	8
Acid from:								
glucose	+	+	−	+	+	+	+	+
fructose	+	+	−	+	+	+	+	+
lactose	−	+	−	d	+	+	−	−
maltose	−	+	−	+	+	+	−	+
mannitol	+	+	−	d	−	+	−	d
salicin	−	+	?	−	d	+	−	−
sucrose	−	d	?	d	+	−	−	−
xylose	+	+	−	+	d	+	+	+

1 **Pseudomonas aeruginosa;** *'P. pyocyanea'*
2 **Pseudomonas cepacia;** *'P. multivorans'; 'P. kingii'*
3 **Pseudomonas diminuta**
4 **Pseudomonas fluorescens**
5 **Pseudomonas maltophilia;** *Xanthomonas maltophilia*
6 **Pseudomonas pseudomallei;** *'Loefflerella pseudomallei', 'L. whitmor(e)i'; 'Pfeifferella whitmori';*
    'Malleomyces pseudomallei'
7 **Pseudomonas putida**
8 **Pseudomonas stutzeri**

Symbols used in the Table are explained in Tables 5.1 and 5.2 on p.47.

high typability as there is considerable overlapping of patterns and lysis by some phages is particularly frequent. It is nevertheless a useful adjunct to O-serological typing.

The acid production from carbohydrates shown in Table 7.6a occurs when the organisms are grown in media without peptone (ASS, Appendix A2.5.5). Media containing only a small amount of peptone (e.g. Hugh & Leifson base, Appendix A2.5.1) may also be used. Acid may be produced from more carbohydrates in the buffered single substrate tests of Pickett & Pedersen (1970b, c) in which a heavy suspension of the test organism is added to the carbohydrate+buffer+indicator+bacteriostatic-agent mixture. The differences between the results of the two kinds of test can be seen by comparing Tables 7.6a and b.

Pseudomonas aeruginosa produces alkali on Christensen's urea medium and, more slowly, on the base without urea. Many pseudomonads break down arginine but Møller's method is not always satisfactory with these organisms; Sherris *et al.* (1959) and Thornley (1960) have described suitable methods. For detecting lysine and ornithine decarboxylases of pseudomonads, Richard's (1968) methods are more sensitive than those of Møller (Snell *et al.*, 1972).

Nutritional requirements can also provide diagnostic characters for some pseudomonads: thus *Pseudomonas maltophilia* requires methionine, and *P. diminuta* (Section 7.5.3.) needs cysteine for growth.

Pseudomonas maltophilia, originally described by Hugh & Ryschenkow (1961) as an *Alcaligenes*-like species, is unusual in producing acid from maltose in Hugh and Leifson sugars before it is seen in glucose, which often remains negative in ASS media. Park (1967) found that the glucose was attacked even though acid was not produced. *P. maltophilia* is also unusual for a pseudomonad in that different strains give different results in the oxidase test. Hugh & Ryschenkow found that 10 of 26 strains gave positive results and Holmes, Lapage & Easterling (1979) likewise found 25 of 117 strains positive, but Pickett & Pedersen (1970b) had only 3 positive reactions among their 27 strains; the variability, apart from the actual strains, may be due to differences in sensitivity of the reagents used for the test (Snell, 1973).

Species described more recently include *P. pickettii* (Ralston, Palleroni & Doudoroff, 1973) and *P. paucimobilis* (Holmes *et al.*, 1977), comprising strains from clinical material and hospital equipment. The latter organism and the so-called '*Agrobacterium* yellow group' (7.6.2.) are closely related. *P. men-*

docina closely resembles *P. stutzeri* but we do not include it in Table 7.6*a* as it is thought to occur only rarely in clinical material; the characteristics for differentiating them are given by Holmes (1986*a*). *P. vesicularis* is phylogenetically closely related to *P. diminuta* (Table 7.5) but it differs from the latter organism in being orange-pigmented and in producing acid from a wider range of carbohydrates.

Also included in Table 7.6*a* are the yellow-pigmented oxidase-negative organisms of 'Group Ve-1' and 'Group Ve-2' of Clark *et al.* (1984): although generally regarded as *Pseudomonas*-like with the names *Pseudomonas luteola* and *Pseudomonas oryzihabitans* proposed for them (Kodama, Kimura & Komogata, 1985), they are now named respectively *Chryseomonas luteola* and *Flavimonas oryzihabitans* (Holmes *et al.*, 1987).

> **Minidefinition**: *Pseudomonas (oxidizers). Gram-negative rods; motile (by polar flagella). Aerobic. Catalase-positive; oxidase-positive. Attack sugars by oxidation. Fluorescent, diffusible yellow pigment may be produced by some species. Type species: P. aeruginosa; NCTC strain 10332.*

7.6.5 Flavobacterium (Table 7.6*c*).

Flavobacterium has long been regarded as an unsatisfactory genus, made up of a heterogeneous collection of species which formed yellow colonies. Although the type species is no longer regarded as a flavobacterium, the genus has been re-defined (Holmes, Owen & McMeekin, 1984*a*) and now comprises seven well-defined taxa that fall into three natural groups which are rather different to the groups previously described by Pickett & Pedersen (1970*a,b,c*). The first group comprises three saccharolytic, indole-positive species; the second a single non-saccharolytic indole-negative species; and the third group three saccharolytic, indole-negative species. As the last three species contain novel sphingophospholipids in their cell walls, a new genus *Sphingobacterium* has been proposed for them (Yabuuchi *et al.*, 1983). We feel, however, that this characteristic alone is insufficient to warrant a new genus and so we retain these three species in *Flavobacterium*. The three taxa comprising the first natural group are not easily differentiated from each other and one of them, *Flavobacterium* species Group IIb, is heterogeneous in conventional biochemical tests. The name *F. indologenes* has been proposed for the whole of Group IIb but it is also heterogeneous by DNA-DNA hybridization; the name *F. gleum* has been proposed for certain strains of Group IIb showing a high degree of relatedness (Holmes *et al.*, 1984*b*). Until this nomenclatural problem is resolved we prefer to use the original designation *Flavobacterium* species Group IIb. *F. meningosepticum* is the species of major clinical interest (Holmes, 1987).

Colonies of *Enterobacter sakazakii* and *Erwinia herbicola* (known in the USA as *Enterobacter agglomerans*) characteristically produce yellow colonies. In other fields some species of *Pseudomonas* and *Xanthomonas* produce yellow pigments, and neglect to determine the Gram reaction of isolates may cause some difficulty with a few Gram-positive species.

Indole production by those species that do so is weak and for demonstration of this character extraction with xylene followed by the addition of Ehrlich's reagent is recommended.

The indole-producing but non-pigment-forming taxa, Groups IIf and IIj, often regarded as *Flavobacterium* – like organisms which could have formed a fourth natural group in that genus, have been transferred recently to a new genus, *Weeksella*, by Holmes *et al.* (1986*a,b*). We deal with the species in this genus in Section 7.6.6 but it should be noted that they do not attack carbohydrates.

> **Minidefinition**: *Flavobacterium. Gram-negative rods; non-motile. Aerobic. Catalase-positive; oxidase-positive. Colonies yellow-pigmented. Carbohydrates attacked slowly by oxidation or not at all. Resistant to most antimicrobial agents. Type species: F. aquatile; ATCC 11947.*

7.6.6 Weeksella (Table 7.6*c*).

This new genus was proposed by Holmes *et al.* (1986*a,b*) to accommodate the two indole-producing, non-saccharolytic *Flavobacterium*-like taxa, Group IIf, isolated mostly from the female genital tract (Mardy & Holmes, 1988), and Group IIj, commonly associated with animal bites (Rubin, Granato & Wasilauskas, 1985). Unlike *Flavobacterium* taxa, however, they do not form yellow-pigmented colonies and they are highly susceptible to most antimicrobial agents. The name

Table 7.6c. *Second–stage table for* Flavobacterium *and* Weeksella

	1	2	3	4	5	6	7	8	9
Carbohydrates [in ammonium salt media], acid from:									
glucose	+	+	+	−	+	+	+	−	−
adonitol	−	−	−	−	−	−	+	−	−
arabinose	−	−	d	−	+	d	+	−	−
cellobiose	−	−	−	−	+	+	+	−	−
ethanol	−	d	d	−	−	+	−	−	−
glycerol	−	d	d	−	+	+	+	−	−
lactose	−	d	−	−	+	+	+	−	−
maltose	+	+	+	−	+	+	+	−	−
mannitol	−	d	−	−	−	+	−	−	−
raffinose	−	−	−	−	+	+	+	−	−
rhamnose	−	−	−	−	d	−	+	−	−
salicin	−	−	−	−	+	+	+	−	−
sucrose	−	−	d	−	+	+	+	−	−
trehalose	−	+	+	−	+	+	+	−	−
xylose	−	−	d	−	+	+	+	−	−
Aesculin hydrolysis	−	+	+	−	+	+	+	−	−
Casein hydrolysis	+	+	+	+	−	−	−	+	d
Gelatinase production	+	+	+	+	−	+	+	+	+
Growth at 42 °C	−	−	d	−	−	−	+	+	−
Indole production (Ehrlich reagent)	+	d	+	−	−	−	−	+	d
Nitrate reduced to nitrite	−	−	d	−	−	−	+	−	−
Nitrite reduced	−	d	d	+	−	−	−	−	−
ONPG	−	+	d	−	+	+	+	−	−
Starch hydrolysis	−	−	d	−	−	−	−	−	−
Urease	−	d	d	+	+	+	+	−	+

1 Flavobacterium breve
2 Flavobacterium meningosepticum
3 Flavobacterium species Group IIb; *F. gleum; F. indologenes*
4 Flavobacterium odoratum; Group M–4f
5 Flavobacterium multivorum; Group IIk–2; *Sphingobacterium multivorum*
6 Flavobacterium spiritivorum; *Sphingobacterium spiritivorum*
7 Flavobacterium thalpophilum
8 Weeksella virosa; Group IIf
9 Weeksella zoohelcum; Group IIj

Symbols used in the Table are explained in Tables 5.1 and 5.2 on p.47.

Weeksella virosa has been proposed for Group IIf and *W. zoohelcum* for Group IIj organisms (Holmes *et al.*, 1986a,b). *W. virosa* produces extremely mucoid colonies and, unlike *W. zoohelcum*, grows on MacConkey agar.

> **Minidefinition:** *Weeksella. Gram-negative rods; non-motile. Aerobic. Catalase-positive; oxidase-positive. Do not produce yellow-pigmented colonies. Carbohydrates not attacked. Sensitive to most antimicrobial agents. Type species: W. virosa; NCTC strain 11634.*

7.7   The Pasteurella and pasteurella-like group
(*Pasteurella, Actinobacillus, Cardiobacterium, Francisella*)

Characters common to members of the group: **Gram-negative rods; non–motile at 37 °C. Aerobic and facultatively anaerobic. Oxidase-positive. Attack sugars fermentatively.**

This group of organisms is still heterogeneous and relatively uncommon as pathogens of man despite the transfer of the plague organism and its close relations to the genus *Yersinia*. However, when they do cause infection, they pose a challenge to both microbiologist and clinician in terms of diagnosis and treatment. We describe the *Yersinia* species in Section 7.9.20 and give their characters in Table 7.9g but show them also in Table 7.7 for comparison with *Pasteurella*.

Actinobacillus and *Pasteurella* have much in common and suggestions have been made for their fusion. *Cardiobacterium* was named in 1964 by Slotnick & Dougherty as an agent causing endocarditis (Wormser & Bottone, 1983) though it was first described as a *Pasteurella*–like organism by Tucker *et al.* (1962).

Francisella, unlike the other genera in this group, requires specially enriched media for isolation (Berdal & Søderlund, 1977). The original species of this genus, previously regarded as *Brucella*-like or as *Yersinia*-like, was placed in the genus *Pasteurella* in the 7th edition of *Bergey's Manual* (1957). Following taxonomic work (Owen, 1974), it was placed in a new genus and renamed *Francisella tularensis* to commemorate the pioneering work of Edward Francis on tularaemia. The genetic identity of this genus and its subdivision have since been confirmed (Olsufiev & Meshcherykova, 1983).

In Table 7.7 we include two organisms, *Actinobacillus actinomycetemcomitans* and *Haemophilus aphrophilus*, which have much in common with each other. They are both small Gram–negative coccobacilli which grow in broth as 'granules' adherent to the tubes; on plates, colonies of *A. actinomycetemcomitans* stick to the medium. Growth of both is improved by CO_2; and neither of them needs X or V factors although *H. aphrophilus* has an apparent X factor requirement on first isolation. The latter is probably placed correctly in the genus *Haemophilus* where we discuss it more fully. Recent taxonomic work (Potts, Zambon & Genco, 1985) suggests that *A. actinomycetemcomitans* could also be transferred to *Haemophilus* though its lack of X or V factor requirements would conflict with this genus as currently defined. We therefore show both these organisms in Table 7.7 as well as with *Haemophilus* in Table 7.10b.

Lastly, as before, we again include *Aeromonas salmonicida*, previously called *Necromonas*, in Table 7.7 as its characters seem to fit quite well in this group. Although it has no known medical significance, it can be isolated from fish and, despite the validity of its current name, we suspect that it will not remain in the genus *Aeromonas* for ever.

7.7.1 Pasteurella (Table 7.7). Several species have been described for this genus, which at one time also included the 'plague bacillus' – now named *Yersinia pestis* – together with *Y. pseudotuberculosis* and *Y. enterocolitica*. *Pasteurella multocida* represents an 'umbrella' species which includes numerous strains that were originally named after the animals from which they had been isolated; sensibly, however, the single epithet *multocida* was later applied to the commoner strains which caused haemorrhagic septicaemia and abscesses in animals of all kinds, including man. Cutaneous infections in man also occur following animal scratches and bites, particularly from cats and dogs. Subsequently, subdivisions of this unified species were again made and these included *P. haemolytica* (Newsom & Cross, 1932) and *P. pneumotropica* (Jawetz, 1950; Henriksen, 1962) as well as *P. haemolytica* var. *ureae* (Henriksen & Jyssum, 1960) which was later elevated to species rank as *Pasteurella ureae* (Jones, 1962; Smith & Thal, 1965). The biochemical characters of these species are shown in Table 7.7.

The principles of the CAMP test (Appendix C3.7) were used by Bouley (1965) to differentiate between *P. multocida* (negative) and *P. haemolytica* (positive). Dye sensitivity tests, included in the second edition of this *Manual*, were also used previously not only to distinguish *Pasteurella* from *Yersinia* but also to differentiate between *Pasteurella* species (Midgley, 1966). As they are not often used for these purposes and now have little taxonomic value, we do not tabulate the test results but mention that thionin (1: 25 000), malachite green (1:50 000) and safranin O (1:25 000) in media should inhibit the growth of *Pasteurella* but not of *Yersinia* species. *P. haemolytica* was divided into serotypes by Biberstein, Gills & Knight, (1960) and into biotypes A (arabinose fermenters) and T (trehalose fermenters) by G.R. Smith (1961); the latter biotype is also catalase-negative (Biberstein & Gills, 1962). Freshly isolated strains of *P. haemolytica* produce clear zones of β–haemolysis on Blood Agar but this haemolytic ability may be reduced after several subcultures.

Several serological schemes have been proposed

Table 7.7. *Second-stage table for* Pasteurella, Actinobacterium, Cardiobacterium, Yersinia *and* Francisella

	1	2	3	4	5	6	7	8	9	10	11	12	13	14	15	16	17	18	19
Motility at 22 °C	–	–	–	–	–	–	–	–	–	–	–	–	–	–	–	+	+	–	–
Catalase	+	+	+	+	–	+	w	+	+	+	+	–	–	–	+	+	+	+	+
Oxidase	d	+	+	+	+	+	+	+	+	?	–	–	+	+	–	–	–	+	d
Growth on MacConkey Agar	–	–	–	+	+	–	+	+	+	+	–	–	–	–	+	+	+	?	–
Growth improved by CO_2	?	?	?	?	?	?	–	–	–	+	+	+	+	+	?	?	?	?	w
Growth in KCN	+	–	–	d	–	–	–	–	–	?	?	?	?	?	–	–	–	–	?
Carbohydrates, acid from:																			
arabinose	d	d	–	d	–	–	d	–	+	+	–	–	–	–	+	+	+	+	?
lactose	d	(d)	–	d	–	d	(+)	+	+	–	–	+	+	–	–	–	(d)	–	–
maltose	d	+	+	+	+	+	+	+	+	–	+	+	+	+	+	+	+	+	d
mannitol	+	–	+	+	+	–	+	+	–	+	d	–	–	d	+	+	+	+	+
raffinose	–	+	–	+	+	–	–	+	+	–	–	+	–	?	–	–	–	–	?
salicin	–	–	–	–	+	–	–	–	+	–	–	–	–	–	+	+	–	+	?
sorbitol	d	–	d	+	+	–	d	–	–	?	–	–	–	+	–	–	+	–	?
sucrose	+	+	+	+	+	+	+	+	+	–	+	+	+	–	–	+	–	–	d
trehalose	d	+	–	–	+	+	–	+	+	+	d	–	+	+	+	+	+	d	?
xylose	d	d	–	+	–	d	+	+	+	+	d	–	–	–	+	+	(+)	–	?
ONPG	d	+	–	d	–	d	+	+	+	?	–	+	+	–	+	+	+	–	?
Aesculin hydrolysis	–	–	–	d	+	–	–	–	+	?	–	–	–	–	+	+	–	+	?
Nitrate reduced	+	+	+	+	+	+	+	+	+	+	+	+	+	–	+	+	+	+	?
Nitrite reduced	d	–	+	+	+	–	?	?	?	?	?	+	+	?	?	?	?	–	?
Indole	+	+	–	–	–	–	–	–	–	?	–	–	–	+	–	–	d	–	?
Gelatin hydrolysis	–	–	–	–	(+)	–	–	(+)	–	–	–	?	?	–	–	–	–	+	–[a]
Urease	d	+	+	–	–	–	+	+	+	+	–	–	–	–	+	+	–	–	?
H_2S	–	–	–	–	(+)	–	+	+	+	+	+	+	–	+	+	–	–	–	+
Ornithine decarboxylase	+	d	–	–	–	d	–	–	–	?	–	–	–	–	–	–	+	–	?

1 **Pasteurella multocida**; *'P. septica'*
2 **Pasteurella pneumotropica**
3 **Pasteurella ureae**; *'P. haemolytica var. ureae'*
4 **Pasteurella haemolytica** type A; *P. haemolytica*
5 **Pasteurella haemolytica** type T; *P. trehalosi*
6 **Pasteurella gallinarum**
7 **Actinobacillus lignieresii**
8 **Actinobacillus equuli**; *'Shigella equuli'; 'S. equirulis'; 'Bacterium viscosum-equi'; 'B. nephritidis-equi'*
9 **Actinobacillus suis**

10 **Actinobacillus from sow's vagina** (Ross *et al.* 1972); *A. rossi*
11 **'Actinobacillus' actinomycetemcomitans**
12 **Haemophilus aphrophilus**
13 **Haemophilus paraphrophilus**
14 **Cardiobacterium hominis**
15 **Yersinia pestis**; *'Pasteurella pestis';* plague bacillus
16 **Yersinia pseudotuberculosis**; *'Pasteurella pseudotuberculosis'*
17 **Yersinia enterocolitica**; Pasteurella X
18 **Aeromonas salmonicida**; *'Necromonas salmonicida'*
19 **Francisella** spp.

[a] *F. philomiragia* often positive

Other symbols used in the Table are explained in Tables 5.1 and 5.2 on p.47.

for the subdivision of *P. multocida* (Steel, 1963); and Frederiksen (1971) divided this species biochemically into six and *P. pneumotropica* into three biotypes. There is a close relation between *P. multocida* and *P. pneumotropica* and it seems probable that changes in the taxonomic status of the latter may follow from current DNA hybridization work. *P. ureae* was isolated originally from respiratory infections in man. A new species, *P. aerogenes*, was proposed by McAllister & Carter (1974) for a group of organisms that produced gas from sugars and which were isolated from human infections following pig bites. These organisms are non-haemolytic, indole-negative and urease-positive.

> **Minidefinition:** *Pasteurella. Gram–negative rods. Non–motile. Aerobic and facultatively anaerobic. Usually catalase-positive; oxidase-positive. Sugars are attacked by fermentation. Type species: P. multocida; NCTC strain 10322.*

7.7.2 Actinobacillus (Tables 7.7; 7.10b) consists of species that seem to have no obvious home. Organisms of at least two kinds are represented: the

119

actinobacilli proper based on the type species *Actinobacillus lignieresii* and another organism, *A. actinomycetemcomitans*, usually but not always associated with *Actinomyces israelii* in material from patients with actinomycosis. Cowan suggested that the latter organism, *A. actinomycetemcomitans*, was only placed in this genus by Topley & Wilson (1929) in the first edition of their book *Principles of Bacteriology and Immunity* because they could not think where else to put it, and it has since remained there. It closely resembles *Haemophilus aphrophilus* and would be more satisfactorily placed in that genus if the definition would allow it, but as it is not satisfactory in *Actinobacillus* we show it also in Table 7.10*b* for comparison with *Haemophilus*. *A. lignieresii*, found in cattle and sheep, is very similar to *A. equuli* and Wetmore *et al.* (1963) proposed that they should be amalgamated. *A. equuli* causes joint-ill and nephritis in foals. Colonies of both species are sticky and difficult to remove from the surface of agar media. Both of these non-motile, urease positive species have been associated with human infections and can be differentiated by trehalose and melibiose fermentation. *A. suis* strains usually produce a clear haemolytic zone on Blood Agar and hydrolyse aesculin.

Minidefinition: *Actinobacillus. Non-motile Gram-negative rods. Aerobic and facultatively anaerobic. Catalase-positive; oxidase-positive (except A. actinomycetemcomitans). Sugars are attacked fermentatively without gas production. Nitrate reduced. Type species: A. lignieresii; ATCC strain 4189.*

7.7.3   Cardiobacterium (Table 7.7). This pleomorphic organism is Gram-negative but it may retain sufficient crystal violet stain to give the appearance of metachromatic granules (Slotnick & Dougherty, 1964); the bacilli also usually have swollen bulbous ends resembling 'teardrops', which form characteristic rosette clusters. Like *Haemophilus*, it prefers a high humidity for growth, so incubation in a jar is advisable. Carbon dioxide improves growth but is not essential though it may appear so on first isolation; growth under strictly anaerobic conditions is good. Only one species, *C. hominis*, has been identified: it is probably part of the normal flora of the nose and throat of man but may occasionally cause endocarditis in sus-

ceptible persons with cardiac lesions (Weaver, Tatum & Hollis, 1972; Wormser & Bottone, 1983).

Minidefinition: *Cardiobacterium. Non-motile, pleomorphic Gram-negative rods sometimes with Gram-positive traces. Aerobic in a humid atmosphere and facultatively anaerobic. Catalase negative; oxidase-positive. Sugars fermented. Type species: C. hominis; NCTC strain 10246.*

7.7.4   Francisella (Table 7.7) currently contains two species of medical importance, *F. tularensis* (McCoy & Chapin, 1912) and *F. novicida* (Larson, Wicht & Jellison, 1955). *F. tularensis*, the cause of the plague-like illness tularaemia in man, was previously placed in the genus *Pasteurella*. It contains at least two biotypes with differing geographical spread and pathogenicity (Olsufiev, Emelyanova & Dunaeva, 1959; Olsufiev, 1970; Eigelsbach & McGann, 1984); in addition, despite some phenotypic differences between *F. tularensis* and *F. novicida*, Hollis *et al.* (1989) regard the latter as a further biotype of *F. tularensis*. These organisms are transmitted to man from a variety of zoonoses in wild animals, including rabbits, beavers, squirrels and game birds, either through direct contact or by biting insects.

For isolation and growth, which is relatively slow, *F. tularensis*, the most exacting, requires media enriched with blood, cysteine and glucose (Berdal & Søderlund, 1977; Eigelsbach & McGann, 1984). In fresh cultures, the organisms are small, non-motile, often capsulated and cocco-bacillary in form; in older cultures, they show marked pleomorphism. They are catalase-positive, oxidase-negative, produce H_2S and form acid but not gas from glucose and several other sugars. The possession of a citrulline-ureidase system distinguishes virulent strains of *F. tularensis* from the less virulent (Marchette & Nicholes, 1961).

These organisms must be handled with respect and precautions taken to avoid laboratory-acquired infections; indeed serological procedures such as slide agglutination reactions and fluorescent microscopy with specific antisera are usually used for identification. For these reasons, although we include the collective reactions for *Francisella* in Table 7.7, we do not recommend the use of conventional characterization tests for their identification in routine laboratories.

The organism isolated from water and the muskrat by Jensen, Owen & Jellison (1969), previously included in *Yersinia*, is genetically similar to *Francisella* but is oxidase-positive and salt-tolerant. Hollis *et al.* (1989), who have isolated similar organisms from clinical infections in man, accordingly suggest that it should be transferred to *Francisella* as *F. philomiragia*.

> **Minidefinition:** *Francisella. Gram-negative rods. Non-motile. Aerobic and facultatively anaerobic. Catalase-positive; oxidase-negative. Sugars attacked fermentatively. Type species: F. tularensis; ATCC strain 6223.*

7.7.5   Yersinia (Tables 7.7; 7.9g) is an offshoot of *Pasteurella*. It is now included among the enterobacteria and we deal with it in Section 7.9g. To show the similarities to and differences from *Pasteurella*, the characters of *Yersinia* are given also in Table 7.7.

We repeat the Minidefinition here.

> **Minidefinition:** *Yersinia. Gram-negative rods; motile or non-motile (temperature dependent). Aerobic and facultatively anaerobic. Catalase-positive; oxidase-negative. Sugars attacked fermentatively, occasionally with production of gas. Grow on MacConkey agar. Type species Y. pestis: NCTC strain 5923.*

7.7.6   'Necromonas', a single-species genus created by I.W. Smith (1963) for the organism causing furunculosis of fish and previously included in this *Manual*, is no longer *extant*. This organism has now been transferred to the genus *Aeromonas* and we deal with it in Sections 7.8 and 7.8.2.

7.7.7   'Haemophilus' aphrophilus (Tables 7.7; 7.10b) seems to be X-factor-dependent on first isolation (Boyce, Frazer & Zinnemann, 1969) but loses this requirement rapidly on subculture. King & Tatum (1962) thought this species had much in common with *Actinobacillus actinomycetemcomitans* but doubted if it would be any better placed in that genus than in *Haemophilus*; however, Potts, Zambon & Genco (1985) suggest that they are both more akin to haemophili and should be transferred to that genus. For comparison of these two species we show *Haemophilus aphrophilus* in Table 7.7a and the actinobacillus in Table 7.10b.

7.8   The Vibrio and vibrio-like group
(Vibrio, Aeromonas, Plesiomonas, Chromobacterium violaceum)

> ***Characters common to members of the group:*** **Gram-negative rods. Aerobic and facultatively anaerobic. Motile; catalase-positive; oxidase-positive. Attack sugars fermentatively. Nitrates are reduced by most species.**

This group of organisms is fairly homogeneous so that, apart from the pigment produced by *Chromobacterium violaceum*, it is easier to cite characters in common than those by which the genera can be distinguished. Knowledge about the taxonomy, ecology and pathogenicity of this group has now increased considerably and, as forecast in the last edition of this *Manual*, the generic names *Beneckea* and *Lucibacterium* have been abolished and their species incorporated within *Vibrio*; the genus *Photobacterium* remains intact but we do not include it here as no pathogenic species are known. Several new *Vibrio* species have also been described, many of which are regarded as opportunist pathogens for man or aquatic animals. The microaerophilic species previously included in *Vibrio* and exemplified by '*V. fetus*' have now been transferred to the genus *Campylobacter*.

Based on 5S rRNA sequencing, MacDonell & Colwell (1985b) have suggested that *Vibrio* species pathogenic for fish should be placed in a new genus, *Listonella*, but as this awaits ratification, we continue to regard them as vibrios. The genus *Allomonas*, with a single species, *A. enterica*, proposed by Kalina *et al.* (1984) is probably identical with *V. fluvialis*.

The taxonomy of *Aeromonas* still remains far from satisfactory. The case for placing the salmon-disease organism in a separate genus, '*Necromonas*', has not been accepted although in contrast to the other *Aeromonas* species it is non-motile, grows at 5 °C but not at 37 °C, is fermentative and can produce small amounts of gas from glucose; the species name *A. salmonicida* is therefore retained. The genus *Plesiomonas* remains well defined with a single species, *P. shigelloides*, though many strains are agglutinated by phase 1 *Shigella sonnei* antiserum and it may be more closely related genetically to the Enterobacteriaceae than to *Vibrio* and *Aeromonas*. Similarly, RNA sequencing suggests that *Aeromonas* could be separated from the Vibrionaceae into a new family, Aeromonadaceae (Colwell *et al.*, 1986). Under these proposals, the Vibrionaceae would contain *Vibrio* and *Photobacterium* as well as the new genera *Listonella* and *Shewanella*. The latter genus, *Shewanella*, would contain no pathogens but include some species previously placed in *Alteromonas*. However, unlike the other genera in this family, strains of *Alteromonas* are not active fermenters and we suspect their inclusion in such a new genus may not meet with general approval (but see Section 7.5). Taxonomists will no doubt continue to debate the generic allocation of species but for identification purposes and for convenience we still prefer to consider *Vibrio*, *Aeromonas* and *Plesiomonas* together because they share so many routine laboratory test characteristics; we also continue, for the same reasons, to consider *Chromobacterium violaceum* in this group since the production of a diffusible pigment may be no more than a species characteristic.

7.8.1 Vibrio (Table 7.8*a*, *b*, *c*).

At present, some 34 species of *Vibrio* have been validly described, though knowledge of those recently approved is limited and many of them have not been isolated from clinical material. They all require NaCl for growth, the optimum concentration varying with the species; the requirement of some, such as *V. cholerae*, *V. metschnikovii* and *V. mimicus*, as well as some strains of *V. fluvialis*, *V. furnissii* and *V. anguillarum*, is so low that they are able to grow, albeit suboptimally, in Tryptone Water without added NaCl. In contrast, halophilic marine species such as *V. alginolyticus* and *V. parahaemolyticus* can tolerate concentrations of NaCl as high as 6–8%. All the medically important species will, however, grow in isolation and identification media containing 1% NaCl, as indeed do virtually all pathogenic bacteria. The differentiation of arginine-positive *Vibrio* species from *Aeromonas*, however, depends on this salt requirement. The name *Vibrio* usually implies gastrointestinal infection caused by *V. cholerae* or by the marine organism *V. parahaemolyticus*, which is commonly associated with food-poisoning from sea-foods; but many other

Vibrio species may also cause sporadic cases of diarrhoea as well as opportunist superficial eye, ear or wound infections.

For the isolation of cholera and other vibrios from faeces, both direct plating and enrichment methods should be used. All the known enteropathogenic species, (except *V. hollisae*) grow on Thiosulphate Citrate Bile-salt Sucrose medium (TCBS) which is the selective agar medium of choice. After overnight incubation on TCBS Agar at 37 °C, large or medium-sized yellow (sucrose-fermenting) colonies should be subcultured onto Nutrient Agar, checked for purity, and tested for agglutination with *V. cholerae* O1 antiserum and for the oxidase reaction. This may be sufficient for recognition of an epidemic strain but otherwise biochemical characterization should be used for generic confirmation and species identification. With seafood and related environmental samples associated with food-poisoning, large yellow (sucrose-fermenting) colonies with a tendency to spread or swarm are more likely to be *V. alginolyticus*, a widespread halophilic and chitinolytic marine organism. Green (sucrose non-fermenting) colonies on TCBS medium should be regarded as probable strains of *V. parahaemolyticus* (Barrow & Miller, 1976).

Enrichment in Alkaline Peptone Water containing 1% NaCl with early subculture from the surface to TCBS or other selective agar media is suitable for all vibrios. For *V. parahaemolyticus* in food and environmental samples, however, selective enrichment in media such as Glucose Salt Teepol Broth or Polymyxin Salt Broth can be used (Barrow & Miller, 1976; Ayres & Barrow, 1978; Joseph, Kaper & Colwell, 1982). Isolation of vibrios from clinical material other than faeces is relatively easy as they all grow well on Blood Agar and other non-selective media.

We show the characters useful for distinguishing *Vibrio* species from each other as well as from related genera in Tables 7.8*a*, *b*: the species listed have all been encountered in clinical material or in associated food and environmental samples. For provisional identification vibrios are motile Gram-negative rods which ferment glucose without gas production, are sensitive to the vibriostatic agent O/129 (2-4-diamino-6,7-diisopropylpteridine) and, except for *V. metschnikovii* which is atypical, are oxidase-positive.

Table 7.8a. *Second–stage table for* Vibrio, Aeromonas, Plesiomonas, Chromobacterium *and* Janthinobacterium

	1	2	3	4	5	6	7	8	9
Growth at 37 °C	+	+	+	+	+	–	+	+	–
Motility	+	+	+	+	d	–	+	+	+
Oxidase	+	+	–	+	+	+	+	+	+
Nitrate reduced	+	+	–	+	+	+	+	+	+
Møller's decarboxylases									
arginine	–	+	+	–	+	+	+	+	–
lysine	+	d	d	–	d	d	+	–	–
ornithine	d	–	–	–	–	–	+	–	–
Gas from glucose	–	d	–	–	d	w/–	–	–	–
Resistance to									
O/129 10 µg	d	d	–	d	+	+	d	–	–
O/129 150 µg	–	–	–	d	+	d	d	–	–
Growth with 0% NaCl	d	d	d	–	+	+	+	?	?
Growth with 6% NaCl	d	d	+	+	–	–	–	–	?

1 **Vibrio** spp. including *V. cholerae, V. mimicus, V. vulnificus, V. parahaemolyticus, V. alginolyticus, V. harveyi, V. cincinnatiensis*
2 **Vibrio** spp. including *V. fluvialis, V. furnissii, V. anguillarum, V. damsela*
3 **Vibrio** spp. including *V. metschnikovii*
4 **Vibrio** spp. including *V. hollisae, V. natriegens*
5 **Aeromonas** spp.
6 **Aeromonas salmonicida**
7 **Plesiomonas shigelloides**
8 **Chromobacterium violaceum**
9 **Janthinobacterium lividum**

Symbols used in the tables are explained in Tables 5.1 and 5.2 on p.47.

Although not taxonomically valid, Barrow & Miller (1976) found the catalase reaction and the methylene blue sensitivity test of Yan (1969) helpful for screening purposes. All vibrios have a DNA G+C mole% ratio of between 38 and 51 compared with 57–60 for *Aeromonas* (Véron, 1966; Hugh & Sakazaki, 1972) and most of them possess a single polar flagellum; these characters are of little use for differentiation in the routine laboratory where the key tests for this purpose include the O–F, VP and sugar reactions, Moeller's arginine, lysine and ornithine tests and those for nitrate reduction and salt tolerance.

Taxonomically *V. cholerae* is a homogeneous species, comprising organisms that are similar to each other biochemically, share a common H antigen and are closely related genetically. Based on the somatic O antigen scheme of Sakazaki *et al.* (1970) more than 80 serogroups are now recognised within the species (Donovan, 1984), serogroup O1 representing the causal organism of epidemic and pandemic cholera. The cholera toxin (CT) responsible for the 'rice water' stools of cholera has been characterized, the gene concerned identified and a DNA probe developed for its recognition (Mekalanos, 1985). Although not yet applicable in routine laboratories, such a gene probe would enable the rapid screening of strains for toxigenicity. Some strains of other serogroups, termed 'non-O1 *V. cholerae*', can also produce cholera toxin. In contrast, in countries where cholera is not endemic, O1 strains, particularly from environmental sources, usually lack the CT gene.

V. cholerae serogroups occur, sometimes in large numbers, in brackish and estuarine waters throughout the world; most of these environmental strains are incapable of producing CT, and they probably do not cause diarrhoea. Toxigenic strains may however also survive in such waters for many years (Miller, Feachem & Drasar, 1985; Bourke *et al.*, 1986). Strains of 'non-O1 *V. cholerae*' may be isolated from sporadic cases of diarrhoea: indeed in countries where cholera is not endemic, such strains are more likely to be isolated than O1 strains from those

Table 7.8b. *Third–stage table for* Vibrio

	1	2	3	4	5	6	7	8	9	10	11	12	13	14
Swarming	–	–	–	d	+	–	?	–	–	–	?	–	?	–
Growth with 0% NaCl	+	+	–	–	–	–	–	d	d	d	–	+	–	–
Møller's decarboxylases:														
arginine	–	–	–	–	–	–	–	+	+	+	+	+	–	–
lysine	+	+	+	+	+	+	+	–	–	–	d	d	–	–
ornithine	+	+	+	+	d	+	–	–	–	–	–	–	–	–
Nitrates reduced	+	+	+	+	+	+	+	+	+	+	+	–	+	+
Oxidase	+	+	+	+	+	+	+	+	+	+	+	–	+	+
Gas from glucose	–	–	–	–	–	–	–	–	+	–	–	–	–	–
Indole	+	+	+	+	+	+	–	d	–	+	–	+	+	–
ONPG	+	+	+	–	–	d	+	+	+	+	–	+	–	d
VP	+	–	–	–	+	–	+	–	+	+	d	–	–	–
Resistance to														
0/129 10 µg	–	–	d	+	+	d	+	+	+	d	–	–	–	+
0/129 150 µg	–	–	–	–	d	d	–	–	–	–	–	–	–	–
ampicillin 10 µg	–	–	–	+	+	+	–	+	+	+	?	d	?	–
polymyxin B 50 i.u.	+	–	d	d	–	–	–	–	–	–	–	–	–	–
Hydrolysis of:														
starch	+	–	+	+	+	+	+	+	d	+	?	+	?	+
urea	–	–	—	d	d	d	–	–	–	–	–	–	–	d
Acid from:														
L–arabinose	–	–	–	d	–	–	+	+	+	d	–	–	+	+
arbutin	–	d	+	–	–	d	+	d	–	–	?	d	–	+
salicin	–	–	+	–	d	+	+	d	–	–	–	d	–	+
sucrose	+	–	d	–	d	d	+	+	+	+	–	+	–	+
xylose	–	–	–	–	–	–	+	–	–	–	–	–	–	–
Growth on:														
ethanol	–	–	–	d	d	–	–	+	+	–	?	–	?	d
propanol	–	–	–	+	d	–	?	+	+	–	?	–	?	d
D–galacturonate	–	–	–	–	–	–	?	+	+	–	?	–	?	d
D–glucosamine	+	+	+	+	d	–	?	+	+	+	?	d	?	+

1 **Vibrio cholerae;**
  V. comma'; cholera vibrio
2 **Vibrio mimicus**
3 **Vibrio vulnificus**
4 **Vibrio parahaemolyticus;**
  '*Beneckea parahaemolytica*';
  '*Oceonomonas parahaemolytica*';
  '*Pastemella haemolytica*';
  '*Pseudomonas enteritis*'

5 **Vibrio alginolyticus;**
  '*Oceonomonas alginolytica*'
6 **Vibrio harveyi**
7 **Vibrio cincinnatiensis**
8 **Vibrio fluvialis;**
  V. fluvialis biotype I
9 **Vibrio furnissii;**
  V. fluvialis biotype II
10 **Vibrio anguillarum**

11 **Vibrio damsela**
12 **Vibrio metschnikovii**
13 **Vibrio hollisae**
14 **Vibrio natriegens**

Data for *V. cincinnatiensis* from Brayton et al. (1986). Data for *V. damsela* and *V. hollisae* from Farmer, Hickman-Brenner & Kelly (1985). Remaining data from Bryant *et al.* (1986a,b)

Symbols used in the table are explained in Tables 5.1 and 5.2 on p.47.

returning from warm climates. Although occasional non-O1 strains can produce cholera toxin most of them have a different enteropathogenic mechanism, as do non-CT-producing O1 strains which are occasionally isolated from patients with diarrhoea. Only O1 strains that produce cholera toxin seem to be associated with cholera epidemics whereas the majority of those isolated from the environment, whatever their serogroup, appear to be incapable of causing diarrhoea.

Thus, within the species *V. cholerae* as now defined, there is a continuous spectrum from enteropathogenic epidemic O1 strains at one extreme to non-pathogenic strains present in the environment at the other extreme. Taxonomists accordingly argue that the colloquial terms 'non-cholera vibrio' (NCV) and 'non-agglutinable vibrio' (NAG) often applied in the past to non-O1 strains should no longer be used because of the variability in their toxigenicity, and because they are of course agglutinated by their homologous antisera. Also these terms have previously been used wrongly by the inclusion of other *Vibrio* species and even aeromonads within them. We certainly agree that the term 'non-agglutinable vibrio' (NAG) is inappropriate though we still think that 'non-cholera vibrio' (NCV) has as much if not more meaning medically (and microbiologically) than the awkward term 'non-O1 *V. cholerae*'. However, the clinical and epidemiological significance of vibrio isolates should in any case always be explained to clinicians.

The epidemic cholera strains, *V. cholerae* O1, can be divided into two variants commonly called the 'Classical' or *cholerae* biotype and the *eltor* (or El Tor) biotype. The *eltor* biotype was largely responsible for the pandemic in Asia which began in the 1960s and replaced the classical strains, until the latter reappeared. In general, *eltor* strains are VP-positive: they haemolyse sheep erythrocytes in Thioglycollate Cysteine Agar (Sakazaki, Tamura & Murase, 1971) or in the tube test of Feeley & Pittman (1963); agglutinate chicken erythrocytes in the slide test of Finkelstein & Mukerjee (1963); are sensitive to polymyxin B (50iu disc test of Gan & Tija, 1963); resistant to classical phage IV (Mukerjee, Guha & Guha-Roy, 1957); and sensitive to *eltor* phage V (Basu & Mukerjee, 1968). Classical strains have the opposite reaction in each of these tests. As they require careful standardization and adequate controls, these tests are more suitable for reference laboratories. The majority of non-O1 strains and O1 environmental isolates are strongly haemolytic and show the other characteristics of *eltor* strains except that they are usually resistant to both phages.

Strains of *V. cholerae* O1 may be subdivided with absorbed sera into antigenic variants or subtypes called Ogawa, Inaba and Hikojima which share three somatic antigens (a, b and c) in different proportions. Absorption of O1 antiserum with Ogawa organisms produces a serum which agglutinates Inaba and Hikojima but not Ogawa strains. Similarly O1 antiserum absorbed with Inaba organisms agglutinates only Ogawa and Hikojima strains. Unabsorbed *V. cholera* O1 antiserum is still commonly but confus-

ingly described as 'polyvalent *V. cholerae* antiserum' because it agglutinates all three of these O1 variants although it does not agglutinate strains of non-O1 serogroups. As there are only three antigenic variants, more than one of which may be isolated from the same patient (Sakazaki & Tamura, 1971), they have only limited, if any, value for epidemiological purposes. Nor are the fermentation groups of Heiberg (1936) of any use as they do not correlate with anything and they cannot distinguish between *Vibrio* and *Aeromonas* (Sakazaki, Gomez & Sebald, 1967).

Infection with *V. parahaemolyticus*, a marine organism widely distributed in temperate and warm coastal waters throughout the world, is usually associated with inadequately cooked or raw seafoods; indeed, it is the commonest cause of food poisoning in Japan. First described by Fujino in 1951 (see Fujino, 1974) and regarded as a species of *Pasteurella*, it was later placed in the genus *Pseudomonas* and finally, following taxonomic studies, in *Vibrio* (Sakazaki, Iwanami & Fukumi, 1963; Fujino *et al.*, 1965). Most strains isolated from patients with diarrhoea are Kanagawa-positive – that is, they are able to lyse human erythrocytes in Wagatsuma agar – in contrast to less than 1% of isolates from seafoods and environmental samples (Miyamoto *et al.*, 1969; Peffers *et al.*, 1973). Despite much research, the correlation between haemolysin production and pathogenicity is still unclear, although a laboratory infection and volunteer feeding tests convinced Sakazaki and his colleagues (1968) that Kanagawa–positive strains are potentially pathogenic. For epidemiological purposes, some strains may be further differentiated by their O and K antigens (Sakazaki & Balows, 1981) and commercial sets of antisera are available. Serologically, *V. parahaemolyticus* and *V. alginolyticus* have a common H antigen and there is some overlapping of O antigens (Sakazaki *et al.*, 1968).

V. mimicus (Davis *et al.*, 1981) has the same H antigen as *V. cholerae* and strains of this species were originally regarded as sucrose-negative variants of it. However, DNA hybridization and phenotypic characterization confirm its separate identity. Unfortunately, true sucrose–negative strains of *V. cholerae* do occur occasionally but, unlike *V. mimicus*, they are VP–positive and resistant to Polymyxin B (50 iu). *V. mimicus* has been isolated occasionally from sporadic

125

cases of diarrhoea usually following the consumption of seafood; its enterotoxgenicity is similar to that of strains of non-O1 *V. cholerae*.

V. fluvialis (Lee *et al.*, 1981), previously described as 'group F' and as 'CDC group EF6' (Huq *et al.*, 1980) halophilic vibrios, comprises two biovars: I (anaerogenic) and II (aerogenic). However, based on DNA hybridization biovar II was assigned to a new species *V. furnissii* (Brenner *et al.*, 1983). The anaerogenic *V. fluvialis* occurs in fresh, brackish and estuarine waters throughout the world (Lee *et al.*, 1981). The circumstantial evidence for its enteropathogenicity is strong but, like *V. parahaemolyticus*, the mechanism has yet to be elucidated (Huq *et al.*, 1980; Lockwood, Kreger & Richardson, 1982).

V. furnissii (Brenner *et al.*, 1983) is similar in habitat to *V. fluvialis* and has been isolated occasionally from patients with diarrhoea, though usually together with recognised pathogens; there is no direct evidence of its pathogenicity. Gas production from sugar differentiates it from *V. fluvialis* (Table 7.8c). The recently described halophilic species *V. hollisae* (Hickman *et al.*, 1982) isolated from faeces on Sheep Blood Agar may be missed because it does not grow on TCBS or MacConkey agar or on other commonly used media selective for intestinal pathogens; its pathogenic role is uncertain (Morris *et al.*, 1982). Other species, such as *V. alginolyticus* and *V. metschnikovii*, have also been detected occasionally in faeces but there is no evidence to implicate them as the causal agents of diarrhoea.

Except for *V. anguillarum*, *V. harveyi* and *V. natriegens*, all the *Vibrio* species in Table 7.8b, including the halophilic species *V. alginolyticus* (Furniss, Lee & Donovan, 1978) and *V. damsela* (Love *et al.*, 1981; Morris *et al.*, 1982) have been isolated occasionally from opportunist tissue infections, which are usually superficial. *V. vulnificus*, previously known as 'Lactose–positive (L+) *Vibrios*' (Farmer, 1979) and briefly as '*Beneckea vulnifica*' (Reichelt, Baumann & Baumann, 1976), has been implicated occasionally in severe wound infections and septicaemia (Tison & Kelly, 1984). As it is similar to *V. parahaemolyticus*, reports prior to 1979 of such infections caused by the latter should be viewed with caution. Unlike *V. parahaemolyticus*, *V. vulnificus* ferments arbutin and salicin. *V. cincinnatiensis*

(Brayton *et al.*, 1986) was isolated from the blood and CSF of a patient with meningitis; similar organisms have also been isolated from animal faeces.

Recent reviews on the identification and characterization of *Vibrio* species and related genera include those of Sakazaki & Balows (1981), Joseph, Kaper & Colwell, (1982), Lee & Donovan (1985) and Bryant *et al.* (1986a, b).

> **Minidefinition:** *Vibrio. Gram–negative rods, motile. Aerobic and facultatively anaerobic. Catalase-positive. Oxidase-positive and reduce nitrate to nitrite (except V. metschnikovii). Attack sugars by fermentation; gas not produced. NaCl (Na+ ions) essential for growth. Type species: V. cholerae; NCTC strain 8021.*

7.8.2 Aeromonas (Tables 7.8a, c).

In contrast to *Vibrio*, the subdivision of *Aeromonas* into species still remains controversial, especially as the fish pathogen previously classified as '*Necromonas salmonicida*' is now retained within it. Excluding the latter, Cowan, in the previous edition of this *Manual*, agreed with Ewing, Hugh & Johnson, (1961) that there should only be a single species, *A. hydrophila*, although Eddy (1960, 1962) had distinguished two species, the aerogenic, VP–positive, gluconate positive '*A. liquefaciens*', and the anaerogenic VP-negative, gluconate-negative '*A. formicans*'. Schubert (1967a,b), however, regarded anaerogenic strains as varieties of three aerogenic species, which he labelled *A. punctata*, *A. hydrophila*, and *A. salmonicida*. Later, Schubert (1971) argued that the aerogenic species, '*A. liquefaciens*', should be abandoned as it was not recognizable, and that the VP–positive *A. hydrophila*, which he described, should become the type species. The main difference between *A. hydrophila* and *A. punctata* (which Schubert had previously favoured as the type species) seemed to be only the production of acetoin (VP–positive) by the former. The strain described as a new species, '*A. proteolytica*', by Merkel *et al.* (1964) is not an aeromonad but a *Vibrio* species correctly named *V. proteolyticus*.

The current division of *Aeromonas* is based on motility and optimum growth temperature. The non–motile strains, which do not grow at 37 °C and are pathogenic for fish, fall into the genetically

Table 7.8c. *Third-stage table for* Aeromonas, Plesiomonas *and* Vibrio *(V. fluvialis and V. furnissii)*

	1	2	3	4	5	6	7	8
Motility	+	+	d	d	d	+	+	+
Growth in 0% NaCl	+	+	+	+	+	d	d	+
Growth in 6% NaCl	−	−	−	−	−	+	+	−
Møller's decarboxylases:								
arginine	+	+	+	+	+	+	+	+
lysine	+	+	−	+	d	−	−	+
ornithine	−	−	−	−	−	−	−	+
Gluconate oxidation	+	d	−	−	−	−	−	−
Gas from glucose	d	d	−	d	−	−	+	−
Indole	+	+	d	d	d	d	−	+
VP	+	d	−	−	d	−	−	−
Resistance to								
O/129 10 µg	+	+	+	+	+	+	+	+
O/129 150 µg	d	+	+	d	d	−	−	−
Hydrolysis of:								
aesculin	+	−	d	d	−	d	−	−
lecithin	d	+	d	+	−	+	+	−
Acid from:								
L–arabinose	d	−	+	?	d	+	+	−
arbutin	+	−	d	+	−	d	−	−
inositol	d	−	−	−	−	−	−	d
salicin	+	d	d	d	d	d	−	−
sucrose	+	+	+	d	+	+	+	−
Growth on:								
ethanol	−	−	−	−	−	+	+	−
propanol	−	−	−	−	−	+	+	−
D–galacturonate	−	−	d	−	−	+	+	−
D–glucosamine	+	+	+	−	−	+	+	+

1 **Aeromonas hydrophila**; *'A. liquefaciens', 'A. punctata';* *'A. formicans'*
2 **Aeromonas sobria**
3 **Aeromonas caviae**
4 **Aeromonas salmonicida** subspecies **salmonicida**; *'Necromonas salmonicida'*
5 **Aeromonas salmonicida** subspecies **masoucida** and **achromogenes**; *'Necromonas salmonicida'*
6 **Vibrio fluvialis**; *Vibrio fluvialis* biovar I
7 **Vibrio furnissii**; *Vibrio fluvialis* biovar II
8 **Plesiomonas shigelloides**; C27; *'Aeromonas shigelloides';* *'Vibrio shigelloides'; 'Fergusonia shigelloides'; 'Pseudomonas michigani'*

Symbols used in this table are explained in Tables 5.1 and 5.2 on p.47.

homogeneous species, *A. salmonicida*, which has three phenotypic subspecies: *salmonicida, masoucida* and *achromogenes*. A proposed new species, *A. media*, found in the environment is also non–motile and is described as intermediate between *A. hydrophila* and *A. salmonicida* (Allen, Austin & Colwell, 1983). As neither *A. salmonicida* nor *A. media* causes disease in man we disregard them,

although for comparison with other species we include the former in Table 7.8*b*.

The majority of motile strains, which grow well at 37 °C, fall into three phenotypic groups corresponding to those described by Popoff & Véron (1976) called *A. hydrophila, A. sobria* and *A. caviae*: they can be differentiated by the production of acid from salicin and gas from glucose. DNA hybridization has demonstrated other groups but these cannot be otherwise distinguished (Popoff *et al.*, 1981). However, in the *Approved Lists of Bacterial Names* (1980) *A. punctata* is listed with two subspecies: *caviae* and *punctata*; and the DNA studies of Popoff *et al.*, (1981) also revealed two hybridization groups in the 'caviae–punctata' group. We therefore leave it to taxonomists to resolve the nomenclatural complexities in this area and refer only to *A. caviae* in Table 7.8*c*.

The motile aeromonads are common in freshwater environments where they are frequently the dominant aerobic bacteria. They have been isolated from a wide range of clinical infections of wounds and soft tissues, sometimes following exposure to water, and from some patients with diarrhoea in the absence of recognised pathogens as well as from septicaemia in immunocompromised patients. Their possible enteropathogenic role has received much recent attention (Pitarangsi *et al.*, 1982; Burke *et al.*, 1983) and a number of selective media have been described for their isolation from faeces (von Graevenitz & Bucher, 1983; Lee & Donovan, 1985).

Aeromonas species, in particular *A. caviae*, may be confused with strains of *Vibrio fluvialis* and *V. furnissii* but resistance to the vibriostatic agent O/129 (150µg disc) and growth in the absence of NaCl as well as growth of the vibrios in the presence of 6% NaCl should resolve the matter.

> **Minidefinition:** *Aeromonas. Gram-negative rods. Motile and non-motile. Aerobic and facultatively anaerobic. Catalase-positive; oxidase-positive. NaCl (Na⁺ ions) not required for growth. Sugars are attacked fermentatively and gas may be produced. Type species: A. hydrophila; NCTC strain 8049.*

7.8.3 Plesiomonas (Tables 7.8*a,c*). The existence of this genus was due almost entirely to uncertainty about the allocation of its single species, *P.*

shigelloides, which has been placed previously in *Aeromonas*, *Vibrio* and *Pseudomonas*. Originally referred to as the C27 organism of Ferguson & Henderson (1947), it was moved to the now valid genus *Plesiomonas* created for it by Habs & Schubert (1962) and supported by Eddy and Carpenter (1964). Its specific name is based on the observation that many strains are agglutinated by phase 1 antiserum to *Shigella sonnei*, from which they can be distinguished by their motility and positive oxidase reaction. They can be differentiated readily from aeromonads and vibrios by O/129 resistance, fermentation of inositol and the production of ornithine decarboxylase and DNase. Most *P. shigelloides* strains are isolated from patients with diarrhoea, often in the absence of known pathogens (Pitarangsi *et al*, 1982); other infections in children have been summarized by Pathak, Caster & Levy (1983).

> **Minidefinition:** *Plesiomonas. Gram-negative rods; motile. Aerobic and facultatively anaerobic. Catalase-positive; oxidase-positive. Sugars attacked by fermentation; gas is not produced. Inositol is fermented and gelatin not liquefied. Ornithine decarboxylase-positive (Møller). Type species: P. shigelloides; NCTC strain 10360.*

7.8.4   Chromobacterium (Table 7.8a) is a genus with a single mesophilic species, *C. violaceum*, that may be isolated occasionally in the clinical laboratory. Like the psychrophilic organism, *Janthinobacterium lividum*, it produces a violet pigment, violacein, that is soluble in ethanol, acetone and amyl alcohol, but is insoluble in chloroform and in water and therefore does not diffuse through the medium. Production of violacein is encouraged by the presence of mannitol and yeast extract in the medium but the pigment makes the oxidase test difficult to read; it is produced only in the presence of abundant oxygen (Sneath 1960).

The older descriptions of *C. violaceum* are confusing because the name was given to nearly all cultures that produced a violet pigment. Sneath (1956) applied the name correctly to the mesophiles; but Leifson (1956) and Eltinge (1956, 1957) used it for the psychrophile now called *Janthinobacterium lividum*. Apart from differing in the temperature range for growth, *J. lividum* has an oxidative metabolism and

we think it is therefore correctly placed with the other oxidizers in Table 7.5; for comparison with the mesophilic organisms, however, we include its characters also in Table 7.8a.

C. violaceum may occasionally be pathogenic for man (Sneath, 1960; Johnson, Disalvo & Stener, 1971) causing abscesses, urinary tract and systemic infections and possibly diarrhoea. The likely source is from soil or water but this has never been clearly demonstrated.

> **Minidefinition:** *Chromobacterium. Gram-negative rods, motile. Aerobic and facultatively anaerobic. Catalase-positive (usually); oxidase-positive. Attack sugars fermentatively. Type species: C. violaceum; NCTC strain 9757.*

7.9   The enterobacteria
(*Buttiauxella, Cedecea, Citrobacter, Edwardsiella, Enterobacter, Erwinia, Escherichia, Hafnia, Klebsiella, Kluyvera, Morganella, Proteus, Providencia, Salmonella, Serratia, Shigella, Tatumella, Yersinia* and others)

***Characters common to members of the group*: Gram-negative rods. Aerobic and facultatively anaerobic. Oxidase-negative. Attack sugars fermentatively. Nitrate reduced to nitrite.**

The enterobacteria grow readily on simple media, on which they will survive for years in tubes sealed with paraffin wax. The majority of species, being easy and 'safe' to handle, provide students, biochemists, geneticists, and even bacteriologists with suitable experimental material. Nevertheless, laboratory infections do occur, especially with *Shigella*, which has a very low infective dose. Because some strains are important pathogens for man and animals and cause intestinal and other infections as well as food-poisoning, the group has considerable epidemiological importance and means are available to 'fingerprint' the members precisely. They have been studied exhaustively by numerous bacteriologists and have introduced many to taxonomy; they have provided feasts for the splitters and banquets for the geneticists. As a result they have been divided into a large number of genera and species, some of which have been further subdivided into countless serotypes and phage types, but, as Kampelmacher (1959) pointed out, there are no antigenic frontiers among the enterobacteria and there is a great deal of overlapping.

The whole group corresponds to what was 'Bacterium' before that genus became the dumping ground for bacteria that could not be assigned readily to some other genus. Nowadays it it usual, if not meaningful, to split the enterobacteria first into tribes and then into genera. In a review of the group, Cowan (in Bergey's Manual, 1974) speculated that what are now regarded as tribes may become the genera of the future as he considered that there had been an excessive subdivision of the group into genera and species; however, recent DNA data now largely confirm the validity of these subdivisions. In this Manual we do not make the division into tribes; we have taken genera and species that will be accepted by most (but not by all) bacteriologists and show some characters (not important in themselves) by which they can be distinguished. A second-stage table (7.9a) leads on to four third-stage tables (7.9b, c, d, e) by which an unknown strain of the group can be identified down to species level in the group. The classification of the enterobacteria is by no means final and the divisions we make do not always correspond to those made by others. Numerous synonyms are given to assist the reader in relating current names to older literature.

To emphasize that this arrangement is devoid of phylogenetic or hierarchical implications, the notes for the genera have been arranged in alphabetical order. Although the tables are useful in aiding identification down to species level as it is understood in this group, this level is well below that of species in many other large groups of bacteria such as the corynebacteria and streptococci. This picture may well change, however, as other large bacterial groups are studied as intensively as the enterobacteria. We do not proceed to biotypes or to the finer subdivisions made by serological and phage-typing methods since few clinical laboratories will have a sufficiently wide range of antisera or phages for such work. Fortunately, reference laboratories are available in many countries, and even if they are national, the services are usually international.

An entirely different means of arriving at an identification of enterobacteria in stages was described by

Baer & Washington (1972). In this method individual characters are scored (e.g. acid from mannitol = 5; gas from mannitol = 10; acid from lactose = 20; growth in KCN medium = 320), and the total score is looked up in one or more identification tables. Such numerical diagnostic keys are discussed in Chapter 8; they have also been extensively reviewed by D'Amato, Holmes & Bottone, (1981).

During the course of intestinal infections, the enterobacteria may be isolated from the bloodstream, intestinal contents (bile or faeces), often from urine, and occasionally from marrow biopsies. In the intestine they form part of a mixed bacterial flora, and are usually isolated by means of enrichment and selective media, from which pure cultures for identification must be obtained by plating on non-inhibitory media.

7.9.1 **'Aerobacter'** is a name that has caused much confusion because it has been applied to several different organisms. Originally used by Beijerinck (1900) for organisms (motile or non-motile) that had optimal growth temperatures about 28 °C but which would not grow at 37 °C, it was later used extensively for organisms that grew at 37 °C or higher, and were usually non-motile. In 1958 Hormaeche & Edwards, who wanted to distinguish klebsiellas from motile bacteria with similar IMViC reactions, used the name for a motile organism that grew at 37 °C; when they realized the difficulties arising from the use of the same name for two different organisms, they changed the name of the group of motile bacteria to Enterobacter (Hormaeche & Edwards, 1960).

Carpenter and many others (1970) asked the Judicial Commission to give an opinion on the use of the name 'Aerobacter' and in Opinion 46 (1971) the Commission declared the name rejected.

7.9.2 **'Bacterium'**, as a generic name, has been outlawed for many years (Opinion 4, revised, 1954) and it is now no longer used. The reason for its rejection was the different usage in different countries, although in any one country its use was probably well known and understood. In British practice it was traditionally used for Gram-negative rods that essentially comprised the enterobacteria; in the sixth edition of Bergey's Manual (1948), which was typical of American practice at that time, the genus 'Bacterium'

Table 7.9a. *Second-stage table for differentiation of the enterobacteria*

	1	2	3	4	5	6	7	8	9	10	11	12	13	14	15[c]	16[d]	17	18[c]
Motility	+	+	+	+	+	+	+	d	−	+	+	d	d	D	+	−	−	D
Yellow pigment	−	−	−	−	D	d	D	−	−	−	−	−	−	−	−	−	−	−
Red pigment	−	−	−	−	−	−	−	−	−	−	−	−	−	−	D	−	−	−
MacConkey growth	+	+	+	+	+	+	+	+	+	+	+	+	+	+	+	+	+	d
Simmons' citrate	d	D	+	−	+	d	D	d	D	+	−	D	d	D	+	−	−	D
Christensen's citrate	+	+	+	+	+	+	D	+	+	+	d	d	+	+	+	−	+	D
Urease	−	−	d	−	D	−	−	−	D	−	+	+	D	−	D	−	−	D
Gelatin hydrolysis	−	−	−	−	D	d	D	−	D	−	−	+	−	D	+	−	−	−
Growth in KCN medium	+	D	D	−	D	d	D	+	d	+	+	+	+	D	d	−	−	D
H₂S (PbAc paper)	−	−	d	+	−	−	−	d	−	d	+	+	d	d	D	−	−	−
H₂S from TSI	−	−	D	+	−	−	−	−	−	−	−	d	−	d	−	−	−	−
Gluconate	−	D	−	−	+	−	−	+	D	−	−	−	−	−	+	−	−	−
Malonate	+	D	D	−	d	d	D	d	D	+	−	−	−	D	D	−	−	−
ONPG	+	+	+	−	+	+	+	+	D	+	−	−	−	D	+	d	−	+
Phenylalanine	−	−	−	−	−	−	−	−	−	−	+	+	+	−	−	−	−	−
Arginine dihydrolase	−	+	+	−	D	−	D	−	D	−	−	−	−	d	−	d	−	−
Lysine decarboxylase	−	−	−	+	D	−	D	+	D	d	−	−	−	D	D	−	−	−
Ornithine decarboxylase	+	D	d	+	+	−	D	+	−	+	+	D	−	D	D	d	−	D
Selenite reduction	−	D	+	d	+	−	+	+	d	+	d	d	d	+	d	d	−	D
Casein hydrolysis	−	−	−	−	−	−	−	−	−	−	−	D	−	−	d	−	−	−
DNase production	−	−	−	−	D	−	−	−	−	−	−	+	d	D	D	−	−	−
Carbohydrates [in Peptone Water medium], gas from glucose	−	D	+	+	+	−	+	+	D	+	+	+	D	D	D	−	−	−
acid from:																		
adonitol	−	−	D	−	D	−	D	−	+	−	−	−	D	−	D	−	−	−
arabinose	+	−	+	d	+	+	+	+	+	+	−	−	−	D	D	+	−	+
cellobiose	+	+	+	−	+	d	D	d	+	+	−	−	−	D	d	−	−	D
dulcitol	−	−	D	−	−	−	D	−	D	−	−	−	−	D	−	−	−	−
glycerol	d	D	d	d	d	d	D	+	+	d	d	+	d	D	+	d	−	+
inositol	−	−	−	−	D	−	−	−	+	−	−	−	D	D	+	−	−	D
lactose	+	D	+	−	+	d	d	−	D	+	−	−	−	D	D	−	−	D
maltose	+	+	+	+	+	d	+	+	+	+	−	D	−	D	+	d	−	+
mannitol	+	+	+	−	+	+	+	+	+	+	−	−	D	+	+	+	−	+
raffinose	+	D	D	−	+	d	D	−	+	+	−	−	−	−	D	d	−	D
rhamnose	+	−	+	−	+	+	+	+	+	+	−	−	D	D	D	D	−	D
salicin	+	+	D	−	+	+	d	d	+	+	−	D	D	D	+	−	+	D
sorbitol	−	D	+	−	D	d	D	d	+	d	−	−	−	D	D	D	−	D
sucrose	−	D	d	−	+	+	D	−	d	+	−	D	d	−	D	−	+	D
trehalose	+	+	+	−	+	+	+	+	+	+	−	d	D	D	+	+	+	+
xylose	+	D	+	−	+	+	+	+	+	+	−	+	−	D	D	−	−	+
starch	−	−	−	−	−	−	−	−	d	−	−	−	−	−	−	−	−	−
MR test (37 °C)[a]	+	+	+	+	D	d	+	d	d	+	+	+	+	+	d	+	−	+
MR test (RT)[b]	+	D	+	+	−	d	+	−	d	+	+	d	+	+	−	+	+	+
VP test (37 °C)[a]	−	D	−	−	d	−	−	d	D	−	−	−	−	−	D	−	−	−
VP test (RT)[b]	−	D	−	−	d	d	−	+	D	−	−	D	−	−	D	−	−	D
Indole	−	−	d	+	−	−	D	−	D	d	+	D	+	−	−	D	−	D
Further details in Table			7.9b						7.9c				7.9d			7.9e		

1 **Buttiauxella agrestis**
2 **Cedecea** spp.
3 **Citrobacter** spp.; *Levinea* spp.
4 **Edwardsiella tarda;** Asakusa biotype; Bartholomew group
5 **Enterobacter** spp.
6 **Erwinia herbicola;** *Enterobacter agglomerans*
7 **Escherichia** spp.
8 **Hafnia alvei**
9 **Klebsiella** spp.
10 **Kluyvera** spp.
11 **Morganella morganii;** *Proteus morganii*
12 **Proteus** spp.
13 **Providencia** spp.
14 **Salmonella** spp. and serotypes
15 **Serratia** spp.[c]
16 **Shigella** spp.[d]
17 **Tatumella ptyseos**
18 **Yersinia** spp.[c]

RT, room temperature (18–22 °C); [a] incubation for two days; [b] incubation for five days. [c] Some strains nitrate-negative. [d] Some strains catalase-negative.

Other symbols used in the table are explained in Tables 5.1 and 5.2 on p.47.

included both Gram-positive and Gram-negative rods.

Most organisms that were formerly called '*Bacterium this-or-that*' in medical laboratories will be found in this *Manual* in Section 7.9 among the enterobacteria. Of the few exceptions, '*Bacterium anitratum*' will be found in Section 7.4.2 under the awkward name of *Acinetobacter calcoaceticus*; and '*Bacterium typhiflavum*' is now placed in *Erwinia* (Section 7.9.8) as *Erwinia herbicola* (Graham & Hodgkiss, 1967).

7.9.3 Buttiauxella (Tables 7.9a, b).

There is but a single species, *B. agrestis*, strains of which have been isolated mostly from water and soil but also from the throat and from urine. They resemble those of *Citrobacter freundii* in their IMViC reactions but differ from them in utilizing malonate, hydrolysing aesculin and usually in failing to ferment sorbitol (Ferragut *et al.*, 1981). Strains of *B. agrestis* also closely resemble those of *Kluyvera* (see Section 7.9.12 and Tables 7.9a, c) but the DNA characteristics show that they should be maintained as separate genera, which Gavini *et al.* (1983) claim can be differentiated on the basis of indole and lysine decarboxylase production and fermentation of sucrose.

> **Minidefinition**: *Buttiauxella. Gram-negative rods, motile. Aerobic and facultatively anaerobic. Catalase-positive; oxidase-negative. Attack sugars fermentatively; gas is not produced. Sucrose-negative. KCN-positive; arginine-negative. Type species: B. agrestis; NCTC strain 12119.*

7.9.4 Cedecea (Tables 7.9a, b).

Originally two named species, *C. davisae* and *C. lapagei*, were described together with three unnamed species referred to as *Cedecea* species 3, 4 and 5 (Grimont *et al.*, 1981). The name *C. neteri* was later proposed for species 4 leaving species 3 and 5 unnamed (Farmer *et al.*, 1982). All strains have been isolated from clinical material, mostly from patients with bacteraemia (Farmer *et al.*, 1982) and from a cutaneous ulcer (Hansen & Glupczynski, 1984). In their biochemical reactions strains of *Cedecea* do not resemble any other member of the Enterobacteriaceae. They do not ferment arabinose or rhamnose or liquefy gelatin nor do they produce extracellular deoxyribonuclease;

they are also resistant to colistin and cephalothin.

> **Minidefinition**: *Cedecea. Gram-negative rods; motile. Aerobic and facultatively anaerobic. Catalase-positive; oxidase-negative. Attack sugars fermentatively. Arabinose-negative. Arginine-positive. Type species: C. davisae; NCTC strain 11645.*

7.9.5 Citrobacter (Tables 7.9a, b).

The common water and soil forms, mainly *Citrobacter freundii*, are rapid lactose fermenters; less common varieties produce indole and may belong to *C. freundii* or more likely to *C. amalonaticus* (originally described as *Levinea amalonatica* by Young *et al.*, 1971) or to *C. koseri* (see below). The Ballerup and Bethesda groups were non- or late-lactose fermenters of the citrobacter group, and in plate cultures could be recognized by the characteristically foul odour they produced.

Sedlák and his colleagues (1971) in a review of 8000 strains of the genus regarded them as 'conditional' or opportunist intestinal pathogens when conditions were suitable for their growth in an unusual situation.

The genus has an unusual history. It was created by Werkman & Gillen (1932) for bacteria that produced trimethylene glycol from glycerol; as tests for this substance were complicated, no-one ever used them but paid attention instead to the character (utilization of citrate as a source of carbon) after which the genus was named. Sedlák *et al.* (1971) recognized two species: *Citrobacter freundii*, H_2S positive, indole-negative, and malonate-positive, and '*C. intermedius*' with the opposite characters; there were also many intermediate forms, which account for the seven species listed by Werkman & Gillen. Of those seven species, only *Citrobacter freundii* became established. Ewing & Davis (1972a) would revive *C. diversus* for the organism named *C. koseri* by Frederiksen (1970) and *Levinea malonatica* by Young *et al.* (1971). We have never been happy with this proposal, however, as the description of *C. diversus* given by Ewing & Davis (1972a) differs in several respects from the original description (Holmes *et al.*, 1974). We prefer to use the name *C. koseri*. Moreover, '*C. intermedius*' is no longer recognized as a separate species.

Chemical analysis of the lipopolysaccharides of

the O antigens indicates that citrobacters are 'closely related to *E. coli*' and that, of twenty citrobacter chemotypes identified, eleven were 'identical with chemotypes occurring in *Salmonella* and *E. coli*' (Keleti *et al.*, 1971). Perhaps citrobacters should be considered as a connecting link uniting *Escherichia* and *Salmonella*; if that is a fair description of the situation then bacteriologists can be excused for wanting a simple test for differentiating *Citrobacter* from *Salmonella*. Catsaras & Buttiaux (1963) thought that the lysine decarboxylase and KCN tests were useful for this purpose; citrobacters were lysine-negative and generally KCN-positive; salmonellas were lysine-positive (with a few exceptions) and KCN-negative. Pickett & Goodman (1966) suggested the ONPG test, but this also had its exceptions. We still think, however, that lactose fermentation is useful (Table 7.9*a*).

> **Minidefinition**: *Citrobacter. Gram-negative rods; motile. Aerobic and facultatively anaerobic. Catalase-positive; oxidase-negative. Attack sugars fermentatively; gas is produced. Citrate-positive; lysine-negative. Type species: C. freundii; NCTC strain 9750.*

7.9.6 Edwardsiella (Tables 7.9*a,b*).

The taxon was first described by Sakazaki & Murata in 1962 (in Japanese) and by Sakazaki (1967), in English, as the 'Asakusa group'. It was redefined by King & Adler (1964) as the 'Bartholomew group', and elevated to a genus by Ewing *et al.* (1965) who also proposed the type species *E. tarda*. A new combination, *Edwardsiella anguillimortifera*, has been proposed for an organism formerly known as '*Paracolobactrum anguillimortiferum*' and considered to be an earlier synonym of *E. tarda* (Sakazaki & Tamura, 1975); they have the same type strain. We continue to use the name *E. tarda* because it has been in common usage for so long.

The features that distinguish *Edwardsiella* from *Escherichia* are mainly quantitative; it produces H_2S in TSI whereas *Escherichia coli* is negative (but may be H_2S-positive if tested by a more sensitive method). *Ewardsiella tarda* ferments fewer sugars more slowly (hence the species name), and a greater proportion of strains decarboxylate lysine and ornithine. In terms of DNA relatedness, however, *Edwardsiella tarda*

forms a distinct homogeneous group (Brenner, 1973). Other biotypes of *E. tarda* and other *Edwardsiella* species have not been isolated from clinical material; for their descriptions see, for example, Holmes & Gross (1983, 1990).

> **Minidefinition**: *Edwardsiella. Gram-negative rods; motile. Aerobic and facultatively anaerobic. Catalase-positive; oxidase-negative. Attack glucose fermentatively; produce gas. H_2S produced on TSI medium. Type species: E. tarda; NCTC strain 10396.*

7.9.7 Enterobacter (Tables 7.9*a,b*)

was the name proposed by Hormaeche & Edwards (1960) for a group of motile organisms with IMViC reactions $- - + +$, and *Enterobacter cloacae* ('*Bacterium cloacae*' Jordan, 1890; '*Cloaca cloacae*' Castellani & Chalmers, 1919) was designated as the type species. Other organisms including *Enterobacter aerogenes*, *E. gergoviae*, *E. sakazakii* and *E. taylorae* have since been placed in the genus. Despite its motility, numerical taxonomic studies of biochemical characteristics (Bascomb *et al.*, 1971) and DNA relatedness (Izard *et al.*, 1980) both indicate that *E. aerogenes* is related more closely to *Klebsiella* species than to the other *Enterobacter* species. The name *Klebsiella mobilis* has therefore been proposed for *E. aerogenes* but it has not been widely accepted. *E. gergoviae* strains were recognized by Richard *et al.* (1976) as a distinct group most similar to *E. aerogenes* though differing from it in producing urease, not growing in KCN medium and in not fermenting adonitol, inositol and sorbitol; the species name *gergoviae* was proposed for them later by Brenner *et al.* (1980b). The name *E. sakazakii* was given to yellow-pigmented strains which failed to ferment sorbitol; such strains were for long regarded as variants of *E. cloacae* until genetic studies showed that they should be recognized as a separate species (Farmer *et al.*, 1980). Although *E. taylorae* occurs occasionally in clinical material, we have not examined representative strains and so do not record its characteristics in the Tables. They are described (Farmer *et al.*, 1985*a*) as giving positive results in the following tests: motility, citrate, KCN, malonate, arginine, ornithine, Voges–Proskaüer and fermentation of glucose (with gas production), arabinose, cellobiose, maltose, mannitol, rhamnose, trehalose and xylose; and negative results for indole,

Table 7.9*b*. *Third-stage table for the enterobacteria (part 1)*

	1	2	3	4	5	6	7	8	9	10	11	12	13	14	15
Motility	+	+	+	+	+	+	+	+	+	+	+	d	+	+	+
Yellow pigment	–	–	–	–	–	–	–	–	–	–	–	–	–	+	d
Red pigment	–	–	–	–	–	–	–	–	–	–	–	–	–	–	–
MacConkey growth	+	+	+	+	+	+	+	+	+	+	+	+	+	+	+
Simmons' citrate	d	–	+	+	+	–	+	+	+	–	+	+	+	+	d
Christensen's citrate	+	+	+	+	+	+	+	+	+	+	+	+	+	+	+
Urease	–	–	–	–	–	–	d	d	d	–	–	d	+	–	–
Gelatin hydrolysis	–	–	–	–	–	–	–	–	–	–	–	d	–	+	d
Growth in KCN medium	+	+	+	+	–	–	+	+	–	–	+	+	–	+	d
H₂S (PbAc paper)	–	–	–	–	–	–	d	+	+	+	–	–	d	–	–
H₂S from TSI	–	–	–	–	–	–	–	+	–	+	–	–	–	–	–
Gluconate	–	–	+	d	+	–	–	–	–	–	+	+	+	+	–
Malonate	+	+	+	+	+	–	–	–	+	–	+	+	+	d	d
ONPG	+	+	+	+	+	+	+	+	+	–	+	+	+	+	+
Phenylalanine	–	–	–	–	–	–	–	–	–	–	–	–	–	–	–
Arginine dihydrolase	–	+	+	+	+	+	+	d	+	–	–	+	–	+	–
Lysine decarboxylase	–	–	–	–	–	–	–	–	–	+	+	–	d	–	–
Ornithine decarboxylase	+	+	–	–	–	+	+	d	d	+	+	+	+	+	–
Selenite reduction	–	d	+	+	+	–	+	+	+	d	+	+	+	+	–
Casein hydrolysis	–	–	–	–	–	–	–	–	–	–	–	–	–	–	–
DNase production	–	–	–	–	–	–	–	–	–	–	–	–	–	+	–
Carbohydrates [in Peptone Water medium],															
gas from glucose	–	–	+	d	+	–	+	+	+	+	+	+	+	+	–
acid from:															
adonitol	–	–	–	–	–	–	–	–	+	–	+	d	–	–	–
arabinose	+	–	–	–	–	–	+	+	+	d	+	+	+	+	+
cellobiose	+	+	+	+	+	+	+	+	+	–	+	+	+	+	d
dulcitol	–	–	–	–	–	–	–	d	–	–	–	–	–	–	–
glycerol	d	d	d	d	+	–	d	+	+	d	+	d	+	d	d
inositol	–	–	–	–	–	–	–	–	–	–	+	–	–	d	–
lactose	+	–	d	d	+	–	+	+	+	–	+	d	d	+	d
maltose	+	+	+	+	+	+	+	+	+	+	+	+	+	+	d
mannitol	+	+	+	+	+	+	+	+	+	–	+	+	+	+	+
raffinose	+	–	–	d	–	+	–	d	–	–	+	d	+	+	d
rhamnose	+	–	–	–	–	–	+	+	+	–	+	+	+	+	+
salicin	+	+	+	+	+	+	+	–	+	–	+	+	+	+	+
sorbitol	–	–	–	d	+	+	+	+	+	–	+	+	–	–	d
sucrose	–	+	–	+	+	+	–	d	d	–	+	+	+	+	+
trehalose	+	+	+	+	+	+	+	+	+	–	+	+	+	+	+
xylose	+	+	–	+	+	+	+	+	+	–	+	+	+	+	+
starch	–	–	–	–	–	–	–	–	–	–	–	–	–	–	–
MR test (37 °C)[a]	+	+	d	+	+	+	+	+	+	+	d	d	+	–	d
MR test (RT)[b]	+	+	–	–	–	–	+	+	+	+	–	–	–	–	d
VP test (37 °C)[a]	–	–	+	–	–	–	–	–	–	–	d	d	–	d	–
VP test (RT)[b]	–	–	+	d	–	–	–	–	–	–	d	d	d	d	d
Indole	–	–	–	–	–	–	+	d	+	+	–	–	–	–	–

1 **Buttiauxella agrestis**
2 **Cedecea davisae**
3 **Cedecea lapagei**
4 **Cedecea species 3**
5 **Cedecea neteri;** *Cedecea* species 4
6 **Cedecea species 5**
7 **Citrobacter amalonaticus;** *'Levinea amalonatica'*
8 **Citrobacter freundii** *'Escherichia freundii';* *'Salmonella coli';* *'S. ballerup';* *'S. hormaechei';* Bethesda-Ballerup group

9 **Citrobacter koseri;** *C. diversus; Levinea malonatica*
10 **Edwardsiella tarda;** *E. anguillimortifera;* Asakusa group; Bartholomew group
11 **Enterobacter aerogenes;** *Klebsiella mobilis;* (NOT *'Aerobacter aerogenes'* Beijerinck)
12 **Enterobacter cloacae;** *'Cloaca cloacae';* *'Aerobacter cloacae'*
13 **Enterobacter gergoviae**
14 **Enterobacter sakazakii**
15 **Erwinia herbicola;** *'Bacterium typhiflavum'*, Enterobacter agglomerans; *Pantoea agglomerans;*

RT, room temperature (18–22 °C); [a] incubation for two days; [b] incubation for five days.

Other symbols used in the table are explained in Tables 5.1 and 5.2 on p.47.

urea, gelatin, H₂S (TSI agar), phenylalanine, lysine, methyl red and fermentation of adonitol, inositol, raffinose and sorbitol. In American literature, the name *Enterobacter agglomerans* is generally used for the organism we describe below (Section 7.9.8) as *Erwinia herbicola*.

The characters of *Enterobacter* species are very similar to those of *Hafnia* and *Serratia*, and Edwards & Ewing (1972) include *Hafnia alvei* (7.9.10) in *Enterobacter*. The two best-known species, *E. cloacae* and *E. aerogenes*, are only weakly urease-positive, thus enabling Matsen's (1970) ten-minute paper-strip test to distinguish between *Enterobacter* (negative) and *Klebsiella* (positive), since it depends on the relative inactivity of the *Enterobacter* species.

> **Minidefinition**: *Enterobacter. Gram-negative rods; motile. Aerobic and facultatively anaerobic. Catalase-positive; oxidase-negative. Attack sugars fermentatively; gas is produced. VP-positive; gluconate-positive. Gelatin may be liquefied slowly. Produce ornithine decarboxylase. Type species: E. cloacae; NCTC strain 10005.*

7.9.8 Erwinia (Tables 7.9a,b).

This genus was named by Winslow *et al.* (1917) after Erwin F. Smith, a plant pathologist who did not agree with and continually argued against the idea of using plant pathogenicity as the keystone for creation of a new genus. We think that certain bacteria isolated from human and other animal sources are so similar to organisms isolated from plants that they should all be included in the same genus; as the plant organisms are part of a recognized genus, *Erwinia*, and since the strains from mammals were never properly classified (until the proposal of the name *Enterobacter agglomerans* by Ewing & Fife, 1972; see below) they should all be regarded as *Erwinia* species. Moreover, Lakso & Starr (1970) found that about a third of the animal strains they tested were as pathogenic for plants as some of the species considered to be natural phytopathogens.

Strains previously labelled 'Bacterium typhiflavum' (Cruickshank, 1935), which for many years could not be placed satisfactorily among the usual 'medical' bacteria, are now regarded as *Erwinia herbicola* (Graham & Hodgkiss, 1967). Similar organisms have been isolated in many clinical laboratories but the characterizations do not always agree with those of the plant pathologists. Such discrepancies may be due to differences in media and temperature of incubation; for example, Ewing & Fife (1972) found that about a quarter of their strains produced gas from glucose, and their characterizations made them allocate their strains instead to *Enterobacter* as *Enterobacter agglomerans*. However, other workers report the human and animals strains as anaerogenic and these results point less clearly to *Enterobacter*. In any case, we are reluctant to accept the proposal of *Enterobacter agglomerans* because the description of the species differs from the original description of 'Bacillus agglomerans' in several important features; in particular, the latter was described as having polar flagella. Although Ewing & Fife (1972) recognized seven anaerogenic and four aerogenic biotypes within *E. agglomerans* this classification showed little correlation with DNA data, by which 10 or more groups could be identified within the species (Brenner *et al.*, 1984). Additional studies are therefore needed before definite proposals for the classification and nomenclature of these organisms can be accepted. Until then we prefer to regard this heterogeneous group as a single species with the name *Erwinia herbicola*.

Although we are not here concerned with the classification and identification of the phytopathogenic erwinias, it should be noted that not all is neat and tidy; indeed Starr & Mandel (1969) are agnostic about the genus. Fermentation end-products merely support the argument that *Erwinia* is a member of the Enterobacteriaceae (White & Starr, 1971), but for the phytopathogens they do not provide any better guide to species than they do for the animal strains. One unusual character not shown in the tables is the symplasmata (sausage-shaped aggregates of bacteria) seen in hanging-drop preparations of the water of condensation from slope cultures (Gilardi, Bottone & Birnbaum, 1970a).

> **Minidefinition**: *Erwinia. Gram-negative rods; motile. Aerobic and facultatively anaerobic. Catalase-positive; oxidase-negative. Attack sugars fermentatively, usually without producing gas. Urease-negative; phenylalanine-negative; KCN-negative. Type species: E. amylovora; ATCC strain 15580.*

7.9.9 Escherichia (Tables 7.9a,c). *Escherichia* is the 'type genus' for the family Enterobacteriaceae and *Escherichia coli* is the type species for the genus. *E. coli* is possibly the most studied as well as one of the more important bacterial pathogens. In addition, the genus includes the less important species *E. adecarboxylata*, *E. blattae*, *E. fergusonii*, *E. hermanii* and *E. vulneris*.

Escherichia coli, like many other enterobacteria, contains numerous serotypes some of which are associated with certain infections in man and in animals. Some are particularly associated with diarrhoeal disease (Gross & Rowe, 1985; Morris & Sojka, 1985) while others cause a variety of extra-intestinal infections (Ørskov & Ørskov, 1985). The species includes a wide range of biochemical varieties, from the 'typical' motile, aerogenic, lactose-fermenting strains to the much less reactive and frequently non-motile strains that closely resemble *Shigella*. Such strains may be difficult to distinguish from shigellas and tests for the utilization of citrate (Christensen's medium) and the decarboxylation of lysine are particularly useful for this purpose. These problematic strains also include the Alkalescens–Dispar (A–D) group, a term previously used for organisms named '*B. alkalescens*' and '*B. dispar*' by Andrewes (1918) and which were once thought to be shigellas. They are now regarded as anaerogenic (non-motile) biotypes of *E. coli* (Ewing, 1949b); the old term A–D is no longer used.

It is not surprising that the distinction between *E. coli* and *Shigella* may be difficult as Brenner *et al.* (1982c) have shown by DNA hybridization that the two organisms belong to a single genetic species. To make the distinction even more difficult, there is considerable antigenic overlap between *E. coli* and *Shigella* so that virtually every *Shigella* serotype has a corresponding *E. coli* O group that is either related or identical to it (Edwards & Ewing, 1972; Rowe, Gross & Guiney, 1976).

An operational classification based on indole and gas production from lactose at 44 $^\circ$C together with other IMViC reactions, despite its limitations, is still used for water examination purposes (Report, 1956c, 1969, 1983).

On first isolation many strains of *Escherichia* are non-motile or only feebly motile and for this reason motility is shown as a 'd' character in Table 7.9c.

Escherichia adecarboxylata was described by Leclerc (1962). Strains are indole-positive, lysine decarboxylase-negative and usually produce a yellow pigment. The species has received little attention but strains are occasionally isolated from clinical specimens. Ewing & Fife (1972) included *E. adecarboxylata* in *Enterobacter agglomerans* (= *Erwinia herbicola*) (see Section 7.9.8); the species is certainly misplaced in *Escherichia* and a new genus *Leclercia* has been proposed to accommodate it (Tamura *et al.*, 1986).

Escherichia blattae, isolated from the intestinal tract of cockroaches, has not been reported in clinical material and therefore we do not include it in Table 7.9c. The species, which is indole-negative and non-motile, was described by Burgess, McDermott & Whiting, (1973); we suspect that it is probably misplaced in *Escherichia*.

Escherichia fergusonii, isolated from animals and human clinical material, was proposed by Farmer *et al.* (1985b) to include a group of motile, non-lactose-fermenting strains which are indole- and lysine decarboxylase-positive. They differ from *E. coli* in their ability to ferment cellobiose.

Escherichia hermanii, isolated particularly from wounds, was described by Brenner *et al.* (1982a) to include motile, indole-positive strains which ferment cellobiose, grow in KCN and may produce a yellow pigment on suitable media; lactose fermentation and lysine decarboxylase production vary from strain to strain.

Escherichia vulneris was also described by Brenner *et al.* (1982b) as a new species to include a group of strains many of which were isolated from human wounds. They are motile, indole negative, lysine decarboxylase positive and ferment cellobiose; lactose fermentation is either delayed or absent.

Minidefinition: *Escherichia. Gram-negative rods; often motile. Aerobic and facultatively anaerobic. Catalase-positive; oxidase-negative. Attack sugars fermentatively; gas normally produced. Usually citrate-negative (Simmons' medium) (except some E. blattae strains). Type species: E. coli; NCTC strain 9001.*

7.9.10 Hafnia (Tables 7.9a, c). The Hafnia group was described by Stuart & Rustigian (1943a) as their

Table 7.9c *Third-stage table for the enterobacteria (part 2)*

	16	17	18	19	20	21	22	23	24	25	26	27	28	29	30
Motility	+	d	+	+	+	d	–	–	–	–	–	+	+	+	d
Yellow pigment	d	–	–	–	–	–	–	–	–	–	–	–	–	–	–
Red pigment	–	–	–	–	–	–	–	–	–	–	–	–	–	–	–
MacConkey growth	+	+	+	+	+	+	+	+	+	+	d	+	+	+	+
Simmons' citrate	–	–	d	–	–	d	+	+	d	+	–	+	–	d	–
Christensen's citrate	–	d	+	d	–	+	+	+	+	+	d	+	d	+	d
Urease	–	–	–	–	–	–	+	+	d	+	–	–	+	+	+
Gelatin hydrolysis	d	–	–	–	–	–	d	–	–	–	–	–	–	+	+
Growth in KCN medium	+	–	–	+	–	+	+	+	d	d	d	+	+	+	+
H₂S (PbAc paper)	–	–	d	–	–	d	–	–	–	–	–	d	+	+	+
H₂S from TSI	–	–	–	–	–	–	–	–	–	–	–	–	–	+	d
Gluconate	–	–	–	–	–	+	+	+	–	–	–	–	–	d	–
Malonate	+	–	–	–	+	d	+	+	–	+	+	+	–	–	–
ONPG	+	d	+	+	+	+	+	+	+	+	–	+	–	–	–
Phenylalanine	–	–	–	–	–	–	–	–	–	–	–	–	+	+	+
Arginine dihydrolase	–	d	d	–	+	–	–	–	d	–	–	–	–	–	–
Lysine decarboxylase	–	d	+	d	+	+	+	+	d	+	–	d	–	–	–
Ornithine decarboxylase	–	d	+	+	–	+	–	+	–	–	–	+	+	+	–
Selenite reduction	+	d	+	+	+	+	+	+	–	d	–	+	d	+	d
Casein hydrolysis	–	–	–	–	–	–	–	–	–	–	–	–	–	d	+
DNase production	–	–	–	–	–	–	–	–	–	–	–	–	–	d	+
Carbohydrates [in Peptone Water medium], gas from glucose	+	d	+	+	+	+	+	+	d	+	–	+	+	+	+
acid from: adonitol	+	–	+	–	–	–	+	+	+	+	+	–	–	–	–
arabinose	+	+	+	+	+	+	+	+	+	+	+	–	–	–	–
cellobiose	+	–	+	+	+	d	+	+	+	+	+	–	–	–	–
dulcitol	+	d	–	+	–	–	d	d	–	+	–	–	–	–	–
glycerol	–	+	–	–	–	+	+	+	d	+	d	d	d	+	+
inositol	–	–	–	–	–	–	+	+	d	+	+	–	–	–	–
lactose	+	d	d	d	d	–	+	+	d	+	–	–	–	–	–
maltose	+	+	+	+	+	+	+	+	+	+	+	–	–	–	+
mannitol	+	+	+	+	+	+	+	+	+	+	+	–	–	–	+
raffinose	d	d	–	–	+	–	+	+	+	+	+	–	–	–	–
rhamnose	+	+	+	+	+	+	+	+	d	+	+	–	–	–	–
salicin	+	d	+	d	+	d	+	+	+	+	+	–	–	–	–
sorbitol	–	+	–	–	–	d	+	+	+	+	+	d	–	–	–
sucrose	d	d	–	d	–	–	+	+	+	+	+	+	–	–	+
trehalose	+	+	+	+	+	+	+	+	+	+	+	–	–	+	d
xylose	+	+	+	+	+	+	+	+	+	+	+	–	–	+	+
starch	–	–	–	–	–	–	d	d	d	+	d	–	–	–	–
MR test (37 °C)[a]	+	+	+	+	+	d	d	d	+	+	+	+	+	d	d
MR test (RT)[b]	+	+	d	+	+	–	d	d	+	+	+	+	+	d	d
VP test (37 °C)[a]	–	–	–	–	–	d	d	d	–	–	–	–	–	–	–
VP test (RT)[b]	–	–	–	–	–	+	d	d	–	–	–	–	–	d	–
Indole	+	+	d	+	–	–	+	–	–	–	–	d	+	–	–

16 **Escherichia adecarboxylata**
17 **Escherichia coli**
18 **Escherichia fergusonii**
19 **Escherichia hermannii**
20 **Escherichia vulneris**
21 **Hafnia alvei**; *'Enterobacter alvei'*
22 **Klebsiella oxytoca**
23 **Klebsiella pneumoniae** subsp. **aerogenes**; *'K. aerogenes'*; *K. pneumoniae (sensu lato)*; (NOT *'Aerobacter aerogenes'* Beijerinck)
24 **Klebsiella pneumoniae** subsp. **ozaenae**; *K. ozaenae*
25 **Klebsiella pneumoniae** subsp. **pneumoniae**; *K. pneumoniae (sensu stricto)*; Friedländer's pneumobacillus
26 **Klebsiella pneumoniae** subsp. **rhinoscleromatis**; *K. rhinoscleromatis*
27 **Kluyvera** spp.
28 **Morganella morganii**; *'Proteus morganii'*; Morgan's no. 1 bacillus
29 **Proteus mirabilis**
30 **Proteus penneri**; *P. vulgaris* biogroup 1

RT, room temperature (18–22 °C); [a] incubation for two days; [b] incubation for five days

Other symbols used in the table are explained in Tables 5.1 and 5.2 on p.47.

biotype 32011. Sakazaki (1961) and Ewing (1963) have both suggested that *Hafnia* should be included in *Enterobacter*, as '*E. alvei* 'and '*E. hafniae*', respectively. DNA studies, however, show that *H. alvei* deserves separate generic status (Brenner, 1978); they also revealed three groups within the species, each of which may eventually be recognized as separate species. As with *Serratia*, the biochemical characters are subject to temperature variations, and the most typical results are best obtained at 25–30 °C.

> **Minidefinition**: *Hafnia. Gram-negative rods; motile. Aerobic and facultatively anaerobic. Catalase-positive; oxidase-negative. Attack sugars fermentatively and gas is produced. Gelatin is not liquefied; urea is not hydrolysed. Type species: H. alvei; NCTC strain 8105.*

7.9.11   Klebsiella (Tables 7.9*a, c*). For many years the main problem in identifying Friedlander's bacillus (to which the name *K. pneumoniae* was later applied) was to distinguish it from '*Aerobacter aerogenes*' (later to be called '*K. aerogenes*') which was considered to be a non-motile organism. Much less difficult was its separation from the motile organism now known as *Enterobacter aerogenes* but which for a short time was also known as '*Aerobacter aerogenes*' (Hormaeche & Edwards, 1958); by means of a paper-strip test for urease, Matsen (1970) claimed to be able to make the distinction in ten minutes. This contrasts with the lengthy DNA reassociation experiments of Brenner, Steigerwalt & Fanning, (1972) and Brenner (1973) which provided much more convincing (but not routine) evidence for the distinction.

Other naming problems now enter the arena since '*Klebsiella aerogenes*' (Report, 1956*b*), currently without standing in nomenclature is, by many workers, also named *K. pneumoniae*. In addition, the subdivision of the klebsiellas in previous editions of this *Manual* was excessive. The maintenance of '*K. atlantae*' and '*K. edwardsii*' as separate species was not supported either by numerical taxonomy of biochemical characters (Bascomb *et al.*, 1971) or by DNA–DNA hybridization studies (Brenner, Steigerwalt & Fanning, 1972), so these two names have now fallen into disuse. The latter study also revealed that organisms appearing in the last edition of this *Manual* under the names '*K. aerogenes*', *K. ozae-*

nae, *K. pneumoniae* (*sensu stricto*) and *K. rhinoscleromatis* are, in effect, only biotypes, or subspecies, of a single species with the name *K. pneumoniae*. What we regarded as *K. pneumoniae* was a more closely defined taxon than the *K. pneumoniae* of many other workers (e.g. Ørskov in *Bergey's Manual*, 1974; Edwards & Ewing, 1972) so we accepted the term used by Bascomb *et al.* (1971) for our species as *K. pneumoniae* (*sensu stricto*) because it helped to contrast with the *K. pneumoniae* (*sensu lato*) of Ørskov and others. *K. pneumoniae* (*sensu lato*) includes the organisms we previously referred to as '*K. aerogenes*', '*K. atlantae*' and '*K. edwardsii*'. Against this scientific background and two differing opinions about the classification of the klebsiellas, it is difficult to draw up a compromise solution. The prevailing view is to accept *K. pneumoniae* (*sensu lato*) and reject *K. pneumoniae* (*sensu stricto*) as judged by the inclusion of *K. pneumoniae* in the *Approved Lists of Bacterial Names* (1980) and the omission of '*K. aerogenes*'. In the interests of uniformity we shall accept the name *K. pneumoniae* for the species as a whole and we foresee that the most widely accepted classification will effectively be *K. pneumoniae* subspecies *pneumoniae* (= *K. pneumoniae sensu lato*), *K. pneumoniae* subsp. *ozaenae* (= *K. ozaenae*) and *K. pneumoniae* subsp. *rhinoscleromatis* (= *K. rhinoscleromatis*). As a temporary measure, we propose amending this classification so that *K. pneumoniae* subsp. *pneumoniae* = *K. pneumoniae sensu stricto* and we shall retain '*K. aerogenes*' as a fourth subspecies, *K. pneumoniae* subsp. *aerogenes*. We have followed this uneasy compromise in the Tables but it must be remembered that as these four taxa are effectively a single species there are bound to be numerous intermediate forms that do not correspond neatly to any of the taxa.

The correlation between the subspecies and capsule serotypes is: *K. pneumoniae* subsp. *pneumoniae* (*K. pneumoniae sensu stricto*), type 3; *K. pneumoniae* subsp. *rhinoscleromatis*, type 3; *K. pneumoniae* subsp. *ozaenae*, types 3, 4, 5, and 6; and *Klebsiella pneumoniae* subsp. *aerogenes*, all types. *K. pneumoniae* subsp. *pneumoniae* is associated with acute infections and *K. pneumoniae* subsp. *ozaene* with chronic lung disease, but *K. pneumoniae* subsp. *aerogenes* is seldom pathogenic (Fallon, 1973). Like most enterobacteria, the reactivity of klebsiella antigens extends beyond the klebsiella group.

Indole-positive forms are probably not uncommon and strains that produce indole and liquefy gelatin have been named *K. oxytoca*; Ørskov (1955, 1957) and Ewing (1963) prefer to retain them in the genus, but Lautrop (1956*b*) and Hugh (1959) think that these strains should be excluded from *Klebsiella*. DNA–DNA relatedness studies suggest, however, that *K. oxytoca* strains should be placed in a genus separate from *Klebsiella* (Jain, Radsak & Mannheim, 1974). In Table 7.9*c K. oxytoca* is included for the indole- and often gelatin-positive forms. Other indole-producing strains have been placed in *K. planticola* (Bagley, Seidler & Brenner, 1981) and *K. trevisanii* (Ferragut *et al.*, 1983). Strains of these two species (which may well be synonymous) were isolated from non-clinical sources, and hence are not included in the Tables. However, Freney *et al.* (1986) reported that 18% of the clinical isolates they examined and which had been identified initially as *K. oxytoca*, proved to be strains of *K. trevisanii*.

Some strains of *Klebsiella pneumoniae* (*sensu lato*) are able to fix atmospheric nitrogen (Mahl *et al.*, 1965) but this character does not seem to have any known taxonomic value and cannot be used in the identification of *Klebsiella* species.

Minidefinition: *Klebsiella. Gram-negative rods; non-motile. Aerobic and facultatively anaerobic. Catalase-positive; oxidase-negative. Attack sugars fermentatively, usually with the production of gas. KCN- and VP-positive (important exceptions). Ornithine decarboxylase not produced. Urea generally hydrolysed. Phenylalanine-negative. Type species: K. pneumoniae; NCTC strain 9633.*

7.9.12 Kluyvera (Tables 7.9*a*, *c*). This genus was proposed by Asai *et al.* (1956) with two species, 'K. citrophila', to accommodate citrate-utilizing strains and 'K. noncitrophila' for strains not utilizing citrate, the principal feature differentiating them from *Escherichia* being their apparent polar flagella. In 1962, Asai *et al.* published evidence showing that their strains were peritrichously flagellated and they proposed transferring them to the genus *Escherichia*. These species names, which had been little used, were not included in the *Approved Lists of Bacterial Names* (1980). However, the generic name *Kluyvera* was revived by Farmer *et al.* (1981) with two species,

K. ascorbata (whose strains gave a positive result in the ascorbate test and failed to produce acid from glucose after incubation for 21 days at 5 °C) and *K. cryocrescens* (whose strains gave the opposite results in the above tests). As it is impracticable to differentiate between the two species routinely by biochemical tests we combine them in the Tables as a single taxon *Kluyvera* spp. However, strains of *K. cryocrescens* generally display large zones of inhibition around discs of carbenicillin and cephalothin whereas strains of *K. ascorbata* fail to do so. *Kluyvera* strains can easily be confused with strains of *Buttiauxella* and *Citrobacter*.

Most of the reported strains have been isolated from sputum and smaller numbers from urine, faeces and blood cultures; diarrhoea possibly caused by *Kluyvera* species has also been reported (Fainstein *et al.*, 1982; Aevaliotis *et al.*, 1985).

Minidefinition: *Kluyvera. Gram-negative rods; motile. Aerobic and facultatively anaerobic. Catalase-positive; oxidase-negative. Attack sugars fermentatively; gas is produced. Sucrose-positive. Generally citrate-positive; generally KCN-positive. Arginine-negative. Type species: K. ascorbata; ATCC strain 33433.*

7.9.13. Morganella (Tables 7.9*a*, *c*). Bacteriologists have for long been fascinated by Morgan's number 1 bacillus (Morgan, 1906), a quite unimportant organism in spite of his belief that it was the cause of 'summer diarrhoea' in infants. Thjotta (1920) thought that it was a 'metacolon' (*Escherichia coli* in today's terms); Jordan, Crawford & McBroom, (1935) doubted whether there was a species well enough characterized to be recognized and preferred to think of it as a large and variable group. To Rauss (1936) it was a member of the *Proteus* group, and he showed that on a solid medium of low agar content it would swarm as *Proteus* did on ordinary Nutrient Agar media. Fulton (1943) proposed a separate genus, *Morganella*, for it. Richard (1965) found that it had four to ten times the urease activity of other *Proteus* species, and he thought that this put it into a category of its own. Meanwhile, Rauss & Vörös (1959) had joined the ranks of the separatists and supported the creation of *Morganella*.

Convincing evidence for a difference between

Morganella morganii and *Proteus* species has come from research. The urease and phenylalanine deaminase enzymes are said to be serologically distinct from those of *Proteus* species; and the G+C content of the DNA for *Morganella morganii* is 50% and for *Proteus* species 40% (Penner, 1984a,b). Such a wide difference is unlikely to be found between members of the same genus. Unfortunately this kind of information is obtained by methods that are not yet available in routine clinical laboratories; we must make the distinction and identification from the results of routine tests and include sufficient characters in the tables to show up differences in as convincing a manner as possible. From a strictly medical viewpoint, it is doubtful if the effort to distinguish these organisms is worthwhile, for neither *Morganella* nor *Proteus* species appear to be convincing pathogens though as laboratory nuisances they both hold high places.

> **Minidefinition**: *Morganella. Gram-negative rods; motile. Aerobic and facultatively anaerobic. Catalase-positive; oxidase-negative. Glucose is fermented with the production of a small bubble of gas. Phenylalanine-positive; urease-positive. Citrate-negative; gelatin-negative. Type species: M. morganii; NCTC strain 235.*

7.9.14   Proteus (Tables 7.9a, c, d). The collection of species in the genera *Proteus* and *Providencia* and the various proposals to combine them and then to separate them again have the monotonous sounds of much taxonomic argument; we shall summarize this and give references for those who wish to pursue it. Rustigian & Stuart (1945) proposed that four species of the genus *Proteus* should be recognized, *P. vulgaris*, *P. mirabilis*, *P. morganii*, and *P. rettgeri*; this arrangement gained wide acceptance, though a few preferred to combine the first two species as '*Proteus hauseri*'. Because the '29911 group' of organisms of Stuart, Wheeler & McGann, (1946) was phenylalanine-positive it was added to *Proteus* by Singer & Bar-Chay (1954), Buttiaux *et al.* (1954) and Shaw & Clarke (1955) as the 'Providence group' or as *Proteus inconstans*.

In the opposite direction, several splittings and new genera were proposed: *Morganella* by Fulton (1943) for Morgan's No. 1 bacillus; Proom & Woiwod (1951) suggested the exclusion of Rettger's bacillus

from *Proteus*, and Kauffmann (1953) created a new genus for it ('*Rettgerella*'). Kauffmann & Edwards (1952) listed a new genus *Providencia*; Ewing (1962) described it and named two species, *P. alcalifaciens* and *P. stuartii*. Rauss & Vörös (1959) and Rauss (1962) supported the proposals for new genera (*Morganella*, '*Rettgerella*', and *Providencia*) but Richard (1966) thought that Rettger's bacillus should be included in *Providencia*. Lautrop, in *Bergey's Manual* (1974), reviewed the situation as it existed early in the 1970s and discussed the possible taxonomic treatments. His general conclusion was that Morgan's bacillus, with its G+C content of DNA of 50%, compared with 40% for the other *Proteus* species, seemed the best candidate for separate recognition. Since then, DNA–DNA hybridization studies have confirmed that *Morganella morganii* deserves separate generic status as it is more closely related to other Enterobacteriaceae than to *Proteus* or *Providencia* (Brenner *et al.*, 1978). These studies also confirmed that the two biotypes A and B of *Proteus inconstans* deserve separate generic status and should also be classified as separate species: *Providencia alcalifaciens* and *Providencia stuartii* respectively. Despite its ability to produce urease, which served as a useful test to distinguish *Proteus* and *Providencia*, DNA studies also showed that *Proteus rettgeri* should be transferred to *Providencia* as *Providencia rettgeri* leaving only *P. vulgaris* and *P. mirabilis* as distinct species in the genus *Proteus*. However, more detailed DNA–DNA hybridization studies revealed that *P. vulgaris* can be subdivided into three biogroups, each of which should probably be recognized as separate species (Hickman *et al.*, 1982). Biogroup 1 strains do not produce indole and fail to ferment salicin (the name *Proteus penneri* has been proposed for them); biogroup 2 strains produce indole and ferment salicin; biogroup 3 strains produce indole but do not ferment salicin. The type strain of *P. vulgaris* belongs to biogroup 3 so this name may ultimately be reserved for strains of biogroup 3 and yet another new name may be proposed for biogroup 2. We have followed this current classification in the Tables. The usual biochemical characterizing tests often reveal aberrant strains as, for example, the indole-positive *Proteus mirabilis* strains reported by Matsen *et al.* (1972), and lactose-fermenting strains of *Providencia rettgeri* (Sutter & Foecking, 1962).

In the medical laboratory, *Proteus* species, because of their swarming property, are a nuisance and rarely a subject for identification. Various tricks have been devised to inhibit swarming: the inclusion of bile salts in the medium (as in MacConkey Agar) is one of the most successful, though it may make the medium unsuitable for the growth of the organisms we want to isolate. Other measures include exposure to ether vapour (Bray, 1945), chloral hydrate (Gillespie, 1948); increased concentrations of agar (Hayward & Miles, 1943) or NaCl (Kopper, 1962); and deletion of added salts as in the Cystine-Lactose-Electrolyte Deficient (CLED) medium of Mackey & Sandys (1966).

We have not yet mentioned Proteus OX strains; these are strains of *Proteus vulgaris* which form the basis of the Weil–Felix reactions in patients with typhus infections. Such strains do not need to be identified among laboratory isolates of *P. vulgaris* from clinical material; their importance lies solely in their use as diagnostic agents. Although they are not connected in any way with the infecting agents (*Rickettsia prowazekii* or *R. mooseri*), they are, in the O (non-motile) form, agglutinated by the sera of typhus patients, a titre of 1 in 50 or more suggesting a rickettsial infection which should be confirmed by a rise in titre during the course of the clinical illness. *Proteus* OX19 is agglutinated by sera from patients with classical typhus (*R. prowazekii* infection) and *Proteus* OXK by sera of patients with tsutsugamushi fever (*R. orientalis* infection). These tests, however, are likely to become less useful in future with the application of specific sero-diagnostic methods.

> **Minidefinition:** *Proteus. Gram-negative rods; motile. Aerobic and facultatively anaerobic. Catalase-positive; oxidase-negative. Attack sugars fermentatively, usually with gas production. Phenylalanine-positive; urea hydrolysed. Gelatin hydrolysed. Type species: P. vulgaris; NCTC strain 4175.*

7.9.15 Providencia (Tables 7.9a, d). The history of the genera *Morganella*, *Proteus* and *Providencia* is so inextricably interlinked that, having already covered *Morganella* and *Proteus* in detail, there now remains little further to add on *Providencia*. Although three species, *P. alcalifaciens*, *P. rettgeri*

and *P. stuartii*, are generally recognised and are included in the Tables, DNA–DNA hybridization data show that *P. alcalifaciens* can be further subdivided (Hickman-Brenner *et al.*, 1983), so that strains fermenting galactose though not adonitol should now be classified as *Providencia rustigianii*.

> **Minidefinition:** *Providencia. Gram-negative rods; motile. Aerobic and facultatively anaerobic. Catalase-positive; oxidase-negative. Attack sugars fermentatively, generally without gas production. Phenylalanine-positive; gelatin not hydrolysed. Type species: P. alcalifaciens; NCTC strain 10286.*

7.9.16 Salmonella (Tables 7.9a, d). The identification of a bacterium as a salmonella is not difficult but, with that done, two problems arise. The first is the complex antigenic analysis and often phage typing needed to identify strains in sufficient detail to be helpful in tracing the source of infection; the second is how to label (by name or antigenic formula) the strain in the report that must be made to the clinician and to public health officials. The Salmonella Subcommittee (1934) thought that serology was the ultimate criterion in the classification (and, by implication, identification) of the group though they did not suggest that it should be based on serology alone. Complete antigenic analysis and phage typing are not routine procedures for clinical laboratories, but reference laboratories are available in most countries. Simplified diagnostic schemes using a limited number of antisera are usually used (Edwards & Kauffman, 1952; Spicer, 1956) permitting the presumptive serotyping of many salmonellas isolated from clinical material. It should be noted that many of the serotypes are also known by well-established names, which have no formal standing in nomenclature, such as 'S. pullorum', 'S. gallinarum' and 'S. paratyphi A'.

A polyvalent salmonella phage was of some use in distinguishing salmonellas from other enterobacteria but it was not a substitute for classical methods (Talley, 1968). More recently, DNA hybridization methods have been described to detect salmonellas in foods (Fitts *et al.*, 1983) and to identify *Salmonella typhi* in stools (Rubin *et al.*, 1985); such probes are likely to become widely used in the future.

One serotype, *S. typhi*, is distinct both serologically and biochemically and warrants separate description; it differs from most other salmonellas in being citrate negative (Simmons' medium), in not producing gas from glucose and in producing only small amounts of H_2S. 'S.gallinarum', which causes disease in poultry, does not produce gas and other serotypes may occasionally yield anaerogenic variants. 'S. paratyphi A' is also not typical in several characters: few strains produce H_2S from TSI slopes; it does not use citrate as a carbon source or produce acid from xylose; and it does not decarboxylate lysine. In addition, the type species of the genus, Salmonella choleraesuis, is biochemically atypical and does not ferment arabinose or trehalose. Lactose-fermenting strains that are otherwise biochemically typical are rare but do occur among several serotypes (Threlfall, Hall & Rowe, 1983). Members of the Arizona group (S. arizonae) often ferment lactose although this reaction may be delayed; in addition they are ONPG-positive, liquefy gelatin and are usually malonate-positive (Shaw, 1956). Most other Salmonella serotypes are biochemical variants with a fairly stable pattern, and Borman, Stuart & Wheeler (1944) proposed that they should all be called 'Salmonella kauffmannii'. For a similar all-embracing species Kauffmann & Edwards (1952) suggested the name 'Salmonella enterica', which would have been unusually meaningful and has recently found favour (see below); Ewing (1963) proposed that the name Salmonella enteritidis should be followed by the serotype name (when it had one) or the antigenic formula; this system has been tried in the USA but failed to gain acceptance elsewhere.

Kauffmann (1963a) divided the Salmonella group into what he called sub-genera; these are now widely accepted as distinct groups (though not as subgenera) and we therefore include them in Table 7.9d. If Salmonella is regarded as a genus, then these groups could conveniently be considered as species: 'Salmonella kauffmannii' (subgenus I), 'S. salamae' (II), S. arizonae (III), and 'S. houtenae' (IV) (Le Minor, Rohde & Taylor, 1970). Later Le Minor, Véron & Popoff (1982) proposed on the basis of numerical taxonomy and DNA relatedness that the genus Salmonella should consist of a single species composed of six subspecies. S. choleraesuis was proposed as the type species with the six subspecies as follows: subsp. choleraesuis would include all sub-

genus I strains; subsp. salamae would correspond to subgenus II; subsp. arizonae would include the monophasic serotypes of subgenus III while subsp. diarizonae would include the diphasic serotypes; subsp. houtenae would correspond to subgenus IV and subsp. bongori would consist of ONPG- and KCN-positive strains that fermented dulcitol. A seventh subspecies, indica, has since been proposed for strains that are gelatinase-positive but negative for malonate, tartrate, salicin and sorbitol (Le Minor et al., 1986). More recently, a new proposal to change the type species to 'S. enterica' has been published (Le Minor & Popoff, 1987); this proposal has the advantage that the name has not been used previously for any bioserovar of Salmonella and it is thus less likely to cause confusion. It remains to be seen whether these latest proposals gain wide acceptance. We are sceptical about these proposals and think that, for practical purposes, clinical laboratories are likely to continue to use serotype names such as S. typhimurium rather than the cumbersome equivalent 'S. choleraesuis [or S. enterica] subsp. choleraesuis bioserovar Typhimurium'.

The typically non-motile salmonellas ('S. gallinarum' and 'S. pullorum') from poultry are often combined, but as they differ from each other in several characters we show them separately in Table 7.9d.

Although numerous isolation media are described, they do not seem to have changed much in principle since Hobbs & Allison (1945), after comparing several media, found that of Wilson & Blair (1931) to be the most valuable solid medium with Deoxycholate Citrate Agar a close second; they recommended, however, that both media should be used as the combination gave more Salmonella isolations than either medium alone. For enrichment, Selenite F (F for faeces) gave the best results when plated on Wilson & Blair's Bismuth Sulphite agar medium. Harvey & Thomson (1953) found that cultures incubated at 43 °C yielded more positive results but temperature regulation had to be accurate as 44 °C was inhibitory for salmonellas. Selenite F incubated at 43 °C is also recommended by Georgala & Boothroyd (1965) followed by plating on Brilliant Green Agar. For a summary of available media, see Ewing (1986) and Fricker (1987).

Minidefinition: *Salmonella. Gram-negative rods; motile (a few exceptions). Aerobic and*

Table 7.9d. *Third-stage table for the enterobacteria (part 3)*

	31	32	33	34	35	36	37	38	39	40	41	42	43	44
Motility	d	d	d	+	d	+	−	+	−	+	+	+	+	+
Yellow pigment	−	−	−	−	−	−	−	−	−	−	−	−	−	−
Red pigment	−	−	−	−	−	−	−	−	−	−	−	−	−	−
MacConkey growth	+	+	+	+	+	+	+	+	+	+	+	+	+	+
Simmons' citrate	d	−	d	+	+	d	−	−	−	+	+	+	+	−
Christensen's citrate	+	d	+	+	+	+	+	+	+	+	+	+	+	+
Urease	+	+	−	+	+	−	−	−	−	−	−	−	−	−
Gelatin hydrolysis	+	d	−	−	−	−	−	−	−	−	d	d	d	−
Growth in KCN medium	+	+	+	+	+	−	−	−	−	−	−	−	+	−
H$_2$S (PbAc paper)	+	+	d	+	d	d	+	d	d	+	+	+	+	+
H$_2$S from TSI	d	d	−	−	−	d	d	−	d	+	+	+	+	d
Gluconate	−	−	−	−	−	−	−	−	−	−	−	−	−	−
Malonate	−	−	−	−	−	−	−	−	−	−	+	+	−	−
ONPG	−	−	−	−	−	−	−	−	−	−	d	+	−	−
Phenylalanine	+	+	+	+	+	−	−	−	−	−	−	−	−	−
Arginine dihydrolase	−	−	−	−	−	+	−	+	d	+	+	+	+	+
Lysine decarboxylase	−	−	−	−	−	+	+	−	+	+	+	+	+	+
Ornithine decarboxylase	−	−	−	−	−	+	+	+	+	+	+	+	−	+
Selenite reduction	+	d	d	+	d	d	d	+	+	+	+	+	+	+
Casein hydrolysis	d	−	−	−	−	−	−	−	−	−	−	−	−	−
DNase production	+	+	d	d	d	d	d	−	d	d	d	d	−	−
Carbohydrates [in Peptone Water medium], gas from glucose	+	+	d	−	−	+	−	+	d	+	+	+	+	−
acid from:														
adonitol	−	−	d	+	−	−	−	−	−	−	−	−	−	−
arabinose	−	−	−	−	−	+	+	+	+	+	+	+	+	−
cellobiose	−	−	−	−	−	−	−	−	−	d	d	−	d	−
dulcitol	−	−	−	−	−	d	+	+	−	+	+	−	−	d
glycerol	+	+	d	d	+	d	d	d	−	d	d	−	d	d
inositol	−	−	−	+	+	−	−	−	−	d	d	−	−	−
lactose	−	−	−	−	−	−	−	−	−	−	−	d	−	−
maltose	+	+	−	−	−	+	d	+	+	+	+	+	+	+
mannitol	−	−	−	+	−	+	+	+	+	+	+	+	+	+
raffinose	−	−	−	−	−	−	−	−	−	−	−	−	−	−
rhamnose	−	−	−	d	−	+	d	+	d	+	+	+	+	−
salicin	+	−	−	d	−	−	−	−	−	−	−	−	d	−
sorbitol	−	−	−	−	−	+	d	+	−	+	+	+	+	+
sucrose	+	+	d	d	d	−	−	−	−	−	−	−	−	−
trehalose	d	d	−	−	+	−	+	+	+	+	+	+	+	+
xylose	+	+	−	−	−	+	d	−	d	+	+	+	+	+
starch	−	−	−	−	−	−	−	−	−	−	−	−	−	−
MR test (37 °C)[a]	+	+	+	+	+	+	+	+	+	+	+	+	+	+
MR test (RT)[b]	+	+	+	+	+	+	+	+	+	+	+	+	+	+
VP test (37 °C)[a]	−	−	−	−	−	−	−	⟍	−	−	−	−	−	−
VP test (RT)[b]	−	−	−	−	−	−	−	−	−	−	−	−	−	−
Indole	+	+	+	+	+	−	−	−	−	−	−	−	−	−

31 **Proteus vulgaris biogroup 2**

32 **Proteus vulgaris biogroup 3**

33 **Providencia alcalifaciens**; *Proteus inconstans*; '*Proteus inconstans A*'; '*Proteus providenciae*'; '*Providencia providenciae*'

34 **Providencia rettgeri**; '*Proteus rettgeri*'; '*Rettgerella rettgeri*'

35 **Providencia stuartii**; '*Proteus stuartii*'; '*Proteus inconstans B*'; '*Proteus providenciae* B'

36 **Salmonella choleraesuis**

37 **'Salmonella gallinarum'**

38 **'Salmonella paratyphi A'**

39 **'Salmonella pullorum'**

40 **Salmonella subgenus I**; '*S. kauffmannii*'; '*S. enterica*'; *S. enteritidis* serotype (bioser) xyz

41 **Salmonella subgenus II**; '*S. salamae*'; '*S. dar-es-salaam*'

42 **Salmonella subgenus III**; '*Arizona arizonae*'; '*A. hinshawii*; Salmonella arizonae*

43 **Salmonella subgenus IV**; '*S. houtenae*'

44 **Salmonella typhi**

RT, room temperature (18–22 °C); [a] incubation for two days; [b] incubation for five days

Other symbols used in the table are explained in Tables 5.1 and 5.2 on p.47.

facultatively anaerobic. Catalase-positive; oxidase-negative. Attack sugars by fermentation with production of gas. Simmons' citrate usually positive (S. typhi is an important exception that does not produce gas and is Simmons' citrate-negative). KCN-negative (except subgenus IV); lysine decarboxylase usually positive (with the exception of 'S. paratyphi A'). Type species: S. choleraesuis; NCTC strain 5735.

7.9.17 Serratia (Tables 7.9a, e). Classically, members of certain species of this genus produce a bright pink or red pigment though in culture non-pigmented variants are constantly thrown off; non-pigmented strains occur also in nature and, in some species, all strains are non-pigmented. In a five month period, 92% of *Serratia* strains isolated in a Boston hospital were not pigmented (Wilfert *et al.*, 1970); consequently, bacteriologists must be able to identify this organism in the absence of pigment. However, if pigment is present, identification is much easier, and various media have therefore been devised to encourage its production. Meat extracts seem to inhibit pigment formation but it can be restored by transfer to a medium without meat (Goldsworthy & Still, 1936). Kharasch, Conway & Bloom, (1936) thought that glucose was necessary for pigment production by *Serratia marcescens*; on the other hand, Goldsworthy & Still (1936, 1938) found that glucose inhibited and mannitol stimulated pigment production by their strains. Cowan & Steel (1974) confirmed these findings, which indicate that strains vary in the way in which they respond to glucose in the medium. One of the most satisfactory media for showing pigment potential is medium A of King, Ward & Raney, (1954) (Appendix A2.4.3); Sedlák and his colleagues (1965) reported good results with Dorset Egg medium at 22 °C. As with *Hafnia*, the most characteristic results of biochemical tests are obtained at about 25 °C.

Sometimes the occurrence of serratias in human secretions can be misleading for the unwary; for example, their growth in sputum after expectoration may suggest haemoptysis (Robinson & Woolley, 1957). Serratias may cause occasional infections, especially in children and, with the recognition of non-pigmented strains, reports of their isolation have

become more frequent (see, for example, Brooks, Chambers & Tabaqchali, 1979). *Serratia marcescens* liquefies gelatin rapidly and, in this and other characters, Pederson & Breed (1928) noticed that it closely resembled the liquefying species of '*Aerobacter*' (subsequently '*Enterobacter liquefaciens*') and thought that such non-pigmented strains might be included in *Serratia*. The resemblance extends to deoxyribonuclease activity (DNase) which occurs more frequently and is more active in strains of *Serratia marcescens* and '*Enterobacter liquefaciens*' than in most other enterobacteria (Vörös, 1969). Black, Hodgson & McKechnie, (1971) compared methods for carrying out this test in routine laboratories and preferred that of Jeffries, Holtman & Guse, (1957). A rapid and easily read method (combined with the PPA test) was described by Oberhofer & Maddox (1970). The suggestion of Pederson & Breed (1928), which has been repeated by many others, has been generally accepted and '*E. liquefaciens*' is now included in *Serratia* as *S. liquefaciens*.

Serratia marcescens can be typed for epidemiological purposes by their O and H antigen serology (Traub, 1985), by bacteriocins (Anderhub *et al.*, 1977; Traub, 1980), bacteriophages (Pitt, Erdman & Bucher, 1980), and by biotyping (see Pitt, 1982). Biotyping of *S. marcescens* was described by Grimont & Grimont (1978a,b) who tested strains for the ability to utilise various substrates. Conventional tests used for species identification are not generally suitable for biotyping due to the similarity of biochemical reactions within the species.

Another species, *Serratia rubidaea*, described by Breed in *Bergey's Manual* (1948) as having characters much like those of *S. marcescens*, has been revived by Ewing, Davis & Fife, (1972); although some strains came from human sources the clinical significance was not indicated and presumably was unknown. In several instances the strains described by Ewing and his colleagues, and for which an old name was revived, differ in their characteristics from those on which the original description of the species was based. *S. rubidaea* is no exception and we prefer to use the name *S. marinorubra* for this organism (see Grimont *et al.*, 1977), which is anaerogenic and does not decarboxylate ornithine. *Serratia odorifera* was described from 25 strains isolated mostly from clinical material; of these 17 were designated biotype 1

Table 7.9e. *Third-stage table for the enterobacteria (part 4)*

	45	46	47	48	49	50	51	52[d]	53	54[c]	55	56	57	58	59
Motility	+	+	+	+	+	+	−	−	−	+	+	+	+	−	d
Yellow pigment	−	−	−	−	−	−	−	−	−	−	−	−	−	−	−
Red pigment	−	−	d	−	−	d	−	−	−	−	−	−	−	−	−
MacConkey growth	+	+	+	+	+	+	+	+	+	+	+	+	+		+
Simmons' citrate	+	+	+	+	+	d	−	−	−	−	d	d	−	−	−
Christensen's citrate	+	+	+	+	+	+	−	−	+	d	d	+	+	−	−
Urease	−	d	−	−	−	−	−	−	−	+	+	+	+	−	+
Gelatin hydrolysis	+	+	+	+	+	+	−	−	−	−	−	−	−	−	−
Growth in KCN medium	+	+	d	+	+	d	−	−	−	d	d	+	+	−	−
H₂S (PbAc paper)	−	d	−	d	−	d	−	−	−	−	−	−	−	−	−
H₂S from TSI	−	−	−	−	−	−	−	−	−	−	−	−	−	−	−
Gluconate	d	+	+	+	+	d									
Malonate	−	−	d												
ONPG	+	+	+	+	+	+	+		−	+	+	+	+	+	+
Phenylalanine	−	−	−	−	−	−	−	−	−	−	−	−	−	−	−
Arginine dihydrolase	−	−	−	−	−	−	d	d							
Lysine decarboxylase	+	+	d	+	+	−									
Ornithine decarboxylase	+	+	−	+	−	−	+			+	+	+	+		
Selenite reduction	d	+	+	d	+	d	+	d	−	d	d	d	d	−	d
Casein hydrolysis	d	+	d	d	+	d									
DNase production	d	+	d	d	−	d	−	−	−	−	−	−	−	−	−
Carbohydrates [in Peptone Water medium], gas from glucose	d	d	−	−	−	d	−								−
acid from:															
adonitol	−	d	+	d	+	−				−			−		−
arabinose	+	−	+	+	+	+	+	d	−	+	+	+	+	+	+
cellobiose	d	−	+	+	+	d	−			+	+	+	+		−
dulcitol	−	−	−	−	−	−		d		−		−			−
glycerol	+	+	+	+	+	d	d	d	−	+	+	+	+	d	+
inositol	+	+	+	+	+	d	−	−		d	d	d	−	−	−
lactose	−	−	+	d	+	d						d		−	−
maltose	+	+	+	+	+	+	+	d		d	+	+	+	d	+
mannitol	+	+	+	+	+	+	+	d		+	+	+	+	+	+
raffinose	+	−	+	+	−	d	d	d		−	+	−	+	−	−
rhamnose	−	−	−	+	+	−	+	−		+	+	+	−	−	+
salicin	+	+	+	+	+	+	−	−	+	d	+	+	−	+	d
sorbitol	+	+	−	+	+	d	−	d	−	+	+	+	+	−	−
sucrose	+	+	+	+	−	+	−	−	+	+	+	+	−	−	−
trehalose	+	+	+	+	+	+	+	d	+	+	+	+	+	+	+
xylose	+	−	+	+	+	+	−	−	−	d	+	+	+	+	+
starch	−	−	−	−	−	−	−	−	−	−	−	−	−	−	−
MR test (37 °C)[a]	+	−	d	+	+	d	+	+	−	+	+	+	+	d	+
MR test (RT)[b]	−	−	−	−	−	d	+	+	+	d	+	+	+	+	+
VP test (37 °C)[a]	−	+	d	−	−	d	−	−	−	−	−	−	−	−	−
VP test (RT)[b]	d	+	d	−	−	d	−	−	−	d	d	d	−	−	−
Indole	−	−	−	−	−	−	−	−	d	−	d	+	d	−	−

45 **Serratia liquefaciens;** *'Enterobacter liquefaciens'; 'Aerobacter liquefaciens'*

'46 **Serratia marcescens;** *'Erythrobacillus prodigiosus'; 'Chromobacterium prodigiosum'*

47 **Serratia marinorubra;** *S rubidaea, Serratia* biotype II (Bascomb *et al.,* 1971); *Serratia* Phenon B (Grimont *et al.,* 1977)

48[c] **Serratia odorifera biovar I**

49 **Serratia odorifera biovar II**

50 **Serratia plymuthica**

51 **Shigella sonnei**

52[d] **Shigella spp.** (excluding *S. sonnei*); *S. boydii* ([serotypes] 1–15; Boyd's dysentert bacilli); *S. dysenteriae* ([serotype 1: 'S. shigae'; Shiga's bacillus]; [serotypes 2-10; Large-Sach's group; 2 = 'S. schmitzii'; 'S. ambigua'; Schmitz's bacillus]); *S. flexneri* ([serotypes 1–5: Flexner's dysentery bacilli]; [serotype 6: Boyd 88]; Manchester bacillus; see Table 7.9*f*)

53 **Tatumella ptyseos**

54[e] **Yersinia enterocoliticia; 'Pasteurella X'**

55 **Yersinia frederiksenii**

56 **Yersinia intermedia**

57 **Yersinia kristensenii**

58 **Yersinia pestis;** *'Pasteurella pestis'*; the plague bacillus

59 **Yersinia pseudotuberculosis;** *'Pasteurella pseudotuberculosis'; 'P. rodentium'*

RT, room temperature (18–22 °C); [a] incubation for two days; [b] incubation for five days; [c] Some strains nitrate-negative; [d] Some strains catalase-negative.

Other symbols used in the table are explained in Tables 5.1 and 5.2 on p.47.

and the remaining eight as biotype 2 (Grimont *et al.*, 1978). Strains of biotype 1 decarboxylate ornithine, and ferment raffinose and sucrose whereas those of biotype 2 give the converse results in these tests; their clinical significance is unknown. Other species of *Serratia* reported occasionally in clinical material include *S. ficaria* (normally associated with figs and fig wasps), from respiratory specimens (Gill *et al.*, 1981; Brouillard, Hansen & Compete, 1984) and from a leg ulcer (Pien & Farmer, 1983), as well as *S. plymuthica* from a burn site (Clark & Janda, 1985). *S. fonticola*, isolated from water, was described by Gavini *et al.* (1979) but, after numerical analysis of the genus, Feltham & Stevens (1983) queried its inclusion; we do not therefore show this environmental organism in the tables.

> **Minidefinition**: *Serratia. Gram-negative rods; motile. Aerobic and facultatively anaerobic. Catalase-positive; oxidase-negative. Attack sugars fermentatively, often with gas production in some species. VP usually positive. Gluconate-positive. Strains of some species produce ornithine decarboxylase; deoxyribonuclease-positive. Strains of some species produce a red pigment when grown on suitable media. Type species: S. marcescens; NCTC strain 10211.*

7.9.18   Shigella (Tables 7.9a, e, f). Modern ideas on the classification of this genus owe much to Ewing, who built on the foundations laid by Murray (1918), Andrewes & Inman (1919), and by Boyd (1938) whose recognition of specific and group antigens introduced some system into the serological analysis of shigellas. Ewing (1953) also showed that many strains previously thought to be shigellas are best regarded as non-motile, anaerogenic strains of *E. coli*. More recently, DNA hybridization studies have confirmed that *Shigella* and *E. coli* belong to a single genetic species (Brenner *et al.*, 1982c). It is therefore not surprising that most shigellas are closely related to O groups of *E. coli* (Edwards & Ewing, 1972; Rowe, Gross & Guiney, 1976). The distinction between *Shigella* and *E. coli* in the diagnostic laboratory depends on only a few tests and those for motility, lysine decarboxylase and the utilization of citrate

(Christensen's medium) are of particular value.

Biochemically the *Shigella* group is divided into the mannitol non-fermenters (*Shigella dysenteriae*) and the mannitol fermenters (*S. boydii, S. flexneri* and *S. sonnei*) although exceptions occur with most serotypes. *Shigella dysenteriae* serotype 1 (Shiga's bacillus) differs from all the others in that it is catalase-negative; among other shigellas catalase-negative strains occur occasionally, especially with *S. flexneri* type 4a (Carpenter & Lachowicz, 1959), but it is not a constant character of any serotype except *S. dysenteriae* 1.

Strains of *S. dysenteriae* 2 (Schmitz's bacillus) always produce indole, a character shared among the mannitol non-fermenters by the rarer serotypes 7 and 8. Among the mannitol fermenters the distinction between *Shigella flexneri* (subgroup B) and *S. boydii* (subgroup C) is made entirely on serological grounds; strains of *S. flexneri* possess common group antigens that do not occur in the other subgroups.

Strains of *Shigella flexneri* 6 may differ in some biochemical and immunological characters from serotypes 1 to 5, and Russian workers believe that *S. flexneri* 6 should be transferred to the *S. boydii* subgroup (Petrovskaya & Khomenko, 1979); the special characteristics of the Manchester and Newcastle varieties (Downie, Wade & Young, 1933) of *S. flexneri* 6 are shown in Table 7.9f, which is adapted from that of Carpenter, Lapage & Steel, (1966). It should be noted that some strains do produce gas.

Shigella sonnei (subgroup D) produces colicines which, when tested on 'indicator' strains, can be used to sub-divide strains into epidemiologically significant types (Abbot & Shannon, 1958). Typically *S. sonnei* is indole-negative and most (though not all) strains are late fermenters of lactose and sucrose; Szturm-Rubinsten (1963) recognized different biotypes. The ONPG test confirms their inherent ability to ferment lactose (Le Minor & Ben Hamida, 1962) and with other shigellas many serotypes (especially *S. dysenteriae* 1) also give positive results in this test (Szturm-Rubinsten & Piéchaud, 1963). The antigenic relationship betweeen *S. sonnei* and *Plesiomonas shigelloides* should be borne in mind (Ferguson & Henderson, 1947; Martin, Mock & Ewing, 1968).

Table 7.9f. *Unusual biochemical characteristics of biotypes of* Shigella flexneri 6 *(modified from* Carpenter et al., *1966)*

	1	2	3	4
Glucose (acid)	+	+	+	+
Glucose (gas)	–	–	+	d
Mannitol (acid)	+	+	+	–
Dulcitol (acid)	–	(d)	(d)	(d)
Indole	d	–	–	–

1 **Shigella flexneri** serotypes 1–5
2 **Shigella flexneri** 6; Boyd 88 biotype
3 **Shigella flexneri** 6; Manchester biotype; Denton strains (Downie *et al.*, 1933)
4 **Shigella flexneri** 6; Newcastle biotype; *'Shigella newcastle'*

Symbols used in the table are explained in Tables 5.1 and 5.2 on pp. 47.

For the isolation of shigellas it is preferable to culture freshly passed stools, although if this is not possible rectal swabs showing marked faecal staining may be used. Ideally specimens should be taken during the acute stage of illness before any chemotherapy is given and examined as soon as possible after collection. Enrichment with 'Gram-negative (GN) broth' (Hajna, 1955) may be advantageous but isolation is normally possible by direct plating, especially if blood and mucus is present. Some strains grow poorly on inhibitory media and it is therefore advisable to use a relatively non-inhibitory medium, such as MacConkey or Eosin Methylene Blue (EMB) agar, as well as an inhibitory medium, such as Deoxycholate Citrate Agar (DCA) or Salmonella–Shigella (SS) agar. After overnight incubation at 37 °C, non-lactose-fermenting colonies are selected for further examination, but it should be noted that there may be only a scanty growth of *Shigella*, even with fresh specimens taken during the acute stage of diarrhoea. In preliminary evaluation, a new selective medium containing potassium tellurite performed better than MacConkey and SS agar used together (Rahaman *et al.*, 1986).

Minidefinition: *Shigella. Gram-negative rods; non-motile. Aerobic and facultatively anaerobic. Catalase-positive (one important exception); oxidase-negative. Attack sugars by fermentation without gas production (a few exceptions produce gas). Citrate-nega-tive; KCN-negative; lysine decarboxylase-negative. Type species: S. dysenteriae; NCTC strain 4837.*

7.9.19 Tatumella (Tables 7.9a, e). There is but a single species, *T. ptyseos*, strains of which have been isolated mostly from sputa (Hollis *et al.*, 1981). The organism is unusual among the Enterobacteriaceae in having a small number of flagella (usually only one), in displaying a large zone of inhibition around penicillin discs, and in surviving for only a comparatively short period on some laboratory media. Growth occurs on MacConkey agar and most strains are reported to be motile and to utilize citrate (Simmons' medium) at 25 °C but give negative results in these tests at 35–37 °C. They produce phenylalanine deaminase weakly in a suitable medium. Their clinical significance is uncertain.

Minidefinition: *Tatumella. Gram-negative rods; motile, but with few (usually only one) flagella. Aerobic and facultatively anaerobic. Catalase-positive; oxidase-negative. Attack (fermentatively) only glucose, salicin, sucrose and trehalose; gas is not produced. Type species: T. ptyseos; NCTC strain 11468.*

7.9.20 Yersinia (Tables 7.7; 7.9a, e, g) is a genus originally created for the plague and pseudotuberculosis organisms by van Loghem (1944–5), who separated them from the pasteurellas. Other organisms have since been added: *Yersinia enterocolitica* (Pasteurella X) isolated from animals and man (Mollaret & Chevalier, 1964) and *Yersinia ruckeri* from rainbow trout with red mouth disease (Ewing *et al.*, 1978). As a result of further studies on *Y. enterocolitica* and similar organisms described as *Y. enterocolitica*-like, *Yersinia enterocolitica (sensu stricto)* was redefined by Bercovier *et al.* (1980*a*) and three new species isolated from the aquatic environment and from man were described: *Y. frederiksenii* (Ursing *et al.*, 1980), *Y. intermedia* (Brenner *et al.*, 1980*a*) and *Y. kristensenii* (Bercovier *et al.*, 1980*b*). Subsequently, four further species were described: *Y. aldovae* from fresh water (Bercovier *et al.*, 1984), *Y. rohdei* from human and dog faeces and surface water (Aleksić) *et al.*, 1987); and *Y. mollaretii* and *Y. bercovieri* from human stools and other sources

Table 7.9g. *Third-stage table for* Yersinia

	1	2	3	4	5	6	7	8	9	10	11	12	13	14	15
Motility at 37 °C	−	−	−	−	−	−	−	−	−	−	−	−	−	−	d
Motility at 20 °C	+	+	+	+	+	+	+	+	+	+	+	+	+	−	+
Simmons' citrate	−	−	−	−	−	(d)	(d)	−	(d)	−	−	+	−	−	(+)[a]
Nitrate reduced	+	+	+	d	−	+	+	+	+	+	+	+	+	d	+
Glucose, gas from	−[b]	−	−	−	−	−	−	−	−	−[b]	−[b]	−	−	−	−[b]
Carbohydrates, acid from															
arabinose	+	+	+	+	+	+	+	+	+	+	+	+	+	+	−
cellobiose	+	+	+	+	+	+	+	+	−	+	+	+	−	−	−
fucose	d	d	d	d	−	+	d	d	d	+	−	?	−	?	?
lactose	d	−	−	−	−	(d)	−	(d)	−	−	−	+	−	−	−
maltose	+	+	+	d	+	+	+	+	+	+	+	+	+	+	+
melibiose	−	−	−	−	−	−	+	−	−	−	−	d	+	d	−
raffinose	d	−	−	−	−	−	(+)	−	−	−	−	d	−	−	−
rhamnose	−	−	−	−	−	(+)	(+)	−	+	−	−	−	+	(+)	−
salicin	d	−	−	−	−	+	+	(d)	−	(+)	.(d)	−	(+)	d	−
sorbitol	+	+	+	+	d	+	+	+	+	+	+	+	−	d	−
sorbose	d	d	d	d	d	+	+	+	−	−	+	?	−	−	?
sucrose	+	+	+	+	d	+	+	−	−	+	+	+	−	−	−
trehalose	+	+	+	+	−	+	+	+	+	+	+	+	+	+	+
xylose	(+)	(+)	(+)	−	−	(+)	(+)	(+)	(+)	+	+	+	+	+	−
Mucate	−	−	−	−	−	d	d	−	d	+	+	−	−	?	−
ONPG	+	+	d	d	−	+	+	+	+	+	+	+	+	+	+
Pyrazinamidase	d	d	d	d	−	+	+	+	+	+	+	+	−	−	?
Aesculin	d	−	−	−	−	+	+	(d)	−	(+)	(+)	−	+	+	−
Indole	+	(+)	−	−	−	+	d	d	−	−	−	−	−	−	−
Urease	+	+	+	+	+	+	+	+	+	+	+	+	+	−	−
Lipase at 22 °C	+	−	−	−	−	d	d	d	d	−	−	−	−	−	(d)
Arginine dihydrolase	−	−	−	−	−	−	−	−	−	−	−	−	d	−	−
Lysine decarboxylase	−	−	−	−	−	−	−	−	−	−	−	−	−	−	+
Ornithine decarboxylase	+	+	+	+	d	+	+	+	+	+	+	+	−	−	+
VP at 22–30 °C	+	+	+	+	d	+	+	−	+	−	−	−	−	−	(d)

1 **Yersinia enterocolitica biovar 1**	9 **Yersinia aldovae**
2 **Yersinia enterocolitica biovar 2**	10 **Yersinia bercovieri;** *Y. enterocolitica* biogroup 3B
3 **Yersinia enterocolitica biovar 3**	11 **Yersinia mollaretti;** *Y. enterocolitica* biogroup 3A
4 **Yersinia enterocolitica biovar 4**	12 **Yersinia rohdei**
5 **Yersinia enterocolitica biovar 5**	13 **Yersinia pseudotuberculosis;** *'Pasteurella pseudotuberculosis'*
6 **Yersinia frederiksenii**	14 **Yersinia pestis;** *'Pasteurella pestis'*; plague bacillus
7 **Yersinia intermedia**	15 **Yersinia ruckeri;** red mouth bacterium
8 **Yersinia kristensenii**	

a Positive only at 22–25 °C.
b A few strains produce a small amount of gas.

Other symbols used in the Table are explained in Tables 5.1 and 5.2 on p47.

(Wauters *et al.*, 1988). The so-called *'Yersinia philomiragia'* (Jensen, Owen & Jellison, 1969) was shown not to be a member of *Yersinia* or indeed of the Enterobacteriaceae (Ursing, Steigerwalt & Brenner, 1980a) but probably belongs to the genus *Francisella*. We include *Yersinia* in Table 7.7 for comparison with *Pasteurella* and in Tables 7.9a,e for comparison with the other enterobacteria; we give the characters of *Yersinia* species in Table 7.9g.

It is worth noting that the temperature of incubation is important in tests for the characterization of yersinias. *Y. pestis* produces a capsule (or envelope) at 37 °C but not at 20–22 °C (Schütze, 1932a); *Y. pseudotuberculosis* is motile at 22 °C but not at 37 °C (Preston & Maitland, 1952); and while *Y. enterocolitica* is VP negative at 37 °C, it may be positive at 25–30 °C.

Y. enterocolitica is now divided into five biovars

(Niléhn, 1969; Wauters, 1970) by their biochemical characteristics. As the distribution of some of these biovars is epidemiologically quite distinct, we not only mention them but include them also in Table 7.9g. Biovars 1–4 are ornithine-, urease-, cellobiose- and sucrose-positive; they give a positive VP reaction at 30 °C but are negative at 37 °C. Biovars 1–4 can be differentiated by their reactions for lipase, indole, aesculin, salicin and xylose (Table 7.9g). Although *Y. enterocolitica* has been described as lactose negative, it is not unusual to find biovar 1 strains that are lactose positive; such strains are also likely to ferment raffinose (Cornelis, Luke & Richmond, 1978).

Biovar 5 strains (Mollaret & Lucas, 1965), isolated from hares may often give negative reactions for sucrose, ornithine and acetoin (VP) and they always give a negative reaction for trehalose, whereas the other four biovars give positive reactions in these tests.

Y. frederiksenii and *Y. intermedia* can be distinguished from *Y. enterocolitica* by the production of acid without gas from rhamnose. *Y. intermedia*, in addition, gives positive reactions with α-methyl-D-glucoside, raffinose and melibiose.

Y. kristensenii and *Y. aldovae* can be distinguished by their negative reactions with sucrose. They can be differentiated from each other and from sucrose-negative *Y. enterocolitica* biovar 5 strains by their reactions with cellobiose, rhamnose and the VP test. *Y. mollaretii* and *Y. bercovieri*, formerly known respectively as *Y. enterocolitica* biogroups 3A and 3B, differ from each other in their ability to ferment fucose and sorbose and from *Y. enterocolitica sensu stricto* in the production of acid from mucate. *Y. rohdei* differs from *Y. enterocolitica sensu stricto* in growing in Simmons' citrate medium and in giving negative results in the VP test. *Y. pseudotuberculosis* strains are urease-positive and motile at room temperature but not at 37 °C; they give negative sucrose, cellobiose and ornithine test reactions. Many of these reactions are temperature dependent and are best carried out at 30 °C.

Y. pseudotuberculosis is a homogeneous species with few exceptions. A number of serotypes can be distinguished for epidemiological purposes; strains of serotype III are usually melibiose-negative (Mair, Fox & Thal, 1979).

The plague bacillus, *Yersinia pestis*, which

requires haematin (Lapage & Zinnemann, 1971), grows slowly in Hugh & Leifson's OF medium: acid appears first in the open tube and only later in the sealed tube. We interpret this as fermentation following an initial oxidative stage; consequently we describe the organism as fermentative and include it with the Enterobacteriaceae (Tables 7.9a,e). Membership of this family was confirmed by numerical taxonomy (Sneath & Cowan, 1958) and by the antigenic relationships demonstrated by Schütze (1928, 1932b) between *Y. pseudotuberculosis* and the 'Salmonella' group B, and between *Y. pseudotuberculosis* and *Y. pestis*. DNA–DNA relatedness indicates that *Y. pseudotuberculosis* and *Y. pestis* constitute a single species and it was proposed that the latter should be regarded as a subspecies of the former (Bercovier et al., 1980c). However, the proposal has sensibly been rejected because of the medical dangers that might arise through such a change in nomenclature.

Minidefinition: *Yersinia. Gram-negative rods; motile or non-motile (temperature dependent). Aerobic and facultatively anaerobic. Catalase-positive; oxidase-negative. Sugars attacked fermentatively, occasionally with production of gas. Grow on MacConkey agar. Type species: Y. pestis; NCTC strain 5923.*

7.9.21   Other genera. For the genera of enterobacteria already discussed we have included only those species associated with clinical specimens; however, there are several other species which have not yet been isolated from such material (see Holmes & Gross, 1983; 1990) and these are described in *Bergey's Manual* (1984). For completeness, we mention briefly other genera, the strains of which are mostly few in number and which have been isolated either occasionally or not at all from clinical material. We do not include them in the Tables but give references for those interested.

Budvicia has a single species *B. aquatica*, which has been isolated so far only from fresh water and small wild mammals. The strains have complex growth factor requirements and are reported to produce H_2S, and to hydrolyse urea and O-nitrophenyl-β-D-galactopyranoside. They do not produce acid from glycerol, maltose, sucrose or trehalose, and do not decarboxylate arginine, lysine or ornithine, or produce phenylalanine deaminase (Bouvet *et al.,* 1985).

Ewingella has a single species *E. americana*, isolated from clinical specimens. The few strains reported are said to be anaerogenic, to produce acid from glucose and to give a positive result in the Voges–Proskaüer test. They do not produce deoxyribonuclease, arginine dihydrolase, lysine decarboyxlase, or ornithine decarboyxlase nor do they ferment arabinose, raffinose, sorbitol or sucrose (Grimont *et al.,* 1983). The reference strains we have examined were indistinguishable from *Erwinia herbicola* (see Section 7.9.8).

Koserella has a single species *K. trabulsii*, described from 12 strains isolated from clinical material (Hickman-Brenner *et al.,* 1985*a*). The species, which closely resembles *Hafnia alvei*, is reported to utilize citrate (Simmons' medium), to give positive results in tests for arginine dihydrolase, lysine decarboxylase, ornithine decarboxylase, fermentation of cellobiose and melibiose and in the methyl red test. The strains give negative results for indole, VP, H$_2$S, urease and phenylalanine deaminase production, and do not ferment glycerol, lactose, sorbitol and sucrose.

Leminorella has two species: *L. grimontii* and *L. richardii* (Hickman-Brenner *et al.,* 1985*b*). The first species was described from six strains (four from faeces; two from urine) and the second from four strains from faeces. The former species produces gas from glucose and gives a positive reaction in the methyl red test whereas strains of *L. richardii* give negative results. *Leminorella* strains produce H$_2$S and ferment arabinose and xylose but give negative results in most other tests.

Moellerella has a single species *M. wisconsensis*, described from nine strains isolated from faeces (Hickman-Brenner *et al.,* 1984). They are reported to give positive results in Simmons' citrate medium and the methyl red test and to produce acid from lactose and raffinose, but give negative results in most other tests. Colonies on MacConkey Agar are indistinguishable from those of *Escherichia coli*. We have examined some strains but all of them differed from the original description of the species in fermenting

arabinose and not utilizing citrate (Simmons' medium), presumably due to differences in methods.

Obesumbacterium has a single 'species', *O. proteus*, which Priest *et al.* (1973) divided into groups 1 and 2. Despite their phenotypic similarity and their association with the brewery environment they are phylogenetically different. Indeed, DNA–DNA hybridization reveals that *O. proteus* biogroup 1 is closely related to *Hafnia alvei*; Farmer *et al.* (1985) therefore proposed that it should be classified as a distinct biogroup of *H. alvei* to be known either as *H. alvei* biogroup 1 or as the *H. alvei*–brewery biogroup; *O. proteus* biogroup 2 would retain the name *Obesumbacterium*. Strains of both biogroups are difficult to identify as they are slow-growing and fastidious when incubated at 36 °C. Strains of both biogroups ferment D-glucose and D-mannose, but other sugar reactions may vary between the biogroups.

Pragia with a single species, *P. fontium*, has so far been isolated almost exclusively from water in Czechoslovakia. It is said to be motile, able to grow on Simmons' citrate medium and to produce H$_2$S, oxidize gluconate, ferment glucose and galactose and give a positive result in the methyl red test (Aldová *et al.*, 1988).

Rahnella has a single species *R. aquatilis*, which has so far been isolated only from water and soil (Izard *et al.*, 1979). The reference strains we have examined failed to utilize citrate (Simmons' medium), and did not produce urease, H$_2$S or liquefy gelatin; they were malonate- and ONPG-positive, and fermented several carbohydrates but not adonitol, inositol or starch; gas was not produced from glucose.

Xenorhabdus has two species: *X. luminescens* and *X. nematophilus*, both so far isolated only from nematodes and the insect larvae they parasitise (Thomas & Poinar, 1979). They are unusual members of the Enterobacteriaceae in giving negative results in most biochemical tests used for differentiation. They do not reduce nitrate or ferment most carbohydrates; acid production from glucose is generally weak or delayed. The former species is bioluminescent and the latter does not produce catalase.

Yokenella has a single species *Y. regensburgei*, described from eleven strains of which five were isolated from clinical material and six from insects (Kosako, Sakazaki & Yoshizaki, 1984). The strains are reported to resemble *H. alvei* except for utilizing citrate (Simmons' medium), fermenting cellobiose and melibiose, in giving negative Voges–Proskaüer test results (at 37 °C) and in failing to ferment sorbitol. This organism is probably synonymous with *Koserella trabulsii* (Hickman-Brenner *et al.*, 1985*a*).

The characteristics not only of most of the above species, but also of several as yet unnamed groups of enterobacteria and of particular biotypes of some of the better-known species, are given by Farmer *et al.* (1985).

7.10 A group of difficult organisms
(*Haemophilus, Gardnerella, Campylobacter, Arcobacter, Helicobacter, Anaerobiospirillum, Eikenella, Streptobacillus, Legionella, Mycoplasma*)

***Characters common to members of the group*: Gram-negative rods. Exacting though differing requirements for isolation and continued growth in subculture.**

These organisms have little in common except for the demands they make on the skill and ingenuity of bacteriologists. If, as in the first edition of this *Manual*, we had a chapter on miscellaneous bacteria and those of uncertain taxonomic position all these would have qualified for it, but as we are more concerned with identification than with taxonomic position, we have collected them into a 'group of difficult organisms'. They are difficult in many ways, not least in being fastidious in their nutritional and atmospheric requirements. Neither *Eikenella* nor *Campylobacter* can be isolated from material incubated aerobically, and anaerobic culture is not much more successful. *Eikenella* grows in air with added CO_2 while *Campylobacter* prefers air with only 5–10% oxygen in it, as also do *Arcobacter* and *Anaerobiosprillum* though the latter requires anaerobic conditions for subculture. *Haemophilus* species are not so fussy about their atmospheric surroundings but they are demanding in their X- and V-factor requirements. *Streptobacillus* prefers anaerobic conditions and

requires a medium much richer in protein than is usually provided; like other members of the group its growth is improved by the addition of carbon dioxide. *Legionella* has an absolute nutritional requirement for L-cysteine and iron for primary isolation and often for subculture. And *Mycoplasma* is in a class of its own and requires special methods for characterization.

7.10.1 Haemophilus (Tables 7.10*a,b*) is still defined as Gram-negative coccobacilli or rods that require one or both of the two accessory growth factors X (haemin or other porphyrins) and V (Coenzyme 1: nicotinamide adenine dinucleotide (NAD) or its phosphate). These species will not grow on the media used in conventional biochemical tests, and X and V factor supplements are needed for the indole and carbohydrate tests shown in Table 7.10*b*. The X-factor requirement reflects their inability to synthesise the porphyrins necessary for their respiratory enzymes: it is usually demonstrated by the absence of growth on porphyrin-deficient but otherwise nutritionally adequate media except near paper discs or strips impregnated with X- and, if necessary, V-factor. However, most basic liquid and solid media contain traces of X-factor, as do some brands and batches of peptone. Zinnemann (1960) recommended Yeastrel (Yeast Extract) Agar as a consistently X-free medium for testing this requirement of *Haemophilus* species. Doern and Chapin (1984) found Trypticase Soy Agar to be more reliable than Brain Heart Infusion or Mueller-Hinton agar for this purpose. Kilian (1974) doubted whether any complex medium which otherwise satisfied the growth requirements of haemophili was completely free of X-factor. He claimed that more reliable results for X-factor requirements were obtained by testing the ability of haemophili to synthesize porphyrins from δ-amino laevulinic acid (ALA) and this was confirmed by Tebbutt (1983). A disc method for the ALA porphyrin test (Lund & Blazevic, 1977) and a porphyrin test medium (Gadberry & Amos, 1986) have also been described. V-factor acts as a coenzyme or catalyst in oxidation-reduction reactions and this requirement of strains can be determined either by means of impregnated paper discs or strips, or less specifically by demonstrating satellitism near the growth of *Staphylococcus aureus* which produces V-factor in

Table 7.10a. *Second-stage table for* Haemophilus, Eikenella, Gardnerella, Campylobacter, Helicobacter, Streptobacillus, Arcobacter, Anaerobiospirillum, Legionella *and* Mycoplasma

	1	2	3	4	5	6	7	8	9
Motility	–	–	–	+	–	–	+	+	+
Growth in air	+	w^d	+	–	+	+	+	–	?^{a}
Growth under anaerobic conditions	+	+	+	D	+	+	d	+	.
Catalase	D	–	–	D	–	–	d	–	+
Oxidase	D	+	–	+	–	–	+	–	d
Swelling of microbial cell	–	–	–	–	+	–	–	–	–
Colony adherent to medium	–	+	–	–	–	+	–	–	–
Growth at 42 °C	–	w	w	D	–	?	w/–	+	d
Growth favoured by O$_2$	?	?	?	+^{g}	+	?	+^{h}	–	+
Growth favoured by CO$_2$	D	+	+	+	+	?	+	?	?
Growth improved by blood/serum	D^b	+	–	+	+	+	+	+	?
Growth improved by moisture (closed jar)	+	+	+	+	+^{a}	?	?	?	+
Carbohydrates [F/O/–]	F	–	F	–	F	F/–	–	F	–
Glucose, acid from	+	–	+	–	+	+	–	+	–
Starch hydrolysis	?	–	+	–	+	+^{c}	–	–	–
Nitrate reduced	+	+	–	D	–	?	+	–	–
Indole	D	–	–	–	–	?	–	–	–
Gelatin liquefied	–	–	?	–	–	–	–	–	+
Urease	D	–	–	D	–	D	D	–	NT
H$_2$S	D	(w)/–	–	D	–	?	–	?	?
Arginine dihydrolase	–	–	–	?	+	D	?	?	–
Lysine decarboxylase	D	+	–	?	?	?	?	?	–
Ornithine decarboxylase	D	d	–	?	?	?	?	?	–
Zone of inhibition with metronidazole (50 µg)	?	–	+	d	?	?	+	+	–

1 Haemophilus spp.
2 Eikenella corrodens; HB–1
3 Gardnerella vaginalis; *'Corynebacterium vaginale'*
4 Campylobacter and Helicobacter spp.; *V. fetus*
5 Streptobacillus moniliformis; *'Actinobacillus muris'; 'Actinomyces muris'*
6 Mycoplasma spp.; **Acholeplasma** spp
7 Arcobacter spp.
8 Anaerobiospirillum succiniciproducens
9 Legionella spp.

a Requirement for growth
b Blood requirement is for haematin (X factor)
c False positive reactions can occur due to amylases in serum
d Haemin usually required for growth under aerobic conditions
e Cysteine and iron salts required for growth
f *C. curvus* and *C. rectus* positive in modified test of Tarrand & Gröschel (1982)
g O$_2$ essential for growth but >10% is toxic
h Optimal O$_2$: 3-10%
NT not testable by usual method

Other symbols used in the table are explained in Tables 5.1 and 5.2 on p.47.

excess of its own need. Since V-factor is susceptible to heat, media in which all the constituents have been autoclaved will be reliably free from it. However, consistent results in tests for these growth factor requirements depend on the use of small inocula to avoid any carry-over. Occasional strains in other unrelated taxa sometimes exhibit growth-factor requirements similar to those of *Haemophilus* species; for example, occasional strains of *Eikenella corrodens* have an apparent requirement for X-factor. This can cause confusion and illustrates the danger of basing identification of the genus *Haemophilus* solely on X- and V-factor requirements.

Haemophilus species are fastidious not only in

151

their X- and V- requirements but also in their need for other nutritional factors, which vary among the species. *H. ducreyi* and *H. parasuis* have a requirement for serum; so does *H. paragallinarum*, which also has a requirement for NaCl (Rimler *et al.*, 1977) though it is not halophilic in the usual meaning of the term. Raised carbon dioxide tension improves growth, and may be necessary for a number of species, including *H. aphrophilus*, *H. paraphrophilus*, *H. paraphrohaemolyticus* and *H. paragallinarum*. This apparent need for CO_2 may be fulfilled by incubating cultures in the moist atmosphere of a sealed jar. However under the usual conditions of aerobic incubation recently isolated strains may grow only feebly or not at all; added CO_2 should therefore be used for primary isolation and it may prove beneficial for subsequent subcultures of haemophili (Frazer, Zinnemann & Boyce, 1969). The optimum temperature for growth is 35–37 °C.

For culture, ordinary Blood Agar medium is not suitable unless heated to form 'Chocolate Agar'; this not only releases the V-factor from disrupted erythrocytes but also inactivates any enzymes which might affect X-factor. For primary isolation of haemophili from the respiratory tract, selective media containing for example crystal violet (Turk, 1963), bacitracin (Baber, 1969) and other antibacterial agents (Chapin & Doern, 1983) can be used to inhibit overgrowth by other members of the normal flora.

Some species of *Haemophilus*, notably *H. influenzae* as well as *H. parasuis*, *H. gallinarum* and *H. avium*, can produce polysaccharide capsules which are antigenically type-specific and related to pathogenicity. Occasional capsulated strains of *H. parainfluenzae* have also been described (Sims, 1970). Such strains exhibit iridescence on transparent media such as that of Levinthal (1918) or the peptic digest of Fildes (1920). With *H. influenzae*, six capsular types (a–f) can be identified (Pittman, 1931) of which type b is the most frequent among capsulated strains isolated from infections in man.

Haemophilus species can be differentiated by their growth-factor requirements and cultural characteristics (Table 7.10*b*). The species commonly encountered in medical laboratories can usually be identified satisfactorily by these methods alone. With a difficult strain, or in order to confirm the identity of an unusual species, further biochemical tests may be necessary; these include carbohydrate utilization tests in Phenol Red Broth sugars supplemented with 10 µg/ml each of X- and V-factors (Kilian, 1976). The results can usually be read after 24 hours incubation, though some species, notably *H. segnis*, give weak reactions. As carbohydrate utilization and concomitant acid production by haemophili are, to some extent, dependent on the medium used, the results of these tests should be interpreted with caution. Most strains of *H. parainfluenzae*, *H. haemolyticus*, *H. aphrophilus* and *H. paraphrophilus* produce small amounts of gas (H_2 and CO_2) from glucose (Kilian, 1976); other species of *Haemophilus* do not produce any gas. As facultative anaerobes, all *Haemophilus* species can ferment glucose anaerobically (Sneath & Johnson, 1973) but the exact mode of carbohydrate breakdown is not known so that the description 'fermentation' may simply mean acid production by unknown metabolic means. The catalase activity of haemophili (Table 7.10*b*) may vary with the cultural conditions; for example, some apparently catalase-negative strains may give a positive reaction if provided with sufficient haemin (Biberstein & Gills, 1961). The oxidase reaction is always positive with *H. influenzae* and negative with *H. aphrophilus*; the other species do not give consistent results. Rapid test kits for identification of *Haemophilus* species have also been described (Janda, Malloy & Schreckenberger, 1987; Murphy *et al.*, 1990).

Three biochemical reactions – indole production and urease and ornithine decarboxylase activity – form the basis of a scheme devised by Kilian (1976) for biotyping *H. influenzae* and *H. parainfluenzae*. These tests, which depend on the presence of preformed enzymes, are performed in media heavily inoculated with bacterial growth from an 18 hour agar culture. The results can be read after 5 hours incubation, though the ornithine decarboxylase test may give a clear reaction only after overnight incubation. With *H. influenzae*, Kilian distinguished five biotypes (I–V) which showed some correlation with different infections. Three further biotypes of *H. influenzae* were described subsequently by Oberhofer & Back (1979), Gratten (1983) and Sottnek & Albritton (1984). The majority of clinical isolates of *H. influenzae* belong to biotypes I, II and III; most isolates from low-grade and chronic infections are non-capsulated strains of biotypes II and III whereas those from acute infections such as meningitis are usually caused by capsulated strains of biotype I. Other studies purport to show a correlation between biotype, serotype, antimicrobial susceptibility (Granato, Jurek & Weiner, 1983) and the source of the isolates (Albritton *et al.*, 1978). With *H. parainfluenzae*, eight biotypes have been described (Kilian, 1976; Oberhofer & Back, 1979; Sturm, 1986). It is not clear, however, if biotyping has contributed greatly to our understanding of *Haemophilus* infections.

For epidemiological studies, subtyping schemes based on outer membrane proteins (Loeb & Smith, 1980), on lipopolysaccharides (Inzana, 1983) or on isoenzyme profiles (Musser *et al.*, 1985) are more sensitive than biotyping.

Metabolic adaptations among *Haemophilus* species can occur *in vitro* which, by reducing or abolishing specific requirements, may be responsible for some of the conflicting statements in the literature. *H. aphrophilus* was originally isolated from cases of infective endocarditis by Khairat (1940) and was so named because it needed X-factor and CO_2 for growth, though the X-factor requirement may be lost on subculture. King & Tatum (1962) were unable to confirm the X-factor requirement of strains sent to them, but they pointed out that these strains had been subcultured several times and so may well have lost it. They thought that the strains had much in common with those of *Actinobacillus actinomycetemcomitans*, but had relatively few of the recognized characters of either *Haemophilus* or *Actinobacillus*. White & Garrick (1963) showed that *H. aphrophilus* possessed all the enzymes of the haemin-biosynthetic pathway characteristic of species not requiring X-factor; indeed, it gave a positive but weak reaction in the porphyrin ALA test. The reason for the apparent X-factor requirement on primary isolation is unknown. Boyce, Frazer & Zinnemann (1969) discussed the difficulties of classifying strains that adapt quickly to *in vitro* conditions and concluded that because the majority of bacterial cells in each culture were incapable of synthesising X-factor, *H. aphrophilus* should be regarded as essentially X-dependent. Since we try to show the characteristics of freshly isolated strains, this X-dependence is recorded in Table 7.10*b*. DNA–DNA hybridization studies indicate that *H. aphrophilus* and *H. paraphrophilus* are closely related (Potts *et al.,* 1986; Tønjum, Bukholm & Bøvre,

1990), thus adding weight to the suggestion of Potts & Berry (1983) that one of them could be regarded as a subspecies of the other. However, as *H. aphrophilus* is X-factor and *H. paraphrophilus* V-factor dependent, we continue to regard them as separate species.

There has been much debate as to whether *H. aegyptius* (the Koch-Weeks bacillus) should be regarded as a species separate from *H. influenzae*. The dilemma is not surprising since transformation studies (Leidy, Hahn & Alexander, 1959; Leidy, Jaffee & Alexander, 1965) and DNA hybridization (Casin, Grimont & Grimont, 1986) have shown a high degree of relatedness. Pittman and Davis (1950) differentiated *H. aegyptius* from *H. influenzae* on the basis of acid production from xylose and agglutination of human red cells. Kilian (1976) considered *H. aegyptius* to be synonymous with *H. influenzae* biotype III. In a further taxonomic study of 112 strains of *Haemophilus* isolated from conjunctivae, Kilian *et al.* (1976) again stated that *H. aegyptius* should be regarded as a haemagglutinating variety of *H. influenzae* biotype III. However Mazloum *et al.* (1982), in a study of 29 isolates from cases of acute conjunctivitis in Egypt, claimed that strains of *H. aegyptius* could be distinguished from those of *H. influenzae* biotype III by their inability to ferment xylose or to grow in Trypticase Soy Agar despite added X- and V-factors, and by their susceptibility to troleandomycin. Kilian & Biberstein (1984) stated that only sensitivity to troleandomycin would unequivocally distinguish between them but Carlone *et al.* (1985) regarded this test as unreliable; their studies did however reveal distinct differences in the protein profiles of the outer membranes of the two organisms despite their close genetic relatedness. Brenner *et al.* (1988) accordingly adopted the term '*H. influenzae* biogroup aegyptius' for strains which would formerly have been called *H. aegyptius*. However, the view of Casin, Grimont & Grimont, (1986) that the differences in pathogenicity between the two organisms are of little relevance in classification accords with the probability that they represent one taxon; for this reason, we do not include *H. aegyptius* in Table 7.10*b*. This organism has nevertheless been associated with the infection described recently as 'Brazilian purpuric fever' (Brenner *et al.*, 1988).

Haemophili isolated from swine and fowl have

Table 7.10*b*. *Third–stage table for* Haemophilus, Gardnerella, Actinobacillus actinomycetemcomitans *and* Eikenella corrodens

	1	2	3	4	5	6	7	8	9	10	11	12	13	14*	15	16
V–factor requirement	+	+	−	−	−	+	+	+	+	+	+	+	+	−	−	−
X–factor requirement	+	+	+	+	+[h]	−	−	−	−	−	−	−	−	−	−	+[d]
ALA → porphyrins	−	−	−	−	w	+	+	+	+	+	+	+	+	?	?	?
Catalase	+	+	+	−	−	d	d	+	−	w/−	+	−	+	−	+	−
Oxidase	+	+	+	+	−	+	+	+	−	−	+	−	+	−	+	+
Growth on Chocolate Agar	+	+	+	d[c]	+[e]	+	+	+[e]	+[e]	+	+	+[ef]	+	+	+	+
Haemolysis	−	+[b]	−	d	−	−	+[b]	+[b]	−	−	−	−	−	d[g]	−	−[i]
CO₂ improves growth	−	−	−	d	+	−	−	+	+	−	d	+	−	+	+	+
Indole	D[a]	d	+	−	−	D[a]	−	−	−	−	−	−	−	−	−	−
Urease	D[a]	+	−	−	−	D[a]	+	+	−	−	−	−	−	−	−	−
Ornithine decarboxylase	D[a]	−	−	−	−	D[a]	d	−	−	−	−	−	−	−	−	d
*Carbohydrates, acid from																
glucose	+	+	+	(w/−)	+	+	+	+	+	w	+	+	+	+	+	−
fructose	−	w	−	−	+	+	+	+	+	w	+	+	+	d	+	.
galactose	+	+	−	−	+	+	d	d	−	w	+	−	+	d	d	.
inulin	−	−	−	−	−	−	−	−	−	−	+	−	−	d	−	.
lactose	−	−	−	−	+	−	+	−	+	−	d	−	d	d	−	.
mannitol	−	−	+	−	−	−	−	−	−	−	−	+	d	−	d	.
raffinose	−	−	−	−	+	−	−	−	−	−	−	−	−	d	−	.
ribose	+	+	d	−	+	−	−	−	+	−	+	+	+	d	?	?
sorbitol	−	−	−	−	−	−	−	−	−	−	−	−	+	d	−	.
sucrose	−	−	+	−	+	+	+	+	+	w	+	+	+	d	−	.
trehalose	−	−	−	−	+	−	−	−	+	−	−	−	+	d	−	.
xylose	+	d	+	−	−	−	−	−	−	−	−	−	d	d	d	.

1 **Haemophilus influenzae**
2 **Haemophilus haemolyticus**
3 **Haemophilus haemoglobinophilus;**
   '*H. canis*'
4 **Haemophilus ducreyi**
5 **Haemophilus aphrophilus**
6 **Haemophilus parainfluenzae**

7 **Haemophilus parahaemolyticus;**
8 **Haemophilus paraphrohaemolyticus**
9 **Haemophilus paraphrophilus**
10 **Haemophilus segnis**
11 **Haemophilus parasuis**
12 **Haemophilus paragallinarum**
13 **Haemophilus avium**

14 **Gardnerella vaginalis*;**
   '*Corynebacterium vaginale*'
15 **Actinobacillus**
   actinomycetemcomitans
16 **Eikenella corrodens**

* Note. Phenol red broth sugars supplemented with X and V factors are essential for *Haemophilus* spp. Carbohydrate reactions are not reliable for *Gardnerella*.
a Reactions vary with biotypes
b Haemolysis with bovine or sheep blood; variable with horse blood. May lose haemolytic activity on subculture
c Optimum temperature for growth 33 °C, but very slow. Growth improved with addition of 1% Iso Vitalex (Hammond *et al.*, 1978)
d Haemin usually required for growth under aerobic conditions
e Positive in CO₂
f Serum improves growth
g β-haemolysis with human and rabbit blood; haemolysis variable with horse blood
h Requires haemin–containing media on primary isolation
i Slight greening of medium may occur around colonies

Other symbols used in the table are explained in Tables 5.1 and 5.2 on p.47.

also posed considerable problems of classification and nomenclature, which were discussed at some length by Biberstein & White (1969). '*Haemophilus influenzae suis*' was proposed by Lewis & Shope (1931) for an organism isolated from swine influenza in America. This organism, usually referred to as *H.* *suis*, required both X- and V-factors and was virtually indistinguishable from indole-negative strains of *H. influenzae*. However, the original cultures of Lewis & Shope when re-examined by Matthews & Pattison (1961) were found to be no longer X-dependent, possibly because of adaptation *in vitro*. Biberstein &

White (1969) proposed a new species, *Haemophilus parasuis*, for strains that did not require haemin but which were otherwise identical to *H. suis*. Since then it has become clear that the overwhelming majority of strains isolated from swine require only V-factor and thus, according to the usual convention for naming *Haemophilus* species, should be called *H. parasuis*. Moreover most of the strains in culture collections labelled *H. suis* do not need X-factor and are therefore *H. parasuis* (Kilian & Biberstein, 1984). For these reasons we include only *H. parasuis* in Table 7.10*b*. The organism formerly classified as *Haemophilus pleuropneumoniae* has been transferred recently to the genus *Actinobacillus* (Pohl *et al.*, 1983) on the basis of its phenotypic characters and DNA relatedness to *Actinobacillus lignieresii*; however the emended species *A. pleuropneumoniae* includes both V-factor requiring and V-factor independent biovars.

Haemophili isolated from fowl pose problems similar to those from swine. There are conflicting reports on the growth-factor requirements of *H. gallinarum*, the fowl coryza bacillus. De Blieck (1932) stated that it required both X- and V-factors and this was confirmed by Schalm & Beach (1936) and by Delaplane, Erwin & Stuart, (1938) who showed also that *H. gallinarum* had an obligate requirement for sodium chloride (0.5–2.5%). However later studies have failed to demonstrate any strains of avian haemophili which required X-factor for growth (Page, 1962; Roberts, Hanson & Timms, 1964). Biberstein & White (1969) accordingly proposed the name *Haemophilus paragallinarum* for X-independent haemophili which were otherwise identical to *H. gallinarum*. Piechulla, Hinz & Mannheim (1985) suggested on the basis of DNA homology that *H. paragallinarum* is more closely related to the genus *Actinobacillus* than to *Haemophilus*. Page (1962) divided the avian haemophili into two groups. The first group, *H. paragallinarum*, was catalase-negative, grew in air with 5% CO_2 and caused infectious coryza; the second group of strains, which were catalase-positive, grew in air and were non-pathogenic, was subsequently allocated to a new species, *H. avium*, by Hinz & Kunjara (1977). DNA-DNA hybridization (Mutters *et al.*, 1977) indicated that *H. avium* contained three clusters, which were genetically closer to *Pasteurella multocida* than to *Haemophilus influenzae*. Mutters *et*

al. (1977) accordingly suggested reclassifying *H. avium* into three new taxa, *Pasteurella avium*, *P. volantium* and 'Pasteurella species A'. However, on the basis of their phenotypic characters not all strains of *H. avium* could be assigned to *Pasteurella* in this way (Blackall, 1988). It is thus clear that further work on haemophili from swine and fowl is needed to clarify the present situation.

Casin *et al.* (1985) suggested that *H. ducreyi*, which is phenotypically distinct from other *Haemophilus* species, is misplaced in that genus because of the low level of DNA homology. This is supported by Carlone *et al.* (1988) who found that the respiratory quinone content of *H. ducreyi* differed significantly from that of other haemophili. Indeed Höllander, Hess-Reihse & Mannheim (1981) suggested that *Haemophilus* species should be reclassified on the basis of their respiratory quinones.

The long-standing debate on the correct classification of the organism previously labelled 'Haemophilus vaginalis' and subsequently as 'Corynebacterium vaginale' has been resolved at last by the creation of a new genus with a single species, *Gardnerella vaginalis* (Greenwood & Pickett, 1980; Piot *et al.*, 1980). We describe this Gram-variable rod in Section 7.10.2 but, for convenience, we also record its characteristics in Tables 7.10*a, b*.

Other species have been described, but by present standards they do not warrant inclusion in the genus *Haemophilus* as none of them requires X- or V-factors for growth. They include 'Haemophilus somnus' (Bailie, Coles & Weide, 1973), 'Haemophilus agni' (Kennedy *et al.*, 1958) and 'Haemophilus equigenitalis' (Taylor *et al.*, 1978). An organism requiring V-factor isolated from the small intestine of rabbits with mucoid enteritis was named *Haemophilus paracuniculus* by Targowski & Targowski (1979), but its pathogenic role and correct classification have not yet been confirmed.

Potts, Zambon & Genco, (1985) have proposed that *Actinobacillus actinomycetemcomitans* should be reassigned to the genus *Haemophilus* as *H. actinomycetemcomitans*. DNA–DNA hybridization studies of *A. actinomycetemcomitans*, *H. segnis*, *H. aphrophilus* and *H. paraphrophilus* showed considerable homology consistent with placing them in a single genus. Antigens common to all these species were also found by immunodiffusion. However, '*H. acti-*

nomycetemcomitans' does not require either X- or V-factors and it thus does not easily fit into the genus *Haemophilus* as currently defined, but for comparison we include it in Table 7.10*b*.

> **Minidefinition**: *Haemophilus. Gram-negative rods or coccobacilli; often markedly pleomorphic; non-motile. Aerobic and facultatively anaerobic. Oxidase and catalase reactions vary between species and strains. Nitrate reduced to nitrite: Fastidious; require media containing X- and V-factors and undefined constituents of blood and serum. Attack sugars fermentatively. Type species: H. influenzae; NCTC strain 8143.*

7.10.2 Gardnerella (Table 7.10*a*) has caused much controversy since it was first described by Leopold in 1953. Gardner & Dukes (1954) and Lutz, Grooten & Wurch, (1956) noted that a similar organism was frequently associated with non-specific vaginitis or anaerobic vaginosis; Gardner & Dukes (1955) regarded it as the causal organism and, on the basis of its microscopical appearance and apparent growth requirement for blood, proposed the name *Haemophilus vaginalis*. However, neither X-(haemin) nor V-(nicotinamide adeninine dinucleotide) factor was required for its growth (Edmunds, 1962; Dunkelberg & McVeigh, 1969); one or other of these is essential for inclusion in the genus *Haemophilus* as currently defined. It is, however, fastidious in its growth requirements, needing thiamine or related substances as well as purines and pyrimidines (Dunkelberg & McVeigh, 1969). Lapage (1961) confirmed that it did not require X- or V-factors and suggested it might be a *Corynebacterium*; this was supported on Gram-staining and morphological grounds by Zinnemann & Turner (1963) who recommended its reclassification as *Corynebacterium vaginale*. Although Dunkelberg & McVeigh (1969) agreed with this proposal it failed to gain universal approval. '*C. vaginale*' is catalase-negative, whereas most corynebacteria are positive and the cell wall of '*C. vaginale*', unlike that of corynebacteria, lacks teichoic acid and arabinose (Keddie & Cure, 1978). Not surprisingly, the difficulty receded when Greenwood & Pickett (1979), proposed a new genus, *Gardnerella*, for it based on cell wall composition, DNA homology and electron microscopy.

Subsequent taxonomic studies (Greenwood & Pickett, 1980; Piot *et al.*, 1980) confirmed that *Gardnerella vaginalis* is not related to the genus *Haemophilus* or to *Corynebacterium*, and the name *G. vaginalis* has since been widely accepted.

The precise taxonomic position of *G. vaginalis* remains uncertain; indeed, whether it is Gram-positive or Gram-negative is still unresolved and it is included among both the Gram-positive and the Gram-negative organisms in *Bergey's Manual of Systematic Bacteriology* by Greenwood & Pickett (1984, 1986). Based on the amino acid composition of the cell wall Criswell *et al.* (1971) stated that *G. vaginalis* was Gram-negative but their results were criticised by Easmon & Ison (1984) as they had also failed to detect the diaminopimelic acid known to be present in the cell walls of *Escherichia coli* and *Bacillus megaterium*. Conversely, Harper & Davis (1982) considered the amino acid composition of the cell wall to be that of a Gram-positive organism. Electron microscopy has failed to resolve this dispute, though Reyn, Birch-Anderson & Lapage, (1966) reported that the structure of the cell wall and septa was more like that of Gram-positive organisms; however, Criswell and her colleagues (1971, 1972) observed an unusual trilaminar cell-wall appearance more closely resembling that of Gram-negative bacteria. Greenwood & Pickett (1980) concluded that the cell wall was more like that of Gram-negative than of Gram-positive organisms, but it was not 'typical'. The status of the Gram-reaction has yet to be resolved but in practice, Gram-stained smears of fresh cultures show mostly Gram-positive bacteria and ageing cultures significantly more Gram-negative organisms; in smears from clinical material both forms occur. We have placed it among the Gram-negative organisms in Table 7.10*a* though we refer to it in Section 6.5 and include it also in Table 6.5*b*.

G. vaginalis is aerobic and facultatively anaerobic though obligate anaerobic strains have been reported (Malone *et al.*, 1975); growth is enhanced by the addition of 5–10% CO_2. It produces diffuse β–haemolysis on human or rabbit Blood Agar but not on sheep Blood Agar; haemolysis on horse Blood Agar is variable (Greenwood *et al.*, 1977). This character is exploited for selective isolation of the organism from clinical specimens; and the use of layered human Blood Agar plates, with the addition of Tween

80, has now largely superseded the Peptone Starch Glucose Agar medium described by Dunkelberg & McVeigh (1969) and Totten *et al.* (1982). Smith (1979) and Piot *et al.* (1980) noted, however, that occasional strains of lactobacilli and streptococci from vaginal specimens also produced similar β-haemolysis.

Definitive identification of *G. vaginalis* is difficult as there are no wholly reliable test characters. It ferments carbohydrates without gas production, the major end-product being acetic acid (Moss & Dunkelberg, 1969) but the reported reactions for some carbohydrates vary (Edmunds, 1962; Greenwood & Pickett, 1979; Piot *et al.*, 1980) and are not always reproducible (Taylor & Phillips, 1983) probably because of differences in the test methods and media used. Furthermore, the carbohydrate reactions do not reliably differentiate *G. vaginalis* from lactobacilli among the vaginal flora. We do not therefore recommend their use in routine diagnostic laboratories except for non-genital isolates (Piot, 1985). Yong & Thompson (1982) described a rapid (one hour) micromethod for hippurate hydrolysis and the fermentation of starch and raffinose; the medium described by Dunkelberg, Skaggs & Kellog (1970) modified by Greenwood & Pickett (1979) can also be used for these tests. Heavy inocula may help to minimize the variability of the biochemical results (Piot & van Dyck, 1981).

As simple test characters, β-haemolysis on human, but not on horse Blood Agar, the Gram-reaction, the microscopical appearance, colonial morphology, and negative oxidase and catalase reactions have all been recommended for reliably identifying *G. vaginalis* (Ison *et al.*, 1982; Shaw *et al.*, 1981; Piot *et al.*, 1982). Greenwood and Pickett (1979) used hippurate hydrolysis and β-haemolysis to separate *G. vaginalis* from other catalase- and oxidase-negative organisms; and Jolly (1983) considered them indispensable for the accurate identification of *G. vaginalis* in the routine laboratory. Taylor and Phillips (1983) however found that hippurate hydrolysis did not reliably distinguish between *G. vaginalis* and catalase-negative coryneform organisms. The enzymatic *O*-nitrophenol tests for the detection of α- and β-glucosidase were also recommended by Piot *et al.* (1982) but Taylor & Phillips (1983) found these unhelpful.

G. vaginalis is susceptible to metronidazole and

trimethoprim but resistant to sulphonamides (Bailey, Voss & Smith, 1979; Piot *et al.*, 1980); despite our reservations about such tests, they are helpful in preliminary identification. In addition, Taylor & Phillips (1983) claim that β-haemolysis on human Blood Agar medium, the failure to grow on Nutrient Agar or in the presence of 2% (w/v) NaCl, and the inability to produce lactic acid from glucose will differentiate *G. vaginalis* from lactobacilli and catalase-negative coryneform organisms isolated from vaginal secretions. In routine laboratories, β-haemolysis on human but not horse Blood Agar, the Gram-stain reaction and morphology as well as susceptibility of most strains to discs of metronidazole (50 μg) and trimethoprim (5 μg) should identify satisfactorily more than 90% of isolates. Biotyping schemes for *G. vaginalis* have been described by Piot *et al.* (1984) and by Benito *et al.* (1986).

> **Minidefinition**: *Gardnerella. Gram-negative or Gram-variable rods or coccobacilli; often markedly pleomorphic; non-motile. Aerobic and facultatively anaerobic. Oxidase- and catalase-negative. Fastidious growth requirements. Attacks sugars fermentatively. Gas is not produced. Type species: G. vaginalis; NCTC strain 10287.*

7.10.3   Eikenella (Table 7.10*a*) is the name now given to a group of facultatively anaerobic Gram-negative non-sporing rods that will grow aerobically from the first subculture, though anaerobic conditions may be necessary for isolation (Jackson & Goodman, 1972); these organisms form the HB-1 strains of King & Tatum (1962). The genus was named after Eiken who, in 1958, gave the specific epithet to the organism (which he had placed in *Bacteroides*). According to Jackson & Goodman two rather different organisms, both of which produced 'pitting' on the surface of the medium during growth, have been named *Bacteroides corrodens*; one is a strict anaerobe (and remains so) which is urease-positive; the other (*Eikenella corrodens*) is facultatively anaerobic and urease-negative. A few points of difference between these organisms are shown in Table 7.2*a*. Hill, Shell & Lapage, (1970) did not find any of the strictly anaerobic organisms among the NCTC strains, which had been isolated mostly in the U.K.

In describing these organisms Jackson & Goodman

Table 7.10c. *Third-stage table for* Campylobacter, Helicobacter, Arcobacter *and* Anaerobiospirillum

	1	2	3	4	5	6	7	8	9	10	11	12	13	14	15
Rapid coccal transformation	−	−	−	+	w	+	+	w	−	−	+	w	w	−	w
Spreading surface growth	−	−	−	w	+	+	w	+	−	−	−	+	+^{b}	−	d
Growth at 25 °C	+	+	d^a	−	−	−	−	−	−	−	−	−	−	+^{c}	d
Growth at 43 °C	−	−	w	+	+	+	−	d	d	d^d	d	−	−	−	d
Catalase	+	+	+	+	+	+	d	w/−	−	−	+	+	+	d	−
Growth inhibited by:															
nalidixic acid^e	−	−	−	−	+	+	+	+	d	−	−	+	+	+	−
cephalothin^e	+	+	+	−	−	−	+	+	+	d^d	+	d	+	−	+
Hippurate hydrolysis^f	−	−	−	−	−	+	+	−	−	−	−	−	−	−	−
Indoxyl acetate hydrolysis*	−	−	−	−	+	+	−	+	−	−	−	d	+	+	+
Nitrate reduced^g	+	+	+	+	+	+	−	+	+	+^{d}	−	+	−	+	−
H$_2$S from FBP^h	−	−	−	+/w	−	d	−	−	+	−	−	−	−	−	−
H$_2$S from TSI	−	−	+^{d}	+^{i}	d^i	d^i	−	−	+	+^{d}	−	−	−	−	?
Growth in the presence of:															
triphenyltetrazolium chloride 0.04% (agar)	−	−	−	d	+	+	d	−	−	−	+	+	+	d	?
1% glycine	+	−	+	+	+	+	+	d	+	−	d	+	+	d	?
1.5% sodium chloride (agar)	d	d	d	+	−	−	−	−	+	+^{d}	−	−	−	d	?
Growth under anaerobic conditions	+^{j}	+^{j}	+^{k}	+^{k}	−	−	−	+^{j}	+^{j}	+^{d}	−	−	−	+	+
Urease^l	−	−	−	−^{m}	−	−	−	−	−	−	+	−	−	−	−

1 **Campylobacter fetus** subsp. **fetus**
2 **Campylobacter fetus** subsp. **venerealis**
3 **Campylobacter hyointestinalis**
4 **Campylobacter lari**; *C. laridis*
5 **Campylobacter coli**
6 **Campylobacter jejuni** subsp. **jejuni**
7 **Campylobacter jejuni** subsp. **doylei**

8 **Campylobacter upsaliensis**
9 **Campylobacter sputorum**
  subsp. **sputorum**
10 **Campylobacter concisus**
11 **Helicobacter pylori**
12 **Helicobacter cinaedi**;
  Campylobacter cinaedi

13 **Helicobacter fennelliae**;
  Campylobacter fennelliae
14 **Arcobacter cryaerophilus**;
  Campylobacter cryaerophila
15 **Anaerobiospirillum**
  succiniciproducens

* Rapid disc method of Mills & Gherna (1987)
a Scraped colonies appear yellow
b Smells of hypochlorite
c Growth also at 15 °C
d Requires H$_2$ or formate
e 30 µg disc, any zone of inhibition
f Method of Hwang & Ederer (1975)

g Method 5 – Cook (1950); C3.39
h Method 7 – Lior (1984); C3.30
i Blackening where there is water of synaeresis
j Requires fumarate (0.2%) or nitrate (0.1%)
k Positive in the presence of trimethylamine N–oxide (0.1%)
l Christensen's urea medium without agar (A2.6.41)
m A urease-positive subgroup has been described (Bolton *et al.*, 1985)

Note. Use Mueller–Hinton or Blood Agar for these tests unless otherwise stated. Raising the agar concentration to 2% facilitates reading zones of inhibition by preventing growth spreading. Organisms 7, 8 and 11–15 require blood for reliable growth and plates should be moist.

Other symbols used in the table are explained in Tables 5.1 and 5.2 on p.47.

(1972) and Prefontaine & Jackson (1972) distinguished the facultative anaerobe by its DNA G+C content of 28–30% compared with 57–58% for the strictly anaerobic *B. corrodens*; the fatty acid composition of the organisms as determined by gas chromatography was also different. These are esoteric differences and at present still only of theoretical importance, but they do indicate that there are two colonially similar but otherwise different organisms.

Eikenella corrodens has been isolated alone or in mixed culture from pus from various abscesses, pleural fluids, sputum, tonsils, the ear and the nose; Jackson & Goodman (1972) regard it as an opportunist pathogen but Riley, Tatum & Weaver (1973), with information about 500 strains available to them, thought that it was a normal inhabitant of the pharynx and alimentary canal.

For culture, Blood Agar incubated in an atmosphere enriched with 5–10% CO$_2$ in a closed jar is satisfactory. Jackson & Goodman found growth was improved by 0.1% KNO$_3$, and better with 1% oxygen than under strictly anaerobic conditions. Although anaerobic methods using a closed jar seemed to be essential for isolation, it was not clear whether the anaerobiosis, the moisture, the CO_2, or a combination of these, were the essential factor(s). Haematin seems to be essential for the growth of subcultures in air.

The organism was so named because of the adherent nature of the wrinkled colonies which 'dig' into (corrode) the surface of agar media. Some colonies are not wrinkled, and these are not adherent; they breed true and have the same biochemical characters as the wrinkled colony form. Biochemically, *E. corrodens* is rather inactive and for that reason has been likened to brucellas and even placed in the same family. Like *Campylobacter* (Table 7.10c) *Eikenella* grows better in semisolid than in any liquid medium.

Minidefinition: *Eikenella. Gram-negative rods; non-motile. Facultatively anaerobic on first isolation; soon become aerobic. Catalase-negative; oxidase-positive. Do not attack carbohydrates. Type species: E. corrodens; NCTC strain 10596.*

7.10.4 Campylobacter (Tables 7.10a, c). Since

publication of the second edition of this *Manual*, knowledge of this genus has advanced considerably and *Campylobacter jejuni* is now recognized as a common cause of acute enterocolitis in man. Several new species have been described and the status of earlier named species has been clarified. They formerly occupied a place within the genus *Vibrio* as the so-called microaerophilic members exemplified by the animal pathogen '*Vibrio fetus*', but there is every justification for their inclusion in the genus *Campylobacter* as proposed by Sebald & Véron (1963).

In general, campylobacters do not grow in conventional aerobic or anaerobic culture systems, a fact that undoubtedly delayed their recognition as important human pathogens. They grow best in 5–10% oxygen, though some species, notably *C. sputorum* (Loesche, Gibbons & Socransky, 1965), grow anaerobically in the presence of fumarate or nitrate. Most strains grow satisfactorily in sloppy media (0.16% agar) suitably supplemented and incubated aerobically. The intolerance of most species to atmospheric oxygen is due to their extreme sensitivity to superoxides and free radicals despite their possession of catalase and superoxide dismutase (Hoffman *et al.*, 1979a,b); culture

media must therefore contain agents suitable for neutralizing such toxic substances (George *et al.* 1978). Whole blood is perhaps the most effective agent, but haemin, inorganic iron salts, pyruvate and charcoal among others have a similar effect.

A striking character of campylobacters is their helical or curved shape. Long spiral forms can resemble spirochaetes superficially, but campylobacters have flagella, usually single, at one or both poles (monotrichate or amphitrichate) and are highly motile, spinning around their long axes and frequently reversing direction.

The type species, *C. fetus*, of which there are two subspecies, causes infectious abortion of cattle and sheep, but it rarely infects man. *C. fetus* subsp. *fetus* occasionally causes systemic infection in immunodeficient patients. *C. hyointestinalis* (Gebhart *et al.*, 1985) is closely related to *C. fetus*. Although more usually encountered in the intestinal tracts of pigs and cattle, it is occasionally isolated from patients with diarrhoea (Edmonds *et al.*, 1987).

C. jejuni and *C. coli* – collectively known in obsolete nomenclature as '*C. fetus* subsp. *jejuni*' – are the species most often encountered in medical laboratories as a cause of acute enterocolitis. They are distinguished from *C. fetus* and most other campylobacters by their high optimum growth temperature (42 °C), a feature described by King (1962) who called them 'related vibrios'. *C. jejuni* has two subspecies: subsp. *jejuni* – the familiar cause of enterocolitis in man; and subsp. *doylei* (Steele & Owen, 1988) – a more fastidious and slower growing organism which does not grow at 43 °C or reduce nitrate. *C. lari* (previously termed '*C. laridis*' by Benjamin *et al.*, 1983) is also 'thermophilic' like *C. jejuni* subsp. *jejuni* and *C. coli* but is of low virulence and encountered only occasionally in man. Several biotyping schemes have been described for these 'thermophilic' campylobacters. We mention two: that of Lior (1984), incorporating the modified DNase test of Lior & Patel (1987), which divides *C. jejuni* into four biotypes (I–IV) and *C. coli* and *C. lari* each into two biotypes; and the more complex but more discriminatory combined identification and 'resistogram' typing scheme of Bolton, Holt & Hutchinson (1984). Although serotyping is usually preferred for the differentiation of campylobacter strains, biotyping is a useful alternative or adjunct to it. *C. upsaliensis*, the name for the 'CNW' (catalase-negative/weak) group of Sandstedt, Ursing & Walder, (1983) is related to the 'thermophilic' campylobacters, though not all strains grow at 43 °C. Originally isolated from dogs, *C. upsaliensis* appears to be enteropathogenic for man (Patton *et al.*, 1989; Goossens *et al.*, 1989, 1990). As primary isolation usually requires the use of selective filtration and non-selective media incubated at 37 °C (Bolton *et al.*, 1988; Goossens *et al.*, 1990), it is seldom detected by conventional methods used for *C. jejuni* and *C. coli*. Like *C. jejuni* subsp. *doylei* it is slower growing and more fastidious than *C. jejuni* or *C. coli*.

C. sputorum and *C. concisus* (Tanner *et al.*, 1981), both found in the gingival flora of man, are the principal representatives of the former catalase-negative group of campylobacters, but division of the genus according to catalase activity (Véron & Chatelain, 1973) is unsatisfactory because of wide variation within single taxa; moreover some strains which give negative catalase reactions have been found to possess intracellular catalase. *C. rectus* and *C. curvus*, formerly *Wolinella recta* and *W. curva* (Tanner *et al.*, 1981; Tanner, Listgarten & Ebersole, 1984) but transferred to *Campylobacter* by Vandamme *et al.*, (1991), are also catalase-negative campylobacters found in the mouth. Like *C. concisus* they are often numerous in gingival and periodontal lesions, although their pathogenicity is uncertain. They are phenotypically and genetically close to *C. concisus* (Paster & Dewhirst, 1988); the only simple distinguishing feature is that they are negative in the conventional oxidase test but positive in the modified test described by Tarrand & Gröschel (1982) with the reagent tetramethyl-*p*-phenylenediamine (1%) in dimethyl sulphoxide. Because of this we do not include them in Table 7.10c, but they differ from one another in morphology and in sensitivity to certain dyes and antibiotics (Tanner *et al.* 1984). Nor do we include the genus *Wolinella*, which was proposed by Tanner *et al.* (1981) to accommodate these species as well as the bovine rumen organism originally described by Wolin, Wolin & Jacobs (1961) as '*Vibrio succinogenes*'.

Minidefinition: *Campylobacter. Slender helical or curved Gram-negative rods; highly motile by means of a single polar flagel-*

lum. Coccal forms produced on exposure to air. Optimal oxygen concentration for growth 5–10%; do not usually grow in air or under strictly anaerobic conditions. Capnophilic. Oxidase-positive. Do not ferment or oxidize sugars. Nitrate reduced to nitrite (some exceptions); do not produce indole. Type species: C. fetus; NCTC strain 10842.

7.10.5 Helicobacter (Table 7.10 *a*, *c*). The genus *Helicobacter* (Goodwin *et al.*, 1989) was formed to accommodate the gastric spiral bacterium formerly known as *Campylobacter pylori* and originally as *C. pyloridis* (Marshall *et al.*, 1984). *Helicobacter pylori* commonly colonizes the human stomach mucosa, where it causes superficial 'chronic active' gastritis that probably predisposes to peptic ulceration. Two similar species colonize the stomach of the ferret (*H. mustelae*) and of cats and dogs (*H. felis*). Two other species, *H. cinaedi* and *H. fennelliae*, formerly *Campylobacter cinaedi* and *C. fennelliae* (Totten *et al.*, 1985) were transferred from *Campylobacter* by Vandamme *et al.*, (1991); they are associated with proctitis in homosexual men, although the natural habitat of *H. cinaedi* is apparently the intestine of hamsters (Gebhart *et al.*, 1989).

H. pylori is rarely isolated from specimens other than fresh gastric mucosal biopsy tissue or brushings. It takes 3–5 days to produce visible growth on primary culture. It is strictly microaerophilic and shares many of the cultural characters of campylobacters, but it produces a powerful urease. It has a single polar tuft of up to 7 sheathed flagella (lophotrichate). Cells undergo rapid coccal transformation (Karmali *et al.*, 1981) and die within one or two hours of exposure to air (Appendix C3.13).

Minidefinition: *Helicobacter. Helical or curved Gram-negative rods; motile (by means of single or multiple polar sheathed flagella). Coccal forms produced on exposure to air. Optimal oxygen concentration for growth 6%; do not grow in air or under strictly anaerobic conditions. Capnophilic. Catalase- and oxidase-positive. Do not ferment or oxidize sugars. Type species: H. pylori; NCTC strain 11637.*

7.10.6 Arcobacter (Tables 7.10a, c). This genus was designated by Vandamme *et al.* (1991) to accommodate the aerotolerant and low-temperature-growing organism formerly regarded as a campylobacter, *C. cryaerophila* (Neill *et al.*, 1985). *Arcobacter cryaerophilus* is primarily associated with abortion in pigs and cattle, but strains have also been isolated from patients with diarrhoea, mainly children, in developing countries (Tee *et al.*, 1988; Taylor *et al.*, 1989; Kiehlbauch *et al.*, 1991). Several subgroups of *A. cryaerophilus* are recognized, and species status ('*A. butzleri*') has been proposed for one of them (Kiehlbauch *et al.*, 1991). For the present we group all strains under the one species, *A. cryaerophilus*.

> **Minidefinition:** *Arcobacter. Helical or curved Gram-negative rods; motile by means of a single polar unsheathed flagellum. Aerobic or anaerobic, but optimal oxygen concentration for growth 3–10%. Growth occurs at 15–37 °C. Oxidase-positive. Do not attack carbohydrates. Nitrate reduced to nitrite. Type species: A. nitrofigilis; NCTC strain 12251.*

7.10.7 Anaerobiospirillum (Tables 7.10a, c) is a genus of anaerobic flagellated spiral bacteria with a single species, *A. succiniciproducens*, first isolated from dogs and described by Davis *et al.* (1976). Since then strains have been isolated occasionally from human blood and faeces though some of the faecal isolates differ in their carbohydrate fermentation reactions (Malnick *et al.*, 1983; Park *et al.*, 1986; McNeil, Martone & Dowell, 1987). The faecal strains examined in the UK were all isolated on the campylobacter medium of Skirrow (1977) incubated for more than 48 hours in a microaerophilic atmosphere though they required anaerobic conditions for subculture. *Anaerobiospirillum* is readily distinguished from campylobacters by its negative oxidase and catalase reactions and fermentative activity. We show the essential characters of the genus in Tables 7.10a, c.

> **Minidefinition**: *Anaerobiospirillum. Spiral, often filamentous, Gram-negative rods; motile; non-sporing. Anaerobic. Catalase- and oxidase-negative. Sugars attacked fermentatively. Type species; A. succiniproducens; NCTC strain 11536.*

7.10.8 Streptobacillus (Table 7.10a). A fastidious organism that needs a medium enriched with 20% serum, ascitic fluid or blood, prefers anaerobic conditions for isolation, and for whose growth additional CO_2 is needed; it grows slowly even under optimal conditions and growth is inhibited by sodium polyanethol sulphonate (Liquoid) which is frequently used in blood cultures incubated aerobically. It is thus an organism that must be specially looked for if its presence is suspected.

Only one species is listed, but it may be but one representative of an almost unknown group of organisms. In morphology *Streptobacillus moniliformis* is filamentous in young culture but the filaments subsequently break up into shorter sections in which characteristic swellings (but not spores) occur. Biochemical characters may be determined using media enriched with serum and yeast extract by methods that are also suitable for use with L-forms (L-phase variants) of bacteria (Cohen, Wittler & Faber, 1968).

The organism is pathogenic for mice, which die within a couple of days of intraperitoneal inoculation; in rats it is a member of the normal flora of the mouth. It is one of the causes of rat-bite fever – with a septicaemic papular rash and arthralgia – in man; outbreaks of infection with this organism associated with milk or water contaminated from rats have also occurred (Shanson *et al.*, 1983). The other cause of rat-bite fever, the spirochaete *Spirillum minus*, does not usually cause arthralgia.

> **Minidefinition**: *Streptobacillus. Filamentous Gram-negative rods; non-motile. Non-sporing, but filaments may show swellings. Aerobic and facultatively anaerobic. Needs enriched medium for growth. Catalase-negative; oxidase-negative. Attack sugars fermentatively. Type species: S. moniliformis; NCTC strain 10651.*

7.10.9 Legionella (Tables 7.10a, d) represents a genus of motile, pleomorphic, Gram-negative, non-spore-forming rods identified following the outbreak of respiratory infections (Legionnaire's Disease) among those attending a Legion convention in Philadelphia in 1976. There was a high mortality and the causal organism (and type species) was subsequently named *Legionella pneumophila* (Brenner *et*

161

Table 7.10*d***.** *Second-stage table for Legionella*

	1	2	3	4	5	6	7	8	9	10	11	12	13	14	15	16	17	18	19	20	21	22	23	24	25
Growth on BCYE*	+	+	+	+	+	+	+	+	+	+	+	+	+	+	+	+	+	+	+	+	+	+	+	+	+
Growth BCYE(−CF)**	−	−	−	−	−	−	−	−	−	−	−	−	−	−	−	−	−	−	−	−	−	−	−	−	−
Growth requirement for cysteine	+	+	+	+	+	+	+	+	+	+	+	+	+	+	+	+	+	+	+	+	+	+	+	+	+
Catalase	+	+	+	+	+	+	+	+	+	+	+	+	+	w	+	+	+	+	+	+	+	d	+	+	+
Browning of BCYE with tyrosine	+	w	+	+	+	−	+	−	+	−	−	+	+	+	+	+	+	+	+	+	+	+	+	+	+
Gelatin liquefied	+	−	+	+	+	+	+	−	+	+	+	+	+	+	+	+	+	+	+	+	+	+	−	−	−
Motility	+	+	+	+	+	+	+	+	+	+	+	+	+	+	+	+	+	+	+	+	+	w	w	+	+
Hippurate hydrolysis	+	d	+	+	−	−	+	+	−	−	−	−	w	−	−	−	+	−	−	−	−	−	+	−	+
Oxidase	d	−	+	+	−	−	+	+	d	−	−	+	+	−	−	−	+	−	−	−	−	−	−	−	d
β-lactamase	+	−	d	+	w	+	+	+	d	+	+	+	+	+	+	+	+	+	+	+	+	+	+	+	+
Auto-fluorescence	−	−	−	−	−	−	−	−	W	BW	BW	BW	−	−	−	−	−	BW	BW	BW	R	R	−	BW	YG

1 **Legionella pneumophila**	13 **Legionella spiritensis**
2 **Legionella feeleii**	14 **Legionella hackeliae**
3 **Legionella longbeachae**	15 **Legionella maceachernii**
4 **Legionella jordanis**	16 **Legionella jamestowniensis**
5 **Legionella oakridgensis**	17 **Legionella santicrucis**
6 **Legionella wadsworthii**	18 **Legionella cherrii**
7 **Legionella sainthelensis**	19 **Legionella steigerwaltii**
8 **Legionella micdadei**	20 **Legionella parisiensis**
9 **Legionella bozemanii**	21 **Legionella rubrilucens**
10 **Legionella dumoffii**	22 **Legionella erythra**
11 **Legionella gormanii**	23 **Legionella israelensis**
12 **Legionella anisa**	24 **Legionella tucsonensis**
	25 **Legionella birminghamensis**

W = White fluorescence
BW = Bluish white fluorescence
R = Red fluorescence

YG = Yellow-green fluorescence
* BCYE = Buffered Charcoal Yeast Extract agar
** BCYE (−CF) = Buffered Charcoal Yeast Extract agar without cysteine and iron

Other symbols used in the table are explained in Tables 5.1 and 5.2 on p.47.

al., 1979). The genus at present contains more than 30 validly named species (Brenner et al. 1985; Brenner, 1986) as well as many unamed though several of them have not yet been isolated from clinical infections and some are represented by only a few strains. They are essentially environmental organisms associated with soil and water (Fliermans et al., 1981) which can grow in suitable niches in water-associated plant and supply systems, human infection occurring by inhalation of contaminated aerosols. Although not thermophilic, most species (but not L. micdadei) can tolerate elevated temperatures up to 55–60 °C for periods of time which destroy most other vegetative bacteria, and many are resistant also to mild acid treatment; these features can be used to advantage for selective isolation, particularly for environmental strains (Edelstain et al., 1982; Dennis, 1988).

All Legionella organisms require L-cysteine and possibly iron (in one form or another) in media for primary isolation and most subcultures grow better with them both (Smith, 1982). Buffered Charcoal Yeast Extract (BCYE) agar containing these ingredients as well as α-ketoglutarate and ACES (N-2-acetamido-2-aminoethanesulphuronic acid) buffer is recommended for isolation; it can be made more selective by the addition of antibiotics (Edelstein, 1981, 1982). Generic identification either by conventional characterization tests or by the detection of branched-chain fatty acids in the cell wall by gas-liquid chromatography is usually adequate for clinical purposes; for epidemiology, species and, where possible, serotype identification are essential. We show the characters for genus confirmation in Table 7.10d; some, but not all, species can also be distinguished by them. Legionellas as a group are relatively inert biochemically and do not attack sugars; a few species, notably L. micdadei, L. longbeachae, L. jordanis and some strains of L. pneumophila, are clearly oxidase-positive, whereas the others give either negative or weak and variable reactions. L. pneumophila is the only current species which consistently hydrolyses hippurate (Herbert, 1981). Most species produce a brown pigment around colonies on Buffered Charcoal Yeast-Extract Agar (BCYE) containing tyrosine (Baine, Rasheed & Feeley, 1978), and the colonies of some species fluoresce in UV light (Weaver & Feely, 1979). There is little evidence,

however, to support the proposal (Garrity, Brown & Vickers, 1980; Brown, Garrity & Vickers, 1981) that the latter species should constitute a separate genus, Fluoribacter, or that, based on DNA homology, L. micdadei and related species should form a new genus, Tatlockia, within the family Legionellaceae (Brenner et al., 1985). Species identification depends mainly on fatty acid profiles (Moss et al., 1977) and DNA homology (Thacker et al., 1989) but for routine purposes, differentiation is essentially antigenic and based on serological tests usually by immunofluorescence microscopy; serotypes, biotypes and subtypes can also be distinguished within certain species, notably L. pneumophila (Watkins et al., 1895). A scheme, described by Vesey et al. (1988), utilizing 23 simple tests enabled them to differentiate 21 of 23 recognized Legionella isolates.

We show these species in Table 7.10d together with the clinical isolates L. tucsonensis (Thacker et al., 1989) and L. birminghamensis (Wilkinson et al., 1987). Other recently named species isolated from environmental sources and defined by DNA homology include L. moravica and L. brunensis (Wilkinson et al., 1988), L. quinlivanii (Benson et al., 1989) and L. gratiana (Bornstein et al., 1989). Detailed information on the laboratory aspects of legionellas, including generic and species identification, is given by Harrison & Taylor (1988).

Taxonomically, the genus is firmly established: Legionella is not related to other bacterial genera or to other organisms with a similar (39–43%) G+C content. The division into numerous species is, however, in a state of flux and additions as well as changes are inevitable. It seems likely that genetic differentiation will be essential in future, although we would prefer to see consolidation rather than further splitting.

Minidefinition: *Legionella. Gram-negative rods; usually motile. Require L-cysteine and iron salts for growth; aerobic but prefer 80–90% humidity with 2–5% CO_2. Catalase-positive; do not ferment or oxidize sugars. Type species; L. pneumophila; NCTC strain 11192.*

7.10.10 Mycoplasmas (Table 7.10a) are distinct from bacteria and in a class of their own called Mollicutes (Edward & Freundt, 1967). Three genera

163

are currently recognized: *Mycoplasma*, which requires cholesterol for growth; *Acholeplasma*, which does not; and *Ureaplasma*, which is unique in its ability to hydrolyse urea. Those associated with man include *Ureaplasma urealyticum, Acholeplasma laidlawii* and several species of the genus *Mycoplasma*. These organisms may seem out of place in a book devoted to bacteria, but they deserve mention because they may be isolated from clinical specimens as well as from tissue cultures.

They may be regarded as Gram-negative because they are decolorized and take up the counterstain feebly. With Giemsa, they stain poorly and the cells are best visualized in broth cultures by dark-field or phase-contrast microscopy. The organisms are extremely pleomorphic and can be difficult to distinguish from artifacts in the medium. The cells do not have rigid walls and they thus resemble the cell-wall-deficient L forms of bacteria with which they may be confused. Like L forms, mycoplasmas grow in the presence of antibiotics at concentrations normally regarded as inhibitory for bacteria; unlike L forms, however, they cannot revert subsequently in antibiotic-free media to bacteria with normal cell walls.

Mycoplasmas may be found in so-called normal serum and because of their nature and size (0.2 to 0.3 µm) can pass through some types of bacterial filters; in this way they may thus contaminate media thought to be sterile. However, they are heat-labile so that serum can be made safe for incorporation in media if heated at 56 °C for 30 minutes.

Media for the selective isolation of mycoplasmas and suitable for specimens from the genital and respiratory tract have been described (Clyde, 1983*b*; Shepard, 1983; Taylor-Robinson, 1983) but suspect isolates are best referred to a reference laboratory for confirmation and characterization. Like *Eikenella corrodens*, mycoplasma colonies not only adhere to the surface of the medium but also grow into it and, as the barely visible growth spreads on the surface, the microcolony (10–30 µm) develops a 'fried' or 'poached' egg appearance. Although not necessarily anaerobic, mycoplasmas grow well in closed environments, benefiting from the trapped moisture content.

Individual species are identified by serological growth inhibition tests: the antisera are species-specific and, by using impregnated paper disks, inhibit homologous growth on agar plates (Clyde, 1983*a*).

8

Taxonomy in theory and practice

As a subject, taxonomy is often regarded as dull and uninspiring. With understanding, however, it can be stimulating and exciting, as indeed were the personal and sometimes unorthodox views expressed by Cowan in the previous edition of this *Manual*. Moreover, taxonomy is fundamental to the application and use of the increasingly available commercial identification kits now used so widely for medical (and other) bacteria so that knowledge of the basic principles concerned is perhaps more than ever essential.

The application of taxonomy, as a science, to bacteriology took a long time. Bulloch's (1938) *History of Bacteriology*, Brock's (1961) *Milestones in Microbiology* and Postgate's (1969) *Microbes and Man* epitomise the applied and practical nature of early bacteriology. This was concerned chiefly with 'diseases' of wine, plants and animals, and little thought was given to theoretical aspects such as taxonomy. The main lines of investigation were to determine causes and, if possible, find cures, from which diagnostic bacteriology and preventive medicine developed. To the early medical bacteriologists, the systematic classification of bacteria was not essential. Indeed it was not until botanists who took an interest in these 'new' and strange organisms tried to apply variations of their own classical rules for naming them that bacterial taxonomy first began. By and large medical bacteriologists were content to let bacterial names look after themselves; they used names which were meaningful to them in relation to illness, such as '*Bacillus typhosus*' or more generally 'the typhoid bacillus'. Diagnostic bacteriologists 'named' disease-causing agents in this way so that they could refer to them conveniently again without having to use descriptive summaries; other organisms were discarded as contaminants or commensals.

Cowan referred to the terms classification, nomenclature and identification as the 'Trinity that is Taxonomy'. He likened taxonomy to a cocktail in which these three ingredients were blended so skilfully that they were difficult for non-experts to recognize. Taxonomy describes what a taxonomist does; for bacteriology, it is the theory or science of bacterial classification and its applications.

Classification may be defined as the arrangement or distribution of bacteria into orderly groups (or classes) according to common characteristics.

Nomenclature provides acceptable rules for the scientific naming or labelling of bacteria according to a standard code of nomenclature.

Identification is the assignment of identity to an unknown bacterium with that of a known and named one in a previously made classification.

8.1 Different kinds of classification

As early bacteriologists were concerned essentially with isolation, the first steps in the systematic classification of bacteria were made by botanists, who applied their system of latinized nomenclature. They were followed by increasing numbers of bacteriologists who needed labels or name tags so that they could refer to particular organisms without always having to describe them. Whereas botanists and a few academic bacteriologists classified bacteria along the classical lines of orders, families, genera, and species, practical bacteriologists collected them into groups that were meaningful to those who practised a particular application of bacteriology. Such groupings usually depended then on similarities in what the bacteria did rather than on their physical nature or phylogenetic characteristics, though the latter can now be studied in detail with the development of DNA techniques. Cowan grouped and described the various forms taken by these classifications under the following headings.

8.1.1   Minimal difference classifications. These are subsets extracted from more comprehensive classifications. They form part of the minimal difference identification schemes used by bacteriologists concerned with a limited range of bacteria, often from a particular environment; for example, alkalophilic bacteria, found in highly alkaline pools, require a different classification scheme of their own. Traditional water bacteriology also provides a good example of this type of classification in which coliform organisms are classified according to their morphology, a limited range of sugar reactions and a few biochemical characters. The tests were chosen more from a practical routine laboratory viewpoint rather than because of any special value in species differentiation. The 'water' classification of coliform organisms that developed had little in common with those for enterobacteria but it served a useful purpose for indicating possible contamination of potable water supplies. It is based on a few simple tests, the results of which, together with growth at 44 °C, can be expressed by plus or minus signs using the acronym IMViC (Parr, 1936) for Indole, Methyl Red, Voges Proskaüer and Citrate utilization reactions. Present water bacteriologists may well feel that this is now too simplistic a view as current identification techniques can yield additional information of medical and epidemiological value.

8.1.2   Classification by discipline. Because bacteriology started as an applied science, each discipline developed its own classification of relevant bacteria. With pathologists at the helm, medical bacteriology classified and identified organisms according to the diseases they were thought to cause; other organisms were regarded as contaminants and dismissed as unimportant unless they could be confused with a pathogen in which case they were accorded a place within a scheme of labelled bacteria. Other disciplines took similar attitudes and thus developed along divergent paths. Except between human and veterinary medicine, little exchange of information occurred; thus medical and plant pathologists have worked with similar organisms but, using different

methods of classification and identification, they failed to realize that the organisms were probably the same, as for example, *Erwinia herbicola* and *Enterobacter agglomerans*, and *Pseudomonas cepacia* and '*Pseudomonas multivorans*'.

With the increasing need for precise epidemiological studies to pin-point sources of infection, medical bacteriologists gradually began to systematically split the relatively few 'descriptions' of pathogenic organisms into distinct and identifiable bacterial groups. This trend continued with the development first of serological and then of phage and colicine typing methods and ultimately to the present highly specific monoclonal antibody, DNA and other techniques. Much confusion in classification was caused initially by the 'relationships' of bacteria and their association with clinical syndromes. Indeed, until Topley & Wilson's *Principles of Bacteriology and Immunity* was first published in 1929, medical bacteriologists in the United Kingdom were content to follow the lead of pathologists in considering that bacterial pathogens were related to each other only when the diseases were clinically similar, as with the enteric fevers. For this reason, the pertussis and parapertussis organisms, despite their different test reactions, were originally placed in the same genus, *Bordetella*. It is interesting to note, however, that DNA studies now support this classification of *Bordetella*.

8.1.3   All-purpose classifications. In the USA, fewer bacteriologists had their initial training in medicine or in pathology departments and so developments were rather different. Bacteriologists of all disciplines formed the Society of American Bacteriologists – now the American Society for Microbiology – and to them the concept of a hierarchical system for classifying bacteria as described by Winslow *et al.* (1917, 1920) did not seem so revolutionary as it did to the British. However, the Winslow Committee's reports did not help practical microbiologists to identify cultures and, as Chester's *Manual of Determinative Bacteriology* (1901) was out of date, the Bergey Committee was formed. Since the first edition in 1923, *Bergey's Manual of Determinative Bacteriology* has provided both a classification of bacteria and a scheme to help with their identification. Successive editions became a source of invaluable reference material though the hierarchical system of bacterial classification was abandoned altogether in the last (8th) edition in 1974. The first of four volumes of the current *Bergey's Manual of Systematic Bacteriology*, comprising essentially Gram-negative bacteria of general, medical, and industrial importance, was published in 1984; the second, for Gram-positive bacteria other than actinomycetes, in 1986; and the last two volumes, for archaebacteria, cyanobacteria and the remaining Gram-negative organisms, and for the actinomycetes, were published in 1989. For students of taxonomy, *Bergey's Manuals* probably represent the best and most comprehensive of current thought on bacterial classification.

8.1.4 Classifications of convenience. This refers to those kinds of classification which suit the practical bacteriologist and which were exemplified by Rahn (1929). He said that 'It does not matter very much how we divide [bacteria] and which of the many stages of the fluctuating varieties we chose to represent the species, as long as all bacteriologists agree and use the same symbols and names'. But Rahn was a heretic; in 1937 he created the family Enterobacteriaceae with only one genus, *Enterobacter*, which he did not characterize except by lumping together all the so-called genera that he considered should be included: *Escherichia*, *Salmonella*, *Aerobacter*, *Klebsiella*, *Proteus*, *Erwinia*, *Eberthella*, *Shigella* and the gas-formers of *Serratia*, *Pseudomonas*, *Flavobacterium* and *Achromobacter*, comprising altogether 112 species. This, of course, was even more inclusive than the *Enterobacter* genus of Hormaeche & Edwards (1960). Apart from introducing the pseudomonads, Rahn's idea was good and deserved much more serious consideration than it got from the bacteriologists of the day.

Hierarchical classifications are mainly of theoretical interest whereas identification is a practical exercise. The medical bacteriologist is concerned primarily with day-to-day identification of organisms and not with ranks higher than genus or with any supposed phylogeny; classification is only the means to an end – the hooks on which to hang the bacterial coats. The groupings of bacteria used in this *Manual* are such hooks: they are for *our* convenience and do not form part of any formal classification system. The characteristics of the members of the bacterial groups in the Tables represent *our* choice, and the groupings thus follow from the test characters *we* have chosen as signposts to the next set of identification tables.

8.1.5 Classification by statistical methods and computer. Statistical appraisal of the correlation of characters (as distinct from the representation, or expression, of characters by numerals) is quite old, as is the principle of attaching equal significance to all characters. Levine (1918) used such a method to classify 333 coliform organisms, basing his subdivisions on 13 different characters and excluding those, such as glucose fermentation, that were common to all strains.

Little progress was made along these lines until the reappraisal by Sneath (1957*a,b*) – succinctly described by Sokal (1965) as 'based on observed characters of taxa rather than on phylogenetic speculation' – led to the development of what is now known as numerical taxonomy. The subsequent developments with this method of classification – which, together with that of the computer, have revolutionized bacterial taxonomy – were reviewed by Sneath (1972). Statistical analysis of the characterization data provides an objective, scientific approach which has been used successfully for classifying bacteria from a wide range of sources. The stages necessary for statistical classification involve (a) choice of the bacterial strains and characters to be used; (b) collection and coding of all data in a standard manner; (c) calculation of similarities between strains; and (d) grouping together or clustering the similarities to provide taxonomic groups or taxa.

The successful application of numerical taxonomy requires three points to be satisfied: (i) the test characters of a large number of bacterial strains should be determined; (ii) numerous characters should be examined and, as far as possible, these characters should not be subjectively selected. In practice, however, ease of determination makes some characters more popular than others; and (iii) all the characters must be given equal value or weight in the classification. It is not uncommon with modern computers to analyse the characteristics of 300–400 bacterial strains in one project. In practice, with rapid or automated miniaturised laboratory methods, more than 200 phenotypic characterization tests ranging from morphology and physiology to biochemical reactions can be readily performed.

It was feared at first that numerical methods might result in considerable splitting and the creation of numerous taxa with but small differences. In contrast, Focht & Lockhart (1965) thought that taxa were more likely to be lumped together by showing up spurious differences in orthodox classifications, perhaps because of imperfectly standardized techniques (Lockhart, 1967).

Detailed intra-laboratory studies have demonstrated the considerable extent of innate variation in test results for some widely-used methods when applied to any one species. The objective nature of numerical analyses has shown that the experimental error between tests on replicate cultures of the same strain is about 4–5% when measured over a large number of characteristics. Strict standardization of tests is therefore essential – as it is for all statistical methodology – and any tests that prove difficult to standardize should be discarded. The removal of weighting, however, creates a curious dilemma for the design of diagnostic tables: classifications made by numerical taxonomy do not differ significantly when all sugar reactions except glucose are removed from the numerical analysis. If this is true also for identification, the tables could be much smaller without affecting their usefulness; but like Cowan, we leave this for others to pursue.

Once the test reactions have been completed, the results require coding for statistical or numerical analysis. The commonest way is to divide all the test reactions into positive or negative character states (1 and 0 when used with a computer). However, these qualitative results cannot always be used, especially if quantitative tests are included.

The process of numerical taxonomy when applied to a large number of test characteristics for numerous bacterial strains requires rigorous statistical methods to assign the extent of similarity between them. The similarities are best expressed as proportions or percentages and the commonest statistical value used in bacteriology is the simple matching coefficient where only those results which match precisely are included in the calculation. Other statistical approaches can also be used for calculating similarities but none should be considered to provide the one and only 'correct' classification. Computers have made this iterative process so easy that all the possible combinations of similarity between the strains can be pre-

sented as a table of similarities or 'similarity matrix'. As the tables are symmetrical, it is usual to express or present them simply as the lower left triangular part of the whole table. One further refinement can be applied to the data if the extent of the dissimilarities between the strains are calculated. These extents represent analogues of distance; classifications can sometimes be expressed in the form of distances between clusters or organisms in an imaginary hyperspace, rather like the astronomic distances between different-sized planets.

The taxonomic structure or three-dimensional relationships of the strains can be assessed by carrying out the further stage of cluster analysis or ordination. Again a variety of different statistical approaches have evolved. The two commonest clustering methods are the 'unweighted pair group method with averages' (UPGMA) and the 'single linkage method' (SLM). Principal components analysis with canonical variation is usually used for cluster analysis (ordination) methods so that three dimensional perspective pictures can be presented. The commonest form of representation for cluster analysis is in the shape of a family tree or dendrogram showing the detailed relationships between the various strains analysed.

Numerical methods for bacterial classification have tended to either support or disprove the theoretical and tentative conclusions reached by traditional bacteriological methods. However, the lack of objective criteria for assigning ranks to the groups makes it difficult to use numerical taxonomic methods in isolation; those interested in this form of classification should refer to the reviews of Sneath (1972, 1978) for further information.

8.2   Bacterial nomenclature and coding

However good a classification may seem and however easy its units are to define and identify, its usefulness will be tested by its communicability. To be successful the means of communication must be informative and it should be able to reach and be meaningful to those outside the bacteriological field. Communication is made by some form of label, some of which are descriptive and others non-descriptive; some labels consist of words (names, acronyms), others of figures (accession numbers, codes), or of both letters and figures (codes). We describe the naming process as nomenclature; when numbers or codes form the label we call it numericlature or coding. Names are the most popular form of label although numbers and coded forms are usually used when more precise information is needed, as for example with phage types and serotypes. Names are often believed to be descriptive (which they need not be) and they can confuse the unwary and mislead the ignorant, like the politician who wanted the generic name *Salmonella* to be suppressed because he thought it might affect the sales of salmon. Accession numbers (used in culture collections) do not change with the reclassification of organisms, and neither do descriptive codes; both these have a permanency that a name could never hope to attain.

8.2.1 Aims of nomenclature and coding.

It is convenient to consider the aims of nomenclature and coding under three subheadings which, in order of importance, are: (i) ease of reference and comprehension, (ii) permanence and stability, and (iii) descriptiveness (meaningfulness).

(i) Euphonious words are probably the easiest and briefest form of verbal communication, but words that slip from the tongue of natives of one country may be tongue-twisters to others. Although English is now accepted as the international language for science, Latin – which, as a dead language, has no overt nationalistic overtones – is also used internationally for certain scientific purposes. In speech, however, Latin is far from international: different countries vary widely in the pronunciation of the same spelling. The British, for example, pronounce 'cocci' as 'cock-eye' compared with the North Americans who say 'cocks-eye'. For the hard of hearing the difference in sound may render a name quite incomprehensible. Unfortunately, Latin is understood by a decreasing minority of people and we therefore cite the rules – which obey those of classical Latin – applicable to Latinized bacterial names. Bacterial binomial species names should be printed in italics (underlined in typescripts) with an initial capital letter for the genus name, which is a latinized substantive noun; the second part of the name, the specific epithet, has an initial lower case first letter (e.g. *Escherichia coli*). The epithet is a latinized adjective, with the same gender as the genus name. If further ranks, such as sub-

species or biotypes, are used, then the trinomial form provides an additional subspecific epithet. This name should also be latinized and follow the same rules as for the specific epithet with an initial lower case letter and the same gender as the genus, as for example, *Alcaligenes xylosoxidans* subsp. *denitrificans*. Higher rank names, above genus level, are plural adjectives with a feminine gender, which are printed with an initial capital letter but not in italics (e.g. Micrococcaceae).

Although latinized names should be used on all occasions when scientific accuracy is essential, colloquial or vernacular names are frequently and meaningfully used in verbal communication. We doubt, for example, whether there are many bacteriologists who do not understand the meaning of broad descriptions such as 'coliform organisms' or 'Non-Lactose Fermenters' ('NLF') which embrace many different species in a perspective wider than that of genus.

(ii) Permanence usually applies to bacterial labels only if they are descriptive. When the label is a word that is part of a classification (as Pseudomonadaceae derived from *Pseudomonas*) it may change when there is a change in classification. All bacteriologists understand that classifications, like clothes, can alter with increased knowledge and fashion, and changes in fashion may be accompanied by changes in name.

(iii) Descriptive labels do not usually change with revision of a classification; the organism that causes enteric fever has exactly the same characteristics whether it is called the typhoid bacillus, '*Bacillus typhosus*', '*Bacterium typhosum*', '*Eberthella typhosa*', or *Salmonella typhi*. If it were described by a code, as say 'species 12345', that label could be permanently attached to it. However, numerical coding schemes are neither popular nor practical for global use, though conversely they are eminently suitable for culture collections.

Why should bacterial names change? Mention has already been made of reclassification based on increased scientific knowledge following taxonomic study. This may result, for example, in better definition of the members of a genus so that new species or re-naming of old species may follow; thus *Proteus morganii* is now known as *Morganella morganii* after it was shown to be sufficiently different, taxonomically, from the other members of the genus *Proteus*. However, changes in fashion are far less frequent since the publication of the *Approved Lists of Bacterial Names* (1980). In addition, changes in name do not usually mean changes in identifying characteristics. There is one other method by which a name may be changed: it is also far less frequent now, and involves the principle of priority of publication. If a prior and validly published scientific description of an organism is found to exist with a different name, then this older name may be used to replace the current one. The *Approved Lists* have been accepted as the starting date for future reference and they record all the bacterial names that were both recognizable and in current use on 1st January, 1980. Bacterial species were listed only if they had been adequately and validly described and, where cultivable, if a type, neotype or reference strain was available. A type strain is intended to be the most typical strain chosen to represent and characterize a species so that other (unknown) strains can be compared with it for classification or identification purposes. Type strains sometimes become lost and new strains (neotypes) are selected to replace them. Reference strains are often derived from these two categories but are used to represent a whole array of similar strains in comparative work.

Any names not included in the *Approved Lists of Bacterial Names* in 1980 automatically became 'without standing' although provisions exist in the *International Code of Nomenclature of Bacteria* (1976 revision) for their revival if an exceptional case is shown to be valid. Any subsequent changes or additions are published either as papers or, from time to time, in validation lists in the *International Journal of Systematic Bacteriology* (IJSB). These lists have thankfully put an end to the previous necessity of searching interminably through ever-increasing mountains of literature merely to determine the earliest name used for a taxon in order to make a valid new addition to bacterial nomenclature. Since the starting date in 1980, new names must be published or announced in the *International Journal of Systematic Bacteriology*, which is currently the only publication officially recognized for this purpose. Summaries of the validated additions and changes in nomenclature are published annually in the IJSB. In addition, it is intended to publish compendia of all such changes at longer intervals, the first of which is the index by Moore, Cato & Moore (1985) which

lists all names published in the IJSB or other journals and validated by the Judicial Commission from 1980 to 1985.

8.2.2 Bacteriological codes. All scientific names of bacteria are governed by the *International Code of Nomenclature of Bacteria*, colloquially called the 'Bacteriological Code'. After initial proposals (Lapage *et al.*, 1973), it was revised and published on behalf of the International Committee on Systematic Bacteriology by Lapage *et al.* in 1975; however, as it only became effective on 1st January 1976, it is therefore usually referred to as the '*Bacteriological Code, 1976 revision*'. The *Bacteriological Code*, which was originally based on botanical nomenclature, was first published in 1948 with the aim of providing a set of rules to promulgate some stability, if not fixity, among bacterial names and to avoid confusion by providing a sound basis for systematic bacteriology. It contained precise rules for naming bacteria as well as a judicial procedure for settling disputes about them. However, it was subsequently amended repeatedly and eventually contained so many appendices that it became too complex and unwieldy. Although Cowan (1970a; 1971) did not have too much time for such rules – regarding many of them as pedantic – he did much to promote the climate which led to their revision in 1975. This revision greatly simplified the principles of the *Bacteriological Code*, which he regarded as sound. Although much of it is still devoted to rules governing the spelling of names, which Cowan considered far less important than clear and adequate descriptions of organisms, the revised *Bacteriological Code* has in turn led to the acceptance and application in 1980 of the *Approved Lists of Bacterial Names*. We suspect that Cowan would have given his blessing to these lists though he might well have taken exception to a few of the names. Together, we think that the *Bacteriological Code* and the *Approved Lists of Bacterial Names* will provide a firm basis for classification and nomenclature in the future.

We would not do justice to Cowan if we omitted to say that he took exception to Principle 5 of the *Bacteriological Code*. This concerns the nomenclatural type strain as the means for attaching a name to a taxon. It states that 'The application of the names of taxa is determined by means of nomenclatural types', referred to as 'types'. The designation of such types, whether of species, genera or other taxa, is governed by rules that make it clear that the nomenclatural type is not necessarily the most typical or representative element of any taxon. Cowan, however, in this *Manual* (1974) pointed out that ideally it was an obvious requirement that the strain chosen to represent a species should actually be characteristic of that species. Indeed, he agreed with Gordon (1967) who opposed the designation of a single (type) strain to represent a species. Her concept of a species was that of a microbial population which she defined as 'a group of freshly isolated strains, of strains maintained *in vitro* for many years, and of their variants, that have in common a set of reliable characteristics separating them from other groups of strains'. Cowan also agreed with Gordon's view (which he knew was not generally accepted) that the properties of strains persisting after years of cultivation in the laboratory were useful criteria for defining the species.

8.3   Bacterial identification

An unknown organism cannot be identified as a member of a particular group until that group or taxon has been described, named and established. In this *Manual* we do not consider methods for identifying medical bacteria which cannot be performed in routine clinical laboratories. It should be noted, however, that DNA–DNA hybridization, cell wall composition, fatty acid profiles and other techniques may help to characterize and thus assist in the better classification of a group of strains, though they are of limited use to the bench-oriented users of this *Manual*.

Strict standardization and reliability are essential guidelines for good identification methods. Accurate and clear descriptions of test methods are essential for their communication to and satisfactory establishment in other laboratories. Vague information such as 'positive for utilization of citrate' should play no part in diagnostic test descriptions; the medium, its composition, the method, the time and temperature of incubation and the reading and interpretation of the result all add definition to the basic statement. The demand for speed is sometimes an excuse for poor technique in the laboratory or for the use of rapid but crude methods. Rapid methods, however, are not

inherently erroneous provided they give reliable results. It is only when rapidity leads to shoddy workmanship and thus error in identification that they cannot be tolerated. For reliable characterization, pure cultures must always be the starting point for any identification method. This rules out any method in which the inoculum for a set of tests is a colony taken from a primary plate of a selective medium which suppresses but does not kill unwanted organisms. The routine use of a hand lens to assess purity is an important part of good microbiological practice. Similarly, use of the straight wire (and a plate microscope) when subculturing separate colonies for purity from a mixture is likely to give rise to fewer problems than the wire loop.

Identification has been described variously as the lowest form of taxonomic work or as classification in reverse; Mayr (1968) characterized taxonomy as 'essentially the technique of identification'. Identification consists of characterizing the unknown strain as much as is practicable, and comparing its characters with those of known, classified and named organisms. When they match, the unknown strain will be identified with a known organism. If the number of characters compared is small then a 'perfect' match will be relatively common; but more often, when many characters are compared, a near match with a small number of discrepancies is much more likely than true identity. For reliable identification, we have already considered the choice of bacterial characters and the methods for ascertaining them; in the following sections, we describe briefly the various ways of recording and comparing the characters.

8.3.1   Identification by diagnostic tables. Conn (1900) used tables with +, ± and – signs for the bacterial characters of known organisms. The characters of unknown strains were recorded on slips of paper and moved over the table to obtain the best visual match; indeed Cowan & Steel (1961) used Perspex strips in much the same way.

However, Conn and his colleagues (1907) later commented that 'unless the characteristics of species can be clearly and distinctly *tabulated*, it is almost a hopeless task...to identify a new culture with one previously described.' None the less tables of characters, especially sugar reactions, became fashionable though the symbols varied and were often more complex than necessary even for a simple positive result. Subsequent attempts to combine two characters such as acid and gas production in one symbol eventually resulted in tables too complicated for use and, failing standardization of symbols, they fell into disrepute. Tables returned to favour again when a simple, standardized listing arrangement for each organism together with clear descriptions of characters was introduced in the reports of the Enterobacteriaceae Subcommittee (Report, 1954a,b; 1958). These lists of characters could be combined and they were used by Cowan (1956b) and by Cowan & Steel (1961) in their early work on diagnostic tables which led subsequently to this *Manual*. To be of any use, diagnostic tables must have clear symbols to denote the various possible results.

Despite pressure, we have continued to use symbols rather than percentages in diagnostic tables for this *Manual* because the latter, although perhaps more accurate, are much more difficult to compare and interpret quickly. The main disadvantage of tables, especially if large, is the difficulty in appreciating and interpreting the significance of occasional mismatches with the test reactions of unknown strains.

8.3.2 Dichotomous or diagnostic keys.

Botanists use diagnostic keys extensively, but they have never been popular with clinical bacteriologists, who prefer an established laboratory routine that can be followed for most organisms isolated from specimens. An attempt to use dichotomous keys commercially for identifying the Enterobacteriaceae in the early 1970s was soon abandoned with recourse to tabular formats. Indeed the dichotomous keys in *Bergey's Manual of Determinative Bacteriology* were of little practical help until that of Skerman (1949) was added to the seventh (1957) edition. The main disadvantages lie in the exact nature of the result. Each test has to be done in the correct order and the next test to be performed depends strictly on the result of the previous test. Such keys are most successful when the characters used are stable and give constant, clear-cut results. Their usefulness therefore varies with different kinds of organisms: *Streptomyces* species for example as well as other higher taxa can be identified readily using them (Küster, 1972) but they are unlikely to be used in practice to identify enterobacteria.

8.3.3 Mechanical devices.

Cowan described these as the various 'bits and pieces' and 'Heath Robinson' gadgets – such as the 'Determinator' of Cowan & Steel (1960, 1961) – created as an aid to simplify the identification of bacteria. They all suffer from the same disadvantages as dichotomous keys in that they cannot allow enough leeway for the exceptions that constantly occur among biological material. They have now largely given way to computerized assistance, though mechanical devices were developed to help with the intricacies of profile construction for API and similar products (see Section 10.5).

8.3.4 Identification by cards (polyclaves).

With polyclaves or multiple keys, any character can be chosen at random and further characters can be investigated in any order. Identification is made by excluding all but the final answer. Polyclaves are well suited to punched cards, called the 'Peek-a-boo' system, in which cards of a uniform size are notched at the periphery for each taxon. The position for each notch denotes a specific test result: notched for positive, no notch for negative.

To be practicable, card systems must be based on the most useful distinguishing characters of organisms and they can only be as good as the tables or other information on which they are based. Like the diagnostic tables in this *Manual*, punched cards are suitable, with or without computer sorting, for use with a progressive identification system in which a 'minimal difference' set of cards first identifies the genus (or main group) and other sets (or packs) then identifies the species. If not used in a step-by-step system, the cards for the character information would need to be large with numerous holes; to be sufficiently comprehensive, such cards would be too clumsy for routine use.

In the previous edition of this *Manual*, Cowan described in detail a practical and successful punched card system for identifying to both generic and species level bacterial strains encountered in medical and veterinary laboratories. We reproduce this 'Identicard' system with minor changes in Chapter 9 and Appendix E in this third edition as an aid for laboratories where computer assistance may not be readily available. The data still hold good though a few modifications have been made in line with recent taxonomic changes.

The methodology involved has also been updated and computerized by Feltham, Wood & Sneath. (1984) and is available commercially as a computer program; it includes assistance with finding the relevant bacterial identification tables in the present third edition of this *Manual* and also the relevant pages in the 7th edition of *Bergey's Manual of Determinative Bacteriology*.

8.3.5   Arithmetical summation. Fey (1959) devised an identification system in which each bacterial character was scored with a unique but weighted number: for example, acid from mannitol = 5; gas from glucose = 10; growth in KCN = 320, etc. The scores of all the positive characters of the unknown organism were then added together to give a total score which would correspond to one of the scores in a table for organisms of known identity. In practice, the scheme was not reliable as any test discrepancies resulted in a wrong score with consequent misidentification (Steel, 1962a; Baer & Washington, 1972). As for any identification system, this simply confirmed that standardization of tests with adequate controls is absolutely essential; given this, it has potential though with the advent of commercial identification kits and computerized methods it is unlikely to be used.

8.4   Bacterial taxonomy in the future

The recent application of more objective methods of identification, especially numerical taxonomy, as well as the development of quantitative techniques for the measurement of genetic relatedness and evolutionary divergence among bacteria have impinged on traditional classification and nomenclature as used in this *Manual*, sometimes with untoward consequences. For example, the name *Pasteurella pestis* for the plague organism was well known but there was confusion about its status as a pathogen when it was renamed after transfer to the genus *Yersinia* (Williams, 1983). Review of the various approaches to bacterial systematics in the light of this newer taxonomic understanding was therefore important and an *ad hoc* committee of the International Committee on Systematic Bacteriology met in 1987 to examine the wider implications and consider how the different approaches to bacterial systematics could be reconciled with each other. As its report (Wayne *et al.*, 1987) is of considerable importance for taxonomy in the future, we discuss briefly the essential points and recommendations here; the full report is reproduced with permission in Appendix I.

The committee based its discussions on four aspects of bacterial systematics: (i) *Phylogenetic* studies, which are directed towards understanding the evolutionary paths which taxa have taken from early and more recent ancestors. These pathways can be discerned from analyses and comparison of the evolutionary distances between certain 'semantides': large genetic information-bearing molecules such as nucleic acids and proteins. (ii) *Descriptive* studies, which act as a link between the semantide-based phylogenetic taxonomy and traditional bacterial systematics in which organisms are described in phenotypic terms as in this *Manual*. Such descriptions help to define taxonomic groups of organisms which may also be recognised in phylogenetic terms. (iii) *Diagnostic* perspective, where a selection of phenotypic features or of 'probes' derived from phylogenetic analysis are used to recognize unknown strains and assign labels or names to them. Such names, mostly of genera, species and subspecies, are those familiar to readers of this *Manual*. (iv) *Associative* work, in which vernacular names are used to evoke practical information about strains, such as their medical, industrial or ecological significance.

The committee suggested that a single all-embracing hierarchical scheme should be adequate for the taxonomy of all bacteria provided vernacular groupings are kept for diagnostic purposes. The complete DNA sequence would represent the ultimate ideal reference standard for determining phylogeny, which in turn would determine taxonomy; at present DNA reassociation is the nearest approach to this ideal for species. Taxonomic schemes based on phylogeny must, however, exhibit phenotypic consistency. Hierarchical consistency is also important though the actual demarcation points in RNA dendrograms will vary with different branches and can be influenced strongly by stable phenotypic characterizations. Formal nomenclature should agree with and reflect the genomic relationships and is essential for major groupings such as genera which form the basis of bacterial systematics. It was recognized, however, that there is at present no satisfactory phylogenetic

173

definition of the term genus and that consequently, as with higher taxa, flexibility in approach is necessary because the actual scope of the definitions of different genera will undoubtedly vary. For families, chemotaxonomic and hybridization or sequence data should be consistent with each other.

Species currently represent the only taxonomic units that can be defined in phylogenetic terms. Such phylogenetic species would include bacterial strains with about 70% or more DNA–DNA relatedness at the optimum temperature for reassociation and less than 5% divergence of unpaired bases within related sequences. Phenotypic characters should accord with these criteria and would be allowed to override this phylogenetic concept of species only in exceptional instances. The committee recommend that distinct genospecies that cannot be differentiated from others by any known phenotypic character should not be named until they can be clearly distinguished in this way. The designation of subspecies is, however, acceptable for organisms that are closely related genetically but which have different phenotypic characters. The nomenclature for species should reflect genomic relationships to the greatest extent possible except where to do so rigidly might create a 'nomen periculosum' which, though taxonomically correct, could cause uncertainty, confusion or danger in practice. For example, the name *Yersinia tuberculosis* subsp. *pestis* was proposed instead of *Yersinia pestis* for the plague organism to reflect its close phyloge-

netic relationship with the species *Yersinia tuberculosis*. This was regarded as a '*nomen periculosum*' and rejected because it might cause serious confusion in clinical medicine; the correct name accordingly remains *Yersinia pestis*. Similar reasoning was applied to retention of the species and name *Bacillus anthracis* for the anthrax organism instead of accepting it as a pathogenic variety of *Bacillus cereus*.

Further recommendations are made about other concerns including the special difficulties expected in the taxonomic reorganization of the major phylogenetic taxon referred to as 'the purple photosynthetic bacteria and their relatives'; overcoming the problems inherent in the growth and identification of non- or hardly cultivable bacteria; and the status of organisms only cultivable in ecosystems.

The report of the *ad hoc* committee embodies much of the philosophy and most of the practicalities which Cowan enunciated in this *Manual* in his own inimical style. The recommendations, which we endorse, go a considerable way towards reconciling the divergent scientific approaches to bacterial systematics. We hope they will perhaps stem the tide of new bacterial names – many based purely on phylogenetic characters – which have been appearing since the *Bacteriological Code* (1976 revision) and *Approved Lists of Bacterial Names* (1980) were promulgated. Indeed, the report reinforces the approach to traditional bacterial systematics as used in this *Manual*.

9

Bacterial identification by cards

Identification of bacteria is not always an art. The process of recording, collating and interpreting their common diagnostic characters can be mechanized and used in a visual sorter (Olds, 1966, 1970) based on the Peek-a-boo system (Wildhack & Stern, 1958; Yourassowsky *et al.*, 1965). Hand-sorted punched cards have been used for recording quite varied taxonomic information (Wood, 1957) and, in the first edition of this *Manual*, Cowan & Steel suggested that the 'tables could form the basis of a set of diagnostic punched cards to be used with similar cards on which the characteristics of the unknown [isolates] are punched'. Soon after that was written, Schneierson & Amsterdam (1964) described a punched card used for identifying bacteria at the Mount Sinai Hospital, New York, but unfortunately they did not give details of the 'authoritative reference' sources from which they obtained the characters for their master cards – information which is of course essential for assembling and using tables of characters.

A disadvantage of diagnostic tables is that as more and more detail is included they become less easy to use. For the second edition of this *Manual*, the early drafts of what became Tables 6.1 and 7.1 stretched to more than twenty columns with up to ten lines of characters; to check them Cowan made a set of punched cards with one (or more) cards for each genus. Checks with these punched cards revealed that some of the columns in the tables were in fact similar – though this had not been noticed previously – thus enabling them to be combined and the tables rearranged. Though laborious, this exercise demonstrated how quickly a bacterial identification could be made once the characters had been notched on a card. A new and perhaps better way of using the diagnostic tables was thus confirmed.

9.1 Minimal-difference Identicards for genera

For the identification of bacterial genera encountered in medical and veterinary laboratories, only eleven holes are needed; an additional spare space (hole) can be used also for a favourite or supplementary character that is regarded as useful. Cards are punched as described in Appendix E. A corner is cut off each card so that thet can all be faced correctly for notching. Pre-punched cards available commercially can also be used.

The characters used must include the Gram reaction, which is not shown in the tables; the others comprise the ten used in Table 6.1, which also cover those in Table 7.1 as well as many of those mentioned in the minidefinitions given in Chapters 6 and 7.

The name of the genus is placed in the middle of each master card, together with any relevant information helpful for isolation, subculture (e.g. oxygen requirements of *Campylobacter* or *Eikenella*) or identification.

Some genera need multiple master cards. For example, *Aerococcus*, in which the catalase test may be read as either weakly positive or as frankly negative; *Clostridium*, in which *C. perfringens* is non-motile as well as reluctant to spore; *Gemella*, so easily decolorized, has a card for both the Gram-positive and Gram-negative states; and *Nocardia* is shown separately as acid-fast and as not acid-fast. The enterobacteria are dealt with as one genus but three master cards are needed for the identification of shigellas, including Shiga's bacillus (*Shigella dysenteriae* 1), which is unusual in being catalase-negative.

The notching of the individual master cards is illustrated in Fig. 9.1, which also shows the kind of supplementary information that can be entered in the central area of the card.

Table 9.1. *Aggregations of genera that may occur with the genus Identicard set*

Aggregation	Genera (species) in aggregation
(i)	*Aerococcus* (catalase read as negative) *Gemella* *Pediococcus* *Streptococcus* *Enterococcus*
(ii)	*Actinomyces* *Bifidobacterium* *Clostridium perfringens* (not sporing) *Eubacterium*
(iii)	*Arachnia* *Erysipelothrix* *Lactobacillus*
(iv)	*Mycobacterium* *Nocardia*
(v)	*Leuconostoc* *Peptostreptococcus*
(vi)	Enterobacteria (*Shigella dysenteriae* 1) *Streptobacillus*
(vii)	*Bordetella* *Brucella* *Moraxella*
(viii)	*Actinobacillus* *Pasteurella* *Aeromonas salmonicida*
(ix)	*Aeromonas* *Chromobacterium violaceum* *Plesiomonas* *Vibrio*

To use the Identicard set for genera, first examine the unknown culture for the generic characters used on the card. The acid-fastness and the sporing ability need not be determined for every strain, and it would be surprising if every isolate was tested for anaerobic growth unless the culture failed to grow aerobically at the first attempt. Positive characters of the unknown organism are notched from the appropriate hole of a blank card. Rod-shaped organisms (bacilli, vibrios) are assumed unless hole 5 (coccus) is notched; alternatively, for an actual record for every character, additional holes may be used and notched.

9.1.1   Aggregation of cards. In many instances the characters chosen will be sufficient to identify to genus level most of the bacteria likely to be isolated in medical and veterinary laboratories; however,

because so few generic characters are used in marking up (notching) the cards, some unknown strains will inevitably end up after sorting with more than one card, and the genus identification must then be made by studying the characters given in the second-stage (or third-stage) tables of Chapters 6 and 7, or from using further sets of Identicards (see Section 9.2). The most surprising aggregation of genus Identicards occurred with *Shigella dysenteriae* 1 and *Streptobacillus* (Table 9.1, no.vi) though in practice there would be no difficulty in distinguishing them at the bench; the similarity simply begins and ends with the characters chosen for Table 7.1. In contrast, the other aggregations are of similar organisms such as *Actinobacillus* and *Pasteurella* (*sensu stricto*) that are difficult to separate even by experienced bacteriologists.

9.2   Identicards for species

The user of the Identicard set for genera will probably find species identification easy by consulting the tables of Chapters 6 and 7, but where the tables are large a further set of species Identicards may be helpful. The notching of the master cards for species is complicated by the presence of many 'dee' (d and D) characters and by late reactions recorded in the tables within round brackets. These difficulties are overcome by having two rows of holes in the master cards (Fig. 9.2*a*); characters recorded by + signs in the tables are notched to the second (inner or plus) row of holes, and characters for different or delayed reactions shown by d, (d), or (+) are notched only to the first (outer or dee) row (Fig. 9.2*b*). As an example, the notching of the master cards for the species identification of enterobacteria is shown in Table E5 in Appendix E.

Positive characters of the unknown strain to be identified are notched to the inner row of holes (Fig. 9.2*c*); alternatively special cards with one row of holes in line with the inner row of the master set may be used.

9.2.1   Aggregates of species cards. With salmonellas, aggregation of species is to be expected in the Identicard set as the differences between most members of the group are essentially serological, and such differences are not entered on the cards. To a

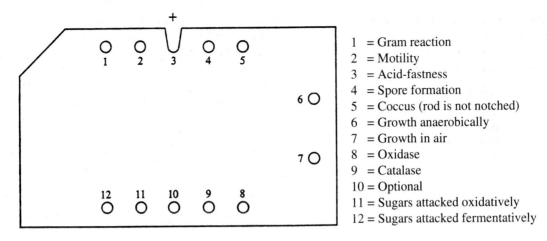

Fig. 9.1. Schematic example of card punched with a single row of holes illustrating notched cut-out for a positive [+] character. Used for master cards (characters of known genera) and as cards for recording the characters of an unknown organism for genus identification.

lesser extent, aggregation applies also to the cards for the *Shigella* group, which Bascomb *et al.* (1973) found difficult to identify by probabilistic methods.

9.2.2   Variants. As the Identicards are based on characters recorded in the tables of Chapters 6 and 7, they are subject to the same limitations. Like the tables, they do not make provision for aberrant strains or the varieties that may occur, sometimes limited to a particular locality: the so-called 'local races'. It should always be borne in mind that a non-motile organism may be a non-motile variant of a motile species, or it may represent technical failure to detect motility. In both motility media and broth cultures, motility is generally most active in cultures incubated below the optimal temperature for growth of the

organism; a temperature between 22 and 25 °C is satisfactory for most mesophilic bacteria.

Anaerogenic variants of *Salmonella* serotypes which normally produce gas may occur and make identification difficult; they can even lead to suspicion that a new 'species' has been isolated.

Reactions that are slow or delayed, as for example gelatin liquefaction by *Enterobacter cloacae*, or lactose fermentation by *Shigella sonnei*, are notched to the first (outer) row of the two-row master cards; by so doing and combining it with the method of probing cards recommended in Appendix E (Tables E5, 6), a reading made before the character has developed (or the test become positive) will not lead to misidentification.

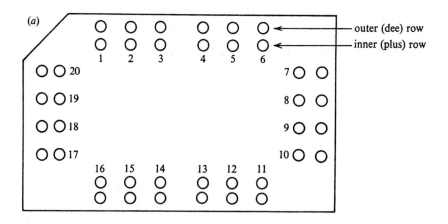

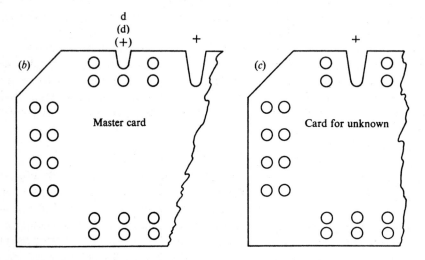

Fig. 9.2(*a*) Card punched with two rows of holes: inner (plus) row for positive (+) characters; outer (dee) row for variable [d, (d) or (+)] characters i.e. different reactions with different strains: positive with some, others negative. Used for master cards (characters of known species) in sets for species identification. May be used as cards for characters of unknown organisms.

(*b*) Master card, showing the method for notching d, (d), (+) and + characters.

(*c*) Card of unknown organism (to be identified) notched for a positive character.

10

Bacterial identification by computer

In 1968, Dybowski & Franklin suggested various theoretical models for using computers to help with the identification of bacteria, but the first practical systems for computer-assisted identification were not introduced until 1973 by Friedman *et al.* and Lapage *et al.*. They depended on a full set of standardized routine tests carried out under strict laboratory control. One such system for strains difficult to identify in diagnostic laboratories has been perpetuated in the Identification Services Laboratory in the National Collection of Type Cultures (NCTC) at Colindale, London. The work of this laboratory was extensively reviewed by Willcox, Lapage & Holmes (1980). Other national culture collections have set up similar services for their own countries. The ranges of the tests applied have increased progressively in order to accommodate new species and genera. Bacterial groups which have been updated recently or examined in this way include the aerobic fermenting and non-fermenting Gram-negative rods (Holmes & Dawson, 1983; Holmes, Pinning & Dawson, 1986), the Gram-positive aerobic cocci (Feltham & Sneath, 1982) and the genus *Bacillus* (Logan & Berkeley, 1984). Other bacterial groups have been investigated elsewhere.

Commercial kit suppliers have constructed large databases for their particular range of tests and organisms. As with the Tables in this *Manual*, the test reactions for identification databases or matrices have often been compiled from a variety of sources. The tables or matrices consist of columns usually showing the percentage of positive test reactions, each row representing a cluster or group of similar organisms. These clusters usually equate to named bacterial species. Each entry in the matrix should be the best estimate for a positive result for that test with that particular group of organisms. This estimate may be obtained from data in the literature which can be combined with the laboratory results given by sample strains and isolates to provide a subjective percentage of positive reactions for the matrix. A more objective database is obtained by aggregating test results for representative strains from each group of organisms with those of recognised type or reference strains. The validity of each entry in the table thus depends on the examination of adequate collections of strains by accepted and suitably controlled tests: the importance of these aspects cannot be over-emphasized.

10.1 Strain collections

The best databases for bacterial identification are those generated from the actual results for particular groups of organisms associated with particular ecological niches and examined by reproducible differentiation tests. Bacterial isolates from patients must be used to construct databases for use in medical laboratories; bacteria from water, soil and fish, for example, should only be used to assist with the identification of aquatic and environmental organisms. As the majority of commercial identification systems currently available have been produced for medical laboratory needs, the tests and databases may thus prove unsuitable for bacteria from other habitats.

Many of the best bacterial identification tables stem from numerical taxonomic studies where the Adansonian concept of large numbers of unweighted tests provide objective clustering of strains. Data from other sources, such as DNA homology and chemotaxonomy, provide additional evidence to help place strains within defined clusters.

The entries in published identification matrices show the probabilities of a positive test reaction expressed as a range usually from 0.01 to 0.99 or alternatively as percentages from 1 to 99%. To be exact, if a test is always negative for a particular bacterial group, the figure should be a probability or percentage of 0 but, to compensate for any conceivable error in the method and to accomodate the single, exceptional isolate that disproves the rule, a slightly greater figure (0.01 or 1%) is used. For example, urease-positive strains of *Escherichia coli* do occur, albeit uncommonly, so that an entry of 0% would be erroneous. To compensate for this modification at the bottom of the scale, a similar adjustment is made at the top end so that entries of 0.99 or 99% are used instead of 1 or 100%.

10.2   Test selection

There is no magic formula for assessing the 'best' tests or the 'right' number for any specified bacterial group. The NCTC uses approximately 60 conventional tests in their scheme whereas commercial kits rarely use more than 24. The 'best' tests are those which are most easily determined and which have a high degree of stability and resistance to operator error. Test reactions can vary depending, for example, on the size of inoculum, the duration and temperature of incubation, the composition and viscosity of the medium and the 'eye of the beholder'. Errors can and do occur when recording results if the end-point is not clearly defined. For example, in the Hugh & Leifson test for Fermentation or Oxidation, the viscosity of the paraffin layer is as important as the definition of the yellow colour produced by acid from the breakdown of glucose. Is the reaction positive if only the top 10 mm is yellow? And was the fermentation tube heated and cooled before inoculation to drive out traces of oxygen? For reasons such as these, computer-assisted identification techniques must be defined precisely and with great care. Indeed colour charts for the end-point of such reactions are extremely useful for their standardization. Variation in test results can be caused also by the selection of characters liable to phage- or plasmid-mediated changes. Such tests would obviously be unsuitable for identification purposes as the variable results would affect the level of identification.

The selection of tests for identification databases must rely on quantifiable reactions which can be used to determine the percentage of positive results. Tests such as pigmentation, colony size or degree of acid-fastness are thus not easily accommodated in computer-assisted identification tables or databases.

The quality of a database can be assessed subjectively by testing a range of known strains. As mentioned already, a number of conditions can affect the database quality but one of the less-defined effects can be caused by geographical variation. Strains isolated in a particular country or even in a region within a country may be phenotypically different from other strains of the same name elsewhere. As examples, some strains of *Yersinia enterocolitica* are virtually continent-specific; and *Serratia* strains are common isolates from urine in the Bordeaux region of France, but exceedingly uncommon in the UK.

Sneath (1979*a, b*; 1980*a, b, c*) and Langham *et al.* (1989) have developed a range of objective techniques for assessing the quality of identification databases by means of computer programs designed either to analyse the degree of spatial overlap of neighbouring imaginary hyperspherical clusters or to rank the characters in order of their separation power. The best tests are those which separate the taxa within the database into two equal parts whereas the worst cannot differentiate between any taxa. Other programs are used to analyse the database for the most typical identification likelihood score for each entry using a range of statistical identification procedures, including taxonomic distance, described in Section 10.4. These techniques were developed to assess the practicality and correctness of particular published databases without the need to obtain strains and test them against the tabulated values. We would advise those who wish to construct their own databases to obtain copies of these programs and ensure that their databases satisfy all the criteria specified.

10.3   Identification of an unknown isolate

The identification of an unknown strain relies on comparison of its test reactions in turn with those of the known species in each column, or test, in the table. This comparison can be quantified in terms of the relationship of the reaction pattern of the unknown strain with that of the statistical nearest pattern among the rows, or species, in the table. If the unknown strain matches a particular species to a defined level, it will identify with that species. If the unknown strain does not match well with any tabulated species, then it would be classified as unidentified with that database. This might be because (i) the database was poorly defined, (ii) operator error occurred in the handling of the unknown strain (e.g. use of an impure culture or unsuitable conditions for growth), (iii) the unknown strain should not have been tested against that particular database but rather a different one: for example, a non-fermenting organism would not identify well with a 'fermenter' database.

10.4   Identification: statistical principles

The statistical process in identification involves calculation of the likelihood or closeness of match of all the characters of the unknown strain with those of each row or species in the relevant table or database; this ensures some degree of ranking or ordering of the identification scores. The principles of many of the various statistical methods which have been applied were described by Sneath (1978); the actual mathematical calculations of those usually used are given in detail by Willcox, Lapage & Holmes, (1980). The commonest approach relies on a taxon-radius model with accumulation of probabilities so that the unknown strain can be compared with a group of imaginary hyperspheres in multi-dimensional space, each test character providing one dimension in that space. The bacterial groups (rows or species) in the table may be perceived as imaginary, hyperspherical clusters separated spatially from other clusters. Each cluster may be defined statistically with a centre of gravity (centroid) and a critical radius that includes a high proportion of the bacterial strains within that group or taxon. Thus each row in an identification table can be defined as a hypersphere with a given position or centroid and radius.

The probabilistic likelihood statistic used involves multiplication of the probabilities that the test reactions of the unknown strain match those for any particular row or species in the table. A hypothetical example will perhaps best illustrate the method which can readily be used with straightforward computer programs such as those published by Sneath (1979a). Consider strains in four hypothetical bacterial groups of taxa (ONE to FOUR) each examined by six characterization tests (A to F). Suppose that the numbers of positive results for each test with each taxon are expressed as percentages, as follows:

Table 10.1. *Percentage of positive test reactions.*

Taxon	Test					
	A	B	C	D	E	F
	Percentage of positive reactions					
ONE	99	1	99	99	50	90
TWO	99	99	99	1	1	1
THREE	1	99	1	90	99	1
FOUR	1	1	1	10	85	50

These percentages can be expressed as probabilities of positive test reactions and the results given by an unknown strain, examined by the same tests, entered thus:

Table 10.2. *Probabilities of positive test reactions and example for an unknown strain.*

Taxon	Test					
	A	B	C	D	E	F
	Probability of positive reactions					
ONE	0.99	0.01	0.99	0.99	0.50	0.90
TWO	0.99	0.99	0.99	0.01	0.01	0.01
THREE	0.01	0.99	0.01	0.90	0.99	0.01
FOUR	0.01	0.01	0.01	0.10	0.85	0.50
UNKNOWN	-	+	-	+	+	Not Tested

The test reactions of the unknown strain are essential for the calculation of the Likelihood scores for matching a particular taxon. To calculate the Likelihood scores, the probabilities of the reactions are multiplied together for each taxon for each test result given by the unknown organism. Any reactions that were doubtful or not tested may be left out of the calculation. If the unknown strain gives a positive test reaction, the actual probability is used, whereas if the reaction is negative, then 1 minus the taxon probability is used to give Likelihood score values thus:

181

Table 10.3. *Likelihood score values for the unknown strain.*

Taxon	Likelihood scores for unknown strain	
ONE	$(1-0.99) \times 0.01 \times (1-0.99) \times 0.99 \times 0.50$	$= 4.95E^{-7*}$
TWO	$(1-0.99) \times 0.99 \times (1-0.99) \times 0.01 \times 0.01$	$= 9.89E^{-9}$
THREE	$(1-0.01) \times 0.99 \times (1-0.01) \times 0.90 \times 0.99$	$= 0.864536$
FOUR	$(1-0.01) \times 0.01 \times (1-0.01) \times 0.10 \times 0.85$	$= 8.33E^{-4}$
	Sum of all Likelihoods	$= 0.8653699$

$*E$ = Exponential; thus $4.95E^{-7} = 0.000000495$

Normalization or standardization of these Likelihood score values is then necessary to provide a true comparison and to compensate for the effects of using 0.01 and 0.99 (or 1% and 99%) for the lower and upper entries in the table. This is achieved by dividing each Likelihood score in turn by the sum of the Likelihood scores for all the taxa, which gives Taxon THREE the high score of 0.999 instead of an apparently mediocre score of 0.864536:

Table 10.4. *Normalized likelihood scores for the unknown strain.*

Taxon	Normalized Likelihood score for unknown strain	
ONE	$4.95E^{-7} \div 0.8653699$	$= 5.72E^{-7}$
TWO	$9.89E^{-9} \div 0.8653699$	$= 1.14E^{-8}$
THREE	$0.864536 \div 0.8653699$	$= 0.999037$
FOUR	$8.33E^{-4} \div 0.8653699$	$= 9.62E^{-4}$

As an alternative to the normalization procedure for finding the nearest match or 'best fit', the Most Typical Likelihood value for each row or taxon giving the most likely result for each reaction may be determined. This is calculated as follows:

Table 10.5. *Most typical likelihood scores for the unknown strain.*

Taxon	Most Typical Likelihood scores for unknown strain	
ONE	$0.99 \times (1-0.01) \times 0.99 \times 0.99 \times 0.5$	$= 0.480298$
TWO	$0.99 \times 0.99 \times 0.99 \times (1-0.01) \times (1-0.01)$	$= 0.950990$
THREE	$(1-0.01) \times 0.99 \times (1-0.01) \times 0.9 \times 0.99$	$= 0.864536$
FOUR	$(1-0.01) \times (1-0.01) \times (1-0.01) \times (1-0.1)$ $\times 0.85$	$= 0.742279$

Instead of using the normalization procedure, the previous Likelihood score values calculated for the unknown strain may be divided by these Most Typical Likelihood scores for each taxon to give Modal Likelihood scores for the unknown strain thus:

Table 10.6. *Modal likelihood scores for the unknown strain.*

Taxon	Modal Likelihood score for unknown strain	
ONE	$4.95E^{-7} \div 0.480298$	$= 1.03E^{-6}$
TWO	$9.89E^{-9} \div 0.950990$	$= 1.04E^{-8}$
THREE	$0.864536 \div 0.864536$	$= 1.00000$
FOUR	$8.33E^{-4} \div 0.742279$	$= 1.12E^{-3}$

From these Modal Likelihood scores it is now apparent that the unknown strain matches completely with taxon THREE, whereas with the normalization procedure the Likelihood score was lower although it was still the highest. For the identification of unknown strains, both of these statistical techniques are frequently used either alone or together with other variants and data such as estimates of the frequency of occurrence of each taxon in the database (Willcox, Lapage & Holmes, 1980).

10.5 Profile numbers

Direct access to computers with relevant identification programs is not always necessary for identifying an unknown strain by means of these statistical methods. Lists of the most commonly occurring patterns of results which have been processed by specially written computer programs can be obtained from commercial sources : these patterns of test reactions are compared with the relevant database table by means of the commercial computer program which uses one of the two statistical identification techniques described to calculate identification scores (Stevens, 1980). Other relevant information such as serology or additional tests can also be appended to the presumptive identity for better differentiation.

Test results for given organisms can be aggregated to give unique profile numbers which denote the particular patterns of positive and negative test results. To form such profiles, the characterization tests are arranged in groups of three (triplets) and positive results score either 4, 2 or 1 in each triplet of tests as follows:

Table 10.7. *Profile numbers from 0–7 for triplets of tests.*

Profile digit	Result given by		
	Test 1	Test 2	Test 3
0	−	−	−
1	−	−	+
2	−	+	−
3	−	+	+
4	+	−	−
5	+	−	+
6	+	+	−
7	+	+	+
Test score	4	2	1

The various combinations of positive and negative test reactions yield a total of eight different patterns of triplet results which may be fully described by unique 'octal' set of single profile digits from 0 to 7 with profile scores of 4, 2 and 1. The majority of commercial and home-produced test kits use this octal format, though API uses the reverse by scoring 1, 2 and 4. The full Bacterial Identification Profile (BIP) is constructed from the individual profile digits for each set of three tests: thus 21 tests give a 7 digit profile. If there are less than three tests in the last group of tests, only the corresponding scores are used; for two tests, 4 and 2 are used for the positive results; and for one test, only 4 or 0 can be scored. Bacterial Identification Profiles are thus a very concise way to express many results precisely but briefly and conveniently.

The profiles can be listed in numerical order to form indices or registers of characterized organisms. Each entry can simply have the name of a specific organism attached to it or, in fuller registers, an abbreviated identification calculation with scores together with the names and scores of two or three of the closest possible species. Further information is usually provided about useful additional tests which could be carried out to yield a better identification score as well as on any tests which have given unexpected results and so count against a better identification score.

Commercial firms are not unique in producing lists of identification profiles for common bacteria. This can be done in routine diagnostic laboratories as exemplified by Clayton *et al.* (1986), who generated such a profile list from the work described in their paper for the routine identification of Gram-negative rods by using a multi-point inoculation method.

The methods described briefly in this Chapter illustrate the basic principles concerned with the data collation and recovery necessary for current 'expert' bacterial identification systems (Valder *et al.*, 1987; Gavini *et al.*, 1990). Such methods will probably be used increasingly in the future as computer hardware becomes more powerful and software more complex.

11
Quality control in microbiology

From the beginning, this *Manual* has preached consistently not only about the importance of pure cultures for identification but also of the need for standardization of test methods both within and between laboratories. We reinforce these views here with a brief outline of the current concepts of quality control and laboratory proficiency which must be understood and put into practice for good identification procedures to succeed. As before, we emphasize the importance of controlling characterization tests with organisms known to give positive and negative results; the test organisms recommended are given in Appendix D together with media and conditions suitable for their propagation short-term and storage.

11.1   Laboratory quality control

Quality control can be regarded as the continual monitoring of equipment, reagents and working practices as well as the provision of training with specified details of laboratory methods and procedures to ensure proficiency. The lack of test reproducibility both within and between laboratories, discussed in previous editions of this *Manual*, has now been well documented (Sneath & Johnson, 1972; Lapage *et al.*, 1973; Sneath, 1974; Sneath & Collins, 1974; Snell, DeMello & Phua, 1986). Variation in test results between laboratories may be due to differences in the sensitivities of the methods used. Such differences are of considerable practical importance as the results given in the diagnostic tables and keys may be applicable only if the methods stated are used. This applies also to micromethods and diagnostic kits. Variation in test results within a laboratory may be caused by several factors and can result in misidentification if the test in question is a key one in a limited set. The prime aim of quality control for bacterial characterization tests is therefore to eliminate or reduce to a minimum the extent of test variation both within and between laboratories.

In a comprehensive approach to laboratory quality control, several factors must be considered, including the standardization of procedures; provision of a laboratory 'manual' of detailed written methods; stock control of media; purity checks on test strains and on media for contaminants; record keeping; and checks of test procedures and controls with known strains.

11.1.1   Standardization of methods is essential to reduce test variation to a minimum. One quality control survey, for example, revealed 21 methods or variations of them for testing for bacterial motility. In general, laboratories use particular methods either because of long experience and confirmed reliability, or with some, simply because of inertia. In the latter case, the methods must be critically evaluated. Details such as inoculum size, time and temperature of incubation, composition of media and the ingredients used including the particular brands can all affect some test results. All such details must be standardized within each laboratory.

11.1.2   A laboratory manual containing full details of all methods and procedures used in a laboratory is essential to avoid the drift which inevitably occurs when methods are passed verbally from one person to another. Such a compendium or manual should be written by staff with many years of practical experience in order to be authoritative, and it should be kept up to date. The instructions should relate to what is expected in practice rather than to a theoretical ideal and they should be reviewed regularly.

The methods should be readily available for daily use and reference within every laboratory, so more than one copy is necessary.

11.1.3 Stock control and shelf life are not easy to define and quantify but some general points will suffice to illustrate the necessary requirements.

An estimate of the likely shelf life of media is valuable. A turnover period of about one calendar month is a reasonable compromise for most characterization media. Storage space, batch size and preparation times can be planned accordingly. After this period, unused media should be discarded to prevent accumulation of older batches. This permits the date marking of batches of media rather than of individual tubes or bottles.

The temperature of storage must be cool and evaporation should be prevented by using either sealed plastic bags or Bijoux bottles, Universal containers or the like with screw caps.

Humidity can cause deterioration of dehydrated products, especially if hygroscopic. If stored in the refrigerator, such products should be allowed to reach room temperature before opening to prevent the condensation of water vapour with subsequent hydration of the material.

Long-term storage media may be necessary for those used for tests performed infrequently: in cool conditions some media can be stored in sealed tubes for up to 6 months. However, these media must be checked with known positive and negative control strains each time they are used. Media or reagents not suitable for extended storage times include for example V factor discs, ONPG broth, Selenite broth, hydrogen peroxide and some carbohydrate media.

Ingredients, such as peptones, which are liable to deteriorate, should be purchased in small quantities and the bottles marked with the dates of receipt and opening. They should be discarded if there is any evidence of change caused by moisture.

11.1.4 Purity checks for contaminants should be carried out on all batches of freshly prepared media. Gross contamination will usually be apparent after 5 days at room temperature. Media should be incubated also at the temperature used for the test before each batch is released. Media for characterization tests should be inoculated only with cultures known to be pure. Subculture directly from selective media significantly increases the risk of mixed growths and, despite the delay, it is safer to follow the procedures for purity described in Section 3.2.

11.1.5 Simple record-keeping not only provides assurance that quality control procedures have been carried out, but enables faulty batches to be identified and discarded, encourages a methodical approach and helps to emphasize the concept of accountability.

11.1.6 Test procedures and controls. All characterization tests should be controlled with organisms known to give clear-cut positive or negative results under appropriate conditions. The suitability of both media and reagents should be checked with known test strains immediately after preparation as well as during any period of extended storage. Misreading of test results due to lack of familiarity is an important cause of error and control organisms are useful for instructing staff in the correct appearance of such reactions. For these purposes, lists of the species and strains recommended are given in Appendix D.

Many laboratories maintain small culture collections of their own. Such stock collections, especially of pathogens encountered infrequently, are invaluable both for teaching purposes and for comparison with field isolates. Strict safety precautions must be observed with such laboratory strains and the description 'teaching organisms' must not be taken to mean 'harmless' (Blaser et al., 1980). For the long-term storage of laboratory strains, several procedures are available. Freeze-drying is the method of choice as it virtually ensures long-term stability of characters and freedom from contamination with simple storage conditions for the ampoules. The necessary apparatus is, however, expensive for small laboratories and as an alternative the simple method of drying described by Rhodes (1950) which needs only a vacuum pump and phosphorous pentoxide can still be used. Storage in liquid nitrogen (-196 °C) guarantees survival and stability but the nitrogen requires constant replenishment. Most medically-important bacteria can be stored satisfactorily in Glycerol Broth at temperatures below -20 °C (typically -70 °C) for several years (Feltham et al., 1978; Jones et al., 1984). Desiccation of bacterial strains on gelatin discs also provides a convenient storage method (Snell, 1984a). Regular subculturing is the least suitable method because of the potential instability of test characters and the possibility of contamination (Snell, 1984b). Frequently-used strains may be kept on nutrient media for convenience but at the end of their storage life (Table D4) they should be replaced from stock cultures preserved by one of the more secure long-term storage methods (e.g. –70 °C or freeze drying). A more comprehensive list is given by Lapage, Shelton & Mitchell, (1970). Cooked meat is a good maintenance medium for many organisms, including anaerobes. Dorset egg is also a good general purpose storage medium; salmonellas retain their antigenic structure well on it though shigellas become rough. In general, media that are less nutrient-rich are better for keeping cultures than richer media in which they die out more quickly. Media containing fermentable carbohydrates should be avoided for maintaining cultures and selective media should never be used. Cultures must not be allowed to dry out and tightly closed screw-capped containers are preferable to waxed or corked tubes.

11.2 Laboratory proficiency and quality assessment

Quality assessment, known also as proficiency testing in some countries, acts as a check on the efficiency of quality control procedures by the introduction of simulated and occasionally real specimens of known but undisclosed content into the laboratory for examination and reporting. This may be done internally within the laboratory and/or externally but in either case the specimens should be examined by the same staff that would normally examine similar clinical material.

When organized internally, specimens of known content are introduced into the routine system by senior staff who intercept and evaluate the reports (Estevez, 1980). This offers the advantage that assessment specimens can be more easily 'disguised' as part of the routine intake and thus offer a more realistic appraisal of the standard of work.

With external assessment, an organizing laboratory sends specimens of known and undisclosed content to participating laboratories for examination and receives the completed reports for analysis. These specimens are more difficult to camouflage and laboratory staff tend to give them special treatment. However, an external assessment scheme offers several advantages including stability of the specimens, the availability of repeat samples in cases of failure and the opportunity to compare individual performance with the general standard of other participants.

National and regional external quality assessment schemes for microbiology have been developed and now exist in several countries. For clinical material national assessment schemes are perhaps preferable to international schemes because the microbes encountered, the reporting and referral practices, as well as the methods and antimicrobial agents used will vary between countries. International assessment schemes are, however, important for harmonisation as well as for public health and regulatory control purposes, especially for perishable produce imported or exported for human or animal consumption. For those considering implementing a national monitoring service we describe briefly the United Kingdom National External Quality Assessment Scheme for microbiology (UKNEQAS) administered by the Public Health Laboratory Service (PHLS).

The scheme is comprehensive and is not limited simply to the isolation and identification of bacterial pathogens but includes viruses, fungi and parasites. It embraces diagnostic microscopy and serology as well as antibiotic assays. The working principles were described by Snell, DeMello & Gardner (1982) and Snell (1984c). On joining the scheme, each participating laboratory is given a unique code number by which it is identified in all transactions so as to maintain confidentiality. Simulated clinical specimens are prepared in the Quality Assurance Laboratory, Division of Microbiological Reagents and Quality Control (DMRQC) at the PHLS Central Public Health Laboratory (CPHL), Colindale, London. All specimens are distributed to participants together with 'request' details and 'report' forms. After examination of the specimens, each participating laboratory reports its findings to the organizing DMRQC laboratory following which a brief outline of the intended results is issued. The reports are then analysed and all participants receive a summary of the overall results for each distribution and a computer-derived analysis of individual results on current as well as recent specimens. Twelve distributions, each of three specimens, for assessing isolation and identification procedures are issued each year. Participation is free to all health care microbiology laboratories in the UK and almost 500 laboratories are included.

Although the great majority of specimens are straightforward and contain bacteria likely to be found in clinical practice in the UK, more unusual specimens are occasionally distributed for educational purposes or where recognition of an unusual pathogen – such as *Corynebacterium diphtheriae* or *Vibrio cholerae* – could be of concern for public health or to persons from abroad. The proportion of 'positive' material is obviously higher than in normal clinical practice. Specimens may contain fully virulent pathogens other than those regarded as highly dangerous in Hazard Group 4 (Advisory Committee, 1990) so that due regard must be paid to safety and hygiene in the laboratory.

Detailed information on the preparation of such specimens is given by DeMello & Snell (1985). Freeze-dried mixtures of bacteria are usually used as simulated specimens. They are chosen to provide a realistic challenge to media and technical skill in the isolation and identification of pathogens from the mixed flora associated with the clinical site in question.

Rigorous quality control tests on the specimens are carried out by DMRQC with checks before, during and after the distribution including the return of duplicate specimens through the post from various geographically dispersed laboratories. If the quality control checks reveal unexpected and unacceptable changes in the content of a specimen, it is regarded as void and the participating laboratories are informed. In such instances, the results are not included in the calculation of laboratory performance statistics.

Three weeks are allowed between distribution of the specimens and return of the final reports on them from the participating laboratories. After this period repeat samples are available for those laboratories which did not obtain the expected result with the original specimen. The performance statistics distributed to each laboratory include scores for the most recent distribution and an analysis of performance ratings over an inclusive six-month period. This gives details of the specimens supplied, the number of specimens reported as 'not examined', the number of reports not returned and the number of reports received too late for analysis.

The analysis gives the total laboratory score, derived by addition of the individual scores for each specimen, the total possible score and the average score. The participating laboratory can use this information for direct comparison with other laboratories and can see whether their performance is better or worse than the average. Laboratories can thus use the

data to monitor their own performance and to take any action required if problems are revealed. Confidential help and advice to participants with continuing problems is available from a national Advisory Panel for Microbiology.

Most participants appear to find the UKNEQAS useful and good relationships are maintained, perhaps because the scheme is seen as educational rather than as regulatory.

11.3   Laboratory safety and hygiene

We include a few elementary precepts on safety and hygiene in the microbiology laboratory in order to reinforce their importance even in taxonomic work. As well as general and statutory considerations concerning safety in the laboratory, particular care and a high standard of personal hygiene are essential in microbiological work because pathogenic organisms may always be encountered. In addition, media not necessarily designed for pathogens may support their growth so that great care is needed in the handling and disposal of all cultures. Sound technique is the basis of safe microbiological procedures and it is important that all individuals concerned with microbiological work should have received adequate training. It is also important that the necessary laboratory equipment and facilities should conform to accepted codes of safety and good laboratory practice (Advisory Committee, 1991).

Certain precautions are essential in the microbiology laboratory not only to prevent contamination of samples and culture media but also to avoid infection hazards to personnel:
- observe strict personal hygiene; keep nails short; and use hair and beard protection if necessary;
- wash hands with soap and warm water both before and after microbiological work as well as after use of the toilet;
- always wear protective clothing in the laboratory;
- sterilize all cultures by autoclaving, and sterilize or disinfect associated apparatus and materials before disposal or reuse;
- do not eat, drink or smoke in the laboratory;
- report any accident, spillage or unusual occurrence to senior staff;
- if in doubt, ask for advice.

APPENDIX A
Preparation and control of culture media

A1 General considerations
A2 Formulae of media
A3 Media control

A1 GENERAL CONSIDERATIONS

The ability of some bacteria to grow on media that are inhibitory to other bacteria gives the former organisms additional special characteristics that may help in their identification. The media themselves, with their selective and differential qualities, are of particular interest in diagnostic bacteriology and for this reason we have sometimes included a few notes on the isolation of certain bacteria and have referred occasionally to enrichment and other media used in culturing organisms from clinical material. We emphasize, however, that this *Manual* is concerned with how to identify organisms that have been isolated and not with how to isolate them.

In this appendix, media are listed under the following section numbers and headings:

A2.1 Basic media
A2.2 Enriched and enrichment media
A2.3 Differential and selective media
A2.4 Media for enhancing pigment production
A2.5 Media for carbohydrate studies
A2.6 Miscellaneous media

A1.1 Cleaning and sterilization of glassware

Glassware for media such as Koser's citrate, in which there is a single source of an element such as carbon or nitrogen must be chemically clean to be free from it. A recommended method of ensuring this is to boil all tubes in 20% nitric acid for 5–10 minutes and then wash and rinse well with with glass-distilled water. Tubes are dried in an oven in the inverted position in baskets lined with filter or blotting paper to prevent the mouths of the tubes touching the metal.

Glassware such as Petri dishes and test tubes with metal caps or cotton-wool plugs are sterilized in a hot air oven, preferably with a fan, at 160–170 °C for one hour. The efficiency of the oven and the even distribution of heat should be checked each day by placing Browne's green spot type III[*] indicator tubes on each shelf (Darmady, Hughes & Jones, 1958; Brown & Ridout, 1960). Overheating of tubes plugged with cotton-wool must be avoided; several workers

(Wright, 1934a; Drea, 1942; Pollock, 1948) have drawn attention to the inhibitory effect of substances volatilized from cotton during dry heat sterilization. Tubes and flasks capped with polypropylene covers (Varney, 1961) and screw-capped bottles (with caps loose) are sterilized by autoclaving.

A1.2 Indicators

The pH indicators used in bacteriology are shown in Table A1; some, such as phenolphthalein, are not readily soluble in water and are dissolved in dilute alkali or ethanol. The preparation of Andrade's indicator and litmus solution are more complex and details are therefore given in Sections A1.2.1 and A1.2.2.

A1.2.1 Andrade's indicator (modified from Andrade, 1906)

Acid fuchsin	5 g
Distilled water	1000 ml
N-NaOH (as required)	150–180 ml

Dissolve the acid fuchsin in the distilled water and add 150 ml of alkali solution. Mix and allow to stand at room temperature with frequent shaking for 24 h; the colour should change from red to brown.

If the dye has not been sufficiently decolorized add a further 10 ml of alkali solution, mix thoroughly and leave for another 24 h. Subsequent additions of alkali may have to be made until a straw-yellow colour is ultimately attained with the minimum of alkali.

To test the final indicator, add 1% of the indicator solution to Peptone Water at pH 7.2, mix thoroughly and determine the pH; note and record the rise in pH due to the alkalinity of the indicator. Should for example the increase in pH be 0.2, all batches of medium to which this batch of indicator is to be added must have an initial pH value 0.2 lower than the desired final reaction.

---

[*] Albert Browne Ltd., Chancery House, Abbey Gate, Leicester LE4 0AA, UK.

Table A1. *Indicators and their characteristics*

Indicator	Usual concentration (%)	ml 0.05 N-NaOH per g indicator	Solvent	pH range	Colour change (acid to alkaline)
Methyl red	0.2	–	50% ethanol	4.2–6.3	red–yellow
Chlorphenol red	0.2	47	water or 50% ethanol	4.8–6.4	yellow–purple
Andrade's	(See A1.2.1)	–	water	5–8	pink–yellow
Litmus	(See A1.2.2)	–	40% ethanol	5–8	red–blue
Bromcresol purple	0.2	37 }	water or	5.2–6.8	yellow–purple
Bromthymol blue	0.2	32	50% ethanol	6.0–7.6	yellow–blue
Neutral red	0.1	–	50% ethanol	6.8–8.0	red–yellow
Phenol red	0.2	57	water	6.8–8.4	yellow–red
Cresol red	0.2	53 }	or	7.2–8.8	yellow–red
Thymol blue	0.2	43	50% ethanol	8.0–9.6	yellow–blue
Phenolphthalein	0.1	–	50% ethanol	8.3–10.0	colourless–red

A1.2.2 Litmus solution (modified from McIntosh, 1920)

Litmus, granular	250g
Ethanol (40%)	1000ml

Grind the litmus and place in a flask with 500 ml of the ethanol; boil for 1 min, decant and keep the liquid; add the remainder of the ethanol to the residue, boil for 1 min, decant and add this liquid to that retained.

Centrifuge and adjust the volume of the supernatant to 1000 ml with ethanol (40%); add N-HCl drop by drop until the solution becomes purple.

To test for the correct reaction, boil 10 ml of distilled water, cool, and add one drop of litmus solution; after mixing the water should become mauve in colour.

This indicator solution is used at a concentration of about 2.5%.

A1.3 Carbohydrates

'Sugars' used in bacteriology are shown in Table A2, where they are grouped by their chemical structure.

A1.4 Clarification of media

Liquid media may be clarified by filtration through paper, sintered or fibre glass, or, if still available, asbestos fibre (Seitz filtration). To prevent adsorption of any constituents, it is better to avoid the use of a filter aid such as kieselguhr or talc. Wright (1934b) found that filtration of broth through a thick filtering layer resulted in marked reduction in its growth-promoting capacity.

The grades of material suitable for clarification of media are shown in Table A3.

Agar-containing media must be clarified while in the molten state; for this purpose use paper pulp or a grade of filter paper especially designed for the filtration of agar sols. To prevent solidification during filtration, a steam or hot-water jacketed funnel is used; alternatively, use a Buchner funnel and filter rapidly through paper of greater wet strength. A method for the filtration of agar-containing media during sterilization in an autoclave was described by Brown (1961).

Gelatin-containing media used to be clarified with the aid of egg-white or horse serum; gelatin for bacteriological use is now of such quality that this step is unnecessary and gelatin media may be clarified by the same methods as those containing agar.

A1.5 Sterilization of media

The method of sterilization recommended for each medium is included with the details of preparation.

A1.6 Storage of media

Although freshly prepared media are usually desirable for the cultivation of most bacteria, with some, such as Wilson and Blair's (1927, 1931) Bismuth Sulphite Agar, maturation or 'ageing' is necessary for satisfactory selectivity; nor should egg-based media be used new. Many media can be safely kept at room temperature or in a refrigerator for several weeks, or even months, before use. Stability varies with the individual medium and it is not possible to fix a universally applicable storage life. The important point is that moisture should be retained. To prevent evaporation and concentration of the constituents during storage, media should be kept in screw-capped rather than in cotton-plugged containers. Appreciable evaporation can occur in a refrigerator but this can be prevented by putting tubed media and plates in polythene bags. If nutrient agar slopes appear to be dry, they should be melted and re-solidifed though not on more than one or two occasions.

Strong light is detrimental to most media and storage in

Table A2. *Carbohydrates used in bacteriology*

Class	Carbohydrate	Convenient concentrations in water (w/v) at 20 °C for stock solutions
Pentoses	Arabinose (L+)	40
	Xylose	50
Methyl pentose	Rhamnose (*iso*dulcitol)	40
Hexoses	Fructose (laevulose)	50
	Galactose	30
	Glucose (dextrose)	50
	Mannose	50
	Sorbose	40
Disaccharides	Cellobiose	10
	Lactose	15
	Maltose	50
	Melibiose	10
	Sucrose (saccharose)	50
	Trehalose	25
Trisaccharides	Melezitose	10
	Raffinose	10
Polysaccharides	Glycogen	5; dissolves to produce an opalescent solution
	Inulin	20 at 70 °C; solution may be slightly opalescent
	Starch, soluble	– soluble in hot water
Glycosides	Aesculin (esculin)	0.1; 7.5 on heating
	Amygdalin	7.5
	Arbutin	10
	Salicin	3
Alcohols	Adonitol	40
	Dulcitol	5; readily soluble on heating
	Erythritol	40
	Glycerol	miscible in all proportions
	Mannitol	15
	Sorbitol	50
Non-carbohydrate	Inositol	15

Table A3. *Filtration materials, and grades, suitable for clarifying media*

	Liquid media	Agar-containing media	
		Simple funnel	Buchner funnel
Papers:			
Green's	798 $^1/_2$; 904 $^1/_3$	500 $^1/_2$; 904 $^1/_3$	960; 993
Whatman	1; 30; 52	15	52
Postlip	633E	agar-agar	agar-agar
Schleicher & Schüll	520B $^1/_3$; 598 $^1/_3$	520A $^1/_2$; 520B $^1/_2$	520B
Delta	317 $^3/_4$		376
Munktell	5		0
Sintered glass:			
Jena	} 1; 2		
Pyrex			
Asbestos pads (if available):			
Seitz	K3; K4; K5		
Sterimats	FCB		
Carlson	K3; K5		

Table A4. *Usual volumes of media (in ml) for tubes of various sizes*

Medium	Tube size			
	75 × 12 mm (3 × ¹/₂ in)	100 × 12 mm (4 × ¹/₂ in)	125 × 12 mm (5 × ¹/₂ in)	150 × 16 mm (6 × ⁵/₈ in)
Liquids	1–2	2–2.5	3	4–5
Slopes (slants)	1	1.5–2	2.5–3	5
Slopes with butts	2.5	2.5	3.5–4	7
Stabs	2.5	2.5	4	7

Table A5. *Concentration (%) of agar in media for different purposes*

Type of Medium	Agar			
	Japanese	New Zealand	Ionagar no. 2*	American
Solid (normal)	1.5–2.0	1.0–1.2	1.0	1.5
Solid (to inhibit spreaders)	7	4		
Semisolid	0.1–0.5	0.05–0.3	0.7	0.3–0.4
'Motility media'				0.1–0.4

*Ionagar no. 2 was a special purpose agar used only when a defined medium was needed. It has been replaced by Purified Agar (Oxoid L28).

the dark is preferable, especially for those containing dyes or indicators.

Egg media should be kept for a long period (e.g. two weeks) before use in order to give contaminants that grow only at room temperature the opportunity to develop into visible colonies.

Cotton-plugged tubes are a potential source of contamination as the moisture absorbed even by 'non-absorbent' cotton wool is sufficient to permit development of fungi, and hyphae may penetrate a cotton plug.

Media that have been kept in a refrigerator should be allowed to attain room temperature before use. Because the solubility of gases in liquids decreases with increase in temperature, it is essential to check that gas bubbles do not appear in the inverted inner (Durham) tubes of carbohydrate media as they warm up from cold storage to room temperature. Liquid media to be used for anaerobic cultivation (particularly those containing thioglycollate) should be heated in a boiling water bath to remove dissolved air and allowed to cool undisturbed before use.

Poured plates may be kept at 4–15 °C, but they should not be put close to the cooling unit of a domestic-type refrigerator. Excess water of condensation can be avoided by allowing the medium to cool to about 55 °C before pouring it into Petri dishes. If plates are to be stored in an exposed position they should be stacked with the lid uppermost; in canisters they should be inverted. Plates for anaerobic use may be pre-reduced by storing in an anaerobic atmosphere either in jars or in a cabinet.

Higher forms of life, including insects, beetles and mites, can also be troublesome in a laboratory. Indeed, 'footprints' left by mites crossing agar media inoculated with cultures have been observed on plates kept on the bench or incubated at 22 °C and in medical laboratories this is potentially dangerous. Dehydrated media are particularly liable to insect attack; the eggs laid by adults hatch into larvae which can then feed upon carbohydrate material.

A1.7 Volumes of media

The volumes of media suitable for dispensing into Petri dishes vary with the size of the dish. For routine bacteriological purposes in the United Kingdom, there is a current British Standard specification (BS 611) for glass Petri dishes (1978) and for those made from 'plastics' (1990) though the former is about to be withdrawn as obsolete. Media volumes of 15–20 ml are recommended for these dishes which have an internal diameter of 90 mm (3.5 in).

Volumes suitable for media in tubes are shown in Table A4.

A2 FORMULAE OF MEDIA

Two terms which refer to all formulae need explanation.

Agar. In this Appendix the agar concentration relates to Japanese agar; when New Zealand agar is used the amount stated in the formulae should be multiplied by 0.6 to give approximately the same gel strength. Concentrations of agar for different types of gel are shown in Table A5. Agar is made from seaweed from many parts of the world but the origin is seldom stated on the label of commercial preparations; consequently Table A5 and others like it are not as useful as they appear. Regard should be paid to the information supplied by the manufacturer and the concentrations advised for different purposes.

Agar is a poor conductor of heat (Bridson & Brecker, 1970) and time must be allowed for heat penetration both in media making and for safety purposes to ensure that cultures on agar plates are properly sterilized before disposal. The altitude of a laboratory may affect the ease with which agar goes into solution and it may not be practicable to dissolve agar in a steamer; above 2000–3000 feet, autoclaving at about 0.36 kgf/cm^2 (5 lbf/in^2) may be essential for melting agar.

Water. The term water, used in all formulae, implies potable tap water. When distilled water is specified in a formula, de-ionized water may be used.

A2.1 Basic media

A2.1.1 Nutrient Broth

Meat (beef) extract	10 g
Peptone	10 g
NaCl	5 g
Water	1000 ml

Dissolve the ingredients by heating in the water. Adjust to pH 8.0–8.4 with 10 N-NaOH and boil for 10 min. Filter while hot through thick filter paper to remove phosphates which are precipitated in alkaline solution at this stage. Adjust to pH 7.2–7.4, and sterilize at 115 °C for 20 min.

Notes. Nutrient Agar is nutrient broth gelled by the addition of 2% agar.

Semisolid Nutrient Agar (Craigie agar, sloppy agar, slush agar) is Nutrient Broth containing 0.4% shredded agar.

Double-strength Nutrient Agar follows the same formula as nutrient agar but the volume of water is reduced to 500 ml.

Layered plates consist of two layers of solidified medium; in layered Blood Agar (Section A2.2.1) the bottom layer consists of Blood Agar base, Peptone Water Agar (Section A2.1.2) or Saline Agar (Section A2.1.11) and the top layer is Blood Agar base with 5% blood added.

The thin top layer may contain other substances under test; some, such as chitin, are insoluble and the suspension is made either in Water Agar (Section A2.1.12) or Saline Agar (Section A2.1.11).

A2.1.2 Peptone Water

Peptone	10 g
NaCl	5 g
Water	1000 ml

Dissolve the solids by heating in the water. Adjust to pH 8.0–8.4 and boil for 10 min. Filter, adjust to pH 7.2–7.4, and sterilize at 115 °C for 20 min.

Peptone Water Agar is Peptone Water gelled by the addition of 2% agar.

A2.1.3 Robertson's Cooked Meat medium (modified from Lepper & Martin, 1929)

Minced meat	1000 g
0.05 N-NaOH	1000 ml

Add the minced meat to the alkali solution, mix well and heat to boiling; simmer for 20 min with frequent stirring. Skim off the fat and check the pH, which should be about 7.5. Strain through gauze or muslin, squeeze out excess liquor, and dry the meat particles at a temperature below 50 °C. For use, place sufficient dried meat in a screw-capped container to a depth of about 2.5 cm and add sufficient Nutrient Broth to give a depth of about 5 cm. Sterilize at 115 °C for 20 min; avoid rapid release of pressure in the autoclave after sterilization.

Note. Although called Robertson's Cooked Meat medium, the method of preparation differs considerably from the original description (Robertson, 1916).

Cooked Meat medium (alternative formula)

Horse meat, fat-free and minced	450 g
Distilled water	1000 ml
Sodium thioglycollate, 45% aq. soln	1 ml
NaCl	5 g
Peptone	10 g

Boil the meat in the water for 1 h. Filter through muslin and press the meat dry. Add the NaCl and peptone to the filtrate, adjust to pH 8.4 with 10 N-NaOH and bring to the boil. Filter and add the thioglycollate solution.

Distribute the dry meat particles to a depth of 2.5 cm into screw-capped bottles, add the prepared broth to a level of 5 cm. Sterilize at 115 °C for 20 min; allow the pressure to fall slowly after sterilization.

A2.1.4 Digest Broth (modified from Hartley, 1922, and Pope & Smith, 1932)

Meat, finely minced	600 g
Na$_2$CO$_3$ anhydrous	8 g
Water	1000 ml
Pancreatic extract, Cole & Onslow's	20 ml

CHCl$_3$	20 ml
HCl, conc.	16 ml

Add the alkali and the meat to the water, heat to 80°C, stir well and cool.

Heat the infused mixture to 45–50 °C, add the pancreatic extract (A2.1.5) and chloroform, and maintain at 45–50 °C for 4–6 h with frequent stirring. Follow the course of digestion with the biuret test (Section A3.2).

Add the acid, boil for 30 min and filter. Adjust to pH 8, boil for 30 min and filter. Adjust to pH 7.6, determine the amino acid nitrogen content (Section A3.3.2) and dilute the broth to contain 700–750 mg amino acid N$_2$ per litre. Sterilize at 115 °C for 20 min.

Notes. Cole & Onslow's pancreatic extract may be replaced by a commercial trypsin extract or powder.

Pope & Smith recommend fractional addition of the enzyme during the digestion process.

Digest Agar is Digest Broth gelled by the addition of 2% agar.

A2.1.5 Pancreatic Extract (Cole & Onslow, 1916)

Fresh pig pancreas	250 g
Distilled water	750 ml
Industrial methylated spirit	250 ml

Add the water and spirit to the fat-free and minced pancreas in a 2 l flask and stopper tightly. Shake thoroughly and leave at room temperature for 3 days with frequent shaking. Filter, add 0.1% conc. HCl to the filtrate and mix well. Store at 4 °C. The cloudy precipitate which settles in a few days may be filtered off. The extract may be expected to retain its activity for several months when stored at 4 °C.

Note. A satisfactory extract should have a tryptic content of at least 50 units per ml (Section A3.1.8).

A2.1.6 Infusion Broth (modified from Wright, 1933)

Meat, minced	450 g
Water	1000 ml
Peptone	10 g
NaCl	5 g

Allow the meat to infuse in the water overnight at 4 °C. Skim the fat from the infused mixture, add the peptone and salt and boil for 30 min. Filter, adjust to pH 8.4 and boil for 20 min. Filter, adjust to pH 7.6, and sterilize at 115 °C for 20 min.

Infusion agar is Infusion Broth gelled by the addition of 2% agar.

A2.1.7 CYLG Broth (Marshall & Kelsey, 1960)

Casein digest	10 g
Marmite* (yeast extract)	5 g
Sodium glycerophosphate	10 g
Potassium lactate, 50% aq. soln	10 ml
Glucose	2 g
Inorganic salts soln	5 ml
Distilled water	1000 ml

Dissolve the ingredients by heating, mix, filter, and sterilize at 115 °C for 20 min.

Inorganic salts solution:

10 N-H$_2$SO$_4$	0.1 ml
MgSO$_4$·7H$_2$O	4 g
MnSO$_4$·4H$_2$O	0.4 g
FeSO$_4$·7H$_2$O	0.4 g
Water	100 ml

Add the acid to the water and dissolve the salts without heating.

Note. This basal medium may be supplemented by the addition of blood or serum, gelled by the addition of agar, and can form the basis of many standard media. It is reproducible, does not require pH adjustment, and can be prepared and stored in concentrated form.

A2.1.8 Thioglycollate Broth (modified from Brewer, 1940)

Peptone	15 g
Yeast extract	0.05 g
NaCl	0.05 g
Agar	0.01 g
Thioglycollic acid	0.01 g
Glucose	5 g
Methylene blue, 1% aq. soln	0.02 ml
Water	1000 ml

Dissolve the solids in the water with gentle heat. Add the thioglycollic acid and adjust to pH 8.5 with N-NaOH. Autoclave at 115 °C for 10 min. To prevent darkening of the medium, screw-caps should be loosened during autoclaving.

Adjust to pH 7.2, add the glucose and dye solution, mix well and sterilize at 115 °C for 10 min.

Notes. This medium should be stored in screw-capped containers in the dark at 4 °C (Cook & Steel, 1959*b*).

If more than 20% of the medium shows a green colour before use, it should be heated in a boiling water bath or steamer for 5–10 min and allowed to cool undisturbed; this treatment must not be repeated. Media containing thioglycollate tend to become inhibitory to anaerobes with prolonged storage.

---

* Beecham Bovril Brands, P.O. Box 18, Burton-on-Trent, DE14 2AB, UK.

A2.1.9 Dorset Egg medium

Egg yolk and white (about 16 hen eggs)	800 ml
NaCl, 0.9% sterile aq. soln	200 ml

Wash the eggs in 70% ethanol and lay on a sterile surface. Break the shells with a sterile knife and let the contents fall into a sterile flask; add the saline aseptically. Shake thoroughly to break up the yolks and produce a homogeneous mixture. Distribute 2 ml volumes into sterile 5 ml screw-capped (bijoux) bottles or 5 ml volumes into sterile 30 ml screw-capped (1 oz Universal or McCartney) bottles. Slope the containers in an inspissator and heat slowly to 75 °C. Maintain at this temperature for 1 h and repeat the process on each of the following two days.

Note. As an alternative to inspissation for egg and serum media, several workers have described methods of auto-claving which give uniform slopes free from air bubbles. The following procedure may be used with manually operated autoclaves : place the tubes in the autoclave in an inclined position and close the door and all valves of the autoclave; allow steam to enter the chamber rapidly until the pressure reaches 1.1 kgf/cm^2[†]. Maintain this pressure for 10 min; as the air has not been expelled, the temperature will rise slowly, preventing the formation of air bubbles during coagulation. After 10 min, open the air exhaust valve very slowly ensuring that a pressure of 1.1 kgf/cm^2 is maintained until the valve is fully open; rapid pressure changes will cause disruption of the slopes. Maintain the steam pressure for 15 min and then close both the steam supply and air exhaust valves. Allow the autoclave to cool slowly and do not open it until at least 5 min after the pressure has fallen to atmospheric.

A2.1.10 Nutrient Agar

Nutrient Broth (A2.1.1) gelled by the addition of 2% agar.

A2.1.11 Yeast Extract Agar (Report, 1956c, 1983)

Yeast extract	3 g
Peptone	5 g
Agar	12 g
Distilled water	1000 ml

Dissolve the yeast extract and peptone in the water. Adjust the reaction to pH 7.3. Add the agar and steam to dissolve. Distribute in 15 ml amounts in tubes or universal containers and larger volumes in screw-capped bottles. Autoclave at 115 °C for 10 minutes.

Like Yeastrel Agar (Zinnemann, 1960), this medium is free from X and V growth factors and can be used as a base for testing for them.

[†]15 lbf/in^2

A2.1.12 Mueller–Hinton Agar (Mueller & Hinton, 1941)

Meat infusion	6 g
Casein hydrolysate	17.5 g
Starch	1.5 g
Agar	10 g
Water	1000 ml

Bring to the boil to dissolve the ingredients completely. Adjust pH, if necessary, to 7.4. Sterilize at 121 °C for 15 min.

This medium, which was originally designed for *Neisseria*, contains starch to adsorb toxic substances produced during growth.

A2.1.13 Saline Agar

NaCl	8.5 g
Agar	20 g
Water	1000 ml

Dissolve by steaming; sterilize at 115 °C for 20 min.

A2.1.14 Water Agar

Agar	20 g
Water	1000 ml

Dissolve by steaming; sterilize at 115 °C for 20 min.

A2.2 Enriched and enrichment media

Basic culture media may be made more suitable for the growth of many organisms, especially if fastidious or slow-growing, by the addition of nutritious substances such as blood, serum or sugars. Such enriched media are essentially non-selective. Substances may also be added to media in order to encourage the growth of particular organisms or groups of organisms and isolation procedures often use such enrichment media. Their distinction from selective media, which inhibit the growth of unwanted organisms, is often blurred so that several of the media in Section A3 could also be described and used as enrichment media. Many such media have been developed for these purposes. Some have but a brief trial and are then discarded; those that are successful may be further developed and produced commercially.

It should be noted that *Salmonella choleraesuis* is inhibited by selenite media commonly used for enrichment and isolation of enteric bacteria.

A2.2.1 Blood Agar

Defibrinated blood	50 ml
Nutrient Agar	950 ml

Melt the Nutrient Agar, cool to 50 °C and add the blood aseptically. Mix and distribute in tubes or plates.

Notes. Haemolysis can be seen better in layered Blood Agar plates. For such plates, a layer of Peptone Water Agar is poured into the Petri dish, allowed to set, and the blood-containing medium is poured on top. Alternatively, a simple agar solution without nutrients may be used as the lower layer; it must however be made isotonic to prevent haemolysis of the blood in the upper layer.

The inclusion of glucose in the basal medium for Blood Agar is not recommended as its presence inhibits haemolysin production by streptcocci (Fuller & Maxted, 1939).

Blood Broth is prepared by the aseptic addition of 5% sterile defibrinated blood to the appropriate volume of Nutrient Broth.

A2.2.2   Chocolate Agar

Place a Blood Agar plate (medium down) in an incubator set at 65 °C for 1–1^1/$_2$ h until the medium assumes a uniform 'chocolate' colour.

Alternatively, melt Nutrient Agar and cool to 50 °C. Add 5% sterile blood, mix and heat in a water bath to 80 °C with frequent mixing. Maintain at 80 °C until the medium has a 'chocolate' colour and distribute aseptically.

A2.2.3   Fildes' peptic digest of blood (Fildes, 1920)

Defibrinated sheep blood	25 ml
NaCl, 0.9% sterile aq. soln	75 ml
HCl, conc.	3 ml
Pepsin	0.5 g

Mix the blood and saline in a glass-stoppered bottle and add the pepsin and acid. Shake thoroughly and place in a water bath at 55 °C for 4 h with occasional shaking. Add 6 ml 5 N-NaOH and check that the pH is 7.0. Add 0.25 ml CHCl$_3$ as a preservative and shake thoroughly. The digest will keep for at least 12 months but should be stored at 4 °C. It is better to leave it too acid rather than too alkaline.

Note. Before use the chloroform must be removed by heating gently in a water bath.

A2.2.4   Fildes' Digest Agar

Fildes' peptic digest of blood	50 ml
Nutrient Agar	950 ml

Maintain the Fildes' digest at 55 °C for 30 min to volatilize the chloroform. Then aseptically add it to the Nutrient Agar, previously melted and cooled to 55 °C. Mix and distribute aseptically.

A2.2.5   Serum Agar

Sterile serum	50 ml
Nutrient Agar	950 ml

Melt the Nutrient Agar, cool to 50–55 °C and aseptically add the serum. Mix and distribute.

Serum Broth is prepared by the aseptic addition of 5% sterile serum to Nutrient Broth.

A2.2.6   Serum Glucose Agar (Jones & Morgan, 1958)

Peptone	10 g
Meat extract	5 g
NaCl	5 g
Agar	20 g
Water	1000 ml

Prepare this base as for Nutrient Agar (A2.1.10) and sterilize at 115 °C for 20 min..

Sterile horse serum	50 ml
Glucose, 20% aq. soln	50 ml
Nutrient base	1000 ml

Add the serum and sterile glucose solution to the base, previously melted and cooled to 50–55 °C. Mix and distribute aseptically.

A2.2.7   Glucose Broth

Glucose, 20% aq. soln	50 ml
Nutrient Broth	950 ml

Sterilize the glucose solution by filtration and add aseptically to the Nutrient Broth. Mix and distribute aseptically.

A2.2.8   Glycerol Agar

Glycerol	50 ml
Nutrient Agar	1000 ml

Melt the Nutrient Agar, add the glycerol, mix and sterilize at 115 °C for 20 min.

Note. Gordon & Smith (1953) used 7% glycerol in Soil Extract Agar (A2.6.35).

A2.2.9   Tomato Juice Agar
(modified from Kulp & White, 1932)

Tomatoes	250 g
Distilled water	500 ml

Cut up the tomatoes and steam in the water for an hour or until they are pulped. Clarify through gauze and filter through paper.

Peptone	10 g
Peptonized milk	10 g
Agar	20 g
Tomato juice	400 ml
Distilled water	600 ml

Dissolve the solids in the water by heating. Add the tomato juice, mix, and sterilize at 115 °C for 20 min. The final pH value of the medium should be 6.0–6.2.

A2.3   Differential and selective media

A2.3.1   Acetate Agar (Whittenbury, 1965a)

Meat extract (powder)	5 g
Peptone	5 g
Yeast extract (powder)	5 g
Tween 80	0.5 ml

Glucose	10 g
Agar	15 g
Distilled water	850 ml

Dissolve the ingredients by heating, adjust to pH 5.4 with 2 M-acetic acid and sterilize at 115 °C for 20 min.

Before dispensing, add 100 ml of 2 M-acetic acid with sodium acetate buffer (pH 5.4) to the molten medium. Bottle and sterilize at 115 °C for 20 min.

Note. Prepare the acetate buffer by adjusting a 2 M-solution of sodium acetate to pH 5.4 with 2 M-acetic acid.

A2.3.2   Bile Agar

Ox bile, dehydrated	10 g
Nutrient Agar	1000 ml

Melt the Nutrient Agar, add the bile (equivalent to 10% bile), mix and dissolve. Sterilize at 115 °C for 20 min. Cool to about 55 °C and distribute. For fastidious organisms, serum (5%) may be added after cooling to 55 °C.

Notes. For 40% Bile Agar, use 40 g dehydrated ox bile per litre. Bile Agar can be used as whole plates, or as ditches in plates of Blood or Serum Agar.

A2.3.3   Blood–Tellurite Agar

K$_2$TeO$_3$, 2% aq. soln	16 ml
Sterile blood	50 ml
Infusion Agar	1000 ml

Melt the Infusion Agar medium, cool to 50 °C and aseptically add the blood and sterile tellurite solution. The medium must not be heated after addition of the tellurite. Mix and distribute.

Notes. Sterilize the tellurite solution by filtration, not by heat. The final concentration of tellurite in this medium is approximately 0.03% (1/3333).

Several tellurite media have been described; Anderson *et al.* (1931) and Barksdale (1981) used a 'chocolate' (heated blood) agar base, and laked (lysed) blood was used by Wilson (1934) and Hoyle (1941).

A2.3.4   Bordet–Gengou Agar (modified from Bordet & Gengou, 1906)

Peptone	10 g
NaCl	5 g
Glycerol	10 ml
Soluble starch	2.5 g
Agar	3 g
Water	1000 ml

Make a smooth paste of the soluble starch with a few ml of the water. Dissolve the peptone, NaCl, and glycerol in the remaining water, heat, and add the starch suspension. Adjust to pH 7.5, add the agar and dissolve by heating. Sterilize this base at 115 °C for 20 min.

For use, aseptically add 500 ml horse blood (warmed to 45 °C) to 1000 ml of base melted and cooled to 55–60 °C. Mix and distribute.

Notes. Medium in plates should be thick, at least 5 mm in depth, and must not be overdried; it should be bright red in colour (Bailey, 1933); a dark medium indicates old or overheated blood.

Some brands of peptone are markedly inhibitory to the growth of *Bordetella pertussis* and the original formula of Bordet & Gengou did not include peptone. Dawson *et al.* (1951) consider that 30% blood is the minimum for a satisfactory product; however, haemolysis is not usually seen when the blood concentration exceeds 30%; the original medium contained 50%.

Bacteriological charcoal can be used instead of or as well as blood (Ensminger *et al.*, 1953; Brumfitt, 1959) and antibiotics may be added to inhibit the competing flora (Lacey, 1954; Regan & Lowe, 1977).

A2.3.5   Bromthymol Blue Salt Teepol Agar (BTBST)
(Kobayashi *et al.*, 1963; Sakazaki, 1965*b*)

Meat extract	3.0 g
Tryptone	10.0 g
Sucrose	10.0 g
Teepol 610	2.0 ml
NaCl	30.0 g
Bromthymol blue	0.08 g
Agar	15.0 g
Distilled water	1000 ml

Dissolve by steaming; adjust pH to 7.8 and pour as plates for immediate use. Sterilize stock medium at 121 °C for 15 min. For use, melt by steaming.

Note. Plates should not be overdried.

A2.3.6   Buffered Charcoal Yeast Extract Agar (BCYE) with a-ketoglutarate for *Legionella*
(Edelstein *et al.*, 1981)

N-(2-acetamido)-2-aminoethane-sulphonic acid buffer (ACES)	10 g
KOH	2.8 g
Activated charcoal	1.5 g
Yeast extract	10 g
Agar	17 g
α-ketoglutarate	1 g
L-cysteine hydrochloride 4% (w/v) sterile aq. soln	10 ml
Ferric pyrophosphate 28% (w/v) sterile aq. soln	10 ml
Distilled water	1000 ml

Add the ACES buffer to 900 ml of distilled water in a flask and warm to 50 °C until dissolved. Add the KOH pellets to the buffer. Mix together the activated charcoal, yeast extract, agar and α-ketoglutarate and add them to the flask,

CULTURE MEDIA

rinsing with a further 80 ml of water. Sterilize at 121 °C for 15 min.

Cool to 50 °C and add separately the filter-sterilized solutions of ferric pyrophosphate and L-cysteine hydrochloride. Adjust the pH if necessary to 6.9 ± 0.2 with N-HCl or KOH. Cool to 45 °C and distribute aseptically. The plates will keep for 2 weeks at 5 °C in plastic bags.

A2.3.7 Glucose Salt Teepol Broth (Akiyama *et al.*, 1963)

Meat extract	3 g
Tryptone	10 g
NaCl	30 g
Glucose	5 g
Methyl violet	0.002 g
Teepol 610	4 ml
Distilled water	1000 ml

Dissolve in the cold and adjust the pH to 9.4. Sterilize at 121 °C for 15 min. Dispense aseptically as needed.

A2.3.8 MacConkey Agar (modified from MacConkey, 1908; Report, 1956c, 1983)

Peptone	20 g
NaCl	5 g
Sodium taurocholate	5 g
Agar	20 g
Lactose	10 g
Neutral red, 1% aq. soln	10 ml
Water	1000 ml

Dissolve the peptone, NaCl and bile salt in the water by heating. Adjust to pH 8.0, boil for 20 min, cool and filter. Add and dissolve the agar by boiling and adjust to pH 7.4. Add the lactose and indicator solution, mix and sterilize at 115 °C for 20 min.

Notes. The exact quantity of indicator depends on the depth of colour preferred.

Sodium taurocholate, sodium tauroglycocholate or other satisfactory bile salt, including ox gall, may be used (see Section A3.1.5).

The use of 0.1% Teepol 610 (an anionic detergent) in place of bile salt in MacConkey Agar was recommended by Jameson & Emberley (1956).

For *MacConkey Broth* see Section A2.6.9.

A2.3.9 Salt Colistin (Polymyxin) Broth (Sakazaki, 1972; Nakanishi & Murase, 1974)

Yeast extract	3 g
Tryptone	10 g
NaCl	20 g
Colistin sulphomethate sodium (Colomycin)	0.5×10^6 i.u
OR (Polymyxin B)	(2.5×10^5 i.u.)
Distilled water	1000 ml

Dissolve the yeast extract, tryptone and salt in the water. Adjust to pH 7·0. Autoclave at 121 °C for 15 min and allow to cool. Add the Colomycin or Polymyxin aseptically. Keep at 4 °C and dispense as required.

A2.3.10 Thiosulphate-Citrate-Bile salt-Sucrose (TCBS) Agar (Akiyama *et al.*, 1963; Sakazaki, 1965b)

Yeast extract	5 g
Peptone	10 g
Sodium thiosulphate	10 g
Sodium citrate	1 g
Ox bile	8 g
Sucrose	20 g
Sodium chloride	1 g
Ferric citrate	1 g
Bromthymol blue	0.04 g
Agar	15 g
Distilled water	1000 ml

Add all the ingredients to the water and bring to the boil to dissolve. Do NOT autoclave. Dispense and allow to cool.

A2.4 Media for enhancing pigment production

A2.4.1 Potato slopes.

Take several large potatoes and scrub them thoroughly under running water. Cut cylinders with an 18–20 mm cork borer, rejecting any that are bruised or diseased. Cut each cylinder obliquely into two and place each half in a 30 ml screw-capped bottle or 25 mm diameter tube with the thick end resting on a small plug of absorbent cotton. Fill the containers with water and steam for 30 min. Pour off the water and sterilize at 115 °C for 20 min.

A2.4.2 Mannitol Yeast-Extract Agar

Peptone	2.5 g
NaCl	2.5 g
Agar	20 g
Water	1000 ml

Dissolve the solids in the water by heating. Adjust to pH 8.0, boil for 30 min and filter.

Mannitol	5 g
Yeast extract	2.5 g

Adjust to pH 7.0, add the mannitol and yeast extract. Mix, dissolve, and sterilize at 115 °C for 20 min.

A2.4.3 King's media – for pseudomonads (King, Ward & Raney, 1954)

Medium A – for pyocyanin

Peptone	20 g
Glycerol	10 g
K_2SO_4, anhyd.	10 g
$MgCl_2$, anhyd.	1.4 g

197

Agar	20 g
Water	1000 ml

Dissolve the constituents except agar by heating in the water. Adjust to pH 7.2 if necessary. Add the agar and dissolve and sterilize by autoclaving at 115 °C for 10 min.

Medium B – for fluorescin

Proteose peptone	20 g
Glycerol	10 g
K_2HPO_4	1.5 g
$MgSO_4 \cdot 7H_2O$	1.5 g
Agar	20 g
Water	1000 ml

Proceed as for medium A above.

A2.5   Media for carbohydrate studies

A2.5.1   Hugh and Leifson's OF medium (Hugh & Leifson, 1953)

Peptone	2 g
NaCl	5 g
K_2HPO_4	0.3 g
Agar	3 g
Distilled water	1000 ml
Bromthymol blue, 0.2% aq. soln	15 ml

Dissolve the solids by heating in the water. Adjust to pH 7.1, filter, and add the indicator. Sterilize at 115 °C for 20 min.

Add a sterile solution of glucose or other appropriate carbohydrate aseptically to give a final concentration of 1%. Mix and distribute aseptically in 10 ml volumes into sterile tubes of not more than 16 mm diameter.

A2.5.2   Peptone Water sugars. The method of preparation will depend on the indicator:

Andrade's indicator. Adjust the reaction of 900 ml Peptone Water to pH 7.1–7.3 so that the addition of 10 ml of Andrade's indicator will bring it to pH 7.5. Sterilize at 115 °C for 20 min; this medium is pink when hot but the colour fades on cooling. Dissolve 5–10 g of the appropriate sugar in 90 ml of water and steam for 30 min or sterilize by filtration. Aseptically add this to the sterile Peptone Water with indicator, distribute into sterile test tubes with inverted inner (Durham) tubes and steam for 30 min.

Other indicators. To 900 ml Peptone Water add 10 ml indicator solution (Bromcresol purple, bromthymol blue, or phenol red) and sterilize at 115 °C for 20 min. Dissolve 5–10 g of the appropriate sugar in 90 ml water and steam for 30 min or sterilize by filtration. Add this to the sterile Peptone Water with indicator, distribute into sterile tubes with inverted inner (Durham) tubes and steam for 30 min.

Notes. The addition of some carbohydrates may cause an acid reaction; in these instances add sufficient 0.1 N-NaOH to restore the original colour.

Where the solubility of a carbohydrate is low (Table A2), the required amount of solid material may be added to the base and, when dissolved, the complete medium is sterilized.

A2.5.3   Broth sugars

Broth-based sugars are used extensively in the USA and are recommended by the international subcommittee on Enterobacteriaceae (Report, 1958). They are also recommended for haemophili and streptococci.

Peptone	10 g
Meat extract	3 g
NaCl	5 g
Distilled water	1000 ml
Andrade's indicator *OR*	
Phenol red aq. soln	10 ml

Dissolve the solids in the water, add the indicator and adjust to pH 7.1–7.2. Sterilize at 115 °C for 20 min. Aseptically add 0.5–1% of the appropriate carbohydrate (sterilized by membrane filtration), mix, distribute into sterile tubes containing inverted inner (Durham) tubes, and steam for 30 min.

Note. A small amount of agar (e.g. 0.1%) may be included.

A2.5.4   Serum Water sugars

Peptone	4 g
Na_2HPO_4	0.8 g
Distilled water	800 ml
Sterile serum	200 ml
Bromcresol purple, 0.2% aq. soln	10 ml

Dissolve the peptone and phosphate in the water, steam at 100 °C for 15 min and filter. Add the serum and steam for a further 15 min. Adjust pH to 7.5–7.8 and add the indicator. Sterilize at 115 °C for 10 min.

Aseptically add 0.5–1% of the appropriate sugar as a sterile solution and distribute into sterile tubes.

Note. It is an advantage to have perfectly clear media. Different batches of serum differ in their coagulability by heat, and occasionally the medium is cloudy when serum in the amount given above is used. It is a good plan to add varying amounts of each batch of serum (e.g. in concentrations of 10–25%) to tubes of the basal medium, to autoclave them, and to choose the highest concentration that does not show marked cloudiness after sterilization.

A2.5.5   Ammonium Salt Sugars (ASS)(Smith, Gordon & Clark, 1952)

$(NH_4)_2HPO_4$	1 g
KCl	0.2 g
$MgSO_4 \cdot 7H_2O$	0.2 g
Yeast extract	0.2 g

Agar	20 g
Distilled water	1000 ml
Bromcresol purple, 0.2% aq. soln	4 ml
OR Bromythmol blue	0.04 g

Add the solids to the water and dissolve by steaming. Add the indicator and sterilize at 115 °C for 20 min. Allow the basal medium to cool to about 60 °C and add the appropriate carbohydrate as a sterile solution to give a final concentration of 0.5–1%. Mix and distribute aseptically into sterile tubes which are inclined so that the medium sets as slopes.

A2.5.6 Sugars for neisserias (Thompson & Knudsen, 1958)

Digest Broth	1000 ml
Agar	3 g
Phenol red, 0.2% soln	10 ml
Sterile rabbit serum	50 ml
Sugar, sterile 10% soln	100 ml

Dissolve the agar in the broth by heating, add the indicator solution and sterilize at 115 °C for 20 min. Cool to about 55 °C and aseptically add the serum and sugar solution. Distribute into sterile tubes.

Notes. The four sugars used to differentiate *Neisseria* species are glucose, lactose, maltose, and sucrose.

Wilkinson (1962) recommends a solid medium containing hydrocele fluid for detecting acid production by *Neisseria* species.

A2.5.7 Sugars for lactobacilli (de Man, Rogosa & Sharpe, 1960)

MRS broth, modified	1000 ml
Carbohydrate	20 g
Chlorphenol red, 0.2% soln	20 ml

Prepare the basal MRS broth as in Section A2.6.25, omitting the meat extract and glucose; adjust to pH 6.2–6.5, add the indicator, and sterilize at 115 °C for 20 min. Add the carbohydrate (mannose, xylose, and maltose should be filter-sterilized and added aseptically), mix, and distribute; steam for 30 min.

A2.5.8 Nutrient sugar media with agar

(1) *For utilization tests*
Lactose (or Glucose) 10% Agar

Peptone	5 g
Meat extract	3 g
Lactose (or glucose)	100 g
Agar	20 g
Distilled water	1000 ml
Bromcresol purple, 0.2% soln	10 ml

Dissolve the solids in the water by heating, adjust to pH 6.8 with 10 N-NaOH, filter, and add the indicator solution.

Sterilize at 115 °C for 20 min and distribute as plates or slopes.

(2) *Media for 3-ketolactose production from lactose*
Medium 1

Yeast extract	10.0 g
Glucose	20.0 g
Calcium carbonate	20.0 g
Agar	11.0 g
Distilled water	1000 ml

Mix ingredients well to produce an even suspension. Adjust pH to 7.0–7.2 and sterilize at 115 °C for 20 min. Distribute in plates.
Medium 2

Yeast extract	1.0 g
Lactose	10.0 g
Agar	11.0 g
Distilled water	1000 ml

Dissolve ingredients, adjust to pH 7.0–7.2 and sterilize at 115 °C for 20 min. Distribute in plates.

A2.5.9 MacConkey Broth (Report, 1956c, 1983)

Peptone	20 g
NaCl	5 g
Sodium taurocholate[*]	5 g
Water	1000 ml
Bromcresol purple, 0.2% soln	5 ml
Lactose	20 g

Dissolve the peptone, NaCl and bile salt in the water by heating. Adjust to pH 8.0 and boil for 20 min. Cool, filter, and adjust to pH 7.4. Add the lactose and indicator solution, mix and distribute into tubes containing inverted inner (Durham) tubes. Sterilize at 115 °C for 15 min.

Note. See MacConkey Agar (Section A2.3.8) for remarks on bile salts.

A2.5.10 MR–VP test medium

Glucose–phosphate medium

Peptone	5 g
K_2HPO_4	5 g
Distilled water	1000 ml

Steam until the solids are dissolved, filter, and adjust to pH 7.5.

Glucose	5 g

Add the glucose, mix and distribute 1.5 ml volumes into tubes. Sterilize at 115 °C for 10 min.

Notes. For sterilization, the tubes must be placed in a solid-bottomed container to protect them from contact with steam; if this is neglected, the medium becomes straw-yellow in colour.

Workers in the USA generally use 7 g peptone.

This medium is also used for the VP test; other media for the VP test are shown below.

A2.5.11 VP test media

Glucose–peptone medium (Abd-el-Malek & Gibson, 1948b)

Peptone	10 g
Glucose	5 g
Distilled water	1000 ml

Mix and dissolve by gentle heating. Filter, adjust to pH 7.6, and distribute into tubes. Sterilize at 115 °C for 10 min in a solid-bottomed container.

Glucose-salt medium (Smith, Gordon & Clark, 1946)

Proteose peptone	7 g
NaCl	5 g
Glucose	5 g
Distilled water	1000 ml

Dissolve the solids in the water, distribute into tubes, and sterilize at 115 °C for 20 min in a solid-bottomed container.

Semi-solid VP medium (Furniss, Lee & Donovan, 1978)

Tryptone	10 g
Yeast extract	5 g
NaCl	5 g
K_2HPO_4	5 g
Glucose	5 g
Agar	3 g

Dissolve ingredients by heating. Dispense in 2.5 ml volumes in bijoux bottles and sterilize at 115 °C for 10 min.

A2.5.12 Media for dextran and levan production

Sucrose Agar

Sterile serum	50 ml
Sucrose	50 g
Digest agar	1000 ml

Melt the Digest Agar, add the sucrose, and steam for 30 min. Cool to 55 °C, aseptically add the serum, and distribute into Petri dishes.

Sucrose Broth

Sucrose	50 g
Infusion Broth	1000 ml

Dissolve the sucrose in the broth, distribute in tubes and steam for 1 h.

A2.5.13 Starch Agar

Potato starch	10 g
Distilled water	50 ml
Nutrient agar	1000 ml

Triturate the starch with the water to a smooth cream, and add to the molten Nutrient Agar. Mix, and sterilize at 115 °C for 10 min. Distribute into Petri dishes.

Notes. This medium should not be filtered after adding the starch suspension.

Overheating may hydrolyse the starch.

A2.6 Miscellaneous media

A2.6.1 Aesculin Broth

Aesculin	1 g
Ferric citrate	0.5 g
Peptone Water	1000 ml

Dissolve the aesculin and iron salt in the Peptone Water, and sterilize at 115 °C for 10 min.

Aesculin Agar is Aesculin Broth gelled by the addition of 2% agar.

A2.6.2 Aesculin–bile Agar (Williams & Hirch, 1950; Swan, 1954)

Ox bile, dehydrated	40 g
Aesculin	1 g
Ferric citrate	0.5 g
Agar	15 g
Nutrient Broth	1000 ml

Dissolve all the ingredients except aesculin by heating. Allow to cool and then add the aesculin. Dispense in screw-capped bottles, sterilize at 115 °C for 20 min and allow to set as slopes.

A2.6.3 Aesculin Blood Agar (Phillips, 1976) for anaerobic work

Prepare an aqueous solution of aesculin (2% w/v) and ferric citrate (1% w/v) and steam at 100 °C for 5 minutes. Since aesculin at this concentration is completely soluble only when the solution is warm, spread pre-dried Blood Agar plate with 1.0 ml of the aesculin–ferric citrate solution at about 50 °C; this gives a final concentration of about 0.1% aesculin in the medium. Spot-inoculate plates and incubate anaerobically for 48 hours. Aesculin hydrolysis is indicated by blackening of the medium under and around bacterial growth.

A2.6.4 Arginine media

Arginine Broth (Niven, Smiley & Sherman, 1942)

Peptone (tryptone)	5 g
Yeast extract	5 g
K_2HPO_4	2 g
Glucose	0.5 g
Arginine monohydrochloride	3 g
Distilled water	1000 ml

Dissolve by heating, adjust to pH 7.0, boil, filter, and sterilize at 115 °C for 20 min.

Note. L-arginine monohydrochloride is dextro-rotatory and in consequence was incorrectly called D-arginine monohydrochloride in the original paper of Niven *et al.*

Arginine Agar (Thornley, 1960)

Peptone	1.0 g
NaCl	5.0 g

K$_2$HPO$_4$	0.3 g
Phenol red, 1.0% aq. soln	1.0 ml
L(+)arginine hydrochloride	10.0 g
Agar	3.0 g
Distilled water	1000 ml

Dissolve the solids in the water, adjust to pH 7.2, distribute into tubes or screw-capped (6 mm) bottles to a depth of about 16 mm (3.5 ml) and sterilize at 121 °C for 15 min.

A2.6.5 Bicarbonate Agar with Serum (Burdon, 1956; Burdon & Wende, 1960) for encapsulation of *B. anthracis*

Nutrient Broth (without added salt)	100 ml
Yeast extract	0.3 g
Glucose	0.5 g
Agar	2.5 g

Make up with gentle heating, in distilled water. Sterilize by autoclaving at 115 °C for 10 minutes. Add 7% solution of NaHCO$_3$, sterilized by filtration, to the sterile molten agar medium to give a final concentration of 0.7% bicarbonate. Then add sterile bovine serum albumin, fraction V, to give a final concentration of 0.7% (w/v); alternatively, in order of preference, add human, sheep, calf or horse serum to a final concentration of 20% (v/v). Pour into plates.

A2.6.6 Casein Agar (Milk Agar) (modified from Hastings, 1903)

Milk, skim	500 ml
Nutrient Agar, double-strength	500 ml

Prepare the skim-milk as in Section A2.6.23 and sterilize by heating at 115 °C for 10 min. Cool to about 50 °C and add to the double-strength Nutrient Agar (Section A2.1.1) melted and cooled to 50–55 °C. Mix and distribute in Petri dishes or tubes.

Note. As the acid produced by lactose fermentation had an inhibitory effect on the hydrolysis of casein, Eddy (1960) recommended dialysis of milk before adding to the basal medium.

Alternatively, a 10% aqueous solution of skimmed milk powder may be used. This is distributed in screw-capped bottles and autoclaved at 121 °C for 5 min. For use, add 50 ml of the skimmed milk solution to 100 ml of a melted sterile Nutrient Agar solution (2.5% in distilled water), mix and pour into Petri dishes.

A2.6.7 Citrate media

Christensen's medium (Christensen, 1949)

Sodium citrate	3 g
Glucose	0.2 g
Yeast extract	0.5 g
L-cysteine hydrochloride	0.1 g
Ferric ammonium citrate	0.4 g

KH$_2$PO$_4$	1 g
NaCl	5 g
Na$_2$S$_2$O$_3$	0.08 g
Agar	20 g
Phenol red, 0.2% aq. soln	6 ml
Distilled water	1000 ml

Dissolve the solids in the water by heating and filter; adjust to pH 6.8–6.9, add the indicator, and sterilize at 115 °C for 20 min.

Note. This medium is also suitable for demonstrating H$_2$S production; if it is not to be used for this purpose the Na$_2$S$_2$O$_3$ and ferric ammonium citrate can be omitted.

Koser's medium (modified from Koser, 1923; Report, 1983)

NaCl	5 g
MgSO$_4$·7H$_2$O	0.2 g
NH$_4$H$_2$PO$_4$	1 g
K$_2$HPO$_4$	1 g
Citric acid	2 g
Distilled water	1000 ml

Dissolve the salts in the water.

Add the citric acid to the salts solution and adjust to pH 6.8 with N-NaOH. Dispense in 5 ml volumes in screw-capped containers and autoclave at 115 °C for 20 min. The medium should be colourless.

All glassware must be chemically clean and alkali-free (see Section A1.1).

Note. In his original paper, Koser (1923) used 2 g sodium citrate or 2.77 g of the hydrated salt in place of the citric acid in the formula given above; it is not known which of the three sodium salts of citric acid was used although Koser stated that it had 5½ molecules of water of crystallization.

Simmons' medium (modified from Simmons, 1926)

This is the modified Koser's Citrate medium (above) incorporating 0.008% bromthymol blue (i.e. 20 ml of 0.4% aqueous solution per litre), and gelled by the addition of 2% agar. The colourless or faintly green medium is rendered blue by bacterial growth if citrate is utilized.

A2.6.8 Organic acids as carbon sources (Gordon & Mihm, 1957)

NaCl	1 g
MgSO$_4$·7H$_2$O	0.2 g
(NH$_4$)$_2$HPO$_4$	1 g
KH$_2$PO$_4$	0.5 g
Organic acid (sodium salt)	2 g
Phenol red, 0.2% aq. soln	4 ml
Agar	20 g
Distilled water	1000 ml

Dissolve the agar by steaming in about 800 ml of the water. Dissolve the salts in the remainder of the water and add to the agar solution. Adjust to pH 6.8 and add the indicator solution. Sterilize at 115 °C for 20 min.

Notes. Organic acids used as their sodium salts include: acetate, benzoate, citrate, lactate, oxalate, propionate, pyruvate, succinate and tartrate; malate is used as its calcium salt, and mucate as the free acid.

This medium resembles the modified Simmons' Citrate medium (above) but contains less NaCl and a different indicator.

A2.6.9 Decarboxylase media

Møller's medium (Møller, 1955)

Peptone	5 g
Meat extract	5 g
Pyridoxal	5 mg
Glucose	0.5 g
Bromthymol purple 0.2% aq. soln	5 ml
Cresol red, 0.2% aq. soln	2.5 ml
Distilled water	1000 ml

Dissolve the solids in the water by heating. Adjust to pH 6.0. Add the indicators, mix, and distribute into four equal volumes. Sterilize at 115 °C for 20 min.

For use make the following additions and then re-adjust to pH 6.0 if necessary:

1. L-arginine hydrochloride	1%
2. L-lysine hydrochloride	1%
3. L-ornithine hydrochloride	1%
4. No addition	

Distribute the four media in 1–1.5 ml volumes into small rimless tubes (67 × 10 mm or 3 × ³/₈ in) containing sterile medicinal grade liquid paraffin to a height of about 5 mm above the medium. After distribution sterilize at 115 °C for 10 min or by steaming at 100 °C for 30 min on three successive days.

Notes. Møller specified Orthana Special peptone but other peptones are satisfactory.

When DL-amino acids are used, the concentration should be 2%. If glutamic acid decarboxylase activity is also to be investigated, the basal medium should be divided into five portions, to the fifth of which 1% L-glutamic acid is added.

Falkow's medium (modified from Falkow, 1958)

Peptone	5 g
Yeast extract	3 g
Glucose	1 g
Bromcresol purple, 0.2% aq.soln	10 ml
Distilled water	1000 ml

Dissolve the solids in the water, adjust to pH 6.7, and add the indicator solution. Sterilize at 115 °C for 20 min. Divide into four equal volumes and make the following additions:

1. L-arginine hydrochloride	0.5%
2. L-lysine hydrochloride	0.5%
3. L-ornithine hydrochloride	0.5%
4. No addition	

Re-adjust pH to 6.7 if necessary. Dispense in 2 ml volumes in small tubes and sterilize at 115 °C for 10 min.

A2.6.10 DNA Toluidine-blue Agar media

(Modified from Schreier, 1969) *for DNase Method 2.*

Tryptose	20 g
Deoxyribonucleic acid	2 g
NaCl	5 g
Toluidine blue	0.1 g
Agar	20 g
Distilled water	1000 ml

Dissolve constituents in the distilled water, autoclave at 121 °C for 15 min. and pour into Petri dishes.

(Lior & Patel, 1987) *for DNase Method 3*

Deoxyribonucleic acid	0.3 g
0.01 M-calcium chloride	1 m
Sodium chloride	10 g
Agar	6.5 g
0.05 M-Tris buffer pH 9.0	1000 ml

Add all the ingredients to the buffer solution and heat to boiling until the DNA and agar are completely dissolved. Cool to 50 °C, add 2.5 ml of 3% toluidine blue '0' and mix well. Does not require sterilization. Store in the dark.

Note. Tris buffer requires a pH electrode with calomel reference. Tris buffers are available commercially which do not require adjustment.

A2.6.11 Ferric Bisulphite Pyruvate (FBP) medium for rapid H₂S test (method 7)

Nutrient Broth	100 ml
Na₂HPO₄ (anhydrous)	1.18 g
KH₂PO₄ (anhydrous)	0.23 g
Agar	2 g
Water	900 ml

Dissolve the ingredients in the water by heating, sterilize at 121 °C for 15 min and cool to 48 °C. Add the following ingredients in the manner described below:-

FeSO₄·7H₂0, 10% soln	10 ml
Sodium metabisulphite, 10% aq. soln	10 ml
Sodium pyruvate, 10% aq. soln	10 ml

Add the ferrous sulphate solution to the metabisulphite solution, mix well, then add to the pyruvate solution, mix again and add to the basal medium. Adjust to pH 7.3 with 1 N-NaOH. Store at 4 °C and prepare fresh every few weeks.

A2.6.12 Ferrous chloride Gelatin medium (Report, 1958) for H₂S test (Method 2)

Meat extract	7.5 g
Peptone	25 g

NaCl	5 g
Gelatin	120 g
Distilled water	1000 ml
FeCl$_2$, 10% aq. soln	5 ml

Prepare the base as for Nutrient Gelatin (A2.6.14). After sterilization and before the medium gels, add the freshly prepared FeCl$_2$ solution. Dispense into narrow tubes, cool immediately, and seal the tubes with corks that have been soaked in hot paraffin wax.

A2.6.13 Fluorescence–denitrification medium
(FN medium of Pickett & Pedersen, 1968)

Proteose peptone	10.0 g
MgSO$_4$·7H$_2$O	1.5 g
K$_2$HPO$_4$	1.5 g
KNO$_3$	2.0 g
NaNO$_2$	0.5 g
Agar	15.0 g
Water	1000 ml

Dissolve by heating. Adjust pH to 7.2; dispense in 4 ml volumes in 12 mm tubes or about 10 ml in 28 ml (Universal or McCartney) screw-capped bottles. Sterilize at 121 °C for 10 min. Set at an angle to give a slope and butt of approximately equal length.

For fluorescence, inoculate the surface; for denitrification, stab-inoculate the butt.

A2.6.14 Gelatin media
Gelatin Agar (Frazier, 1926)

Gelatin	4 g
Distilled water	50 ml
Nutrient Agar	1000 ml

Soak the gelatin in the water and, when thoroughly softened, add to the melted Nutrient Agar. Mix, and sterilize at 115 °C for 10 min. Distribute into plates.

Note. After growth, gelatinase activity is demonstrated by treating with a solution of 15% mercuric chloride in 1 N-HCl. Zones of clearing develop around gelatinolytic colonies.

For safety reaons, 30% trichloroacetic acid is preferable to use of the acid mercuric choloride solution.

Nutrient Gelatin

Meat extract	3 g
Peptone	5 g
Gelatin	120 g
Water	100 ml

Add the gelatin to the water and allow to stand for 15–30 min. Heat to dissolve the gelatin; add and dissolve the other constituents. Adjust to pH 7.0, and sterilize by heating at 115 °C for 20 min.

Note. This medium must not be overheated.

A2.6.15 Gluconate Broth (Shaw & Clarke, 1955; Carpenter, 1961)

Peptone	1.5 g
Yeast extract	1 g
K$_2$HPO$_4$	1 g
Potassium gluconate	40 g
Distilled water	1000 ml

Dissolve in the water by heating. Adjust to pH 7.0. Filter, and sterilize at 115 °C for 20 min.

Note. The potassium gluconate may be replaced by 37.25 g of sodium gluconate.

A2.6.16 Glucose Phenolphthalein Broth (Clarke, 1953b)
Glycine buffer

Glycine	0.6 g
NaCl	0.35 g
Distilled water, freshly boiled	60 ml
0.1 N-NaOH	40 ml

Dissolve the glycine and NaCl in the water and add the alkali.

1% Glucose Broth (A2.2.7)	900 ml
Glycine buffer	100 ml
Phenolphthalein, 0.2% aq. soln	5 ml

Mix and keep overnight at 4 °C in a stoppered flask. Sterilize by filtration and aseptically distribute into sterile 5 ml screw-capped bottles leaving as little air space as possible. Incubate overnight to check sterility and discard any bottles not showing a definite pink colour.

Note. This medium should be used as soon as possible after preparation.

A2.6.17 Hippurate media
Hippurate Agar (modified from Hajna & Damon, 1934; Thirst, 1957a)

NaCl	5 g
MgSO$_4$·7H$_2$O	0.2 g
NH$_4$H$_2$PO$_4$	1 g
K$_2$HPO$_4$	1 g
Sodium hippurate	3 g
Agar	20 g
Distilled water	1000 ml
Phenol red, 0.2% soln	5 ml

Dissolve the solids in the water by heating, adjust to pH 6.8–7.0, and add the indicator. Sterilize at 115 °C for 20 min.

Hippurate Broth (Hare & Colebrook, 1934)

Sodium hippurate	10 g
Infusion Broth	1000 ml

Dissolve the hippurate in the broth and sterilize at 115 °C for 20 min.

Alternatively, for streptococci, add sodium hippurate

(10% solution sterilized by membrane filtration) to Nutrient Broth containing 0.1% glucose to give a final concentration of 1% hippurate.

A2.6.18 KCN Broth (modified from Møller, 1954b; Rogers & Taylor, 1961)

Peptone	3 g
NaCl	5 g
KH$_2$PO$_4$	0.225 g
Na$_2$HPO$_4$·2H$_2$O	5.64 g
Distilled water	1000 ml

Dissolve the solids in the water and distribute in 100 ml volumes in screw-capped containers. Sterilize at 115 °C for 20 min.

For use, add 1.5 ml of a freshly prepared 0.5% KCN solution in sterile water to 100 ml of base. Mix and distribute aseptically in 1 ml volumes in sterile 5 ml screw-capped (bijoux) bottles.

Note. Store at 4 °C and use within 4 weeks of preparation.

A2.6.19 Loeffler serum slopes

Glucose	5 g
Nutrient Broth	250 ml
Serum, sterile	750 ml

Dissolve the glucose in the Nutrient Broth and steam for 10 min. Cool and add aseptically to the filtered serum. Distribute 2.5 ml volumes into sterile tubes and heat at 75 °C for 2 h on each of 3 successive days, keeping the tubes in such a position that a slope is made.

Notes. It is essential that during the first period of heating the temperature is raised slowly, otherwise the surface serum will be coagulated before the dissolved air has been driven off and the finished medium will have an uneven surface.

For an alternative sterilization procedure see Section A2.1.9.

A2.6.20 Lowenstein–Jensen medium (modified from Lowenstein, 1931; Jensen, 1932)

Mineral Salt solution

KH$_2$SO$_4$	2.4 g
MgSO$_4$·7H$_2$O	0.2 g
Glycerol	12.0 ml
Distilled water	600 ml

Dissolve the ingredients in the water and autoclave at 110 °C for 15 minutes.

Malachite Green solution

Malachite green	0.2 g
Distilled water	10 ml

Mix and incubate at 37 °C or place in water bath at 56–60 °C to dissolve. Autoclave at 115 °C for 10 min. or sterilize by membrane filtration.

Egg Mixture

Immerse twenty hens' eggs in 70% ethanol and leave for 15 min. Remove to a clean tray and allow to dry. Break into a sterile jar containing glass beads and shake well to mix the white and yolks. Strain through sterile gauze into a sterile beaker and add the mineral salt and malachite green solutions. Mix thoroughly and distribute in 5.0 ml volumes in 30 ml screw-capped (Universal or McCartney) bottles. Screw caps tightly, place the bottles almost horizontally in a hot-air oven and inspissate by a single heating; raise the temperature to 75 °C and hold it between 75 °C and 85 °C for 45 minutes.

For characterization tests distribute in 2 ml volumes in 7 ml bottles and inspissate as above.

Lowenstein–Jensen medium with TSC (Thiosemi-carbazone; thiacetazone)

0.5% TSC in dimethylformamide	0.6 ml
Lowenstein–Jensen Medium	300 ml

Dissolve the TSC (thiosemicarbazone; thiacetazone) in the dimethylformamide solvent (0.6 ml), dilute with twice its volume of sterile distilled water and add to 300 ml of liquid LJ medium. Mix and dispense before inspissation. Final concentration of TSC = approximately 10 mg/ml.

Lowenstein – Jensen medium with PNB (p-nitrobenzoic acid)

Add 300 mg PNB (p-nitrobenzoic acid) to 10 ml sterile distilled water. Add 1 drop 0.4% aqueous phenol red solution and 2 ml of 1 N-NaOH. Stir or shake until dissolved. With continuous shaking, add 1 N-HCl drop by drop until the indicator just turns yellow when the PNB will precipitate out. Back titrate with a small amount of 1 N-NaOH until the indicator just turns pink when the precipitate will redissolve. Add to 600 ml liquid LJ medium, mix and distribute before inspissation. Final concentration of PNB = approximately 500 mg/ml.

A2.6.21 Lecithovitellin (LV) Agar (Macfarlane, Oakley & Anderson, 1941)

Lecithovitellin solution (egg-yolk saline)

Hen eggs	4
NaCl, 0.85% soln	1000 ml

Separate the yolks from the whites and beat the yolks in the saline to form a homogeneous mixture. Add 25 g kieselguhr (diatomite), mix and clarify by filtration through paper. Sterilize the clarified material by filtration.

Notes. If not for immediate use, distribute the solution aseptically into sterile containers and keep in a refrigerator; it may decrease in sensitivity slightly over a period of 2 weeks or so, but most batches remain unaltered in sensitivity for months; if a precipitate appears, the batch should be discarded.

Yolks vary in size and in order to overcome the variations in egg-yolk saline due to this, McGaughey & Chu (1948) used 5% w/v egg-yolk.

Billing & Luckhurst (1957) claim that filtration is easier when distilled water is used in place of saline.

Lecithovitellin Agar

Lecithovitellin solution (or Egg Yok Emulsion)	100 ml
Nutrient Agar	900 ml

Melt the Nutrient agar and cool to about 55°C. Add the lecithovitellin solution aseptically, mix and pour plates.

A2.6.22 Malonate–phenylalanine medium (Shaw & Clarke, 1955)

$(NH_4)_2SO_4$	2 g
K_2HPO_4	0.6 g
KH_2PO_4	0.4 g
NaCl	2 g
Sodium malonate	3 g
DL-phenylalanine	2 g
Yeast extract	1 g
Distilled water	1000 ml
Bromthymol blue, 0.2% aq. soln	12.5 ml

Dissolve the solids in the water by heating. Filter, add the indicator solution, and sterilize at 115 °C for 20 min.

Notes. When L-phenylalanine is used, only 1 g is needed. Another medium, Phenylalanine Agar, for detecting phenylalanine deaminase is described in Section A2.6.30.

A2.6.23 Milk media

Litmus Milk. Stand fresh whole milk in a refrigerator overnight and remove the milk below the cream layer by siphoning, taking care to avoid the cream layer. Steam for 1 h and cool in a refrigerator. Filter and measure the volume of filtrate. Add sufficient litmus solution (Section A1.2.2) to give a bluish-purple colour and sterilize at 115 °C for 10 min *or* by steaming for 30 min on each of 3 successive days. After heating, this medium is colourless but the colour returns on cooling.

Notes. Overheating must be avoided to prevent caramelization.

Homogenized milk is unsuitable.

Purple Milk, as above but replace litmus solution with 10 ml 0.2% aqueous bromcresol purple solution per 1000 ml skim-milk.

Ulrich's Milk (Ulrich, 1944) as litmus milk but use chlorphenol red (0.0015%) as the pH indicator, and methylene blue (0.0005%) as a redox potential indicator. To 1000 ml skim-milk, add 7.5 ml 0.2% aqueous chlorphenol red solution and 2.5 ml 0.2% aqueous methylene blue solution.

A2.6.24 Motility media

Peptone	10 g

Meat extract	3 g
NaCl	5 g
Agar	4 g
Gelatin	80 g
Distilled water	1000 ml

Soak the gelatin in the water for 30 min, add the other ingredients, heat to dissolve, and sterilize at 115 °C for 20 min.

Note. Hajna (1950) modified this formula to permit the simultaneous detection of H_2S production by the addition of 0.2 g cysteine and 0.2 g ferrous ammonium sulphate; 2 g sodium citrate was added to clarify the medium and provide an extra nutrient for citrate-utilizing bacteria.

Sulphide–indole-motility (SIM) medium

Tryptone	30 g
Meat extract	3 g
$Na_2S_2O_3 \cdot 5H_2O$	0.5 g
Cysteine hydrochloride	0.2 g
NaCl	5 g
Agar	5 g
Distilled water	1000 ml

Add the constituents to the water and heat to dissolve. Dispense into bottles or tubes and sterilize by autoclaving at 121 °C for 15 minutes. For use, stab-inoculate cultures and incubate for 18–24 hours at 37 °C. Diffusion of growth from the line of inoculum indicates motility; blackening, H_2S production; and the development of a red colour within one hour after the addition of Kovacs' reagent (Section C1.7) indicates indole production.

A2.6.25 MRS Lactobacillus Broth (de Man, Rogosa & Sharpe, 1960)

Peptone	10 g
Meat extract	10 g
Yeast extract	5 g
Glucose	20 g
Polyoxyethylene sorbitan-mono-oleate (Tween 80)	1 ml
K_2HPO_4	2 g
$CH_3COONa.3H_2O$	5 g
Triammonium citrate	2 g
$MgSO_4 \cdot 4H_2O$	0.02 g
$MnSO_4 \cdot 4H_2O$	0.05 g
Distilled water	1000 ml

Dissolve the ingredients in the water, and sterilize at 115 °C for 20 min or at 121 °C for 15 min.

Notes. This medium may be gelled by the addition of 2% agar.

As a basal medium for carbohydrate studies this formula is modified by the omission of glucose and meat extract (Section A2.5.7).

A2.6.26 Nitrate media

Nitrate–Blood Agar (Cook, 1950)

KNO₃, sterile 20% aq. soln	5 ml
Horse blood	60 ml
Nutrient Agar or Digest Agar	1000 ml

Melt the Nutrient Agar, cool to 50–55 °C, add the sterile KNO₃ solution and horse blood aseptically, mix, and distribute into Petri dishes.

Nitrate Broth

KNO₃	1 g
Nutrient Broth	1000 ml

Dissolve the KNO₃ in the broth, distribute into tubes containing inverted inner (Durham) tubes, and sterilize at 115 °C for 20 min.

A2.6.27 Nitrite Broth

NaNO₂	0.01 g
Nutrient Broth	1000 ml

Dissolve the nitrite in the broth, distribute into tubes and sterilize at 115 °C for 20 min.

A2.6.28 ONPG Broth (Lowe, 1962)

ONPG	6 g
0.01 M-Na₂HPO₄	1000 ml

Dissolve at room temperature the ONPG (*O*-nitro-phenyl-D-galactopyranoside) in the phosphate solution at pH 7.5; sterilize by filtration.

Note. This solution should be stored in a refrigerator at 4 °C and protected from light.

ONPG soln	250 ml
Peptone Water	750 ml

Aseptically add the ONPG solution to the Peptone Water (Section A2.1.2) and distribute in 2.5 ml volumes in sterile tubes.

Notes. The medium is stable for a month when stored at 4 °C.

Sodium Potassium Magnesium (SPM) *Broth* may be used instead of Peptone Water. SPM broth contains: Tryptone, 10 g; NaCl, 10 g; KCl, 1 g; MgCl₂·6H₂O, 4 g; distilled water, 1000 ml.

A2.6.29 Phenolphthalein Phosphate Agar

Phenolphthalein diphosphate, Na salt 1% aq. soln. Sterilize by filtration and store at 4 °C.

Phenolphthalein phosphate soln	10 ml
Nutrient Agar	1000 ml

Melt the Nutrient Agar and cool to 45–50 °C. Add the phenolphthalein phosphate solution aseptically, mix, and distribute into Petri dishes.

A2.6.30 Phenylalanine Agar (Ewing, Davis & Reavis, 1957)

DL-phenylalanine	2 g
Yeast extract	3 g
Na₂HPO₄	1 g
NaCl	5 g
Agar	20 g
Distilled water	1000 ml

Dissolve the ingredients by heating in the water, filter, tube, and sterilize at 115 °C for 20 min. Solidify in a slanting position to give a long slope.

Notes. When L-phenylalanine is used, only 1 g is required.

A combined medium (with malonate) is described in Section A2.6.22.

A2.6.31 Polyhydroxybutyrate (PHB) Agar (Owens & Keddie, 1968)

Basal Medium

K₂HPO₄	0.52 g
KH₂PO₄	0.375 g
(NH₄)₂SO₄	0.5 g
CaCl₂	0.05 g
MgSO₄·7H₂O	0.2 g
NaCl	0.1 g
FeCl₃·6H₃O	0.01 g
MnSO₄·4H₂O	0.002 g
Na₂MoO₄·2H₂O	0.002 g
New Zealand Agar (Davis)	13.0 g
Distilled water	1000 ml

Bring to boil all ingredients except the agar, cool to room temperature and filter. Add the agar and boil to dissolve. Check reaction and adjust to pH 7.0. Dispense in 20 ml volumes in Universal bottles and sterilize by autoclaving at 115 °C for 15 min.

Complete medium

Melt 20 ml of mineral base by heating at 115 °C for 10 min. Allow to cool to 60 °C. Add 0.1 g of the sodium salt of DL-β-hydroxybutyric acid to the molten base, mix gently and distribute into Petri dishes. Store at 4 °C.

A2.6.32 Pyruvate Fermentation medium

Tryptone	10 g
Yeast extract	5 g
Sodium pyruvate	10 g
Bromthymol blue (ethanolic solution, 4 mg/ml)	10 ml
K₂HPO₄	5 g
Agar	10 g
Distilled water	1000 ml

Dissolve the solid ingredients by heat; allow to cool and add the indicator solution. Mix, adjust pH to 7.2–7.4 and dispense in small screw-capped bottles or tubes. Sterilize at 115 °C for 20 min. Allow to cool as slopes.

A2.6.33 Salt Broth. Nutrient Broth (A2.1.1) with the NaCl content increased to 65 g/1000 ml, or the amount needed to give the concentration required.

Note. For halophilic vibrio species the salt concentration of all test media should be 1.5–3%.

A2.6.34 Selenite Broth (Hobbs & Allison, 1945, modified by Lapage & Bascomb, 1968)

Peptone	5 g
Mannitol	4 g
$Na_2HPO_4 \cdot 12H_2O$	4.3 g
$NaH_2PO_4 \cdot 2H_2O$	2.8 g
Water	1000 ml

Dissolve the ingredients in the water with gentle heat. Adjust pH to 7.2; sterilize at 121 °C for 30 min.

Sodium hydrogen selenite, 40% aq. soln
Sterilize by filtration and store at 4 °C.

On the day of use add 1 ml 40% selenite solution aseptically to 99 ml of the broth; mix, and distribute 4 ml volumes into sterile 150 × 16 mm (6 × 5/8 in) test tubes; use metal closure caps.

A2.6.35 Soil-extract Agar (Gordon & Smith, 1953)

Soil extract

Garden soil, air-dried	1000 g
Water	2400 ml

Sift the air-dried soil through a fine (no.9) mesh sieve and add to the water. Mix well and heat the suspension in an autoclave at 121 °C for 1 h or at 126 °C for 20–30 min. Stir and filter through paper.

Notes. If the soil is rich in organic matter, 500 g will suffice. If the soil is insufficiently dry the filtrate will be turbid, but may be clarified by the addition of talc, and then refiltered.

Soil-extract Agar

Peptone	5 g
Meat extract	3 g
Agar	20 g
Soil extract	1000 ml

Heat to dissolve, adjust to pH 7.0, and sterilize at 115 °C for 20 min.

A2.6.36 Medium for preparation of Streptomyces extract for streptococcal grouping (modified from Maxted, 1948)

NaCl	5 g
K_2HPO_4	2 g

$MgSO_4 \cdot 7H_2O$	1 g
$CaCl_2$	0.04 g
$FeSO_4 \cdot 7H_2O$	0.02 g
$ZnSO_4 \cdot 7H_2O$	0.01 g
Yeast extract	5 g
Agar	20 g
Distilled water	1000 ml

Dissolve the agar by steaming in 750 ml of the water. Dissolve the salts and yeast extract in the remaining water and add to the agar solution. Mix and sterilize at 115 °C for 20 min.

Glucose, 20% sterile aq. soln	25 ml

For use, melt and cool to about 60 °C, aseptically add sterile glucose solution, and distribute into sterile Roux bottles.

A2.6.37 Todd-Hewitt Broth (modified from Todd & Hewitt, 1932)

Meat, minced	450 g
Water	1000 ml

Soak the meat in the water overnight at 4 °C; skim the fat from the infused mixture, heat to 85 °C, and maintain at this temperature for 30 min; filter and adjust the volume if necessary to 1000 ml.

Peptone	20 g
10 N-NaOH	2.7 ml
$NaHCO_3$	2 g
NaCl	2 g
$Na_2HPO_4 \cdot 12H_2O$	1 g
Glucose	2 g

Add the peptone to the meat infusion; mix well and add the alkali, followed by the other ingredients; slowly heat to boiling-point and boil for 30 min; allow to cool, adjust to pH 7.8, filter and sterilize at 115 °C for 20 min.

Note. When this medium is to be used for streptococcal type identification, it is essential that the peptone used does not encourage production of the proteinase that destroys the M antigen (Elliott, 1945). Suitable peptones for this medium include Difco Neopeptone and Evans' peptone.

A2.6.38 Triple Sugar Iron Agar (TSI) (Report, 1958)

Meat extract	3 g
Yeast extract	3 g
Peptone	20 g
Glucose	1 g
Lactose	10 g
Sucrose	10 g
$FeSO_4 \cdot 7H_2O$	0.2 g
OR [Ferric citrate]	[0.3 g]
NaCl	5 g
$Na_2S_2O_3 \cdot 5H_2O$	0.3 g
Agar	20 g

Distilled water 1000 ml
Phenol red, 0.2% aq. soln 12 ml

Heat to dissolve the solids in the water, add the indicator solution, mix and dispense into tubes. Sterilize at 115 °C for 20 min and cool to form slopes with deep butts about 3 cm long.

A2.6.39 Tween 80 medium (Sierra, 1957)

Peptone 10 g
NaCl 5 g
CaCl$_2$·2H$_2$O 0.1 g
Agar 20 g
Distilled water 1000 ml

Dissolve by steaming; adjust the pH to 7.4. Volumes of 500 ml are sterilized in flasks, which are cooled to 40–50 °C.

Tween 80 is sterilized at 121 °C and 5 ml added aseptically to each flask to give a final concentration of 1%. Dispense into Petri dishes.

A2.6.40 Tyrosine Agar (Gordon & Smith, 1955)

Peptone 5 g
Meat extract 3 g
Agar 20 g
Distilled water 100 ml
L-tyrosine 5 g

Prepare the base as for Nutrient Agar (Section A2.1.1); add the tyrosine, mix well to produce a uniform suspension of the insoluble tyrosine, and sterilize at 115 °C for 20 minutes and allow to cool to 60 °C. Distribute into Petri dishes.

A2.6.41 Urea media

Christensen's medium (Christensen, 1946)

Peptone 1 g
NaCl 5 g
KH$_2$PO$_4$ 2 g
Agar 20 g
Distilled water 1000 ml

Dissolve the ingredients by heating, adjust to pH 6.8, filter, and sterilize at 115 °C for 20 min.

Glucose 1 g
Phenol red, 0.2% aq. soln 6 ml

Add to the molten base, steam for 1 h, and cool to 50–55 °C.

Urea, 20% aq. soln 100 ml

Sterilize by filtration and add aseptically to the base cooled at 50–55 °C. Distribute the medium aseptically into sterile containers and allow to cool as slopes or plates.

SSR medium (Stuart, van Stratum & Rustigian, 1945)

KH$_2$PO$_4$ 9.1 g
Na$_2$HPO$_4$ 9.5 g
Yeast extract 0.1 g
Urea 20 g

Phenol red, 0.2% aq. soln 5 ml
Distilled water 1000 ml

Dissolve the solids in the water without heating, check and if necessary adjust the pH to 6.8, add the indicator, and sterilize by filtration. Aseptically distribute into sterile, chemically clean tubes.

Alternatively, the base can be prepared and sterilized by autoclaving and the urea added aseptically as a sterile solution.

Maslen's (1952) liquid modification of Christensen's medium

Peptone 1 g
Glucose 1 g
Na$_2$HPO$_4$ 1.2 g
KH$_2$PO$_4$ 0.8 g
NaCl 5 g
Phenol red 0.2% aq. soln 5 ml
Distilled water 1000 ml

Dissolve the solids in the water. Check and if necessary adjust the pH to 6.8. Sterilize at 115 °C for 20 mins. Cool to 55 °C and aseptically add 50 ml sterile 40% urea solution. Mix well and distribute in 2.5 ml volumes.

A2.6.42 Xanthine and Hypoxanthine Agar (Gordon & Mihm, 1957)

Prepared as for Tyrosine Agar (Section A2.6.40), but substituting xanthine or hypoxanthine (4 g/l) for tyrosine.

A3   MEDIA CONTROL

Quality control in the preparation and evaluation of culture media in the laboratory is essential. This is a continuous process extending from the raw materials, through manufacture to the final product used on the bench. In this Section, some of the basic practicalities and ways of monitoring the suitability of media are considered. The wider aspects of quality control and laboratory proficiency are discussed in Chapter 11.

Standardized media are as important as standardized methods and reagents. Commercially prepared media are tested to show that, within certain limits, they conform to stated formulae but, as many of the media contain peptone and other material of biological origin, the analysis may not be particularly helpful and often does not indicate the suitability of the medium for the particular task in hand. In many laboratories, media preparation is still left to junior or unskilled personnel in a 'media kitchen'. However media preparation is far removed from cookery and the work deserves the status of a department. Although media preparation has many features of an art it also has a scientific basis.

The aim of quality control is to ensure that media conform to predetermined standards, whereas evaluation implies the determination of their efficacy under the conditions of intended usage. The results of both quality control tests and bacteriological evaluation must be correlated and discrepancies or unexpected results investigated. For example, if after preparation a batch of Glucose-phosphate medium looks yellow (due to overheating) it is not likely to give satisfactory results in the methyl red test and it must be discarded. The growth of *Escherichia coli*, or other organisms which do not utilize citrate, in Koser's Citrate medium which appears satisfactory on the basis of chemical tests requires further investigation; common causes of such failure include the use of dirty glassware or the presence of organic matter from cotton-wool plugs. And most laboratories have at some time omitted the lactose or bile salts from MacConkey agar, or used a wrong ingredient in media preparation.

A3.1 Raw materials

Chemicals, reagents, and carbohydrates should be of Analytical Reagent (AR) quality or conform to Pharmacopoeial standards. The bacteriological laboratory is generally not equipped to carry out the necessary examination of these materials (which may involve spectrophotometry, flame-photometry, ion-exchange, chromatography, titration in non-aqueous media, or potentiometric titration, besides the more conventional assay methods) and it must rely upon the integrity of the supplier. Materials of biological origin are generally more difficult to standardize and may still vary considerably in composition (Report, 1956a).

Details of chemical and microbiological assays are outside the scope of this *Manual* and reference must be made to appropriate monographs and textbooks.

A3.1.1 Agar. The concentration necessary to produce a suitable gel varies with the geographical source of the seaweed from which the agar was made (Table A5). A method for estimating the gel strength of agar was described by Jones (1956). A good indication of the source of a sample of agar may be obtained by observation of the diatoms present. These are obtained either by centrifugation of a dilute agar sol or by ashing and extracting the residue with dilute hydrochloric acid; silica skeletons of diatoms, sand particles, and sponge spicules are present in the acid-insoluble ash. Examination of granular or powdered agar is less rewarding as undamaged diatoms are seldom found. Forsdike (1950) examined agars from various sources and his paper illustrates many of the different diatoms. The presence of nitrogenous material may be detected by heating with soda lime, when ammonia is evolved; adulteration with gelatin will be detectable in this way or, alternatively,

by the formation of a turbidity or precipitate when a 1% agar sol is mixed with an equal volume of 1% aqueous picric acid.

A3.1.2 Peptone. Although some studies on the constituents of different peptones have been published (Report, 1956a; Habeeb, 1960a, b), much work still remains to be done and until more information is available it is not possible to define standards. All peptones should dissolve completely in water to give clear solutions having a pH value between 5 and 7.

Indole production requires a peptone with a high tryptophan content; a gelatin hydrolysate is deficient in tryptophan as is an acid hydrolysate of casein, although an enzymic casein hydrolysate is suitable. Rosenheim's test is of value in detecting tryptophan: to 2 ml 5% peptone solution add 0.05% $FeCl_3$ solution. Cautiously pour concentrated H_2SO_4 down the side of the tube. A purple colour develops at the junction of the liquids when tryptophan is present. Peptones for use in media for carbohydrate studies must be tested for the presence of fermentable carbohydrates. Soya peptone generally contains carbohydrate and should be avoided in 'sugar' media. The influence of peptone on the methyl red test and carbohydrate reactions are discussed under Evaluation in Section A3.5. It is unlikely that modern peptones will be inhibitory because of a high copper content (O'Meara & Macsween, 1936, 1937) but this possibility should be borne in mind.

A3.1.3 Meat (Beef) extract. In the absence of standards for the product the only simple tests which can be performed are the enumeration of viable organisms (which should be few) and the detection of fermentable carbohydrate (which should be absent).

A3.1.4 Yeast extract, unlike meat extract, has a high carbohydrate content. The moisture content may also be high (about 30%) and considerable quantities of NaCl may be present; samples containing more than about 15% NaCl should be rejected.

A3.1.5 Bile salts. The complex nature of bile salts makes standardization difficult. Of the components present, deoxycholic acid (as its sodium salt) is widely used (Leifson, 1935). In the absence of suitable chemical standardization, biological evaluation is necessary and we recommend the method described by Burman (1955), in which a batch of bile salt is standardized against a batch known to be satisfactory. The inhibitory effect of bile salts can be influenced by other constituents of the medium such as NaCl (Leifson, 1935) and phosphates (Allen, Pasley & Pierce, 1952). The evaluation of sodium deoxycholate for use in inhibitory selective media is discussed by Taylor *et al.* (1964). For some purposes, surfactants such as Teepol or Tergitol can be used instead of bile salts though it should be appreciated that these also are to some extent variable.

A3.1.6 Gelatin comes from many animal sources and undergoes different processes; consequently it is available in several grades. For bacteriology, edible gelatin is generally used, the technical grades being unsatisfactory as they often contain preservatives and may have a high SO_2 and heavy-metal content. Leffmann & La Wall (1911) considered that a standard should be established for SO_2 in gelatin intended for bacteriological use. Some tests for the physical properties of and extraneous matter in gelatin are detailed in a British Standard (757:1959) which gives methods for determining the moisture content, gel strength, viscosity, melting point, water absorption, solubility, keeping quality and pH as well as the amounts of grease, ash, sulphur dioxide, chlorides, arsenic, and heavy metals.

A3.1.7 Carbohydrates and related products Testing is usually restricted to the solubility, clarity and pH reaction of solutions, and to simple tests such as absence of reducing sugar in non-reducing sugars, absence of aglycones in glycosides, and the absence of monosaccharides in higher saccharides. Some samples of sucrose may contain invert sugar, detectable by measuring the optical rotation of a solution or more simply by testing with Fehling's or Benedict's solution (Section C1.3) for the presence of reducing substances. Soluble starch should be free from reducing sugars and when treated with iodine solution should give a deep blue colour; a reddish or purple colour would indicate dextrin. Some tests for other carbohydrates are mentioned in Section A3.3.3.

A3.1.8 Cole and Onslow's or other pancreatic extracts act by their tryptic content which may be estimated as follows:

(i)   *Qualitative.* A 1/100 dilution should digest the gelatin from a used photographic plate or film within 30 min at 37 °C.

(ii)   *Quantitative* (modified from Douglas, 1922). To 50 ml fresh milk, from which the cream has been removed by centrifugation, add 50 ml 0.2 M-$CaCl_2$; mix thoroughly and measure 5 ml volumes of the milk into 150×16 mm (6 $\times$ 5/8 in) tubes. Place the tubes in a water bath at 38–40 °C. Make dilutions of the enzyme from 1/10 to 1/100 and begin testing with the 1/100 dilution.

Add 1 ml of the diluted enzyme preparation to a tube of calcified milk, shake thoroughly, return to the water bath and note the time. Examine the tube at intervals and note the time at which a precipitate or clotting occurs. Continue

to test dilutions of the enzyme until the clotting time is between 1 and 2 minutes.

Calculation. Suppose 1 ml of a 1/60 dilution of the enzyme clots the milk in 80 seconds, then 1 ml of the original solution contains:

$$(60 \times 100) \div 80 = 75 \text{ units.}$$

A satisfactory batch of Cole and Onslow's extract should have a tryptic content of at least 50 units per ml.

A3.1.9 Thioglycollic acid for inclusion in media should be assayed periodically and rejected when its activity falls below 75% (Report, 1953); the acid should be kept in a tightly stoppered bottle at 4 °C. The stability of thioglycollate solutions has been studied by Cook & Steel (1959*a*, *b*) and the assay method of Steel (1958) is recommended.

A3.2 Digest media: Intermediate control

During the preparation of digest media (Section A2.1.4) it is important to follow the course of digestion. Samples are taken at the start and at 30–45 minute intervals; the disappearance of undigested protein is most easily shown by the **biuret test**: heat a 5 ml sample to boiling to stop digestion, cool and add 0.5 ml 10 N-NaOH. Filter and add 0.1 ml 1% $CuSO_4 \cdot 5H_2O$ solution to the filtrate. Proteins give a violet colour, proteoses a reddish-pink colour, and amino acids produce no colour reaction.

A3.3 Digest media: Final control

The final product of digestion should be examined physically and chemically, as well as by bacteriological tests which are discussed under Evaluation (Section A3.5); some of the causes of faulty media are considered later (Section A3.6). Among the physical properties, colour, clarity, pH, viscosity, and gel strength of solid media should be examined. Determination of specific gravity does not appear to be of much value. For the pH determination of solid media a flat electrode is useful and avoids the need to melt the medium and compensate for the increased temperature.

Chemical properties tested may include the presence of the correct ingredients (testing for human error), nitrogen estimations, detection of breakdown products of components (especially those of carbohydrates), and freedom from the end-product(s) which will be looked for after the organism has grown.

A3.3.1 Total nitrogen is usually estimated by the Kjeldahl method or some modification of it. In this, organic nitrogen is converted to ammonium sulphate by sulphuric acid in the presence of sodium sulphate with copper and selenium as catalysts. The digested reaction mixture is steam-distilled with sodium hydroxide to liberate ammonia. The ammonia is absorbed and estimated colorimetrically with Nessler's reagent or by titration. In all cases a blank determination on the reagents must be made. For details of the technique see an appropriate textbook of analytical chemistry or original papers, for example, by Middleton & Stuckey (1951).

Proteose nitrogen is estimated similarly; the proteoses are first separated by precipitation with saturated zinc sulphate solution, and their nitrogen content determined.

A3.3.2 Amino nitrogen

one of two methods may be used but the results given by the two methods may not be identical as they do not estimate exactly the same compounds; formol titration is the simpler method but in dark-coloured solutions the end-point may be difficult to see.

(i) *Sørenson's formol titration method*: in this method, formaldehyde reacts with the NH_2-groups of amino acids to form acidic complexes which are titratable with alkali.

Neutralize 40% formaldehyde solution (formalin) with 0.1 N-NaOH until just pink to phenolphthalein. To a 5 ml sample of the medium, add 0.05 ml of phenolphthalein solution and 0.1 N-NaOH until just pink; then add 5 ml neutralized formalin and titrate with 0.1 N-NaOH until the pink colour reappears.

1 ml 0.1 N-NaOH ≡ 1.4 mg amino nitrogen.

(ii) *Pope & Stevens' (1939) method*: in this method, copper phosphate reacts with amino acids to form soluble copper complexes; the amount of copper in solution is estimated iodometrically.

Copper phosphate suspension:

0.16 M-CuCl$_2$	20 ml
0.18 M-Na$_3$PO$_4$	40 ml
0.075 M-borate buffer (pH 8.5)	40 ml

Mix the three solutions. The suspension should be freshly prepared and discarded after three days.

Place a 5 ml sample of medium in a 50 ml volumetric flask and make just alkaline (blue) to thymolphthalein with 1 N-NaOH. Add one drop of *n*-octanol to prevent foaming and 30 ml copper phosphate suspension. Make up to 50 ml with distilled water, mix well and filter. Acidify 10 ml filtrate with 0.5 ml glacial acetic acid, add 2 ml of 50% KI solution and 10 ml of 10% KCNS solution. Titrate with 0.01 N-Na$_2$S$_2$O$_3$ using starch mucilage as indicator. The Na$_2$S$_2$O$_3$ is standardized by the same method against 0.01 N-CuSO$_4$.

1 ml 0.01 N-Na$_2$S$_2$O$_3$ ≡ 0.28 mg amino nitrogen.

A satisfactory digest medium should contain about a quarter of its total nitrogen in the form of amino nitrogen. Typical results for the amino acid content of Digest Broth (Section A2.1.4) and Infusion Broth (A2.1.6) are in the range 72–91 and 68–84 mg amino nitrogen per 100 ml respectively. To achieve some degree of standardization, it is usual to adjust the amino nitrogen content of both these media to 70 mg per 100 ml by blending weak and strong batches. The amino nitrogen content of Todd–Hewitt broth (Section A2.6.37) is usually about 117–145 mg per 100 ml.

A3.3.3 Other tests.

The methods adopted to detect the presence or absence of particular substances in culture media are mainly the straightforward techniques of classical chemical analysis, such as chloride estimation by Mohr titration, but the *Extra Pharmacopoeia* (1955) is useful for particular tests. Some of the test methods are derived from clinical biochemistry, and a brief selection is given below to illustrate their diversity.

Detection of bile salts in MacConkey Broth (Hay's test for bile salts in urine): sprinkle powdered sulphur on the surface of the medium in a wide tube or beaker – bile salts lower the surface tension and the particles sink.

Presence of nitrate and *absence of nitrite* in Nitrate Broth: to 5 ml medium add 1 ml nitrite solution A and 1 ml nitrite solution B (Section C1.14): a red colour indicates nitrite and the batch should be discarded. In the absence of a colour change add 20 mg powdered zinc: the development of a red colour indicates the presence of nitrate.

Molisch's test for carbohydrates: to 5 ml medium add 0.1 ml 5% ethanolic α-naphthol, mix and cautiously pour concentrated H$_2$SO$_4$ down the side of the tube. A purple colour at the junction of the liquids indicates the presence of carbohydrate.

Individual carbohydrates may be detected by standard biochemical tests; the distinction between galactose, glucose, lactose and maltose ultimately depends upon the formation of crystalline osazones and their identification by microscopical examination. Several multitests have been proposed by which different carbohydrates can be detected by the same reagent (Barakat & Abd El-Wahab, 1951; Love, 1953); the results of such tests should be confirmed by other methods.

Detection of starch in Starch Agar: pour an iodine solution (e.g. Lugol's, Section B1.11) over the medium. A blue colour indicates the presence of starch.

Pentoses may be detected by the orcinol reaction: mix equal volumes of test solution and reagent (orcinol, 0.2 g; concentrated HCl, 100 ml; 10% FeCl$_3$, 0.2 ml) and gently heat to boiling. A green or blue–green colour or precipitate indicates the presence of pentoses.

Detection of citrate in Citrate media: boil a 5 ml sample of medium with 1 ml mercuric sulphate solution (5% HgO in 20% (v/v) H_2SO_4), filter, boil, and add 5 drops 1% $KMnO_4$ solution. Decolorization of the reagent and formation of a white precipitate indicates the presence of citrate.

Detection of hippurate in Hippurate Broth: add 5% $FeCl_3$ solution. A brownish-pink precipitate soluble in excess reagent indicates the presence of hippurate.

Hydrolysis of salicin in 'sugar media' sterilized by heat treatment is shown by the presence of reducing sugar when the medium is boiled with Benedict's reagent, and by a violet colour when $FeCl_3$ solution is added.

Hydrolysis of starch in Starch Serum Water is indicated by a coloured precipitate when a sample of the medium is boiled with Benedict's reagent. Such hydrolysis of starch by the action of amylase may occur when the serum has not been inactivated by heat (Goldsworthy, Still & Dumaresq, 1938).

Many of the tests used are not specific but give a good indication of whether the medium has been correctly prepared. In contrast to the bacteriological control methods described below, chemical tests have the advantage of speed.

Media in tubes plugged with cotton-wool may lose water by evaporation and, by concentration of ingredients, become unsuitable for their intended use; the addition of sterile water to rectify the concentration is not satisfactory (Vera, 1971).

A3.4 Control of equipment

Equipment and apparatus that should be checked at regular intervals include air-filters, autoclaves, hot-air ovens, incubators, water baths, pH meters, deep-freezes, and refrigerators (Vera, 1971), as well as thermometers, other temperature recording devices, filters and filtration techniques, cabinets, anaerobic jars and anaerobic techniques.

A3.5 Evaluation of media

It is by the behaviour of media in routine use that the reputation of a media department stands or falls. Sterility is obviously of paramount importance and sterility testing is discussed below. Bacteriological control depends on the nature of the individual medium. Its purposes are to test: (i) the ability of nutrient media to support growth from small inocula; (ii) media used in biochemical tests for their ability to show the desired reactions; (iii) differential media to ensure that organisms growing on them are characteristic; (iv) selective and enrichment media for growth of the organisms wanted and inhibition of other unwanted bacteria.

A3.5.1 Sterility testing. A sterility test is a limit test and the conventional technique will detect only gross contamination. The sterility of a product cannot be proved unless the whole of the product (or batch) is tested. Bryce (1956) has calculated that there is a 50% chance of failing to detect contamination when 10 samples are tested from a batch of 500 items, 33 (6.7%) of which are contaminated. However, a contaminant is more likely to develop in a nutrient medium than in a simple aqueous solution, and with bacteriological media it is often sufficient to incubate the medium in order to check for sterility. Culture media are not necessarily suitable for the growth of all micro-organisms; the pH value of a medium intended for bacteria may not be suitable for the growth of fungi. The incubation of an inhibitory medium may fail to show contamination; such a contaminated medium could be the start of a mixed culture which would be revealed only on sub-culture to a non-inhibitory medium. Inhibitory media should therefore be well diluted with sterile Nutrient Broth before incubation.

Media likely to be incubated for long periods, such as Dorset Egg and Lowenstein–Jensen, must be free from slow-growing contaminants; however, an adequate turnover is essential as they deteriorate on storage. Many contaminants grow at room temperatures, as do psychrophiles in media stored at low temperatures. In medical bacteriology, however, the presence of thermophiles is much less likely to be a serious problem in media. Theoretically, sterility tests should detect the presence of all living micro-organisms though only bacteria and fungi are usually sought. It is recommended that all samples of media sterilized by filtration or by heat treatment other than adequate autoclaving, should be subjected to the following tests:

Incubation temperature	Incubation time
55–60 °C	7 days in air
37 °C	7 days in air
37 °C	7 days anaerobically
ambient room (15–20 °C)	14 days in air
4 °C	14 days in air

Incubation at 20–25 °C is better than 30–35 °C for showing evidence of inefficient sterilization of materials for injection (Vera, 1971).

A3.5.2 Growth-supporting ability. The nature of the medium determines the choice of test organisms; for example with 'Chocolate' Agar, strains of *Haemophilus* and *Neisseria* species should be used, whereas with Nutrient Agar, less exacting organisms, such as staphylococci and coliform organisms are suitable. The organisms should be cultured in a suitable medium overnight and nine 10-fold serial dilutions prepared in sterile quarter-strength Ringer's solution; 0.02 ml of each dilution is placed on the surface of medium contained in a Petri dish (as in the Miles & Misra (1938) surface-viable counting technique) or added to 5 ml volumes of liquid media. After incubation, the greatest dilution giving growth is noted. The ability of media to support the growth of anaerobic bacteria is determined in a similar manner. *Clostridium perfringens* is not a good test organism for anaerobiosis; more suitable species are *C. chauvoei* (very exacting), *C. novyi*, or *C. tetani*, but the film-like growth of *C. tetani* may be difficult to see. Some fastidious anaerobes (e.g. *Bacteroides*; *Streptobacillus moniliformis*) may be inhibited by oxidized reducing agents or by Liquoid (sodium polyanethol sulphonate) in media (Holdeman & Moore, 1972). Messer (1947) found an inhibitory agent in a batch of Nutrient Agar and traced it to formaldehyde used to increase the wet strength of filter paper used during the preparation of the medium.

With MacConkey Agar, suitable test organisms include *Escherichia coli*, *Salmonella typhimurium*, *Shigella dysenteriae*, and *Shigella sonnei*. In addition to assessing its growth-promoting ability, this test also serves to show whether the medium distinguishes satisfactorily between these enterobacteria. MacConkey Broth should be tested for its ability to show acid and gas formation at 44 °C when inoculated with a strain of *E. coli*.

A3.5.3 Biochemical performance.
Samples of media must be tested with organisms known to produce positive and negative reactions. Examples of such control organisms are given under the individual test methods in Appendix C. Because of strain variation within species, it is essential that the particular strain used for test purposes possesses the desired characters and in Table D1 we list suitable strains, maintained in the National Collection of Type Cultures, of the organisms required.

The need for biological control was shown by Orr Ewing & Taylor (1945) who found that certain batches of peptone were unsuitable for making carbohydrate media as only in some of them did the Newcastle and Manchester biotypes of *Shigella flexneri* 6 produce both acid and gas. Peptone may also affect the results of a finely balanced reaction such as that of the MR (methyl red) test; each batch of peptone should therefore be tried out in tests with known MR-positive and -negative strains (Jennens, 1954).

A3.5.4 Differentiation.
Differential media must be tested to make sure that organisms growing on them exhibit the typical characters by which they are differentiated from other organisms. For example, the testing of MacConkey Agar for its ability to distinguish lactose-fermenting and lactose-non-fermenting bacteria has been noted above. Tellurite media should be inoculated with each of the three varieties of *Corynebacterium diphtheriae* and after incubation these should be examined for their characteristic colonial appearances.

A3.5.5 Selectivity.
A selective or an enrichment medium should be able to support the growth of a particular organism or group of organisms, and at the same time inhibit others. A convenient method of testing this is to mix broth cultures of the organism to be selected with another organism to be inhibited, in varying proportions (e.g. 1:2, 1:4 and so on). A loopful of each mixture is plated on solid media or inoculated into liquid media. After incubation an estimate of the selectivity of a solid medium may be made by inspection of the growth. The efficiency of a liquid enrichment medium cannot be judged until a subculture to a non-inhibitory solid medium has been made.

A3.6   Causes of faulty media

Major sources of trouble include errors in weighing and measuring, inadvertent use of the wrong ingredients (e.g. hydrated instead of anhydrous salts), and incorrect pH adjustment. Some common faults and their possible causes are listed below:

Loss of growth-promoting capacity

Over-sterilization; repeated remelting of solid media; burning or charring; contamination with metallic salts; incorrect molarity due to careless pH adjustment.

Decreased gel strength

Over-sterilization; hydrolysis of agar media of low pH; incomplete solution of agar; repeated remelting.

Darkening

Over-sterilization; caramelization of sugars; local super-heating due to inadequate mixing.

pH change

Over-sterilization; incomplete mixing; use of alkaline containers; hydrolysis of ingredients; repeated remelting.

Precipitation

Chemical incompatibility; failure to remove phosphates; over-sterilization; prolonged holding of melted agar media at high temperature.

APPENDIX B
Staining: reagents and methods

B1   REAGENTS

All staining reagents should be kept in well-closed glass-stoppered bottles (except Loeffler's methylene blue) and protected from direct sunlight. For frequent use, flexible plastic bottles with tube outlets may be used but they must be washed out thoroughly before refilling. They should not be stored in close proximity to concentrated acids or ammonia. Distilled water for reagents should be freshly prepared and neutral in reaction.

Formulae of staining reagents are listed in alphabetical order.

B1.1   Acetone – iodine solution for decolorization

Strong iodine solution

Iodine	10 g
Potassium iodide	6 g
Distilled water	10 ml
Ethanol (90%)	to 100 ml

Dissolve the iodine and potassium iodide in the water and adjust to volume with the ethanol.

Acetone–iodine mixture

Strong iodine soln	3.5 ml
Acetone	96.5 ml

Mix well before use

B1.2   Acid–alcohol

Conc. HCl	3 ml
Ethanol (95%)	97 ml

Mix well before use.

B1.3   Albert's stain

Malachite green	0.2 g
Toluidine blue	0.15 g
Ethanol (95%)	2 ml
Glacial acetic acid	1 ml
Distilled water	100 ml

Dissolve the dyes in the ethanol. Mix the acid with the water and add to the dye solution. Allow to stand for 24 h and then filter.

B1.4   Ammoniacal silver nitrate solution

$AgNO_3$	5 g
Distilled water	100 ml

Dissolve the nitrate in the water; to 90 ml of this solution add strong ammonia solution (sp. gr. 0.880) drop by drop until the precipitate which forms just dissolves; add sufficient of the remaining $AgNO_3$ solution drop by drop until the reagent remains faintly turbid even after shaking. When protected from light, this reagent is stable for several weeks.

B1.5   Ammonium oxalate – crystal violet stain

Solution A

Crystal violet	10 g
Ethanol (95%)	100 ml

Mix and dissolve.

Solution B

Ammonium oxalate	1% aq. soln

For use, mix 20 ml of solution A and 80 ml of solution B.

B1.6   Aqueous solutions

Simple aqueous solutions of each of the following are used in staining.

Bismarck brown	0.2 %
Chrysoidin	0.4 %
Malachite green	0.5 %
Malachite green	5 %
Safranin	0.5 %

B1.7   Carbol fuchsin

Carbol fuchsin, strong

Phenol	85 g

Basic fuchsin	15 g
Ethanol	250 ml
Distilled water	1250 ml

Mix the phenol and fuchsin and if necessary heat gently to dissolve the phenol. Add the ethanol and distilled water and filter into a stoppered bottle. Propanol may be substituted for ethanol.

Carbol fuchsin, weak

Dilute one volume of strong carbol fuchsin with 10–20 volumes of distilled water.

B1.8   Giemsa stain: stock solution

Giemsa stain (powder)	1.0 g
Glycerol	60 ml
Absolute methanol	60 ml

Heat the glycerol to 55–60 °C in a water bath. Add the stain and mix thoroughly. Incubate the mixture at the same temperature for 2 hours. Allow to cool and add the methanol. This stain is best used after 'maturation' on the shelf for about 2 weeks. For use, add 1 part of stock solution to 10 parts of 0.01 M-phosphate buffer (pH 7.0) and allow to stand for 30 minutes.

B1.9   India ink

A dense, homogeneous India ink free from large particles or clumps of particles is necessary. Duguid's (1951) practice is to mix the ink with a quarter of its volume of grade-12 Ballotini glass beads (0.22 mm) and shake for 1 h in a Mickle tissue disintegrator. Thin ink may be improved by evaporation to concentrate it.

B1.10   Kirkpatrick's fixative

Absolute ethanol	60 ml
Chloroform	30 ml
Formaldehyde (40%) soln	10 ml

Mix well before use.

B1.11   Loeffler's methylene blue

(Loeffler, 1884)

Saturated ethanolic solution

Methylene blue	1 g
Ethanol (95%)	100 ml

Staining solution

KOH 1% aq. soln	1 ml
Distilled water	99 ml
Ethanolic methylene blue	30 ml

Mix in order; this reagent must be ripened by oxidation, a process taking several months to complete, but ripening can be hastened by aeration. Bottles should not be more than half-full, the stopper replaced by a light cotton-wool plug and the bottle shaken frequently. The stain improves with keeping and batches sufficiently large to last for 5–10 years may be prepared

Note. The ripened stain is sometimes called polychrome methylene blue.

B1.12   Lugol's iodine

Iodine	5 g
Potassium iodide	10 g
Distilled water	100 ml

Dissolve the iodide and iodine in some of the water, and adjust to 100 ml with distilled water.

Note. This reagent is Aqueous Iodine Solution of the *British Pharmacopoeia* (1963).

For use dilute 1/5 with distilled water.

B1.13   Muir's mordant

HgCl$_2$, saturated aq. soln (about 7%)	20 ml
Potash alum, saturated aq. soln (about 12%)	50 ml
Tannic acid, 20% aq. soln	20 ml

Mix well before use.

B1.14   Neisser's stain

Solution A

Methylene blue	0.1 g
Ethanol (95%)	5 ml
Glacial acetic acid	5 ml
Distilled water	100 ml

Dissolve the dye in the water and add the acid and ethanol.

Solution B

Crystal violet	0.33 g
Ethanol (95%)	3.3 ml
Distilled water	100 ml

Dissolve the dye in the ethanol–water mixture.

For use, mix 20 ml of solution A and 10 ml of solution B.

B1.15   Ryu's flagella stain

(Kodaka, Armfield & Lombard, 1982)

Solution A (mordant)

Tannic acid (powdered)	10 g
Phenol 5% aq. soln	50 ml
Aluminium potassium sulphate (12-hydrate) saturated soln	50 ml

Solution B (stain)

Crystal violet	12 g

215

Ethanol   100 g
(a saturated solution)

Mix 10 parts of solution A with 1 part solution B and store at ambient temperature. The mixture is stable indefinitely and does not require filtration before use. Allow to stabilize by standing for 2–3 days as the freshly prepared stain is often too potent. As a rule of thumb, apply a fairly fresh stain for 5 min, or a stabilized stain for 10 min.

B1.16   Plimmer's mordant

Tannic acid	20 g
$AlCl_3 \cdot 6H_2O$	36 g
$ZnCl_2$	20 g
Basic fuchsin	3 g
Ethanol (60%)	80 ml

Grind the solids together in a mortar and add the ethanol; triturate until dissolved.

Before use, add 1 volume of mordant to 3 volumes of distilled water and mix well.

B1.17   Rhodes' mordant

Tannic acid, 10% aq. soln	60 ml
Potash alum, saturated aq. soln (about 12%)	30 ml
Aniline, saturated aq. soln (about 3.5%)	6 ml
$FeCl_3$, 5% aq. soln	6 ml

Add the alum solution to the tannic acid solution, followed by the aniline solution. Redissolve the curd which forms by shaking. Add the $FeCl_3$ solution and allow the resulting black solution to stand for 10 min before use.

B1.18   Sudan Black

Sudan black B powder	0.3 g
70% ethyl alcohol	100 ml

Shake well and stand overnight before use. Keep in a well-stoppered bottle.

B2   METHODS

In this section, we describe a small selection of staining methods which are usually satisfactory; for a more complete coverage, reference must be made to specialist monographs such as those by Conn, Darrow & Emmel (1960), E. Gurr (1956) and G.T. Gurr (1963).

After microscopical examination, used slides should be sterilized by autoclaving. It must never be assumed that bacteria will have been killed by the application of the staining reagents. Anthrax spores, for example, have germinated in the immersion oil left on a slide, and Soltys (1948) reported cutaneous anthrax in a veterinary student infected from a stained film.

B2.1   Simple stains

Loeffler's methylene blue is perhaps the most valuable reagent available for staining bacteria. It is excellent for bacteria of the genus *Corynebacterium* where beading, barring, and granules may be demonstrated, especially when the organism has been grown on Loeffler serum slopes. With sporing organisms stained with this reagent, the spores appear as unstained bodies within blue cells.

1. Stain for 1 minute.
2. Rinse with water.
3. Drain or blot to dry.

B2.2   Differential stains

B2.2.1   Gram's method. In the USA the method given here is often referred to as Hucker's modification (Hucker & Conn, 1923), and in this country as Lillie's (1928) modification.

1. Apply ammonium oxalate–crystal violet stain for $1/2$ min.
2. Wash in water.
3. Apply Lugol's iodine solution for $1/2$ min.
4. Drain off the iodine solution but do not wash.
5. Decolorize with a few drops of acetone. (Note: acetone decolorizes very quickly and should not be left on the film for more than 2–3 seconds).
6. Wash thoroughly in water.
7. Counterstain with 0.5% safranin for $1/2$ min. (A few Gram-negative organisms such as *H. influenzae* and *Y. pestis* do not stain well with safranin. Films for such organisms should be counterstained with weak carbol fuchsin for $1/2$ min.)
8. Wash and stand slide on end to drain, or blot dry.

Preston & Morrell (1962) modified Lillie's method by retarding decolorization with an acetone-iodine mixture.

1. Apply ammonium oxalate–crystal violet stain for $1/2$ min.
2. Wash off thoroughly with Lugol's iodine soution.
3. Apply Lugol's iodine for $1/2$ min.
4. Wash off thoroughly with acetone–iodine mixture.
5. Apply acetone–iodine solution for $1/2$ min.
6. Wash thoroughly with water.
7. Counterstain with weak carbol fuchsin for $1/2$ min.
8. Wash and drain or blot to dry.

The whole slide must be flooded with each reagent and the previous reagent must be completely removed at each stage. Insufficient reagent may result in uneven staining or decolorization.

Gram-positive organisms are blue or purple; Gram-negative organisms are red.

Some workers prefer to counterstain with Bismarck brown, which they claim gives a better contrast.

B2.2.2   Ziehl-Neelsen's method (Acid-fast stain)

(Ziehl, 1882; Neelsen, 1883)

1. Flood the slide with strong carbol fuchsin and heat until steam rises (but do not boil).
2. After 3–4 min apply more heat until steam rises again; do not let the stain dry on the slide.
3. About 5–7 min after the first application of heat wash the slide thoroughly under running water.
4. Decolorize in acid–alcohol until all traces of red have disappeared from the film. Decolorization should not be attempted in one stage; there should be intermittent washings in water and re-application of acid–alcohol.
5. Wash well in water when decolorization is complete.
6. Counterstain with Loeffler's methylene blue or 0.5% malachite green for 1 min.
7. Wash and stand on end to drain; DO NOT BLOT.

Acid-fast organisms are red; other organisms are blue or green.

Numerous variations have been advocated such as cold staining or the addition of detergents to the fuchsin but they have little if any advantage over the conventional Ziehl-Neelsen method.

B2.3   Special stains

B2.3.1   Spore stains

Method 1 (modified from Moeller 1891)

This is similar to Ziehl-Neelsen's method but ethanol is used for decolorization.

1. Flood the slide with strong carbol fuchsin and steam.
2. After 5 min wash well in water.
3. Decolorize with ethanol until all traces of red have been removed. Decolorization of the vegetative bacilli can best be controlled by examining the wet film under low power microscopy (after the bottom of the slide has been wiped dry).
4. Wash thoroughly in water.
5. Counterstain with Loeffler's methylene blue for 1–2 min.
6. Wash and drain or blot to dry.

Bacterial bodies stain blue, spores red.

Method 2 (Schaeffer & Fulton's 1933)

1. Flood the slide with 5% aqueous malachite green and steam for 1 min.
2. Wash under running water.
3. Counterstain with 0.5% aqueous safranin for 15 seconds.
4. Rinse with water and drain or blot to dry.

Bacterial bodies stain red, spores green.

This method can be used as a cold stain by allowing the malachite green to act for 10 min.

B2.3.2   Capsule stains

Muir's method

1. Flood with strong carbol fuchsin and heat gently for 1 min.
2. Rinse rapidly with ethanol, then wash well in water.
3. Flood with Muir's mordant (B1.13) for 30 seconds.
4. Wash off with water, and then with ethanol for 30 seconds or until the film is pale red.
5. Wash well with water.
6. Counterstain with Loeffler's methylene blue for 30 seconds.
7. Wash and drain or blot to dry.

Bacteria stain red, capsules blue.

Giemsa method

To fix, immerse air-dried films for 3 minutes in absolute methanol or 1:1000 mercuric chloride. Immerse slide in Giemsa stain (B1.8). Wash with 0.01 M-phosphate buffer, pH 7.0 for 30 seconds, blot and allow to dry. Examine under oil immersion lens. Bacterial cells appear as blue-purple rods surrounded, if present, by pink-red capsules.

India ink wet-film method (Duguid, 1951)

This is a 'negative' stain, which is not a stain in the true sense of the word but a means of colouring the background so that the cells are shown in relief as clear objects.

1. Place a large loopful of undiluted India ink on a slide.
2. Mix this with a small portion of the bacterial colony or a small loopful of the deposit from a centrifuged liquid culture.
3. Place a coverslip on top and press down under a pad of blotting-paper. Ideally, the film should be of the same thickness as the capsulate organisms. If the coverslip is not pressed down sufficiently, the organisms will tend to drift in the ink and may be obscured by overlying ink; if pressed down too much, the capsules may be distorted.

The capsule appears as a clear light zone between the refractile cell outline and the dark background.

For demonstrating slime production by enteric organisms, Duguid cultured them on excess Sugar Agar, a medium containing maltose, phosphate, mineral salts, and a low concentration of peptone.

B2.3.3   Stains for metachromatic (volutin) granules

For metachromatic granules make a smear from a culture on Loeffler Serum medium.

Albert's stain, modified (Albert, 1921; Laybourn, 1924)

1. Stain with Albert's stain (B1.3) for 3–5 min.
2. Wash with water and blot to dry.
3. Stain with Lugol's iodine solution for 1 min.
4. Wash with water and drain or blot to dry.

Cytoplasm appears light green, granules blue-black.

Neisser's (1903) stain
1. Stain with Neisser's stain (B1.14) for 10 seconds.
2. Rinse rapidly with water.
3. Stain with 0.2% Bismarck brown or 0.4% chrysoidin for 30 seconds.
4. Wash rapidly in water, drain or blot dry.

Cytoplasm appears light brown, granules blue-black.

B2.3.4 **Flagella stains**. The arrangement of flagella on the bacterial cell has long been used as a taxonomic criterion. Unfortunately it is not one which is easily or unequivocally determined. The most satisfactory method of determining the mode of bacterial flagellation is by electron microscopy but, since a two-dimensional picture of a three-dimensional object is obtained, the electron micrographs must be interpreted with caution.

Flagella staining should not be undertaken lightly, though reasonably satisfactory results can be obtained when care is taken in the preparation of the culture, the film, and the reagents. Known peritrichous and polar flagellate organisms should be used as controls. The interpretation of the results of flagella staining has been discussed briefly by Hodgkiss (1960).

For staining flagellae, Ryu's method modified by Kodaka, Armfield & Lombard, (1982) is recommended. We also repeat the flagella stains given in the previous edition of this *Manual* for those experienced in their use. Use only young cultures grown under optimum conditions for the organism under study on agar media that do not contain fermentable carbohydrates. Touch a colony with the tip of a straight inoculation wire, taking care not to pick up any agar, then dip the wire in the centre of each of 2 drops of distilled water on a microscope slide. The slide should have been previously cleaned by heating in a (blue) Bunsen flame so that the drops of water wet the surface easily and spread out spontaneously. There should be no turbidity – the aim is to transfer only a few bacteria. Leave the preparation to dry without disturbance. After staining, examine microscopically from the periphery of each spot inwards in order to find the areas of optimum staining. The deposition of coarse blobs of stain all over the slide indicates overstaining.

Ryu's method, modified (Kodaka, Armfield & Lombard, 1982)
1. Apply Ryu's stain (B1.15) to the entire slide for 5 min (fresh stain) or 15 min (matured stain).
2. Wash in running water and allow to dry.

Cesares-Gill's method, modified (Plimmer & Paine, 1921)
1. Treat with Kirkpatrick's fixative (B1.10) for 5 min.
2. Wash off the fixative thoroughly with water.
3. Filter the diluted Plimmer's mordant (B1.16) onto the slide and allow to act for 5 min.
4. Wash off with water.
5. Stain for 2 min with weak carbol fuchsin.
6. Wash and allow to dry in air.

Rhodes' (1958) method
This is a modification of Fontana's method of staining spirochaetes.
1. Apply Rhodes' iron tannate mordant (B1.17) for 3–5 min.
2. Thoroughly wash with water.
3. Heat the ammoniacal silver nitrate solution nearly to boiling and apply to the film.
4. Leave to act for 3–5 min.
5. Wash well with water.
6. Drain or blot to dry.

Unless a permanent preparation is made, the stained film disintegrates after about a week on exposure to air.

APPENDIX C
Characterization tests

C1 Reagents
C2 Buffer Solutions
C3 Test Methods

C1   REAGENTS

Formulae of and notes on the reagents are shown below. Standard acids and alkalis, and simple aqueous solutions are not listed.

C1.1   Acid ferric chloride

$FeCl_3 \cdot 6H_2O$	12 g
Conc. HCl	2.5 ml
Distilled water	to 100 ml

Dilute the acid with 75 ml of the water, dissolve the ferric chloride by warming gently, and adjust to volume with water.

C1.2   Acid mercuric chloride
(Frazier, 1926)

$HgCl_2$	12 g
Distilled water	80 ml
Conc. HCl	16 ml

Mix the mercuric chloride with the water, add the acid, and shake well until solution is complete.

Note. For reasons of safety, 30% trichloracetic acid may be used in tests for gelatinase and caseinase activity instead of the acid mercuric chloride solution.

C1.3   Benedict's qualitative solution

Sodium citrate	17.3 g
Na_2CO_3, anhydrous	10 g
$CuSO_4 \cdot 5H_2O$	1.73 g
Distilled water	to 100 ml

Dissolve the sodium citrate and carbonate in 60 ml of the water. Dissolve the copper sulphate in 20 ml of the water and add it, with constant stirring, to the first solution. Adjust to volume with water.

Note. The solution should be stored in a warm place as it is liable to crystallize if cold.

C1.4   Creatine solution

1% creatine in 0.1 N-HCl

This solution avoids the rather vague 'knife-point of creatine' quoted in many textbooks and is relatively stable; a solution of creatine in alkali is often recommended, but is unstable (Levine *et al.*, 1934).

Ethylhydrocuprein (EHC) discs (synonym: Optochin discs), see Section C1.18.

C1.5   Ehrlich's reagent

p-dimethylaminobenzaldehyde	1 g
Ethanol, absolute	95 ml
Conc. HCl	20 ml

Dissolve the aldehyde in the ethanol and add the acid. Protect from light.

C1.6   Hydrogen peroxide

H_2O_2, 3% aq. soln ('10% volume')

Protect from light and store in a cool place. Keep in a brown bottle closed with a glass stopper, paraffined cork or plastic screw-cap.

Peroxide paper test strips are also available commercially.

C1.7   Kovács' reagent for indole
(Kovács, 1928, 1956)

p-dimethylaminobenzaldehyde	5 g
Amyl alcohol	75 ml
Conc. HCl	25 ml

Dissolve the aldehyde in the alcohol by gently warming in a water bath (about 50–55 °C). Cool and add the acid with care. Protect from light and store at 4 °C.

Note. The reagent should be light yellow to light brown in colour; some samples of amyl alcohol are unsatisfactory, and give a dark colour with the aldehyde. A few organisms produce indole weakly and the use of Ehrlich's instead of Kovács' reagent increases the sensitivity of the test.

For micromethods this reagent is prepared with iso-amyl alcohol.

Lugol's iodine solution: see B1.12.

C1.8 Lytic enzyme for streptococcal grouping
(Maxted, 1948).

Streptomyces griseus NCTC 7807, originally stated by Maxted to be *Streptomyces albus*, is grown on a suitable medium (Section A2.6.36) in Roux bottles for 4 to 5 days at 37 °C. After growth, the agar gel is destroyed by freezing in solid CO_2. The fluid which exudes on thawing contains the lytic principle and can be sterilized by filtration but this is not essential; the pH is not adjusted, nor is a preservative added. Store in a refrigerator.

C1.9 Methyl red solution

Methyl red	0.04 g
Ethanol	40 ml
Distilled water	to 100 ml

Dissolve the methyl red in the ethanol and dilute to volume with the water.

C1.10 α-naphthol solution

5% α-naphthol in ethanol
(not 95% ethanol)

The solution should not be darker than straw colour; if necessary the α-naphthol should be redistilled (Fulton, Halkias & Yarashus, 1960).

C1.11 Nessler's reagent

Dissolve 5 g potassium iodide in 5 ml freshly distilled water. Add cold saturated mercuric chloride solution until a slight precipitate remains permanently after thorough shaking. Add 40 ml 9 N-NaOH. Dilute to 100 ml with distilled water. Allow to stand for 24 h.

Alternative formula: dissolve 8 g potassium iodide and 11.5 g mercuric iodide in 20 ml water and adjust to 50 ml. Add 50 ml 6 N-NaOH. Mix and allow to stand for 24 h.

Notes. The water used in its preparation must be ammonia-free. Allow the reagent to settle before use. Protect from light.

C1.12 Niacin test reagents

(i)   4% aniline in 95% ethanol
      OR 1.5% o-tolidine in 95% ethanol
(ii) 10% aq. cyanogen bromide

Store at 4 °C for up to 2 weeks. Cyanogen bromide solution is toxic and must be treated with an equal volume of ammonia solution (sp. gr. 0.880) or 10 N-NaOH before disposal.

C1.13 Ninhydrin reagent
(for hippurate hydrolysis Method 3).

Dissolve 0.35 g ninhydrin in 10 ml of a 1:1 mixture of acetone and butanol. Prepare freshly for each batch of tests. Alternatively, dispense in bijoux bottles and store in the dark (C3.27, Method 4).

C1.14 Nitrite test reagents

Solution A
    0.33% sulphanilic acid in 5 N-acetic acid
Dissolve by gentle heating.
Solution B
    0.6% dimethyl-α-naphthylamine in 5 N-acetic acid
    OR
    0.5% a-naphthylamine in 5 N-acetic acid
    OR
    0.13% 1-naphthylamine-7-sulphonic acid
    (Cleve's acid) in 5 N-acetic acid
Dissolve by gentle heating.
    Zinc dust *or* 10% zinc dust suspended in 1% methylcellulose solution (Steel & Fisher, 1961)

Note. Cleve's acid is preferred to α-naphthylamine, which is regarded as carcinogenic.

C1.15 Oxidase test reagents

Solution 1
Prepare a fresh solution of tetramethyl-*p*-phenylenediamine dihydrochloride each time of use by adding a loopful of it to about 3 ml of sterile distilled water or saline. Do not use if it becomes blue. Autoxidation of the reagent occurs rapidly and although this can be retarded by the addition of 1% ascorbic acid, it is not sufficiently stable in aqueous solution for storage.
Solution 2
    1% α-naphthol in 95% ethanol

Solution 3

1% *p*-aminodimethylaniline oxalate aq. soln (also known as dimethyl-*p*-phenylenediamine oxalate)
As with solution 1, autoxidation may occur; if ascorbic acid is not used to delay the process the solution should be freshly prepared each week and kept at 4 °C.

C1.16   Sodium hippurate solution (1%)

Sodium hippurate	0.1 g
Sterile distilled water	10 ml

Mix in sterile tubes and place 0.4 ml aliquots in sterile bijoux bottles. Freeze at -20 °C until required.

C1.17   Test papers with reagents

Cut filter paper strips 5–10 mm wide and 50–60 mm long, and impregnate with the appropriate solution; dry at 50 to 60 °C. Store in screw-capped containers.

For the detection of H₂S (Clarke, 1953a)

Lead acetate hot saturated aq. soln (10 g lead acetate in 100 ml hot water)

Note: for the micromethod the papers should be 4 to 5 mm wide.

For the detection of indole (Holman & Gonzales, 1923)

Oxalic acid, hot saturated aq. soln

For the detection of indole (Gillies' 1956)

p-dimethylaminobenzaldehyde	10 g
o-phosphoric acid	20 ml
methanol	100 ml

Dissolve the aldehyde in the methanol and add the phosphoric acid.

For the detection of phenylpyruvic acid (PPA)(Goldin & Glenn, 1962)

0.5% phenylalanine in phosphate buffer (pH 7.4)
Dry the papers at room temperature.

For detection of hydrogen peroxide production

Discs or filter paper strips containing peroxide reagent* can be used for the detection of hydrogen peroxide in broth cultures, especially with streptococci.

Note: Commercial preparations with reagents are available for the detection of a variety of bacterial enzymes, metabolites and test-reactions.

C1.18   Sensitivity discs and test papers

Sterile filter paper discs 6 to 8 mm in diameter (e.g. Whatman No.3) are soaked in the appropriate solution, drained, and dried at 37 °C. Dried discs can be stored in small screw-capped bottles and should be kept at 4 °C. Several of them are available commercially.

For sensitivity to O/129 (Bain & Shewan, 1968)

2,4-diamino-6,7-di-*iso*propyl pteridine phosphate*	0.1 g
acetone	100 ml

Note. O/129 discs containing 10 µg and 150 µg of pteridine phosphate are available commercially.

For sensitivity to optochin

0.05% ethylhydrocuprein hydrochloride aqueous solution.

For sensitivity to bacitracin

Discs 6 mm in diameter containing 0.1 unit of bacitracin should produce zones of growth inhibition of at least 12 mm with *Streptococcus pyogenes and Streptococcus pneumoniae.*

For sensitivity to Liquoid

Discs containing 1 mg of the anticoagulant sodium polyanethol sulphonate (Liquoid) give wide zones of inhibition with *Peptostreptococcus anaerobius and Streptobacillus moniliformis.*

For sensitivity to metronidazole

Discs containing 5 µg metronizadole give wide zones of inhibition with many anaerobic organisms.

Pyridoxal requirement

The requirement for this growth factor can be demonstrated with discs containing 20 µl of a solution (1 mg/ml) on a medium that does not contain yeast extract: for example Blood Agar prepared with a Columbia base.

Cysteine requirement

The requirement of some streptococci and other organisms for cysteine over and above that present in ordinary culture media can be tested with discs containing 10 µl of a 40% (w/v) solution of cysteine hydrochloride.

For X-, V-, and X+V factor requirement

Discs soaked with solutions of X-, V-, or a mixture of X- and V-factors are used for confirmation and identification of haemophili.

C1.19   Tween 80-peroxide mixture
(Kubica, 1973)

10% Tween 80 (10%) made by adding 10 ml Tween to 90 ml distilled water. Sterilize at 121 °C for 10 min. If the Tween separates, rotate the flask to ensure mixing.

Before use mix equal volumes of 10% Tween 80 and 30% H_2O_2.

---

* Obtainable from BDH Chemicals Ltd., Broom Road, Poole, Dorset BH12 4NN, UK. Pteridine phosphate (Cat. No. 44169); Peroxide test (Cat. No. 31520 2F).

C1.20 Preparation of X- and V-factors
(Marshall & Kelsey, 1960)

X-factor. Centrifuge the red cells from 40 ml blood and add to them with shaking 100 ml acetone containing 1.2 ml conc. HCl; filter and add 100 to 120 ml water to the filtrate to precipitate the haemin. Collect by filtration and wash with water. Dissolve the crude haemin in 25 ml 0.1 M-Na_2HPO_4 and sterilize at 115 °C for 10 min.

V-factor. Suspend 50 g yeast in 100 ml 0.2 M-KH_2PO_4 and heat at 80 °C for 20 min. Clarify by centrifugation and sterilize the supernatant by filtration. Store in a refrigerator or deep-freeze.

C2 BUFFER SOLUTIONS

All traditional and biological buffer solutions should be stored in well-stoppered plastic or alkali-free glass bottles. The solutions should not be used for more than 2–3 months after preparation; chemically clean bottles should be used for fresh solutions.

C2.1 McIlvaine's buffer

Solution A
> 0.1 M-citric acid
> ($C_6H_8O_7 \cdot H_2O$, mol. wt = 210.15)

Solution B
> 0.2 M-disodium phosphate
> (Na_2HPO_4, mol. wt = 141.97)

To prepare the buffer, mix as follows:

	soln A		soln B
pH 4.0	61.45 ml	+	38.55 ml
pH 6.0	36.85 ml	+	63.15 ml

C2.2 Phthalate buffer, 0.0125 M, pH 5.0

Solution A
> 0.05 M-potassium hydrogen phthalate
> ($C_6H_4(COOH) COOK$, mol. wt = 204.23)

Solution B
> 0.05 N-NaOH (carbonate-free)

To prepare, mix as follows:

	soln A	soln B	
pH 5.0	50 ml	+	23.85 ml

Dilute to 200 ml with distilled water.

In the micromethod for decarboxylases, 5 ml 1% ethanolic bromcresol purple is added to 200 ml buffer.

C2.3 Phosphate buffer, 0.025 M, pH 6.0

Solution A
> 0.025 M-Na_2HPO_4

($Na_2HPO_4 \cdot 12H_2O$, mol. wt = 358.16)

Solution B
> 0.025 M-KH_2PO_4 (mol wt = 136.09)

To prepare the buffer, mix as follows:

	soln A		soln B
pH 6.0	12 ml	+	88 ml
pH 6.8	50 ml	+	50 ml

For the malonate and urease micromethods, 5 ml 0.1% ethanolic phenol red is added to 100 ml buffer.

C2.4 Sørensen's citrate buffer, 0.01 M, pH 5.6

Solution A
> 0.1 M-citric acid
> ($C_6H_8O_7 \cdot H_2O$, mol. wt = 210.15)

Solution B
> 0.1 M-*tri*-sodium citrate
> ($Na_3C_6H_5O_7 \cdot 2H_2O$, mol. wt = 294.11)

To prepare the buffer, mix as follows:

	soln A		soln B
pH 5.6	13.7 ml	+	36.3 ml

dilute to 500 ml with distilled water.

C3 CHARACTERIZATION TEST METHODS

Unless otherwise indicated, cultures are incubated at 37 °C or at their optimum temperature for growth.

Recommended organisms for use as controls are given in Appendix D.

C3.1 Acetylmethylcarbinol production; the Voges–Proskaüer reaction.

Method 1 (Barritt, 1936). After completion of the methyl red test (C3.35) add 0.6 ml 5% α-naphthol solution (C1.10) and 0.2 ml 40% KOH aqueous solution; shake well, slope the tube (to increase the area of the air–liquid interface), and examine after 15 min and 1 h. A positive reaction is indicated by a strong red colour.

Method 2 (O'Meara, 1931). After completion of the methyl red test, add 2 drops (about 0.05 ml) creatine solution (C1.4) and 1 ml 40% KOH aqueous solution); shake, slope, and examine after 1 and 4 h. A positive reaction is indicated by an eosin-pink colour.

Method 3 (Furniss, Lee & Donovan, 1978). Stab-inoculate semi-solid VP medium (A2.5.11); incubate for 1–3 days. Place on the surface 1 drop creatine solution (C1.4) and about 0.5 ml freshly prepared mixture of 3 parts 5% α-naphthol (C1.10) and 1 part 40% KOH; shake gently to aerate, and read after 1 h. A positive reaction gives a red colour.

Note. Motility can also be observed with this medium

after incubation; motile strains show diffuse growth whereas with non-motile organisms, growth is limited to the line of the inoculum.

Method 4 (NCTC micromethod; Clarke & Cowan, 1952). Incubate the culture overnight on 1% Glucose Agar; wash off with water or saline; centrifuge and resuspend the deposit in water or saline so that the density corresponds approximately to 10^9 *Escherichia coli* per ml. Test: using capillary pipettes that deliver 50 drops/ml, pipette into small tubes (e.g. 65×10mm) as follows:

10% glucose	1 drop (0.02 ml)
0.2% creatine	1 drop (0.02 ml)
0.025 M-phosphate buffer, pH 6.8	2 drops (0.04 ml)
Suspension from Glucose Agar	2 drops (0.04 ml)

Incubate in water bath at 37 °C. Test after 2 h. Add 3 drops (0.06 ml) 5% α-naphthol in ethanol (C1.10); shake well to mix; then add 2 drops (0.04 ml) 40% KOH, shake, leave on bench and after 10 min read the result. A positive reaction is indicated by a red or pink colour.

Controls for all methods:

positive – *Enterobacter cloacae; Streptococcus anginosus ('milleri'); Vibrio alginolyticus*

negative – *Escherichia coli; Streptococcus pyogenes; Vibrio parahaemolyticus*

Acid production from sugars: see Carbohydrate breakdown (C3.8.1).

C3.2 Aesculin hydrolysis

Inoculate Aesculin Broth and examine daily up to 5 days for blackening; this indicates hydrolysis of the aesculin. Alternatively, inoculate Aesculin Agar and look for blackening in and around the bacterial growth.

Controls: positive – *Enterococcus faecalis*
negative – *Streptococcus agalactiae*

C3.3 Aesculin–bile test for streptococci

Streak- or spot-inoculate Aesculin–bile Agar (A2.6.2) and incubate for 24 h for growth and blackening of the medium.

Controls: positive – *Enterococcus faecalis*
negative – *Streptococcus agalactiae*

C3.4 Arginine hydrolysis

Method 1 Inoculate 5 ml Arginine Broth (A2.6.4) and after incubation for 24 h add 0.25 ml Nessler's reagent (C1.11). Arginine hydrolysis is indicated by the development of a brown colour. For streptococci, add 0.5 ml of culture to 4.5 ml distilled water, shake and add 0.25 ml Nessler's reagent.

Method 2 (Thornley, 1960). Stab-inoculate into Arginine Agar and pipette on to the surface a layer of molten sterile petrolatum (soft paraffin) to a depth of about 1 cm. Incubate at an appropriate temperature (pseudomonads at 30 °C, streptococci at 37 °C) and examine daily for up to 5 days. A positive reaction is shown by a colour change of the indicator to red.

Controls: positive – *Enterococcus faecalis*
negative – *Streptococcus salivarius*

C3.5 Bile solubility

Method 1. To 5 ml of an 18 hour culture of the test organism in Serum, Digest, or Infusion Broth add 0.5 ml 10% sodium deoxycholate solution and incubate at 37 °C. Pneumococci are lysed within 15 min of adding the bile salt.

Note. A glucose-containing medium is unsatisfactory for this test as the reaction should not be more acid than pH 6.8.

Method 2. Grow the organism in Serum Broth or Todd-Hewitt broth for 24 h. Centrifuge and discard the supernatant. Resuspend the organisms in phosphate buffered saline (pH 7.3). Add 0.5 ml 10% sodium deoxycholate solution and incubate at 37 °C for 15–30 min. Under these conditions, rapid clearing of the suspension occurs with pneumococci and an occasional strain of *E. faecalis*; if clearing has not taken place in 30 min the organisms are not pneumococci.

Method 3 (Hawn & Beebe, 1965). For a rapid presumptive test on the primary plate touch a suspected colony with a loop charged with 2% sodium deoxycholate (pH 7.0) solution. Incubate the plate for 30 min at 37 °C. Colonies of pneumococcus disappear and, on Blood Agar, leave an area of α-haemolysis.

Controls: positive – *Streptococcus pneumoniae*
negative – *Streptococcus agalactiae*

C3.6 Bile tolerance

Inoculate onto 10% and 40% Bile Agar plates and incubate at 37 °C for 24–48 h. Growth indicates resistance to bile. Alternatively, 'ditch' plates comprising Blood Agar on one side and Bile Agar on the other may be used; strains should not be regarded as bile tolerant unless they grow right across the Bile Agar half.

Controls: positive (10% and 40%– *Enterococcus faecalis; Streptococcus agalactiae*
positive (10% only) – *Streptococcus salivarius*
negative – *Streptococcus dysgalactiae; Streptococcus pyogenes*

C3.7 The CAMP test

(Christie, Atkins & Munch-Petersen, 1944)

Wash sheep erythrocytes with physiological saline to remove any antibodies to the CAMP factor and resuspend the cells in saline to the original volume. Prepare CAMP plates by covering a layer of nutrient base (e.g. Oxoid Blood Agar No. 2) with a similar layer containing 10% of the washed sheep erythrocytes. Inoculate the plate with a single diametric streak of a β-toxin-producing strain of *Staphylococcus aureus* (NCTC 7428). Streak-inoculate the test strains at right-angles to but not touching the staphylococcal inoculum and incubate aerobically at 37 °C overnight. Examine the plates while still warm: diffusion of β-toxin will produce a zone of discolouration of the sheep erythrocytes. Production and diffusion of the CAMP factor from organisms under test will yield a completely clear area shaped like an arrow head in the zone of discolouration caused by the β-toxin.

Alternatively inoculate the test culture to obtain discrete colonies. After incubation overnight, and with the plate still warm, place 0.02–0.04 ml (1 or 2 drops) of staphylococcal β-toxin (10 units/ml) on discrete colonies and re-incubate for a further 2 h before examining the plate. A clear zone of the medium around colonies covered by β-toxin is a positive CAMP test.

Controls: positive – *Streptococcus agalactiae*
negative – *Enterococcus faecalis*

C3.8 Carbohydrate breakdown

Acetylmethylcarbinol production: see C3.1

C3.8.1 Acid from carbohydrates

Method 1. Peptone Water (A2.5.2) and Nutrient Broth sugars (A2.5.3). Inoculate and examine daily for 7 days for acid or acid and gas production. Reversion to alkalinity should also be noted. Negative tests should be examined at regular intervals for up to 30 days.

With some organisms the ability to produce visible gas depends on the temperature of incubation, and if equivocal or suspect results are obtained the tests should be repeated at a lower temperature. As some anaerobes can produce gas from proteins, gas production is not reliable as an indicator of fermentation.

When incubated anaerobically, some indicators may be 'bleached' (reduced to a colourless state); in such cases, test for acid production by the addition of fresh indicator solution.

Method 2. Serum Water Sugars (A2.5.4). Inoculate and examine for acid production or acid and clot formation.

Method 3. Media for neisserias and lactobacilli (A2.5.6)

Inoculate and examine for growth and acid production.

Method 4. Phenol-red Broth sugars for haemophili and streptococci (A2.5.3) Inoculate heavily with growth from Blood Agar medium, incubate at 37 °C and examine for acid production daily for up to 7 days (can normally be read after 1–2 days). For streptococci, use media containing 0.1% agar.

Positive – Yellow

Negative – Orange-red

In case of equivocal results, check pH: a decrease to pH 5.0–6.3 indicates fermentation.

Method 5. Blood Agar plate fermentation method for anaerobes (Phillips, 1976). Spread 1.0 ml of a sterile 20% solution of the fermentable substrate over the surface of a dried Blood Agar plate. Allow absorption of the solution to occur, redrying the plate if necessary. Spot-inoculate the test cultures onto the surface, and incubate anaerobically for 48 hours; a plain Blood Agar plate similarly inoculated should also be included as a negative control. To detect fermentation, remove a plug of the agar medium from the area of growth with a drinking straw, and expose it to a few drops of bromothymol blue indicator in a microtitre tray. Obtain and expose similarly negative control plugs both from the negative control plate and from an area of the test plate remote from bacterial growth. Use known positive cultures as controls to validate the test. To avoid false positive reactions in maltose fermentation tests, blood must be omitted from the agar fermentation base; it is conveniently replaced by haemin–menadione solution.

Method 6. MRS Lactobacillus Agar for leuconostocs (A2.6.25). Despite heavy inocula, the production of gas from glucose by leuconostocs cannot always be detected in broth cultures by the traditional inverted inner (Durham) tube. Instead a few drops of a suspension from a fresh agar culture are mixed with 15 ml of melted MRS (glucose) agar in a test tube and cooled; when set, sterile Nutrient Agar is added on top to form a 'plug' about 1 cm in depth. After incubation for 1–2 days, leuconostocs produce sufficient gas to disrupt the MRS medium and force the plug upwards.

Method 7. Ammonium Salt Sugars (ASS). Inoculate slopes of ASS medium (A2.5.5) and incubate at appropriate temperature for up to 7 days. Examine on alternate days for growth and acid production.

β-galactosidase: see ONPG test (C3.42).

C3.8.2 Oxidation or fermentation of glucose (Hugh & Leifson, 1953)

Some workers steam the OF medium to remove dissolved air, and quickly cool just before use.

Stab-inoculate duplicate tubes with a straight wire. To

one of the tubes add a layer of melted soft paraffin (Petrolatum) to a depth of about 3 cm above the medium to seal it from air. Incubate and examine daily for up to 14 days.

Results	open tube	sealed tube
Oxidation	yellow	green
Fermentation	yellow	yellow
No action on carbohydrate	blue or green	green

Note. This medium can also be used for detecting gas production and motility.

Controls: oxidation – *Acinetobacter calcoaceticus*
fermentation – *Escherichia coli*
no action – *Alcaligenes faecalis*

C3.8.3 Production of 3-ketolactose from lactose
(Bernaerts & DeLey, 1963)

Inoculate a plate containing Medium 1 (A2.5.8) and incubate for 1–2 days; then inoculate a loopful of the resulting growth onto a plate of Medium 2 and incubate for 1–2 days. Flood this plate with a shallow layer of Benedict's reagent (C1.3) and leave at room temperature. Development around the growth of a yellow zone (of Cu_2O) 1–2 cm in width within one hour indicates the production of 3-ketolactose. The yellow colour contrasts markedly with the blue reagent solution.

Controls: positive – *Agrobacterium tumefaciens*
negative – *Pseudomonas aeruginosa*

C3.9 Carbon source utilization (CSU) tests

Apart from the citrate utilization tests (C3.9.1) and tests for use of organic acids (C3.9.2), other CSU tests are not yet well enough developed for use in identification. Those interested in their use in classification should consult Stanier, Palleroni & Doudoroff (1966) where the methods are described.

C3.9.1 Citrate utilization

Make a light suspension of the organisms in sterile water or saline; inoculate Citrate media with a straight wire. Incubate at 30 °C (enterobacteria) or optimum temperature (other organisms).

Method 1. Inoculate Koser's citrate medium and examine daily for up to 7 days for turbidity. Confirm positive results by subculture again to Koser's citrate medium.

Turbidity – citrate utilized
No turbidity – citrate not utilized

Method 2. Inoculate as a single streak over the surface of a slope of Simmons' citrate medium. Examine daily for up to 7 days for growth and colour change. Confirm positive results by subculture to Simmons' or Koser's Citrate medium.

blue colour and streak of growth – citrate utilized
original green colour – citrate not utilized

Controls: positive – *Klebsiella pneumoinae* subsp. *aerogenes*
negative – *Escherichia coli*

Method 3. Inoculate Christensen's Citrate Agar by stabbing the butt and then drawing the wire over the surface of the slope. Examine for up to 7 days for colour change.

magenta colour – citrate utilized
yellow colour – citrate not utilized

Note. An organism giving positive results in Koser's or Simmons' test will be positive in Christensen's medium, but an organism giving a positive result in Christensen's test may or may not be positive in Koser's or Simmons' citrate media.

Controls: positive – *Klebsiella pneumoniae* subsp. *aerogenes*
negative – *Shigella sonnei*

C3.9.2 Utilization of other organic acids as carbon sources

Inoculate the appropriate media and examine at intervals for up to 1 month; use of the carbon compound is indicated by alkali production, shown by colour change of the indicator from yellow to red

Controls:	Positive	Negative
Benzoate		
Mucate	*Mycobacterium*	*Mycobacterium*
Oxalate	*smegmatis*	*phlei*

C3.10 Catalase activity

Method 1. Incubate the organism on a slope of Nutrient Agar or other suitable medium; a supplement of 5% serum may be needed for fastidious organisms such as streptococci. Run 1 ml 3–6% H_2O_2 down the slope and examine immediately and after 5 min for evolution of gas, which indicates catalase activity.

Method 2. Culture the organism in Nutrient Broth; after incubation overnight add 1 ml 3–6% H_2O_2 and examine immediately and after 5 min for evolution of gas.

Notes. Blood Agar and other blood-containing media are unsuitable for the test.

The addition of 1% glucose will avoid confusing reactions from pseudocatalase (Whittenbury, 1964).

False positive results can be produced by dirty glassware; all tubes must be chemically clean (see Appendix A1.1).

Cultures should be exposed to air for at least 30 min before adding H_2O_2 (Holdeman & Moore, 1972).

Controls: positive – *Staphylococcus saprophyticus*
negative – *Enterococcus faecalis*

Method 3 for mycobacteria (Kubica, 1973). Inoculate the butts of Lowenstein-Jensen slopes enriched with 0.1 ml of 7-day cultures in Middlebrook 7H-9 broth (BBL or Difco powder with added ADC (albumin, dextrose (glucose) and catalase enrichment); incubate with caps loose for 2 weeks at 37 °C. Include with each batch of tests controls of a strong (*Mycobacterium kansasii*) and a weak (*M. avium*) catalase producer.

Add 1 ml Tween 80-peroxide mixture (C1.19) to each culture and after 5 min measure the height of the column of bubbles above the surface of the medium.

Results: negative – no froth (usually isoniazid-resistant strain of *Mycobacterium tuberculosis* or *M. bovis*)
positive – froth < 45 mm (*M. avium*)
hyperactive – froth > 45 mm (*M. kansasii*)

C3.11 Chitin hydrolysis
(Holding & Collee, 1971)

Purified chitin (Lingappa & Lockwood, 1961) is made by treating crude chitin alternately with 1 N-NaOH and 1 N-HCl several times, and then with ethanol until foreign material is removed. Dissolve the purified chitin in cold conc. HCl, filter through glass wool, precipitate in distilled water, and wash until neutral. Add to melted Water Agar or Salt Agar at a concentration of about 0.25% (the medium should be slightly opaque) and pour as a thin layer on top of Nutrient Agar.

Streak-inoculate the test organism(s) on the surface and incubate at the optimal growth temperature for the organism or at 22, 30 and 37 °C. Chitin hydrolysis is shown by a clear zone around the growth.

Note. For halophilic organisms such as *Vibrio parahaemolyticus* the chitin should be suspended in Salt Agar, and the NaCl concentration of the basal medium increased to 2–3% or more.

Controls: positive – *Vibrio parahaemolyticus*
negative – *Escherichia coli*

C3.12 Coagulase test

In tube tests, a positive result is indicated by definite clot formation; granular or ropy growth is regarded as doubtful and the organism should be retested.

Method 1 (Cowan, 1938b). Mix 0.5 ml undiluted plasma with an equal volume of an 18–24-hour broth culture and incubate at 37 °C for 4 h. Examine after 1 and 4 h for coagulation. If negative, the tubes should be left at room temperature overnight and then re-examined.

Method 2 (Gillespie, 1943). To 0.5 ml of 1/10 dilution of plasma in saline add 0.1 ml of an 18–24-hour broth culture of the organism. Incubate at 37 °C and examine after 1, 3 and 6 h for coagulation. If negative, the tubes should be left at room temperature overnight and then re-examined.

Method 3 (Cadness-Graves *et al.*, 1943; Williams & Harper, 1946). With minimal spreading, emulsify a colony in a drop of water or saline on a microscope slide to produce a thick suspension. Stir the bacterial suspension with a straight wire which has been dipped into plasma. A positive result is indicated by macroscopic clumping within 5 seconds. Delayed clumping does not constitute a positive reaction.

Method 4 (Subcommittee on taxonomy of staphylococci and micrococci, 1965). A single colony from a 24 h Blood Agar plate is emulsified in 1 ml fresh citrated rabbit plasma diluted 1 in 6 with physiological saline. Incubate in a water bath at 37 °C and read after 1, 2, 4, 8 and 14 h. If possible, include among the controls a weakly positive strain (e.g. NCTC 6571). This method detects free coagulase.

Notes. If the plasma has been stored in a refrigerator it may be sufficiently cold to delay coagulation, especially in the slide test; it is advisable to allow the plasma to reach room temperature before use.

The slide test is a valuable presumptive test but as it only detects bound coagulase, negative results should be confirmed in a tube test which will also detect free coagulase.

Known positive and negative strains should always be tested in parallel and, with the tube tests, an uninoculated control should also be set up.

Controls: positive – *Staphylococcus aureus*
negative – *Staphylococcus saprophyticus*

C3.13 Campylobacter tests for species differentation

C3.13.1 Hydrolysis of indoxyl acetate
(Mills & Gherna, 1987)

Add 50 µl of a 10% (w/v) solution of indoxyl acetate in acetone to an absorbent paper disc 6mm in diameter and allow to dry in air. Apply growth from *Campylobacter* colonies directly to disc(s) and then wet with drop(s) of sterile distilled water. Appearance of a blue-green colour within 5–10 minutes indicates a positive result.

Note. Dried discs are stable for at least 12 months if stored at 4 °C in a dark glass bottle with silica gel.

Controls: positive – *Campylobacter jejuni*
negative – *Campylobacter fetus*

C3.13.2 Rapid coccal transformation on exposure to air
(Karmali, Allen & Fleming, 1981).

Transformation to coccal morphology among campylobacters occurs on exposure to atmospheric oxygen and some species are much more prone to this change than others. To perform the test, incubate duplicate cultures on Mueller–Hinton or Blood Agar for 24 h under the microaerobic conditions normally used for campylobacters (5–10% O_2); expose one plate to air and keep the other (control) plate under microaerobic conditions, both at ambient temperature. After 24–48 h compare the growth microscopically. Rapid coccal transformation (most of the cells coccoid) is a feature of the *Campylobacter jejuni* 'thermophilic' group, being most pronounced with *C. lari* and is and least with *C. coli*. Less than 5% of *C. fetus* cells are coccoid after such exposure to air. *Helicobacter pylori* forms cocci within one hour of exposure to air.

Controls: positive – *Campylobacter jejuni*
negative – *Campylobacter fetus*

C3.14 Decarboxylase reactions

Method 1 (Møller, 1955). From a plate culture, heavily inoculate, with a straight wire, tubes of the four media (arginine, lysine, ornithine, and control) through the paraffin layer. Alternatively, inoculate by adding a drop of a suspension of the organism above the paraffin layer and shaking to distribute the inoculum; the paraffin rises to the top on standing. Incubate and examine daily for up to 5 days. The media first become yellow due to acid production from the glucose; later, if decarboxylation occurs, the medium becomes purple. The control should remain yellow. With non-fermentative organisms, no acid (or insufficient acid) is produced from glucose and there is therefore no change of the indicator to yellow.

Note. In the diagnostic tables, plus signs indicate only the production of a purple colour in the medium. When a positive reaction is obtained with arginine, the medium may be tested with Nessler's reagent (C1.11) for the presence of NH_3 in the absence of urease, the formation of NH_3 indicates that the arginine dihydrolase system has taken part in the reaction (Møller, 1955).

Method 2 (Falkow, 1958). Inoculate tubes of the four media with a straight wire. Incubate and examine daily for up to 4 days. Decarboxylation is indicated by a purple colour, whereas the control and tubes with negative reactions are yellow. Falkow's method is not satisfactory with the genera *Enterobacter* and *Klebsiella*.

Method 3 NCTC micromethod (Shaw & Clarke, 1955). Suspension: culture overnight on Nutrient Agar or other suitable medium, wash off in water, centrifuge and resus-

pend in a small volume of water so that the density is at least equal to 10^9 *E. coli*.ml.

Test:	0.03 M-amino acid (pH 5.0)	0.04 ml
	0.0125 M-phthalate buffer, pH 5.0	
	with bromcresol purple	0.04 ml
	Culture suspension	0.04 ml

Place the tubes in a 37 °C water bath. When decarboxylation takes place a colour change occurs; readings are taken after 2, 4 and 24 h. Each set of tests should include a suspension control without amino acid; when this control is alkaline (blue), the same volume of buffer required to render the control tube yellow should be added to all the amino acid tubes before reading them.

This method is not suitable for decarboxylation of glutamic acid.

Controls:

Arginine	Lysine	Ornithine	
–	–	–	*Proteus vulgaris*
+	–	–	*Aeromonas hydrophila*
–	+	–	*Klebsiella pneumoniae* subsp *aerogenes*
–	–	+	*Morganella morganii*
+	+	–	*Salmonella typhi*
+	–	+	*Enterobacter cloacae*
–	+	+	*Enterobacter aerogenes*
+	+	+	*Salmonella typhimurium*

C3.15 Decomposition of tyrosine or xanthine

Inoculate plates of the appropriate media (A2.6.40; A2.6.42) and examine at intervals up to 5 days for dissolution of crystals under and around the bacterial growth.

Controls: positive – *Nocardia brasiliensis*
negative – *Mycobacterium phlei*

C3.16 Digestion of casein

Inoculate plates of Casein Agar and at intervals examine for up to 14 days for clearing of the medium around the bacterial growth.

Note. In a few instances clearing may be due to solution of the milk proteins by acid or alkaline metabolic products (see Hastings, 1903, 1904); this may be distinguished from true proteolysis by the addition of acid mercuric chloride (C1.2), when a decrease in the cleared area shows that the casein has not been digested.

If soluble casein is used instead of skimmed milk, hydrolysis is detected by flooding the plate with acid mercuric chloride solution.

Controls: positive – *Bacillus subtilis*
negative – *Mycobacterium phlei*

Note. For safety reasons, 30% trichloracetic acid may be used instead of acid mercuric chloride.

C3.17 Digestion of egg

Inoculate a slope of Dorset egg and examine at intervals for up to 14 days for liquefaction.

C3.18 Digestion of meat

Inoculate Cooked Meat medium and on the container mark the level of the meat. Incubate and examine at intervals for up to 14 days for diminution in the volume of the meat and for disintegration, or softening of the meat particles. Blackening or reddening of the meat and/or production of small white feathery crystals of tyrosine may also occur.

C3.19 Digestion of inspissated serum

Inoculate a Loeffler serum slope and examine after incubation under appropriate conditions for liquefaction of the medium.

C3.20 DNase (deoxyribonuclease) activity

Method 1 (Jeffries, Holtman & Guse, 1957). Dissolve DNA in distilled water; prepare sufficient to give a concentration of 2 mg/ml in the final medium. Add the DNA solution to Nutrient Agar (or other) base immediately before autoclaving and pour the plates as soon as the medium cools to 50 °C.

Prepare replicate plates; inoculate test culture(s) as streaks on the surface. Incubate at several temperatures such as 25, 30 and 37 °C.

After incubation for 36 h, flood the plates with 1 N-HCl; a positive result shows as a clear zone around the growth; the surrounding medium – and a negative result of the test – is opaque.

Controls: positive – *Serratia marcescens*
        negative – *Enterobacter aerogenes*

Method 2 (Schreier, 1969). Spot-inoculate DNA Toluidine-blue Agar (A2.6.10) with a loopful of growth from a fresh Blood Agar culture and incubate microaerobically at 42–43 °C for up to 48 hours. A clear colourless or pink zone around the inoculum indicates the production of extracellular deoxyribonuclease.

Controls: positive – *Campylobacter jejuni biotype IV*
        negative – *Campylobacter jejuni biotype I*

C3.21 Eijkman test, modified 44 °C fermentation test (Report, 1983)

Inoculate MacConkey Broth (A2.5.9), warmed to 37 °C and incubate in a water bath at 44 ± 0.1 °C for 48 h. Regard the production of both acid and gas as a positive result.

Note. Many alternatives to MacConkey Broth have been suggested, including the chemically defined Improved Formate Lactose Glutamate (IFLG) medium (Report, 1983).

Controls: positive – *Escherichia coli*
        negative – *Enterobacter cloacae*

C3.22 Ethylhydrocuprein (EHC) sensitivity

Place a disc impregnated with EHC (optochin, C1.16) or a tablet containing 0.05 mg optochin on the surface of a Blood Agar plate inoculated with the organism. Incubate and examine after 18–24 h. Sensitivity to the compound is shown by inhibition of bacterial growth around the disc for a distance of at least 5 mm; resistant organisms will grow up to the disc or may show a small inhibition zone of not more than 1–2 mm.

Controls: sensitive – *Streptococcus pneumoniae*
        resistant – *Enterococcus faecalis*

Fluorescence; see A2.4.3 and A2.7.14.

β-galactosidase; see ONPG test (C3.39).

C3.23 Gelatin hydrolysis (or liquefaction)

Method 1. Inoculate Nutrient Gelatin (A2.6.14) with a straight wire and incubate at 22 °C; observe daily up to 30 days for growth and presence of liquefaction.

Method 2. Inoculate Nutrient Gelatin (A2.6.14) and incubate at 37 °C for up to 14 days; every 2–3 days, place in a refrigerator for 2 h and then examine for liquefaction. Set up a control tube of uninoculated medium in parallel.

Method 3 (Frazier, 1926). Inoculate a slope or plate of Gelatin Agar (A2.6.14) and incubate for 3 days. Flood the surface with 5–10 ml acid mercuric chloride solution (C1.2); clear zones indicate areas of gelatin hydrolysis.

When glass Petri dishes are used, metal tops should be avoided; plastic disposable dishes prevent contamination of glassware with mercuric ions.

Note. 30% trichloracetic acid can be substituted for the acid mercuric chloride in Frazier's method (Pitt & Dey, 1970); for reasons of safety, this may be preferable.

Method 4. (Ferrous Chloride Gelatin (A2.6.12) medium may be used for the determination of both gelatin liquefaction and H_2S production (C3.30, method 2).

Method 5. Greene & Larks' (1955) adaptation of Kohn's (1953) gelatin discs to a micromethod, with a consequent increase in speed. Formalized gelatin discs are washed in water, sterilized by steaming for 30 min and stored in a refrigerator. Discs are added to 1 ml volumes of 1% Peptone Water, heavily inoculated with culture from an agar slope and placed in a 37 °C water bath. With positive cultures the discs disintegrate in 2–6 h.

Controls: positive – *Aeromonas hydrophila*

negative – *Escherichia coli*

C3.24 Gluconate oxidation

Inoculate Gluconate Broth (A2.6.15) lightly and incubate at 37 °C for two days.

Method 1. To 5 ml culture add 1 ml Benedict's qualitative solution (C1.3), mix, and boil for 10 min. The formation of a brown, orange, or tan precipitate constitutes a positive reaction.

Method 2 (Carpenter, 1961). Add one Clinitest* tablet instead of the Benedict's reagent and look for the formation of a coloured precipitate as in method 1.

Controls: positive – *Klebsiella pneumoniae* subsp.

aerogenes

negative – *Escherichia coli*

C3.25 Growth on individual media

The ability to grow on a particular medium occurs in several tables. Media are inoculated and incubated for a suitable period in accordance with the growth rate of the bacteria. Growth should not be scored as absent until adequate time has elapsed for it to have occurred.

The media on which this character is recorded in the tables are:

	Tables
Acetate Agar	6.3*a*
BCYE, BCYE (– CF)	7.10*d*
Bile Agar (10%, 20% and 40%)	6.3*a,b*; 6.7; 7.2*a,b*; 7.4*a*
Cetrimide media	7.5; 7.6*a*
Chocolate Agar	7.10*b*
Dye-containing Agar	7.4*b*
Glycine 1%	7.10*c*
MacConkey agar	7.4*a*; 7.6*a*; 7.7; 7.9*a,b,c,d,e*
Media without salt	7.8*a,b,c*
Media with increased salt	6.3*a,b*; 6.5*c*; 6.9; 7.4*a*; 7.8*a,c*; 7.10*c*
Nutrient Agar	7.3; 7.4*a*
Selenite	7.9*a,b,c,d,e*
SS agar	7.5
Triphenyltetrazolium chloride (TTC) 0.04%	7.10*c*

C3.26 Growth in media with increased NaCl concentration

Inoculate broth of the required salt concentration with the organism to be tested and incubate at the optimal temperature for growth. Many salt-tolerant organisms (and most halophiles) have optimal temperatures below 37 °C

For campylobacters, use Mueller–Hinton agar (1941) containing 1.5% NaCl.

C3.27 Hippurate hydrolysis

Method 1 for streptococci. Culture the organism in Hippurate Broth (A2.6.17) for 2–4 days. Centrifuge the culture and, to 2 ml of the supernatant fluid, add 0.5 ml of a 50% solution of concentrated sulphuric acid. A fine white precipitate (of benzoic acid) indicates hydrolysis of the hippurate.

Controls: positive – *Streptococcus agalactiae*

negative – *Streptococcus salivarius*

Method 2 (Thirst, 1957a). Lightly inoculate slopes of Hippurate Agar (A2.6.17) and examine daily for up to 7 days. Hydrolysis of hippurate is indicated by growth and a pink colour due to alkali production.

Controls: positive – *Klebsiella pneumoniae* subsp.

aerogenes

negative – *Enterobacter cloacae*

Method 3 (Hwang & Ederer, 1975). Suspend a loopful of growth from an 18–24 hour Blood Agar culture in 0.4 ml of a 1% solution of sodium hippurate in phosphate buffer pH 7.0 (freshly prepared or stored frozen at –20 °C). Incubate at 37 °C for 2 hours with occasional mixing. Then slowly add 0.2 ml of a freshly prepared solution of 3.5% ninhydrin (C1.13) down the side of the tube to form an overlay. Reincubate at 37 °C for 10 minutes and examine for the development of a deep purple colour which indicates the presence of glycine, an end product of hippurate hydrolysis. Tubes showing a pale purple colour or remaining colourless indicate negative results.

Controls: positive – *Klebsiella pneumoniae* subsp.

aerogenes

negative – *Enterobacter cloacae*

---

* Ames Division, Miles Laboratories Ltd, Stoke Poges, Slough SL2 4LY, UK.

Method 4 for Legionella pneumophila. Thaw the sodium hippurate solution (Section C1.16). Prepare a milky suspension of organisms from the growth (1–4 days) on BCYE medium (A2.3.6) and add a loopful to the hippurate solution. Incubate in air at 35 °C for 18–20 h. Add 0.2 ml of 3.5% ninhydrin solution (C1.13), mix gently, and reincubate at 35–37 °C for 10 min. Observe for development of a purple colour within 20 min. Regard a grey or light yellow colour as negative.

Controls: positive – *Legionella pneumophila*
negative – *Enterobacter cloacae*

C3.28 Growth anaerobically with specific supplements

The ability of campylobacters to grow anaerobically on supplemented media is an aid to identification (Table 7.10c). The basal medium is semisolid Yeast Extract Agar to which the relevant compound(s) is added. Two or three stab inocula from a 24 h Blood Agar culture are made in the medium to about 1 cm below the surface. Incubate anaerobically and examine periodically for up to 7 days for growth throughout the medium.

C3.29 Hydrogen peroxide production

This character is used in the differentiation of streptococcal species. Culture the organism in Infusion Broth (A2.1.6); centrifuge, discard most of the supernatant and resuspend the deposit in the remaining liquid. Immerse a commercial paper strip or disc containing peroxide reagent (C1.17) in the cell suspension: the rapid development of an intense blue colour indicates the presence of hydrogen peroxide.

Controls: positive – *Streptococcus pneumoniae*
negative – *Streptococcus salivarius*

C3.30 Hydrogen sulphide production

Method 1. Inoculate a tube of Triple Sugar Iron Agar (A2.6.38) by stabbing the butt and streaking the slope; observe daily for up to 7 days for blackening of the butt only due to H$_2$S production. Some organisms produce a dark pigment on the slope only and this should not be mistaken for a positive result.

Method 2. Stab-inoculate a tube of Ferrous Chloride Gelatin medium (A2.6.12) and incubate at 22 °C. Read daily for 7 days for blackening due to H$_2$S production. Gelatin liquefaction may also be observed in this medium; for this incubation is continued for up to 30 days.

Method 3. Inoculate the organism in Nutrient Broth or Peptone Water, and insert a lead acetate paper (C1.17) between the cap or plug and the tube. Examine daily for 7 days for blackening of the paper.

Method 4 for *Brucella* species. Inoculate a Serum Glucose Agar slope (A2.2.6) and insert a lead acetate paper strip as in method 3. Examine and change the paper daily for 7 days, recording the results.

Method 5 (Morse & Weaver, 1950). Medium: 2% thiopeptone in distilled water, pH 6.9; dispense in 0.8 ml volumes in 75 × 10 mm tubes; heat to 37 °C before heavy inoculation by means of a swab from a 6-hour culture on a solid medium. A 5 mm wide strip of lead acetate paper (C1.17) is folded 1 cm from the end and inserted into the mouth of the tube. Morse & Weaver say that the method is more sensitive than macrotests and that the 45 min reading gives the best correlation.

Method 6 (Clarke, 1953a). Suspensions are made from growth on Nutrient Agar (see decarboxylase reactions (C3.14).

0.1% cysteine hydrochloride, pH 7.4	0.04 ml
0.025 M-phosphate buffer, pH 6.8	0.04 ml
Suspension of organism	0.04 ml

Place a small lead acetate paper (C1.17) in the mouth of the tube and keep it in position by a loose cotton-wool plug. Do not allow the paper to touch the suspension–reagent mixture. Incubate at 37 °C; read at intervals of 15 min for 1 h.

Controls: positive – *Proteus vulgaris*
negative – *Shigella sonnei*

Method 7 (Rapid test of Skirrow & Benjamin, 1980, modified by Lior, 1984). A large loopful (5mm) of growth from an 18–24 h Blood Agar culture (incubated at 37 °C in not more than 7% O$_2$) is gently suspended, without mixing, in the upper third of 3–4 ml FBP medium (A2.6.11) in a small screw-capped tube or container. Incubate closed at 37 °C for 2 h. Blackening around the bacterial inoculum indicates a positive result.

Controls: positive – *Campylobacter jejuni* (biotype IV)
negative – *Campylobacter jejuni* (biotype I)

C3.31 Indole production

Method 1. Inoculate Peptone Water or Nutrient Broth, place an oxalic acid paper (C1.17) between the plug or cap and the tube. Incubate and examine daily for up to 7 days. Indole production is shown by the development of a pale pink colour at the lower end of the test paper.

Method 2. Inoculate Peptone Water or Nutrient Broth and incubate for 48 h. Add 0.5 ml Kovács' reagent for indole (C1.7), shake well, and examine after about 1 min. A red colour in the reagent layer indicates indole production.

Method 3. To a 48-hour culture in Peptone Water or Nutrient Broth add about 1 ml ether or xylol; shake; run 0.5 ml Ehrlich's reagent (C1.5) down the side of the tube. A pink or red colour in the solvent indicates indole production.

Method 4 (Arnold & Weaver, 1948). *Medium 1*: Tryptone, 1%; meat extract, 0.3%, in distilled water. *Medium 2:* tryptophan, 0.03%; peptone, 0.1%; K_2HPO_4, 0.5% in distilled water. Adjust both media to pH 7.4.

Inoculate medium heavily from a culture in the logarithmic phase; incubate in a 37 °C water bath. Test by adding 4 drops of Kovács' reagent (C1.7), using *iso*-amyl alcohol as solvent. Medium 2 gives positive results more quickly than Medium 1 (but with both media the tests should be complete within 2 hours).

Method 5 NCTC micromethod (Clarke & Cowan, 1952). Suspensions are made from growth on Nutrient Agar (see Decarboxylase reactions, C3.14).

0.1% tryptophan	0.06 ml
0.025 M-phosphate buffer, pH 6.8	0.04 ml
Suspension of organism	0.04 ml

Incubate in water bath at 37 °C and test at 1 h by adding 0.06 ml Kovács' reagent (C1.7) prepared with *iso*-amyl alcohol; shake. Read immediately; red colour indicates indole production.

Controls: positive – *Escherichia coli*
negative – *Enterobacter cloacae*

Indoxyl acetate hydrolysis test for differentation of campylobacters – see *Campylobacter*, C3.13.1

C3.32   KCN test

Inoculate 1 ml KCN Broth (A2.6.18) with one loopful of an overnight broth culture or a light suspension of the organism. Screw the cap of the bottle tight and incubate for up to 48 h. Examine after 24 and 48 h for turbidity indicating growth, which constitutes a positive reaction. Do not use a large inoculum.

After use, care should be exercised in the disposal of cyanide-containing media; add a crystal of $FeSO_4$ and 0.1 ml 40% KOH before sterilization.

Controls: positive – *Klebsiella pneumoniae* subsp.
aerogenes
negative – *Escherichia coli*

C3.33   Lecithovitellin (LV) reaction

Inoculate LV Agar (A2.6.21) and incubate for 5 days. Examine daily for (i) growth, (ii) opalescence within the medium under and around growth, (iii) 'pearly layer' formation over and around the colonies; (ii) and (iii) constitute positive reactions.

Flood the plate with saturated aqueous $CuSO_4$ solution, remove excess reagent and allow the plate to dry in an incubator for 20 min. An insoluble bright greenish-blue copper soap is formed in those areas containing free fatty acid.

Controls: opalescence – *Clostridium perfringens*
pearly layer – *Clostridium sporogenes*
no reaction – *Bacillus subtilis*

C3.34   Malonate utilization

Method 1. Inoculate Malonate–phenylalanine medium (A2.6.22) lightly and incubate for 18–24 h. Examine for colour change and keep the culture for the phenylalanine deamination test (C3.45). A positive malonate reaction is indicated by a deep blue colour, a negative reaction by the unchanged greenish colour of the medium (with some negative strains a yellow colour appears).

Method 2. NCTC micromethod (Shaw & Clarke, 1955). Suspensions are made from growth on Nutrient Agar (see Decarboxylase reactions, C3.14).

1% sodium malonate	0.04 ml
0.025 M-phosphate buffer, pH 6.0 (phenol red)	0.04 ml
Suspension of organism	0.04 ml

Incubate in water bath at 37 °C; read at intervals up to 24 h. Red colour indicates a positive test.

Controls: positive – *Klebsiella pneumoniae* subsp.
pneumoniae
negative – *Proteus vulgaris*

C3.35   Methyl red (MR) reaction

Inoculate Glucose Phosphate (MR) medium (A2.10) and incubate at 30 °C for 5 days (some workers prefer 37 °C for 2 days). Add 2 drops of methyl red solution (C1.9), shake and examine.

A positive MR reaction is shown by the appearance of a red colour at the surface. An orange or yellow colour should be regarded as negative. (After reading the MR reaction the same culture can be used for the VP test (C3.1).)

Controls: positive – *Escherichia coli*
negative – *Enterobacter cloacae*

C3.36   Milk, growth in *(now rarely used diagnostically)*

Inoculate the appropriate medium (A2.6.23) and examine daily for 14 days for colour change and clotting. The following reactions may be seen:
Litmus milk:
acid production indicated by pink colour,
alkali production indicated by blue colour,

reduction of the indicator shown by colourless (white) medium,

acid clot shown by a firm pink clot which does not retract and which is soluble in alkali,

rennet clot shown by a soft clot which retracts and expresses a clear greyish fluid (whey); the clot is insoluble in alkali; peptonization or digestion of the clot may follow,

'stormy fermentation' in which the acid clot is broken up by gas production.

Purple milk:

as above, but acid production is shown by a yellow colour.

Reduction of the indicator is not seen.

Ulrich milk:

the colour changes may be interpreted as follows:

bluish grey – unchanged,

pale yellow green to yellowish orange – acid,

pale bluish purple to reddish purple – alkaline,

bluish green – oxidation,

white – reduction,

acidity or alkalinity are best observed in the lower (reduced) portion of the medium.

Controls:

acid — *Escherichia coli*
alkaline — *Alcaligenes faecalis*
stormy fermentation — *Clostridium perfringens*
no change — *Proteus vulgaris*

C3.37 Motility

Method 1. Young broth cultures of the organism, incubated at or below the optimum growth temperature (e.g. 37 °C and 22 °C), should be examined in 'hanging drop' preparations, using a high-power dry objective and reduced illumination.

Method 2. Stab-inoculate tubes of motility medium (A2.5.24) to a depth of about 5 mm. Incubate at or below the optimum growth temperature.

Motile organisms migrate throughout the medium, which becomes turbid; growth of non-motile organisms is confined to the stab inoculum.

Method 3 (for anaerobes). Take up some of the liquid from a young culture in Cooked Meat medium into the capillary of a Pasteur pipette; cut the capillary and seal both ends. A fine oxygen flame is needed to give a narrow zone of intense heat which melts the glass quickly.

Examine the sealed capillary under the high-power dry objective.

Notes. OF medium (A2.5.1) may be used to test motility but it cannot be relied upon to the exclusion of the methods described above.

For the enhancement of motility inoculate Craigie tubes (Craigie, 1931) or U-tubes containing semisolid nutrient agar; serial passages may be necessary.

C3.38 Niacin test for mycobacteria

Method 1 (Marks & Trollope, 1960). Heavily inoculate the surface of Dorset Egg medium contained in a bijou bottle; add 0.4 ml sterile water and incubate with the cap loose for 2 weeks at 37 °C; a moist atmosphere must be maintained. Transfer the aqueous extract to a test tube and add 0.6 ml 4% ethanolic aniline followed by 0.6 ml 10% aqueous cyanogen bromide (C1.12). The presence of niacin is indicated by a yellow colour.

Method 2 (Gutiérrez-Vázquez, 1960; modified by Collins, Grange & Yates, 1985). Add 0.3 ml sterile water to a 30-day culture on Lowenstein-Jensen medium; autoclave at 115 °C for 15 min. When cool, remove 2 drops of liquor and place on a white tile. Add 2 drops 1.5% ethanolic *o*-toluidine and 2 drops 10% aqueous cyanogen bromide (C1.12). A positive result is shown by a pink to orange colour; negative reactions remain blue-grey.

Note. Cyanogen bromide is toxic; the test must be carried out in a fume cupboard and, after completion, alkali should be added to decompose the reagent before sterilization.

Controls: positive – *M. tuberculosis*
negative – *M. fortuitum*

C3.39 Nitrate reduction

Method 1. Inoculate Nitrate Broth (A2.6.26) lightly and incubate for up to 5 days. Note any gas formation in the inverted inner (Durham) tube. Add 1 ml of nitrite reagent A followed by 1 ml of reagent B (C1.1).

A deep red colour which shows the presence of nitrite and thus shows that nitrate has been reduced, indicates a positive reaction.

To tubes not showing a red colour within 5 min. add powdered zinc (up to 5 mg/ml of culture) and allow to stand. Red colour = nitrate present in the medium (i.e. not reduced by the organism). Absence of red colour = nitrate absent in the medium (i.e. reduced by the organism to nitrite, which in turn was itself reduced).

Note. Incubation for 5 days is unnecessary with many organisms. Daubner (1962) reported that with the exception of two *Erwinia* species all members of the Enterobacteriaceae reduced nitrate to nitrite within 8 hours; it is convenient to test a sample of the inoculated medium daily and re-incubate if nitrate has not been reduced.

Method 2. Brough (1950) used small volumes (1 ml in 75 × 10 mm tubes) of medium (0.1% KNO_3 in Nutrient

Broth) warmed at 37 °C before inoculation with a heavy suspension and rapid return to the water bath at 37 °C. Test after 15 min with 3 drops each of Solution A and Solution B reagents (C1.14).

Method 3 Bachmann & Weaver (1951). Medium: peptone, 1%, meat extract, 0.3%; KNO_3, 0.1% in distilled water; sterilize and store in flasks. Dispense in 1.0 ml volumes into clean, non-sterile 75×10 mm tubes. Heat tubes in 37 °C water bath and then inoculate with two 3 mm loopsful of 6-hour culture (inoculum should not be broken up but allowed to settle). After 15 minutes add 1 drop each of Solution A and Solution B reagents (C1.14). When nitrite is present a pink colour develops in 5 minutes.

Method 4 NCTC micromethod (Clarke & Cowan, 1952). Suspensions are made from growth on Nutrient Agar (see Decarboxylase reactions, C3.14).

0.05% $NaNO_3$	0.04 ml
0.025 M-phosphate buffer, pH 6.8	0.04 ml
Suspension of organism	0.04 ml

Incubate in water bath at 37 °C and test after 1 h. Add 0.06 ml nitrite test solution A and 0.06 ml test solution B (C1.14). Shake and read after 1–2 minutes. A pink colour is indicative of nitrite. In each series of tests a blank without suspension should be made to exclude the presence of nitrite in the substrate.

Method 5 (Cook, 1950). Place a blotting paper strip (about 16×10 mm) containing potassium nitrate in the centre of a Blood Agar plate at the time of inoculation. The strips are prepared by soaking blotting paper in a warm solution of 40% potassium nitrate and then drying. Stab-inoculate test and control organisms near the periphery of the plate and incubate for 24–48 h. A positive result is shown by a dark green-brown zone of methaemoglobin formed by the reduction of haemoglobin by nitrite.

Controls: positive – *Escherichia coli*

negative – *Acinetobacter calcoaceticus*

C3.40   Nitrite reduction

Inoculate Nitrite Broth (A2.6.27) and incubate for 7–14 days. Add nitrite reagent Solutions A and B (C1.14) as for the nitrate reduction test.

Red colour = nitrite present. Absence of red colour = nitrite absent, i.e. reduced by the organism.

Controls: positive – *Escherichia coli*

negative – *Acinetobacter calcoaceticus*

C3.41   O/129 sensitivity

Method 1 (Davis & Park, 1962). Place a few crystals of 2,4-diamino-6,7-di-*iso*-propyl pteridine phosphate* on the surface of a plate previously inoculated with the test culture. Incubate the plate overnight and examine for inhibition of growth around the crystals.

Method 2 (Bain & Shewan, 1968). Place an O/129 disc (C1.18) on the surface of a Nutrient Agar plate sown with the test organism. Incubate the plate overnight and look for a clear zone of inhibition around the disc.

Method 3 (Furniss, Lee & Donovan, 1978). Place discs containing 10 µg and 150 µg respectively of the pteridine reagent on the surface of medium previously inoculated with the test-culture.

Note. These discs are available commercially.

Controls: positive – *Vibrio parahaemolyticus*

negative – *Escherichia coli*

C3.42   ONPG Test
(Lowe, 1962)

Inoculate a tube of ONPG broth (A2.6.28) and incubate for 48 hours; β-galactosidase activity is indicated by the appearance of a yellow colour due to the production of *o*-nitrophenol.

Controls: positive – *Escherichia coli*

negative – *Morganella morganii*

C3.43   Oxidase (cytochrome c oxidase) activity

Method 1 (Kovács, 1956; modified by Cowan & Steel, 1974). A fresh solution of the reagent is prepared each time of use by adding a loopful of tetramethyl-*p*-phenylenediamine dihydrochloride to about 3 ml of sterile distilled water or saline; the reagent is not sufficiently stable for storage in aqueous solution even in the presence of ascorbic acid. However, solutions prepared with 0.1% ascorbic acid can be kept at –20 °C and thawed when needed. For use, wet a filter paper disc in a sterile plastic Petri dish with a few drops of the indicator solution and smear the test culture (grown on a medium free from glucose and nitrate) across the moist paper with a platinum (not nichrome) loop, glass rod or swab stick. The appearance of a dark purple colour on the paper within 30 seconds denotes a positive reaction.

Method 2 (Gaby & Hadley, 1957). Add 0.2 ml α-naphthol (C1.15, solution 2) and 0.3 ml 1% dimethyl-*p*-phenylenediamine oxalate (C1.15, solution 3) to an overnight broth culture. Shake vigorously. A blue colour appearing within 10 to 30 seconds indicates a positive result; weak reactions occurring between 2 and 5 minutes

---

* Obtainable from BDH Chemicals Ltd., Broom Road, Poole, Dorset BH12 4NN, UK

should be ignored. For plate cultures mix equal volumes of the two reagents (C1.15, solutions 2 and 3) and run a few drops over the surfaces of colonies on the plate (Ewing & Johnson, 1960); colour changes and times are similar to the test in broth.

Note. Method 2 is slightly less sensitive than method 1.

Controls: positive – *Pseudomonas aeruginosa*
negative – *Escherichia coli*

C3.44 Oxygen preference of Mycobacteria

This may be determined by the character and rate of growth at the optimum temperature. Aerobes give 'mature' raised and confluent growth within one week on one or more slopes whereas microaerophiles either take considerably longer to attain mature growth or never do so. This differentiation can be determined more accurately with the semi-solid medium of Marks (1976) and it is used to distinguish between *M. tuberculosis* and *M. bovis*.

Liquid Medium base

Na_2HPO_4	7.5 g
KH_2PO_4	2.0 g
$MgSO_4 \cdot 7H_2O$	0.6 g
Sodium citrate	2.5 g
Ferric ammonium citrate	5 mg
Tryptone	5.0 g
Glycerol	20 ml
Distilled water	to 1000 ml

Adjust pH to 7.3 and autoclave at 120 °C for 15 minutes.

Semi-solid agar medium

Add 1 g purified (ion) agar or similar to 1000 ml liquid medium base. Dissolve by steaming and then by autoclaving at 120 °C for 5 minutes. Shake well and dispense in 10 ml volumes in 14 ml screw-capped bottles and autoclave at 120 °C for 10 minutes.

Before use add aseptically 0.5 ml calf serum. Inoculate with a vigorously growing culture and mix by inversion – do not shake. Incubate at the appropriate temperature and inspect weekly. Aerobes grow in the top 1 cm and microaerophiles to a lower depth often giving a dense band of growth between 12 and 20 mm from the surface.

C3.45 Phenylalanine deamination

Method 1 (Shaw & Clarke, 1955). After recording the result of the malonate test (C3.34) acidify with 0.1 N-HCl drop by drop until the medium is yellow. Then add 0.2 ml of a 10% aqueous solution of $FeCl_3$; shake and observe any colour change. Watch immediately; a positive reaction is indicated by a dark green colour which quickly fades.

Note. This method is not suitable for showing phenylala-

nine deaminase in *Moraxella phenylpyruvica* (Snell & Davey, 1971).

Method 2 (Report, 1958). Inoculate heavily a Phenylalanine Agar slope (A2.6.30). Incubate overnight and run 0.2 ml of a 10% aqueous solution of $FeCl_3$ over the growth. A positive result gives a green colour on the slope and in the free liquid at the base.

Method 3 (Goldin & Glenn, 1962). Make a suspension of the test organism in a small tube. Place a phenylalanine test strip (C1.17) in the tube and let the tip of the paper touch the suspension. Place the tube in a water bath at 37 °C for 1 h, then add 1 drop of 8% aqueous $FeCl_3$ solution to the strip. A positive test produces a green colour. *Moraxella phenylpyruvica* is not likely to give positive results unless incubated for more than 4 hours.

Method 4 (Henriksen, 1950). Make a heavy suspension of the organism with the growth from one Nutrient Agar slope in 0.5 ml saline. Add 0.2 ml suspension to 0.2 ml 0.2% DL-phenylalanine in saline. Shake and place the tube in an almost horizontal position in an incubator. After 4 hours acidify the mixture by adding 10% H_2SO_4 using phenol red as indicator. Next add 4–5 drops of half-saturated aqueous $FeSO_4 (NH_4)_2SO_4 \cdot 6H_2O$, shake the tube and watch for a green colour (= positive) within a minute; the colour quickly fades.

Method 5 NCTC micromethod (Shaw & Clarke, 1955). Suspensions are made from growth on Nutrient Agar (see Decarboxylase reactions, C3.14).

0.03 M-phenylalanine	0.04 ml
0.025 M-phosphate buffer, pH 6.8	0.04 ml
Suspension of organism	0.04 ml

Incubate at 37 °C in a water bath. Test after 2 hours by adding 0.04 ml 2% aqueous ferric chloride; shake. Read a minute later; a green colour indicates the presence of phenylpyruvic acid.

Controls: positive – *Proteus vulgaris*
negative – *Klebsiella pneumoniae* subsp
pneumoniae

C3.46 Phosphatase test

Method 1. Lightly inoculate Phenolphthalein Phosphate Agar (A2.6.29) to obtain discrete colonies, and incubate for 18 hours. Place 0.1 ml ammonia solution (sp. gr. 0.880) in the lid of the Petri dish and invert the medium above it. Alternatively the medium may be exposed to ammonia vapour by holding above an open bottle. Free phenolphthalein liberated by phosphatase reacts with the ammonia and phosphatase-positive colonies become bright pink.

Note. Baird-Parker (1963) recommends incubation of

cultures at 30 °C for 3–5 days before applying the test; this gives a greater number of positive results than in cultures incubated at 37 °C for 18 hours.

Method 2 (White & Pickett, 1953). Substrate: dissolve 30 mg phenol-free phenyl disodium phosphate in 100 ml 0.01 M-Sørensen's citrate-NaOH buffer at pH 5.6 (keeps for 3 months at 4 °C in a stoppered bottle).

Indicator: dissolve 50 mg 2:6-dibromo-*N*-chloro-*p*-quinone imine in 10 ml methanol (stable for 2 months at 4 °C in a dark, stoppered bottle).

Test: pipette 0.5 ml substrate into 100 × 13 mm tube. In this make a heavy suspension (10^{10}/ml) of the organism under test; incubate the tube at 37 °C for 4 hours. Add 4 drops of indicator solution; shake and stand the tube at room temperature for 15 minutes. Add 0.3 ml *n*-butanol; shake, stand for 5 minutes. A purple or blue colour in the butanol layer indicates a positive result.

Controls: positive – *Staphylococcus aureus*
  negative – *Staphylococcus saprophyticus*

C3.47   Pigment production

For general purposes, inoculate a Nutrient Agar plate with a drop of a light suspension of the organism, incubate for 24 hours at 37 °C and then transfer to room temperature and observe for up to 5 days. Record the colours as red, orange, yellow, green, violet, brown, or negative i.e. produces none of these pigments.

For *Chromobacterium* species use Mannitol Yeast Extract Agar (A2.4.2). Incubate at 22–30 °C.

For mycobacteria, inoculate two Lowenstein-Jensen slopes directly from the primary isolate. Incubate one in continuous light; the other should be wrapped to exclude light or incubated in a closed box. Continuous light can be provided by placing a 'cold' fluorescent tube (e.g. 18" long) in the incubator (Collins, Lyne & Grange, 1989). For psychrophiles such as *M. marinum* exposure to day light at room temperature is acceptable.

For most *Pseudomonas* species use King's media (A2.4.3). Incubate medium A at 37 °C for 24–96 hours and medium B at 37 °C for 24 hours followed by 22 °C (or room temperature) for 72 hours. Kligler's Iron Agar (KIA) and TSI enhance the pigmentation of *Pseudomonas cepacia*.

Serratia marcescens strains vary in their media requirements for pigment production; try Nutrient Agar, Mannitol Yeast Extract Agar, or King's medium A at 22 °C or 30 °C.

Note. Non-pigmented strains are not uncommon and a suitable medium for inducing pigment production by all recalcitrant strains has not yet been produced. Micrococci produce pigment well on potato, but staphylococci do not seem to grow well enough on it to show any pigment. In general staphylococci produce pigment best in diffuse daylight.

C3.48   Poly-β-hydroxybutyric acid (PHBA) accumulation

Accumulation of poly-β-hydroxybutyrate (PHB) can be seen by phase-contrast microscopy and confirmed by staining with Sudan black (Stanier, Palleroni & Doudoroff, 1966), or with dilute carbol fuchsin; it may be confirmed by chemical extraction (Williamson & Wilkinson, 1958). The methods are hardly routine in clinical laboratories, but if the information can be obtained it will be useful in identifying pseudomonads.

Method: Inoculate Polyhydroxybutyrate Agar (A2.6.31) and examine after incubation for two days at the optimum temperature for growth. For the presence of PHB inclusions, examine films of the growth microscopically by staining with Sudan Black (B1.18). Dry the film in air and fix by flaming. Flood the slide with freshly filtered Sudan Black stain and leave at room temperature for 15 minutes. Drain off excess stain, blot and allow to dry. Rinse with xylol and blot dry. Counterstain lightly with 1% aqueous safranin for 5–10 seconds, rinse in running water and blot dry.

A positive reaction is indicated by some but rarely all of the organisms showing a purple-black appearance under the microscope.

C3.49   Polysaccharide formation on sucrose media

Inoculate Sucrose Broth (A2.5.3) and incubate. Much dextran formation is shown by an increased viscosity of the culture and the dextran may be flocculated by the addition of ethanol. The dextran is best recognized by a precipitin test in which the broth culture is set up against a capsular antiserum to *Streptococcus pneumoniae* type 2.

Inoculate a plate of Sucrose Agar and incubate. Levan-producing organisms grow as large mucoid colonies; dextran-producing organisms (e.g. *Streptococcus sanguis*) may form small glassy colonies on this medium.

Controls: dextran produced– *Streptococcus sanguis*
  levan produced   – *Streptococcus salivarius*
  neither produced – *Enterococcus faecalis*

C3.50   Porphyrin (ALA) test for haemophili
(Kilian, 1974)

Enzyme substrate. Prepare δ-aminolaevulinic acid (ALA) 2 mM and $MgSO_4$ 0.8 mM in 0.1 M-phosphate buffer at pH 6.9 and filter-sterilize. The substrate can be stored in screw-capped glass bottles for several months at +4 °C and for use distribute in 0.5 ml volumes in small glass tubes as required.

Method 1. Add a full loopful of bacterial growth from a 24-hour Chocolate Agar plate to the substrate and incubate for 4 hours at 37 °C. After incubation expose the tube to Wood's lamp (maximum emission 360 nm) in a darkened room.

Red-fluorescence = positive for porphyrins, i.e. X-factor not required.

Method 2. Set up the test as in method 1 and incubate for 24 h at 37 °C. Add 0.5 ml Kovács' reagent (C1.7) and shake well.

Red colour in lower aqueous phase = positive for porphyrins, i.e. X-factor not required.

C3.51 Pyruvate fermentation test for streptococci

Inoculate slopes of Pyruvate medium (A2.6.32) with test strains and incubate at 37 °C for at least 2 days and examine daily. The indicator changes from green to yellow if pyruvate is fermented.

Controls: positive – *Enterococcus faecalis*
negative – *Streptococcus salivarius*

Rapid coccal transformation on exposure of air – see Campylobacter tests C3.13

C3.52 Salt tolerance of streptococci

Inoculate 4% and 6.5% Salt Broth (A2.6.33) containing 0.1% (w/v) glucose with the test organism and incubate at 37 °C for at least 2 days. Examine daily for growth.

Controls: positive (6.5% NaCl) – *Enterococcus faecalis*
positive (4% NaCl) – *Streptococcus agalactiae*
negative – *Streptococcus sanguis*

C3.53 Selenite reduction

Inoculate a tube of 0.4% Selenite Broth (A2.6.34) with a light suspension of the organism and incubate for 2 days. A positive result is indicated by the appearance of a brick-red precipitate of metallic selenium.

Controls: positive – *Salmonella subgenus III*
negative – *Buttiauxiella agrestis*

C3.54 Starch hydrolysis

Inoculate lightly Starch Agar (A2.5.13) or Nutrient Agar (A2.1.1) containing 0.2% soluble starch and incubate plates at 30 °C for 5 days. For streptococci, incubate at 37 °C in air with added CO_2 for two days.

Method 1. Flood the plate with Lugol's iodine solution (B1.12); the medium turns blue where starch has not been hydrolysed; clear colourless zones indicate hydrolysis.

Method 2 (Kellerman & McBeth, 1912). Flood the plate with 95% ethanol; milky-white areas indicate no action on starch, whereas clear zones indicate hydrolysis. This reaction is not instantaneous and is best observed 30 minutes after addition of the ethanol.

Note. Some strains of *Bacillus* species produce only restricted zones of hydrolysis that may not be obvious until the bacterial growth has been scraped away.

Controls: positive – *Bacillus subtilis, Streptococcus bovis,*
biotype 1
negative – *Escherichia coli, Streptococcus salivarius*

C3.55 Streptococcal grouping

Preparation of the extract

1. *Acid extraction* (modified from Lancefield, 1933). Mix the growth from a quarter of a Blood Agar plate or the centrifuged deposit from a culture (10–25 ml) in Todd–Hewitt broth with 0.4 ml 0.2 N-HCl and place in a boiling water bath for 10 minutes. Cool and neutralize the supernatant with 0.2 N-NaOH, using phenol red as the indicator. Centrifuge and use the supernatant.

2. *Formamide extraction* (Fuller, 1938). Mix the growth from a quarter of a Blood Agar plate or the centrifuged deposit from 5 ml of a culture in Todd-Hewitt broth with 0.1 ml formamide and heat in an oil bath at 160 °C for 15 minutes or until the growth is almost completely dissolved. Add 0.25 ml 95% ethanol containing 0.5% HCl, shake and centrifuge. Discard the precipitate and add 0.5 ml acetone to the supernatant. Shake, centrifuge, and discard the supernatant. Dissolve the precipitate in 0.4 ml saline, and neutralize with 0.2 N-NaOH using phenol red as the indicator.

3. *Enzymic extraction* (Maxted, 1948). Suspend a loopful of growth from a Blood Agar plate in 0.25 ml enzyme solution (C1.8) and heat in a water bath at 50 °C until clear (about 1–2 hours).

The test method

Prepare 'grouping pipettes' from 5 mm diam. glass tubing by drawing out one end into a capillary. Cut to a total length of about 3 cm and stand vertically by placing the capillary end in a block of Plasticine (modelling clay) or similar material. Place a drop of antiserum in the pipette and layer the extract on top. The formation of a precipitate at the interface of the two layers within 2–3 minutes indicates a positive reaction.

Alternatively, use Ouchterlony-type double diffusion tests in agar on slides. Place the streptococcal extracts from the test and control strains and also the grouping antisera in approp;riate wells; incubate and observe for lines of identity between the test and control strains.

Notes. While strains of groups A, B, C and G are those most often investigated in medical laboratories, the tests should be made against all available group antisera. Commercial kits are available for groups A, B, C, D, F & G. By Lancefield's method, some strains are better extracted with 0.07 N-HCl; others, particularly group B strains, yield better extracts by heating at 50 °C for 2 hours (Williams, 1958).

Cross-reactions may occur when the extract prepared by the formamide method is too alkaline. This method tends to destroy the group O antigen.

Maxted's enzyme method is suitable for streptococci of groups A, C and G but strains of other groups (especially D) are less easily lysed by the enzyme.

Group D strains do not always give good reactions and, when suspected, should be grown in broth containing 0.5% glucose.

C3.56   Streptococcal enzyme tests

Production of the enzymes leucine aminopeptidase and pyrrolydonylarylamidase (pyroglutamase or PYRA) are important characters for the identification and differentiation of streptococci. To detect their presence, prepare the respective substrates (L-leucyl-β-naphthylamide and L-pyrrolydonyl-β-naphthylamide) as 0.01% solutions in phosphate-buffered saline (pH 7.3) and sterilize by autoclaving at 121 °C for 10 minutes. For use add 200 µl volumes of each substrate to separate small, capped tubes. Inoculate a tube of each substrate with growth from a fresh culture on Blood Agar to give a turbid suspension. Incubate at 37 °C for 4 hours and then add 50 µl of dimethylaminocinnamaldehyde in 10% (v/v) concentrated HCl to each tube. A red colour developing within 30 seconds denotes a positive result.
Controls:

Leucine aminopeptidase
> positive – *Streptococcus agalactiae*
> negative – *Staphylococcus saprophyticus*

Pyrrolydonylarylamidase
> positive – *Streptococcus pyogenes*
> negative – *Streptococcus agalactiae*

C3.57   String of pearls test
(Charlton, 1980)

Bacillus anthracis produces swollen round cells in chains ('strings of pearls') when incubated for 3–6 hours on Tryptose Agar containing 0.05–0.5 units/ml of penicillin.

To 100 ml of molten Nutrient Agar, add 1 ml of a solution of sodium benzyl penicillin containing 50 units/ml and mix carefully. Pour into Petri dishes and allow to set. With a scalpel cut a block about 1.6 cm^2 from the penicillin-agar plate and place it on a microscope slide in a Petri dish containing a small piece of moistened absorbent cotton wool or filter paper to prevent the agar drying out. Use a young colony to streak inoculate the centre of the agar block. Place a clean coverslip marked on one side about 5 mm from one edge on the agar block so that the marked line is face down alongside the streak inoculum. The line acts as a focussing and location guide. With the lid on, incubate the Petri dish at 37 °C. After 2 hours, remove the slide and examine the inoculum microscopicaly by oil immersion for the 'strings of pearls' growth.

C3.58   Tellurite tolerance

Inoculate Blood Tellurite Agar plates (A2.3.3) and incubate at 37 °C for 24 h. Tellurite-resistant organisms show a heavy growth of jet-black colonies; tellurite-sensitive organisms fail to grow or show a very light growth, the colonies usually being visible only with a hand lens.
Control: positive   – *Enterococcus faecalis*
> negative – *Streptococcus agalactiae*

C3.59   Temperature range for growth

The general principle of this type of test is that a suitable medium is lightly inoculated with the organism under test and incubated at different temperatures. For temperatures above 37 °C, a thermostatically controlled (±0.5 °C) water bath is preferable to an incubator, though heating blocks are even better as they avoid the possibility of contamination from the water.

With aerobic spore-forming bacilli, mycobacteria, and actinomycetes, a solid medium (as a slope) is preferable; with other organisms liquid media are used.

For streptococci, Abd-el-Malek & Gibson (1948a) recommended Litmus Milk; for organisms showing little activity in plain milk they add 0.25% each of glucose and yeast extract.

At 22 °C and above examine cultures for growth daily for up to 7 days; at lower temperatures after 7 and 14 days. The exact duration of incubation will depend upon the normal growth rate of the organism. The ability of an organism to grow at a particular temperature should be confirmed by growth at that temperature after subculture.

C3.60   Temperature tolerance (60 °C) for enterococci and similar organisms

Place 1 ml of a 24-hour Nutrient Broth or Serum Broth cul-

237

ture in a small test tube, and place in a water bath at 60 °C for 30 minutes. Cool under cold running water and incubate at 37 °C for 24 hours. Subculture to a Serum Agar slope and incubate for 24 hours. Examine for growth which indicates the ability of the organism to survive the temperature–time conditions.

Controls: positive – *Enterococcus faecalis*
negative – *Streptococcus pyogenes*

C3.61 Tween 80 hydrolysis

Method 1 (Sierra 1957). Streak-inoculate the test culture on the surface of Tween 80 Nutrient Agar (A2.6.39); incubate at the optimal growth temperature of the organism. Look at the plate each day; an opaque halo of precipitation around the growth indicates hydrolysis of the Tween.

Controls: positive – *Pseudomonas aeruginosa*
negative – *Bordetella bronchiseptica*

Method 2 (modified from Wayne, 1962). A solution of Tween 80 (0.5%) in phosphate buffer, pH 7.0, with neutral red as indicator, is distributed in 2 ml volumes in small screw-capped containers and autoclaved. The final colour should be amber. Store at 4 °C, protected from light, and use within 4 weeks.

Inoculate with a large loopful of growth from Glycerol egg medium, incubate at 37 °C and read twice weekly for 3 weeks.

Controls: positive – *Mycobacterium kansasii*
negative – (i) uninoculated medium
(ii) *Mycobacterium fortuitum* group

C3.62 Urease activity

Method 1. Inoculate heavily a slope of Christensen's Urea medium (A2.6.41); examine after incubation for 4 hours and daily for 5 days. Red colour = positive. For *Helicobacter pylori* inoculate heavily 0.5 ml Christensen's Urea medium without agar. Shake well and examine for pink colour after standing for 5 minutes.

Method 2. Inoculate heavily a tube of SSR Urea medium (A2.6.41); incubate and examine daily for 7 days. Red colour = urea hydrolysed.

Method 3 (Stuart, van Stratum & Rustigian, 1945). Medium for rapid test: to 380 ml distilled water add KH$_2$PO$_4$, 364 mg; Na$_2$HPO$_4$, 380 mg; urea, 8 g; yeast extract, 40 mg; 0.02% phenol red, 20 ml; pH 6.8. Filter to sterilize.

Test: pipette 1.5 ml volumes into small tubes and inoculate heavily with growth from a solid medium. Incubate at 37 °C in a water bath. *Proteus* species produce a red colour in 5–60 minutes.

Method 4 (Hormaeche & Munilla, 1957). Test solution: to 100 ml 2% urea solution add 2 ml 0.04% cresol red. Distribute in 1 ml volumes into small tubes; sterilization is not necessary when the test is to be made on the same day. Inoculate the tubes heavily with growth from a 24-hour agar culture (older cultures are too alkaline). Place the tubes in a water bath at 45–50 °C for 2 hours. Urease-positive cultures produce a violet red colour.

Method 5 for haemophili (Maslen, 1952). Inoculate Maslen's Urea Broth (A2.6.41) heavily with growth from a fresh agar culture not more than 18 hours old. Incubate at 37 °C for 5–18 hours. The rapid development of a red colour indicates urease activity.

Method 6. NCTC micromethod. Suspensions are made from growth on either Nutrient or Glucose Agar; the latter usually give stronger reactions.

2% urea aqueous solution	0.06 ml
0.025 M-phosphate buffer, pH 6.0 phenol red	0.06 ml
Suspension of organism	0.04 ml

Place in 37 °C water bath and observe at intervals of 15 minutes for the first hour; leave negative reactions for a final reading at 4 hours. Positive tests show a red colour.

This is better than the test given by Clarke & Cowan (1952).

Controls: positive – *Proteus vulgaris*
negative – *Escherichia coli*

Voges-Proskaüer (VP) reactions: see C3.1.

C3.63 'X' and 'V' factor requirements

Method 1. Inoculate a Blood Agar plate and a Nutrient Agar plate with the organism and spot inoculate a strain of *Staphylococcus aureus* on each plate. Observe each plate for growth and for 'satellitism'.

Growth on Blood Agar plate only	= requires X factor
Growth shows 'satellitism' on Blood Agar	= requires X and V factors
Shows 'satellitism' on both media	= requires V factor
Growth on both media but not showing 'satellitism'	= neither X nor V factor required

Method 2. Inoculate a Nutrient Agar plate and lay an X-factor and a V-factor disc (C1.18) on the surface at a distance of about 2 cm from each other. Examine for growth in the vicinity of one or both discs.

APPENDIX D
Test organisms

Most of the biochemical characterization tests described in this *Manual* should be controlled by organisms that are known to give either positive or negative reactions under appropriate conditions. For this purpose, we list in Table D1 the species recommended together with the accession numbers of suitable strains available from the National Collection of Type Cultures, Central Public Health Laboratory, Colindale Avenue, London NW9 5HT and, in many instances, also from the American Type Culture Collection, 12301 Parklawn Drive, Rockville, Maryland 20852, USA. As controls for the common tests shown in Table D2, the set of four strains given is adequate. For other bacterial characters, the test strains shown in Table D3 may be used. We emphasize, however, that most of the organisms shown in these tables are pathogenic so that due regard must be paid to safety and hygiene in the laboratory.

For the maintenance and storage of test-control strains, freeze-dried (lyophilized) cultures which retain their characters and keep virtually indefinitely are ideal. However, for those who wish to keep frequently used strains for immediate use, we give in Table D4 suggestions for the nutrient media, cultural conditions and short-term storage period in order to be reasonably sure of their survival before they need replacement from stock cultures.

Table D1. *Recommended strains of test organisms*

	NCTC	ATCC
Acinetobacter calcoaceticus	7844	15308
Aeromonas hydrophila	7810	9071
Alcaligenes faecalis	655	
Bacillus stearothermophilus	10003	
Bacillus subtilis	3610	6051
Bordetella bronchiseptica	452	19395
Buttiauxella agrestis	12119	
Campylobacter jejuni biotype I	11168	
Campylobacter jejuni biotype IV	12145	
Campylobacter fetus subsp. *fetus*	10842	
Clostridium perfringens	6719	9856
Clostridium sporogenes	533	10000
Clostridium tetani (toxigenic)	279	19406
Clostridium tetani (non-toxigenic strain)	6336	

	NCTC	ATCC
Enterobacter aerogenes	10006	13048
Enterobacter cloacae	10005	13047
Enterococcus faecalis	8213[a]	
Escherichia coli	9001	11775
Helicobacter pylori	11637	
Klebsiella pneumonial subsp. *aerogenes*	418	15380
Legionella pneumophila	11192	33152
Morganella morganii	10041[b]	
Mycobacterium tuberculosis	7416	9360
Mycobacterium fortuitum	10394	6841
Mycobacterium kansasii	10268	14471
Mycobacterium phlei	8151	19249
Mycobacterium smegmatis	8159	19420
Nocardia brasiliensis	10300	19295
Nocardia otitidis-caviarum	1934	14629
Proteus vulgaris	4175	13315
Pseudomonas aeruginosa	7244	7700
Salmonella typhi	786	
Salmonella typhimurium	74	13311
Serratia marcescens	1377	274
Shigella dysenteriae 1	4837	13313
Shigella sonnei	8220	
Staphylococcus aureus	8532	12600
Staphylococcus saprophyticus	4276[c]	
Streptococcus agalactiae	8181	13813
Streptococcus anginosus ('S. milleri')	10708	
Streptococcus dysgalactiae	4669	
Streptococcus pneumoniae	7465	10015
Streptococcus salivarius	8618[d]	7073
Streptococcus sanguis	7863[e]	10556
Vibrio alginolyticus	12160	17749
Vibrio furnissii	11218[f]	
Vibrio parahaemolyticus	10903	17802

[a] Listed as *Streptococcus faecalis* in NCTC Catalogue (1972, 1989).
[b] Listed as *Proteus morganii* in NCTC Catalogue (1972, 1989).
[c] Listed as *Micrococcus* sp. subgroup 1 in NCTC Catalogue (1972), and as *Staphylococcus epidermidis* in Cowan & Steel (1974).
[d] Listed as *Streptococcus hominis* in NCTC Catalogue (1972) and as *Streptococcus* species Group K in NCTC Catalogue (1989).
[e] Listed as *Streptoccus* species Group H in NCTC catalogue (1972).
[f] Listed as *Vibrio fluvialis* in NCTC Catalogue (1989).

239

Table D2. *Control strains for commonly used tests*

Test	NCTC Strain Positive	NCTC Strain Negative	Test	NCTC Strain Positive	NCTC Strain Negative
Aesculin hydrolysis	11935	11934	Voges Proskaüer	11935	7475
Citrate utilization	7475	11934	Gas from glucose	11936	11935
Decarboxylases			Acid from:		
Arginine	11936	7475	Adonitol	7475	11934
Lysine	11935	7475	Arabinose	11936	11934
Ornithine	11935	7475	Dulcitol	11936	11934
Deoxyribonuclease	11935	11934	Inositol	11935	11934
Gelatin liquefaction	11935	11936	Lactose	11936	11934
Gluconate oxidation	11936	7475	Maltose	11936	7475
Hydrogen sulphide (TSI)	11934	7475	Mannitol	11936	11934
Indole production	7475	11935	Raffinose	11936	11934
KCN tolerance	7475	11934	Rhamnose	11936	11934
Malonate utilization	11936	7475	Salicin	11935	11934
Methyl red	7475	11935	Sorbitol	11936	11934
ONPG	11935	7475	Sucrose	11936	11934
PPA production	7475	11936	Trehalose	11936	11934
Selenite reduction	11936	11934	Xylose	11936	11934
Urease	7475	11935			

NCTC 11935 = *Serratia marcescens*
NCTC 11934 = *Edwardsiella tarda*
NCTC 7475 = *Proteus rettgeri*
NCTC 11936 = *Enterobacter cloacae*

Table D3. *Further tests and recommended control strains*

Test	Control organism	NCTC number	ATCC number	Expected result
Bacitracin sensitivity	*Streptococcus pyogenes*	8198	12344	Sensitive
	Streptococcus viridans	10712 *		Resistant
Catalase	*Staphylococcus aureus*	8532	12600	Positive
	Streptococcus pyogenes	8198	12344	Negative
Coagulase	*Staphylococcus aureus*	8532	12600	Positive
	Staphylococcus saprophyticus	4276		Negative
Deoxyribonuclease	*Staphylococcus aureus*	8532	12600	Positive
	Staphylococcus saprophyticus	4276		Negative
Haemolysis	*Streptococcus pyogenes*	8198	12344	β-haemolysis
	Streptococcus viridans	10712 *		α-haemolysis
	Staphylococcus saprophyticus	4276		No haemolysis
Oxidation/Fermentation	*Pseudomonas aeruginosa*	10662	25668	Oxidative
	Serratia marcescens	11935		Fermentative
	Acinetobacter lwoffii	5866	15309	Alkaline or negative
Motility	*Serratia marcescens*	11935		Motile
	Acinetobacter lwoffii	5866	15309	Non-motile
Nitrate reduction	*Serratia marcescens*	11935		Positive
	Acinetobacter lwoffii	5866	25668	Negative
Optochin sensitivity	*Streptococcus pneumoniae*	10319		Sensitive
	Streptococcus viridans	10712 *		Resistant
Oxidase	*Pseudomonas aeruginosa*	10662	15309	Positive
	Acinetobacter lwoffii	5866	15309	Negative
Phosphatase	*Staphylococcus aureus*	8532	12600	Positive
	Staphylococcus saprophyticus	4276		Negative
Toxigenicity testing of *C. diphtheriae*	*Corynebacterium diphtheriae*	10648		Positive
	Corynebacterium diphtheriae	3984	19409	Weak positive
	Corynebacterium diphtheriae	10356		Negative
X- and V-factor	*Haemophilus influenzae*	10479		Requires X and V
	Haemophilus parainfluenzae	10665		Requires V
	Haemophilus canis	8540		Requires X

* Listed in NCTC Catalogue (1989) as *Streptoccus* species 'viridans' type; probably *S. mitior*.

241

Table D4. *Suggested conditions for subculture and short-term storage of test organisms*

Genus	Medium	Incubation Temp. (°C)	Time (hours)	Storage* (°C)	Maximum storage period (months)
Acinetobacter	Nutrient agar	37	18	5–25	3
Aeromonas	Nutrient agar	37	18	5–25	3
Alcaligenes	Nutrient agar	37	18	5–25	3
Bacillus	Nutrient agar	30	18	5–25	12
Clostridium	Cooked meat	37	18	5–25	12
Enterobacter	Nutrient agar	37	18	5–25	6
Escherichia	Nutrient agar	37	18	5–25	6
Klebsiella	Nutrient agar	37	18	5–25	3
Mycobacterium†	Lowenstein-Jensen	37	48–72†	15–25	3
Neisseria	Chocolate agar	37	18	25–35	7days
Nocardia	Yeast extract glucose agar	37	48–72	15–25	3
Pseudomonas	Peptone water agar	30	18	5–25	3
Salmonella	Dorset egg	37	18	5–25	12
Shigella	Nutrient agar	37	18	5–25	6
Staphylococcus	Nutrient agar	37	18	5–25	3
Streptococcus	Cooked meat or	37	18	5–25	3
Enterococcus	Blood broth	37	18	5	1
Vibrio	Sloppy agar	30	48	22–25	1
Vibrio (marine)	Salt-water agar or 3% NaCl agar	30	48	15–20	1

* In the dark.

† *Mycobacterium tuberculosis* and other slow-growing mammalian pathogens should be incubated for 10–20 days or until growth is apparent to the naked eye.

APPENDIX E
Preparation and use of Identicards

E1   Identicard set for genus identification

Use a card with a single row of holes (Fig. 9.1).

For the master cards, the key to the numbered holes for the characters is shown in Table E1, and the plan for notching the holes in Table E2. All positive characters are notched from the hole to the edge of the card. For certain genera two or more cards may be needed to make provision for different reactions ('dee' characters) or differences in reading a test (e.g. catalase with *Aerococcus*). A guide card with the holes numbered or labelled is useful for the probing (sorting) operation.

Notching the unknown. Positive characters of the strain under test are notched from the appropriate hole (Table E1) to the edge of the card.

Probing. When notching the card for the unknown strain is complete put it at the front of the pack of master cards, correctly faced, and test each hole in turn with a probe such as a knitting needle.

A probe through the hole of a positive character of the unknown strain will, when lifted, remove master cards that are negative for that character and these can be discounted. The card for the unknown strain and master cards of genera in which that character is positive will drop out of the pack; these cards are collected together and tested again for another character, and so on. Conversely, when unnotched holes (negative characters) of the unknown strain are probed, the cards that are lifted out with the probe are retained for further testing, and those that drop out are discounted (Table E3).

The identity of the unknown strain (as far as can be determined by the set of cards used) will correspond with that of the master card that has similar notchings.

E2   Identicard set for species identification

Use cards with two rows of holes (Fig. 9.2*a*). In the master cards for species, the *outer* row of holes is notched for characters recorded as d, (d) and (+) in the tables in Chapters 6 and 7. Characters shown as + in the tables are notched to the *inner* row of holes (Fig. 9.2*b*). As an example, the notching plan for the enterobacteria is given in Tables E4 and E5.

Table E1. *Key for numbered or labelled holes in the Identicard set for Genera (card with single row of holes)*

Hole no.	Character represented
1	Gram reaction
2	Motility
3	Acid fastness
4	Spore formation
5	Coccus (bacillus [rod] is not notched)
6	Growth anaerobically
7	Growth in air
8	Oxidase
9	Catalase
10	Optional
11	Oxidative attack on sugars
12	Fermentative attack on sugars

Notching the unknown. Positive characters of the unknown organism are notched to the second (inner) row of holes in the two-row cards (Fig. 9.2*c*).

Probing. The completed card(s) is placed in front of the pack of master cards, correctly faced, and the probe inserted through the appropriate holes. In species identification, the probing procedure is different from that for genus identification (see Table E6).

Positive characters of the unknown strain are probed in the first (outer) hole, and the probe lifted to remove master cards in which that character is negative. The cards that drop out are retained for probing other characters in sequence on the card.

Negative characters are probed through the second (inner row) hole, and the cards that are retained on the probe are kept for further tests.

As with the cards for generic identification, the probing is continued until only one master card remains or all the holes have been probed.

Table E2. *Notching of master cards for Identicard set for genera*

Hole no.	1	2	3	4	5	6	7	8	9	10	11	12	Examples of notes for centre of cards
Aerococcus (a)	V				V	V	V					V	Catalase = −
Aerococcus (b)	V				V	V	V		V			V	Catalase = w
Aeromonas		V				V	V	V	V			V	Mesophilic
Aeromonas salmonicida						V	V	V	V			V	Psychrophilic (37 °C = no growth). Brown pigment.
Achromobacter		V				V	V	V		V			
Acidaminococcus				V	V								
Acinetobacter (a)				V		V		V		V			Coccobacillus – coccus
Acinetobacter (b)						V		V		V			Coccobacillus – bacillus
Actinobacillus						V	V	V	V			V	Gas not produced
Actinomyces	V					V						V	May branch
Agrobacterium		V				V	V	V		V			
Alcaligenes		V				V	V	V					
Anaerobiospirillum		V				V						V	
Arachnia	V					V	V					V	(Also *Actinomyces odontolyticus*) Branched, filamentous
Arcanobacterium	V					V	V					V	Microaerophilic
Arcobacter		V				V							Curved rods; 3-10% O$_2$
Bacillus (a)	V	V		V			V		V		V	V	Oxidase variable, ?inconstant
Bacillus (b)	V	V		V		V	V	V	V		V	V	Some spp. facultative [Ø]
Bacillus (c)	V	V		V		V	V	V	V		V	V	Carbohydrates: some spp. F some spp. O some spp. − / One sp. (*B. anthracis*) non-motile
Bacteroides (a)						V						V	Catalase variable
Bacteroides (b)						V			V				Most spp. non-motile
Bacteroides (c)		V				V						V	One sp. motile
Bifidobacterium	V					V						V	Tendency to branch
Bordetella							V	V	V				Does not grow on simple media
Branhamella					V		V	V	V				
Brochothrix	V					V	V		V			V	Catalase at RT
Brucella							V	V	V				Carboxyphilic; urease +
Campylobacter (a)		V						V	V				Will not grow under strict [Ø];
Campylobacter (b)		V						V					optimum = 5-10% O$_2$. Catalase = D
Cardiobacterium							V	V				V	Pleomorphic; metachromatic granules?
Chromobacterium		V				V	V	V	V			V	Mesophilic; growth at 37 °C. Violet pigment
Clostridium (a)	V	V		V		V						V	
Clostridium (b) (asporogenous)	V					V						V	*C. perfringens*; non-motile; seldom spores
Corynebacterium	V					V	V		V			V	Pleomorphic
Eikenella (a)						V	V	V					Needs CO$_2$ for isolation; soon [O]
Eikenella (b)						V		V					probably cannot grow [Ø]; ? other anaerobic species
Enterobacteria (a)		V				V	V		V			V	Most produce gas; NO$_3$ reduced
Enterobacteria (b)						V	V		V			V	Non-motile spp.
Enterobacteria (c)						V	V					V	*Shigella dysenteriae* 1 (Shiga's bacillus)
Enterococcus	V				V	V	V			V			Faecal streptococci
Erysipelothrix	V					V	V					V	
Eubacterium	V					V						V	
Flavobacterium							V	V	V	V			Yellow pigment
Francisella							V	V	V				Enriched media required; dangerous
Fusobacterium							V		V	V			Catalase variable
Gardnerella						V				V			Fastidious
Gemella (a)	V				V	V						V	Easily decolorized; usually
Gemella (b)						V						V	regarded as Gram-negative
Haemophilus (a)						V	V		V				Fastidious; needs X and/or V
Haemophilus (b)						V	V						factor; catalase variable
Helicobacter		V						V					Curved spiral rods; capnophilic; O$_2$ 6%
Janthinobacterium		V					V	V	V			V	Psychrophilic (37 °C = no growth). Violet pigment
Kingella							V	V				V	

Table E2. *(contd.)*

Hole no.	1	2	3	4	5	6	7	8	9	10	11	12	Examples of notes for centre of cards
Kurthia	V	V				V		V					Can grow at low temperatures
Lactobacillus	V				V	V						V	Grows best at about pH 6
Legionella (a)					V	V	V	V				V	⎧ Requires cysteine and iron for growth; catalase +
Legionella (b)					V	V						V	⎩ but some strains give weak reaction
Leuconostoc	V			V	V							V	May form dextran
Listeria	V	V			V	V		V				V	Can grow at low temperatures
Megasphaera				V	V								Large cell size (< 2 μm)
Micrococcus	V			V		V		V		V			Colonies often pigmented
Mobiluncus		V			V								Curved anaerobic rods
Moraxella						V	V	V					Growth improved with blood or serum
Mycobacterium	V		V			V				V			Does not branch or produce aerial hyphae
Neisseria				V		V	V	V		V			Prefer added CO_2
Nocardia (a)	V		V			V		V					Feebly acid-fast; produce aerial hyphae
Nocardia (b)	V					V		V		V			Some spp. (strains) not acid-fast
Ochrobactrum		V				V	V	V		V			*Achromobacter* group A
Pasteurella					V	V	V	V				V	Gas not produced
Pediococcus	V			V	V	V						V	Tetrads common
Peptococcus	V			V	V								Metronidazole-sensitive
Peptostreptococcus	V			V	V							V	Gas may be produced; metronidazole-sensitive
Plesiomonas		V				V	V	V	V			V	Gas not produced; indole +; gelatin −
Propionibacterium	V					V			V			V	Club shapes; branching
Pseudomonas		V					V	V	V	V			May produce fluorescent or green pigment
Rothia	V					V		V				V	⎧ Filamentous; no mycelium or hyphae. Will grow under microaerophilic conditions
Shewanella		V				V	V	V		V			Pink pigmentation; copious H_2S
Staphylococcus	V			V	V	V		V			V		
Stomatococcus	V			V	V	V		V			V		
Streptobacillus *				V	V						V		Needs enrichment; sensitive to Liquoid
Streptococcus	V			V	V	V					V		
Veillonella (a)				V	V								⎧ Catalase variable
Veillonella (b)				V	V			V					⎩ Catalase variable
Vibrio		V			V	V	V	V			V		Gas not produced. Arginine −; lysine +; ornithine +

V = notched (positive character)   * Also *Shigella dysenteriae 1*

See Table E1 for key to holes.
See Tables 5.1 and 5.2 on p.47 for explanation of the symbols used in the column of Notes.

Table E3. *Notching and probing of cards (single row) and action after probing*

Character of unknown strain	Card of unknown strain	Cards from probed set	
		remaining on probe	dropping out
Positive	Notched	Discount (ignore)	Keep and retest for other characters
Negative	Not notched	Keep and retest for other characters	Discount (ignore)

Table E4. *Key to numbered holes for species Identicard set (card with two rows of holes) for enterobacteria*

Hole No.	Character represented
1	Growth in KCN medium
2	Utilization of citrate as C source
3	Gas from glucose
4	VP reaction
5	Gelatin hydrolysis
6	Urease
7	Phenylalanine deaminase (PPA test)
8	Motility
9	H_2S production from TSI
10	Malonate
11	Arginine dihydrolase
12	Lysine decarboxylase
13	Ornithine decarboxylase
14	Optional
15	Optional
16	Adonitol, acid
17	Dulcitol, acid
18	Mannitol, acid
19	Lactose, acid
20	Indole produced

Table E5. *Notching of master cards for species Identicard set (card with two rows of holes) for enterobacteria encountered clinically*

Hole No.	1	2	3	4	5	6	7	8	9	10	11	12	13	14	15	16	17	18	19	20
1 *Escherichia coli*			V					O		O	V	O					O	V	V	V
2 *Escherichia adecarboxylata*	V		V		O			V		V				V	V	V	V	V		
3 *Edwardsiella tarda*			V					V	V			V	V					V		
4 *Yersinia pestis*																		V		
5 *Yersinia pseudotuberculosis*						V		V									V	V		
6 *Yersinia enterocolitica*						V		V					V					V		O
7 *Shigella dysenteriae* 1											O									O
8 *Shigella dysenteriae* 2–10																				O
9 *Shigella flexneri* 1–5																				O
10 *Shigella flexneri* 6			O								O						O	V		
11 *Shigella boydii*											O							V		O
12 *Shigella sonnei*													V					V	O	
13 *Citrobacter freundii*	V	V	V				V	V			O		O				O	V	O	
14 *Citrobacter koseri*		V	V			V		V		V	O		V			V	O	V	O	V
15 *Cedecea* spp.	O	V	O	O				V		V	V		O			V	O			
16 *Salmonella typhi*								V	V		O	V					O	V		
17 *Salmonella pullorum*		O	V								V	V	V					V		
18 *Salmonella gallinarum*		O									O	V					V	V		
19 *Salmonella choleraesuis*		O	V					V	O		O	V	V				O	V		
20 *Salmonella* Subgenus I		V	V					V	V		O	V	V				V	V		
21 *Salmonella* Subgenus II		V	V			O		V	V	V	V	V	V				V	V		
22 *Salmonella* Subgenus III		V	V			O		V	V	V		V	V					V	O	
23 *Salmonella* Subgenus IV	V	V	V			O		V	V		V	V	V					V		
24 *Erwinia herbicola*		V			V			V		V								V	O	
25 *Morganella morganii*	V		V			V	V	V					V					V		V
26 *Proteus vulgaris*	V	O	V		V	V	V	V	V											V
27 *Proteus mirabilis*	V	O	V	O	V	V	V	V	V				V							V
28 *Proteus penneri*	V		V		V	V	V	O	O											
29 *Providencia rettgeri*	V	V				V	V	V								V		V		V
30 *Providencia alcalifaciens*	V	V	V					V	V							V				V
31 *Providencia stuartii*	V	V					V	V												V
32 *Hafnia alvei*	V	V	V	V				V			O		V	V				V		
33 *Serratia marcescens*	V	V	O	V	V			V			O		V	V		O		V		
34 *Serratia liquefaciens*	V	V	V	V	V	O		V					O	V				V	O	
35 *Serratia marinorubra*	V	O	O	V	V	O		V			O		O			V		V	V	
36 *Serratia plymuthica*	O	O	O	O	V			V									V	O		
37 *Serratia odorifera*	V	V			V			V				V	O			O		V	O	
38 *Enterobacter cloacae*	V	V	V	V	O	O		V			O	V		V		O	O	V	O	
39 *Enterobacter aerogenes*	V	V	V	V	O	O		V			V		V	V		V	O	V	V	
40 *Klebsiella oxytoca*	V	V	V	V	V	V					O		V			V	V	V	V	V
41 *Klebsiella pneumoniae* subsp. *aerogenes*	V	V	V	V	O	V					V		V			V	O	V	V	
42 *Klebsiella pneumoniae* subsp. *pneumoniae*		V	V		V						V		V			V	V	V	V	
43 *Klebsiella pneumoniae* subsp. *ozaenae*	V	O	O		O						O					V	O	V	O	
44 *Klebsiella pneumoniae* subsp. *rhinoscleromatis*	V									V						V		V		
45 *Kluyvera* spp.	V	V	V					V			V		O	V			V	V		O
46 *Tatumella ptyseos*																				

V = Notched to the inner row (plus line): usually positive   O = Notched to the outer row (dee line): sometimes positive

Blank (no entry) = Negative

See Table E4 for key to holes.

Table E6. *Notching and probing of cards (double row) and action after probing*

Character of unknown strain	Card of unknown strain	Row tested	Cards from probed set	
			Remaining on probe	Dropping out
Positive	Notched to inner row	Outer	Discount (Ignore)	Keep for retest
Negative	Not notched	Inner	Keep for retest	Discount (Ignore)

APPENDIX F
Use of computers

The availability of laboratory-based computers is increasing considerably, not only because of reductions in their price and size but also because programs suitable for epidemiological and microbiological purposes are more readily available. Historically, laboratory computing developed from the work of relatively few laboratories with limited access to the large mainframe computer facilities available in the 1960s. These were the 'first generation' of laboratory computers. They have all been replaced now by second and even third generation computer 'hardware' (the collective term used to describe the computer processor, the magnetic disk or tape storage apparatus as well as the visual display terminals and printer) and the associated 'software' (the programs for various applications). With the development of the 'silicon chip' all the associated hardware and software is available now for small sized micro-computers which have memory power and data storage capacity equivalent to those of their large predecessors. Any detailed description will undoubtedly soon be out of date but computer facilities with visual display terminals, printers, and adequate magnetic disk storage for as much as three years' clinical laboratory workload together with the necessary software (and training) are currently available at a modest cost. Such computer systems are well suited not only for bacterial identification purposes but also for a broad range of other uses in the microbiology laboratory. For those considering the use of computers but without experience of them, we give here brief guidance on how to go about it and list the basic essentials necessary for bacterial identification purposes. As a useful general introduction to the wide variety of computer equipment and applications currently available, *Computers and their Use* by Carter & Huzman (1984) is recommended. Like practical bacteriology, however, there is no substitute for experience. It is therefore important to appreciate that the value of computers depends not only on the programs used to instruct them (and thus on the skills of programmers) but also on the quality of the data used; hence the aphorism 'garbage in, garbage out'.

A complete 'computer package' consists of the actual computer processor – the electronic 'brain' – which is designed to receive and act upon instructions conveyed to it through a keyboard. These instructions and the ensuing results are displayed visually either in colour or in monochrome on a video display unit (VDU) or monitor screen. The means or 'language' by which the computer is instructed or programmed via the keyboard varies according to its use and function. The usual 'languages' used with microcomputers include BASIC (Beginners All-Purpose Symbolic Instruction Code), 'C', PASCAL (named after a French scientist), SQL (Structured Query Language), MUMPS (Massachusetts General Hospital Utility Multi-Programming System), FORTRAN (Formula Translation) and COBOL (Common Business Oriented Language). The various languages available simply mean that different keyboard letters or symbols and different sequences are used to represent specific programming instructions for different computers, many of which are designed for particular functions and objectives. Most of the languages mentioned can be used with many different computers though sometimes a particular model can provide a specific function which might not be available with other computers. Although understanding how to use the keyboard language to instruct the computer is not easy for the inexperienced, all software is supplied with complete and detailed instructions for keyboard use. The American National Standards Institute (ANSI) has promoted standardization of some of these computer languages by providing and updating guidelines for their compliance and use. The 'standardized' languages accepted by ANSI include BASIC, FORTRAN, COBOL, MUMPS and SQL. Provided that written programs keep to the ANSI recommendations, they should be capable of ready conversion so as to be compatible for use with a wide range of computers. Each language has its own particular advantages and disadvantages but they all provide the means for instructing the computer. The languages cited are termed 'high level' because although they use clear English-type keyboard terms such as INPUT, ENTER, PRINT, etc, these instructions have to be 'interpreted' and converted into 'low level' binary code language (termed machine code) either built into the computer or by using a software program called a 'compiler'; similarly, an 'assembler' program may be required to convert 'low level' language into machine code. Low level languages are usually much faster in use as the computer processor has less interpretation to do. However, writing such programs tends to be time consuming because the instructions are not in normal everyday language. Conversely high level languages are usually faster to instruct but slower for the computer to execute. All these and other factors are taken into account by professional computer programmers when selecting the language appropriate for a particular application.

Computers will retain the instructions programmed only as long as they are supplied with electricity. It is therefore usual to have a separate means of storing the computer programs so that the power supply can be turned off between use. These program storage devices range from magnetic tapes in cassettes to specialised magnetic ('floppy') disks. The magnetic coating retains the program until it is changed by another magnetic field which occurs when amending the instructions or when writing new ones. The information is stored in the form of binary digits termed 'bits' which are usually arranged in groups of eight or sixteen to form 'bytes'. Floppy disks are readily available in two inexpensive sizes: the smaller ($3^1/_2$ in; 8.8 cm) – the so-called 'stiffy', and the larger ($5^1/_4$ in; 9.9 cm). The latter holds up to 360 000 characters of information (360 kb or kilobytes), the smaller 'stiffy' up to 1 440 000 characters (1.4 Mb or megabytes). In addition, 'hard' disks are available which can store from 20 000 000 to 100 000 000 characters (20–100 Mb). The computer retrieves information from these storage devices by means of an operating system in the form of a special program contained either on the disk or in the computer thus enabling the user to control the procedures. Suitably instructed, the operating system will display information on the visual monitor screen; print it out; capture and store data 'typed' in from the keyboard; and store, retrieve, delete and amend instructions on the associated storage equipment.

For bacterial identification by computer, a database containing adequate information about the test characters of a suitable range of known species is first necessary. We describe in Chapter 10 how this information is recorded and transcribed into a form suitable for database compilation together with a simple theoretical example to illustrate the usual methods and statistical procedures used for comparing unknown strains with those in the database. With the large databases necessary for confidence in the results, it is obviously more efficient for speedy bacterial identification to use tailor-made programs prepared with detailed computer instructions. Databases suitable for the identification of medical bacteria have been compiled in many countries and are often used now for tabulating the results in scientific papers. Unlike the diagnostic tables as presented in this *Manual* with the test results represented by +, –, d and other symbols, database tables express them as percentages or as probabilities for the characters specified (Bascomb et al., 1973; Kelley & Kellog, 1978; Wayne et al., 1980; Feltham & Sneath, 1982; Williams et al., 1983; Feltham, Wood & Sneath, 1984; Bryant et al., 1986*b*). Diagnostic kit manufacturers have used such computer proformas to generate profile registers or lists of medical bacteria characterized in this way. Some have also provided computer programs and the necessary databases for use with their own diagnostic kits.

Several computer manufacturers designed their computers for this highly competitive market but their numbers reduced gradually until IBM, the largest computer company, dominated the field with its personal computer in the majority of countries. Its personal computer disk operating system, PC.DOS and, for other computers the equivalent disk operating system MS.DOS or Windows 3 (produced by the company Microsoft), are now used universally as a virtual international standard. The programs called GENMAT (general matrix) containing the material tabulated in this *Manual* as described by Feltham, Wood & Sneath (1984) are all written in BASIC language for PC or MS. DOS operation. They are therefore suitable for use with most computers and all those compatible with IBM personal computers. To identify bacteria with an MS.DOS BASIC computer identification program such as GENMAT based on the tables in this *Manual,* the following equipment is suggested: IBM Personal Computer or one compatible with it; 640Kb or greater memory and keyboard; data storage facility with as a minimum dual floppy disks; 80 column dot matrix printer; MS.DOS (3.2 or later version) and BASIC language implementation. Other commercial computer software packages useful in the microbiology laboratory include those for word-processing, spreadsheets, graphics for histograms, pie charts, etc, and databases for literature references, addresses and the like. For clear and simple instructions on how to program a computer in easy stages and in a methodical way with BASIC language, we can recommend '*Computer Programming in BASIC*' by Carter and Huzman (1987).

Computers can also be used in the microbiology laboratory for a broad range of other purposes including the routine data handling requirements of clinical laboratories (Rant, Feltham & Shepherd, 1987). Electronic 'daybooks' together with entry of results and printed reports provide the core of most systems. Quite apart from the classification and identification of bacteria, many laboratories have extended this basic need to monitoring for hospital infection control and surveillance purposes; to the epidemiology and trend analysis of communicable diseases and outbreaks for public health purposes; to the reading and interpretation of manual laboratory procedures such as antibiotic sensitivity testing; and to wide-ranging 'ad hoc' searches on the database for a variety of clinical laboratory purposes. Further, with the increasing use of automated analytical procedures for routine microbiological purposes, such equipment can be connected to or interfaced with computer systems, thus saving transcription time as well as errors.

The amount and scope of information stored depends on the particular computer system, but the introduction of recent software environments (the so called '4th generation languages') together with 'total' hospital and healthcare information systems with relational links between departmental databases provides ready and instant access to information on potential nosocomial as well as other infections. The computer communications information ('informatics') explosion has also led to the wide availability of 'viewdata'

in homes, offices and in general practice. Validated data – for example on infectious agents and antibiotic resistance – can be transmitted electronically from the microbiology laboratory to all out-stations with peripheral display terminals for immediate access by medical practitioners. It should be noted, however, that when personal (including clinical) information is held on file in computer databases (but not in manual data storage systems) then in the UK registration under the Data Protection Act (1984) may be necessary. Advice may be obtained from the Data Protection Registrar, Springfield House, Water Lane, Wilmslow, Cheshire SK9 5AX, UK.

Despite this glimpse of the many applications of computers in microbiology, we emphasize again that simple and practical laboratory methods for bacterial identification described in this *Manual* are bench-orientated and do not require any special equipment or a computer.

APPENDIX G
The Bacteriological Code

For scientific purposes, the naming of living organisms requires rules to ensure standardization and consistency in nomenclature and thus in the unequivocal communication of identity. The necessary scientific rules for naming all living organisms are embodied in international codes of nomenclature. Separate codes have been formulated for animals, plants, bacteria and viruses. The rules governing the application and use of names for bacteria were long overdue before they were promulgated in the first Bacteriological Code approved in 1947 (Buchanan, St. John-Brooks & Breed, 1948). This code, which was largely based on the Botanical Code, was both long and complicated. Subsequent attempts to increase its usefulness resulted in further difficulties despite the accompanying explanations given in the revised versions published in 1958 (Buchanan *et al.*, 1958) and in 1966. Such rules are necessarily framed in legalistic language, which is not always easily understood. The *Bacteriological Code* has two basic guidelines: (i) to avoid translation into different languages, all names must be Latinized so as to be clearly recognized both scientifically and internationally and (ii) the names must have definite positions in the relevant taxonomic hierarchy.

Informal or vernacular names for bacteria such as 'coliform organisms' and the 'tubercle bacillus' are not governed by the Code although it may help to regulate their use by recommendations for good practice. Informal names such as those for organisms which differ only antigenically are governed by separate rules.

Scientific names are used for species, genera and higher ranks. Thus *Mycobacterium tuberculosis* is the scientific species name for the tubercle bacillus; *Staphylococcus* is the generic name for the group of related staphylococcal species; and *Micrococcaceae* the family name for the group of related genera of Gram-positive cocci.

Following initial proposals (Lapage *et al.*, 1973) the most recent revision of the *Bacteriological Code* – formally entitled the *International Code of Nomenclature of Bacteria* – was first published by Lapage *et al.* in 1975. This version, known coloquially as the *Revised Code* or the

'1976 revision' authorised a new starting date (1st January 1980 instead of 1st May 1975) for the names of bacteria to be ratified. An initial document, the *Approved Lists of Bacterial Names* (Skerman, McGowan & Sneath, 1980) listed all names that were nomenclaturally valid from that date. Part of the introduction to this important document is reproduced with permission in Appendix H. Any bacterial names not included in these lists in 1980 lost all nomenclatural standing and therefore official status unless approved and re-instated subsequently in validation lists published as supplements in the *International Journal of Systematic Bacteriology* (IJSB).

Both the *Revised Code* and the *Approved Lists of Bacterial Names* are under the jurisdiction of the International Committee on Systematic Bacteriology, which is assisted by the Judicial Commission in considering alterations to the Code and any exceptions which require amending of specific Rules. All species of bacteria are named in accordance with the principles and rules of nomenclature detailed in the Code. The correct names of species or of higher taxonomic ranks, is determined by three prime criteria:

(i) Valid publication

All variations to the lists of bacteria, including new names as well as revisions to existing names, are governed by the Code and must be published either primarily in the *International Journal of Systematic Bacteriology* (IJSB) or, if validly published elsewhere, an announcement of the publication must be made in the IJSB.

All descriptions of a named taxon or references to previous effectively published descriptions of it must be given in the IJSB. A formal description of a named taxon must be given and, in the case of cultivable organisms, cultures of the designated type strains of newly named species and subspecies must be deposited in recognized culture collections so that they will be available throughout the world.

The essential part of the description of a new organism is a list of characteristic properties that distinguish it from other organisms thus enabling it to be recognized. Minimum criteria for the description of certain groups of bacteria have been formulated by the Judicial Commission subcommittees; those for other bacterial groups have yet to be completed. These criteria set standards which will ensure not only consistency but also that taxa are not defined unnecessarily thus avoiding repetition of the confusion that existed before 1980.

(ii) Legitimacy of the name

This forms the main legalistic part of the Code and covers the Latinization of Surnames and of Greek or Latin words which describe or refer to the organisms, e.g. *Escherichia coli* and *Staphylococcus aureus*.

Taxonomic hierarchy. Each taxonomic level above species is inclusive and the names within it denote successive categories, each of which has a particular position in the hierarchy referred to as its rank. In decreasing order, the main categories of rank are: Kingdom, Phylum, Class, Order, Family, Genus and Species.

Form of Names. The form of the latinized names differs with the rank. The species name consists of two parts, the first denoting the genus name and the second, the specific name. Genus names are latinized substantive nouns which are spelled with an initial capital letter, e.g. *Shigella*. The specific epithet is a latinized adjective spelled with an initial lower case letter, e.g. *dysenteriae*. Thus the binomial name, or binomen, *Shigella dysenteriae* means the 'Shigella of dysentery', so named after the Japanese bacteriologist, Shiga. Above the rank of genus, most names are plural adjectives in the feminine gender, e.g. *Pseudomonadaceae* (Family), *Pseudomonadales* (Order).

Nomenclatural types. These are cultures of bacterial strains which have been deposited in recognized culture collections together with a description of the strain. When a new species is first described the actual strain deposited may not prove subsequently to be typical of the whole group once more members have been identified and characterized. A 'type strain' therefore represents a reference point for the name. There are various categories of 'type strains'. For example, a neotype is a new strain deposited in a culture collection because the original type strain has been lost or is not available. However, not all descriptions of bacteria have a corresponding associated cultural type strain stored for posterity. This applies to many of the medical bacteria that were isolated and categorized in the 19th and early 20th centuries; the original type strain of *Staphylococcus aureus*, for example, is no longer in existence.

(iii) Priority of publication

According to the Rules of the *Revised Code*, the correct name for a taxon must be the first name validly published in a description of that taxon. This rule still causes some argument among taxonomists as the modern characterization methods available sometimes lead to 'new' species being described though subsequently previous published descriptions are found which had been removed from the *Approved Lists* either because of poor or incomplete descriptions or because type cultures to match the 'new' organism were not available. Such disagrements are settled by the Judicial Commission with decisions made to reduce confusion.

Although the Bacteriological Code, the *Approved Lists of Bacterial Names* and the Judicial Commission have together done much to settle the majority of scientific nomenclatural problems, a few anomalies persist. Generic or specific synonymns for example, can be perpetuated by scientific preference and continued use or by medical considerations; thus *Legionella micdadei* is sometimes referred to as '*Tatlockia*', and *Morganella morganii* is still often referred to as *Proteus morganii*. The Code makes provision for these exceptions and the names retained by international agreement are termed 'conserved'. A 'conserved name' is one which must be used instead of all earlier synonyms. For example, *Edwardsiella anguillimortifera* is an earlier synonym for the commonly used name *Edwardsiella tarda* and, according to the rules, the former should be used. However, in view of the common usage of the latter, a proposal has been made to the Judicial Commission to conserve the name *E. tarda* over *E. anguillimortifera*. In the case of *Morganella morganii* and *Proteus morganii*, both names are in the *Approved Lists* and are therefore correct but only actual usage will determine which is to be preferred.

Knowledge of recent additions to or changes in bacterial nomenclature are important. To help disseminate such information, summaries of the validated changes in nomenclature and additions to the *Approved Lists* are published in the IJSB each year. In this way, archaic and non-standard forms of bacterial names are not perpetuated and false nomenclatural trails thus eliminated.

APPENDIX H
The Approved Lists of Bacterial Names

Following the 1976 revision of the Bacteriological Code (see Appendix G), the *Approved Lists of Bacterial Names* was published in the *International Journal of Systematic Bacteriology* (IJSB) on behalf of the Ad Hoc Committee of the Judicial Commission of the International Committee on Systematic Bacteriology (ICSB) of the International Association [now Union] of Microbiological Societies

(Skerman *et al.*, 1980). It took effect on 1st January 1980 and was subsequently reprinted in book form in 1980 by the American Society for Microbiology. For information, and with permission, the explanatory Introduction to the *Approved Lists* is reproduced here. All subsequent valid alterations and additions as well as proposals for change are published in the IJSB.

Approved Lists of Bacterial Names

edited by
V.B.D. SKERMAN,[1] VICKI McGOWAN,[1] AND P.H.A. SNEATH [2]
Department of Microbiology, University of Queensland, St Lucia, Queensland 4067, Australia[1] and MRC Microbial Systematics Unit, University of Leicester, Leicester LE1 7RH, England[2]

on behalf of

The Ad Hoc Committee of the Judicial Commission of the ICSB
(International Journal of Systematic Bacteriology, vol. 30, pp. 225–420, 1980)

INTRODUCTION

At the meeting of the Judicial Commission of the ICSB held in Jerusalem on the 29th March, 1973 an Ad Hoc Committee was appointed (Minute 22) to organize a review of the curently valid names of bacteria with the object of retaining only names for those taxa which were adequately described and, if cultivable, for which there was a Type, Neotype or Reference strain available; to compile these names under the title of **Approved Lists of Bacterial Names**, and to publish the lists in the International Journal of Systematic Bacteriology, to become effective on January 1, 1980. This date would then replace May 1, 1975 (International Code of Nomenclature of Bacteria and Viruses, Rule 10) as the new date for determining priorities for names of new taxa.

The members of the Ad Hoc Committee originally appointed to oversee the task were S.P. Lapage, H.P.R. Seeliger and V.B.D. Skerman (Chairman). Following his

election as President-Elect of IAMS, H.P.R. Seeliger resigned from the Committee and was replaced by J.G. Holt. P.H.A. Sneath, as Chairman of the Judicial Commission, was coopted to the Committee. This Committee was responsible for the editing of the first draft of the Approved Lists of Bacterial Names published in the IJSB (26, 1976, 563–599).

The Ad Hoc Committee was reconstituted by the Judicial Commission during its meetings at the International Congress of the IAMS in Munich in September, 1978, with V.B.D. Skerman (Chairman), P.H.A. Sneath (newly-elected Chairman of the ICSB) and L.G. Wayne (newly elected Chairman of the Judicial Commission) as Committee members. This Committee was assigned wide powers to complete the work on the Lists and arrange publication.

The initial Committee agreed that, as a basis for inquiry, all names which had been included in the eighth edition of *Bergey's Manual of Determinative Bacteriology*, whether listed as recognised species, synonyms, species *incertae sedis*, or under other headings, should be circulated; that all Subcommittees on Taxonomy of the ICSB should be asked for advice on the retention of taxa for which the Subcommittees were responsible and that specialists be approached for advice on other taxa – only a small list of taxa remained to be considered by the Ad Hoc Committee itself. Advice was also sought on additional names of taxa which had been validly published since the publication of the Manual. Special provision had been made in the Code of Nomenclature for the inclusion of names validly published after the 1st January, 1978 (Rule 24a).

A list of specialists was drawn up and approved by the Ad Hoc Committee. Each specialist was asked to associate two others in reaching a decision on name retention. The Chairman accepted the responsibility for coordination of work associated with the selection of generic names and specific and subspecific epithets and P.H.A. Sneath for the names of higher taxa.

Names of Genera, Species and Subspecies:

The Lists of names of species and subspecies were circulated by airmail in April, 1976 and a draft list of names recommended for retention published in the IJSB (**26**, 1976, 563–599) together with the list of those people associated with that stage of the project. Reference may be made to the draft list for details of the procedures adopted in processing the information.

The object of publishing the draft list was to enable microbiologists, in general, to submit opinions to the Ad Hoc Committee. Several were received. Some of these resulted in modification to lists submitted by Subcommittees on Taxonomy and others.

Rule 24a of the Code of Nomenclature provided, *inter alia*, for the publication with each bacterial name the name(s) of the author(s) who originally proposed it, a reference to an effectively published description of each species and its nomenclatural type whenever possible, and a Type, Neotype or Reference strain by its designation.

To conserve space in publication, it was agreed that for all references to the 8th edition of Bergey's *Manual* (Buchanan, R.E. and N.E. Gibbons (eds). 1974. *Bergey's Manual of Determinative Bacteriology*, 8th ed. The Williams and Wilkins Co., Baltimore) be contracted to 'Bergey 8'.

Although these requirements were formally published in the Code on 1st January, 1976 little action was taken by those responsible for various taxa and in order to assist resolution of the problem, the Chairman and his staff produced a document which listed Collections of Cultures of Microorganisms which held Type, Neotype and Reference strains for those species whose names appeared in the draft list and subsequent amendments. This list, which will be published elsewhere as a publication of the World Data Center for Microorganisms, has been used as a guide to the deletion of numerous names for which no cultures could be located.

The requirements of Rule 24a together with the list of strains, were discussed at a meeting of the ICSB with Subcommittees on Taxonomy at the International Congress for Microbiology in Munich in September, 1978 where the decision was made to list only one designation for each strain and preferably that of the American Type Culture Collection, where available. Because of difficulties associated with locating references to publications in which Type strains, Neotype strains or Reference strains had been designated, it was agreed that references would be given only to those publications concerned with the naming of the taxa and to descriptions of the taxa.

The Judicial Commission also determined that publication should be in the January (1980) issue of the IJSB, thus negating the requirement of Rule 24a that publication take place prior to 1st January 1980. This action enabled the inclusion in the Approved Lists of names of all new taxa which had been validated by publication in the October, 1979 issue of the IJSB and so has obviated the need to make any further additions to the Approved Lists of Bacterial Names.

Formal notice of these requirements was circulated, by airmail, to all Subcommittees and specialists on 5th February, 1979, requesting return of the information by 31st August, 1979. Meanwhile, the Chairman and his staff proceeded as far as possible with the compilation of the whole of the required information, subsequently making use of such submissions as were ultimately received from others, to verify compilations already made.

Computer printouts, in the final format of assembled information, were distributed by airmail to all participants in July, 1979 for the purpose of verification and for the provision of information which was still missing.

A final decision to retain or delete some names was based on our ability to obtain the relevant information.

Names of Taxa Above the Rank of Genus:

Compilation of names of higher taxa was undertaken by Sneath and his associates. No draft list was published but a proposal was discussed at some length in an open meeting at the Munich Congress. The format of the list as submitted was modified to conform with the format adopted for the names of the genera and species. References given in this section of the lists are restricted to those relating to the higher taxa. Those to genera will be found in the list of genera and species.

Designation of Strains:

Strains have been designated by accession numbers of Culture Collections in which they have been deposited. Every effort has been made to ensure that the strains are actually available but no guarantee of this can be given. Names, which have been omitted, may be revived if the location of suitable strains can be ascertained.

The following is a list of addresses of institutions, together with acronyms used to assign accession numbers.

AMRC	FAO–WHO International Reference Centre for Animal Mycoplasmas, Institute for Medical Microbiology, University of Aarhus, Aarhus, Denmark.
ATCC	American Type Culture Collection, Rockville, Maryland 20852, USA.
BKM	All-Union Collection of Microorganisms, Institute of Microbiology, USSR Academy of Sciences, Moscow, USSR.
BKMW	Culture Collection, Institute of Microbiology, USSR Academy of Sciences, Moscow, USSR.
CBS	Centraalbureau voor Schimmelcultures, Baarn, The Netherlands.
CCM	Czechoslovak Collection of Microorganisms, J.E. Purkyne University, Brno, Czechoslovakia.
CDC	Center for Disease Control, Atlanta, Georgia, USA.
CIP	Collection of the Institute Pasteur, Paris, France.
DSM	Deutsche Sammlung von Mikroorganismen, Gottingen, Federal Republic of Germany.
IAM	Institute of Applied Microbiology, University of Tokyo, Tokyo, Japan.
IFO	Institute for Fermentation, Osaka, Japan.
IMRU	Institute of Microbiology, Rutgers – The State University, New Brunswick, New Jersey, USA.
IMV	Institute of Microbiology and Virology, Academy of Sciences of the Ukrainian SSR.
INA	Institute for New Antibiotics, Moscow, USSR.
INMI	Institute for Microbiology, USSR Academy of Sciences, Moscow, USSR.
IPV	Istituto di Patologia Vegetale, Milan, Italy.
KCC	Kaken Chemical Company Ltd., Tokyo, Japan.
LIA	Museum of Cultures, Leningrad Research Institute of Antibiotics, 23 Ogorodnikov Prospect, Leningrad L-20, USSR.
LSU	Louisiana State University, Baton Rouge, Louisiana, USA.
LMD	Laboratorium voor Microbiologie der Landbouwhogeschool, Wageningen, The Netherlands.
NCDO	National Collection of Dairy Organisms, National Institute for Research in Dairying, University of Reading, England, UK.
NCIB	National Collection of Industrial Bacteria, Torry Research Station, Aberdeen, Scotland, UK.
NCMB	National Collection of Marine Bacteria, Torry Research Station, Aberdeen, Scotland, UK.
NCPPB	National Collection of Plant Pathogenic Bacteria, Plant Pathology Laboratory, Harpenden, England, UK.
NCTC	National Collection of Type Cultures, Central Public Health Laboratory, Colindale, London, England, UK.
NIAID	National Institute of Allergy and Infectious Diseases, Hamilton, Montana, USA.
NIHJ	National Institute of Health, Tokyo, Japan.
NRC	National Research Council, Ottawa, Canada.
NRL	Neisseria Reference Laboratory, US Public Health Service Hospital, Seattle, Washington, USA.
NRRL	Northern Utilization Research and Development Division, US Department of Agriculture, Peoria, Illinois, USA.
PDDCC	Culture Collection of Plant Diseases Division, New Zealand Department of Scientific and Industrial Research, Auckland, New Zealand.
TC	Thaxter Collection, Farlow Herbarium, Harvard University, Boston, Massachusetts, USA.
UMH	University of Missouri Herbarium, Missouri, USA.
UQM	Culture Collection, Department of Microbiology, University of Queensland, Brisbane, Australia.
VKM	Institute of Microbiology, Academy of Sciences of the USSR, Moscow, USSR.
VPI	Virginia Polytechnic Institute and State University, Blacksburg, Virginia, USA.
WINDSOR	Culture Collection, University of Windsor, Windsor, Ontario, Canada.

Acknowledgements:

Whilst the task of compilation and preparation of manuscripts for publication has been of necessity concentrated in two areas, the successful completion of the task would not have been possible without the associated efforts of a large number of people whose names are recorded here.

T. V. Aristovskaya, P. K. C. Austwick, E. Baldacci, L. Barksdale, E. Barnes, P. Baumann, J. H. Becking, E. L. Biberstein, I. Bousfield, K. Bovre, W. J. Brinley-Morgan, D. Brenner, T. Brock, E. Brockman, M. Bryant, J. C. Burnham, J. Carr, W. Catlin, E. P. Cato, D. Claus, G. Colman, R. R. Colwell, M. J. Corbel, K. T. Crabtree, T. Cross, G. A. Dubinina, P. Dugan, D. W. Dye, K. Eimhjellen, G. Eldering, W. H. Ewing, S. Faine, S. M. Finegold, E. A. Freundt, W. Frederiksen, A. L. Furniss, E. Garvie, N. E. Gibbons, M. Goodfellow, M. Gordon, B. V. Gronov, H. Hatt, A. C. Hayward, M. Hendrie, S. D. Henriksen, A. Henssen, G. J. Hermann, G. Gobbs, L. V. Holdeman, R. Hugh, D. B. Johnstone, D. Jones, L. V. Kalakoutskii, O. Kandler, K.-A. Karlsson, R. M. Keddie, M. Killian, K. Kitahara, J. Knapp, W. Knapp, M. Kocur, N. R. Kreig, S. P. Lapage, J. M. Larkin, H. Lautrop, H. A. Lechevalier, J. DeLey, R. Mocci, S. Maier, N. S. Mair, P. H. Makela, M. Mandel, E. McCoy, H. D. McCurdy; K. McNiel, W. E. C. Moore, N. Nishida, H. Nonomura, R. A. Ormsbee, F. Orskov, I. Orskov, E. van Oye, O. M. Parinkina, N. Pfennig, J. E. Phillips, F. Pichinoty, M. Pittman, T. Pridham, C. I. Randles, J. W. M. LaRiviere, M. Rhodes-Roberts, D. S. Roberts, R. Rohde, B. Rowe, E. B. Rozlycky, E. Runyon, R. Sakazaki, V. Scardovi, D. Schafer, R. J. Sidleer, J. M. Shewan, G. C. Simmons, I. J. Slotnick, R. M. Sibert, P. H. Smith, J. T. Staley, M. Starr, Y. Terasaki, Y. T. Tchan, E. Thal, J. Thompson, H. Truper, G. Tunevall, D. C. Turk, M. Veron, N. Walker, S. W. Watson, G. Wauters, L. Wayne, R. E. Weaver, O. B. Weeks, E. Weiss, H. J. Welshimer, S. Williams, G. A. Zavarzin, J. G. Zeikus, K. Zinneman.

Thanks are also due to Miss Annette McLennan who typed the original manuscripts and to Dr Lindsay Sly, Dr Horst Doelle and Mrs Elizabeth Marden for considerable assistance in the search for Culture Collections maintaining strains of taxa in the Approved Lists and other information and to the numerous other unnamed people who have assisted in various ways in laboratories throughout the world.

The computer programs used in compiling these lists were written and controlled by Mr. Geoffrey Dengate, Systems Programmer, Prentice Computer Centre, University of Queensland. His help and expertise are sincerely acknowledged.

Financial assistance of the following is gratefully acknowledged: Bergey's Manual Trust, Deutsche Gesellschaft für Hygiene und Mikrobiologie, International Association of Microbiological Societies, International Union of Biological Sciences, Society for Applied Bacteriology, Society for General Microbiology, and the United Kingdom Federation of Culture Collections.

SPECIFIC INFORMATION RELATING TO THE APPROVED LISTS OF BACTERIAL NAMES

The names included in these Lists are those selected by Subcommittees on Taxonomy of the ICSB, specialist advisers and, where the former have not been available or have declined to advise, by the members of the Ad Hoc Committee.

With few exceptions (vide infra) names which have been included in the Lists are those which:

were validly published before the 1st January, 1978 and which have been listed by advisers.

have been validly published since the 1st January, 1978 by publication in the IJSB or by inclusion in the lists of new names cited in the IJSB (to and including Volume 29, Part 4, 1979) as having been effectively published in other Journals.

Specific attention is drawn to the following.

1. Names included in the *Approved Lists of Bacterial Names* are the only names which are nomenclaturally valid as at the 1st January, 1980. All other names which have appeared in the literature prior to 1st January, 1980 are nomenclaturally invalid. Names which have been effectively published in Journals other than the IJSB but which have not been cited in the lists of new names published in the IJSB, have not been validly published under Rule 27 of the Code of Nomenclature. Such names may be validated by publication in forthcoming issues of the IJSB and will simply constitute names of new taxa.

2. No name appearing in the Approved Lists of Bacterial Names is conserved in the sense defined under Rule 56b of the Code of Nomenclature (1976 Revision).

3. Any name previously rejected by the Judicial Commission remains a *nomen rejiciendum* and can no longer be used to name a bacterium.

4. By majority decision of the Ad Hoc Committee, supported by an overwhelming majority of the members of the ICSB, all strains of bacteria which were submitted as nomenclatural Type strains, Neotype strains, Proposed

257

Neotype strains or Reference strains have been elevated to the status of Type strains. The few objections which were received to the elevation of reference strains to Type status were based on concern that such reference strains may not prove to be the best choice for Type strains. This objection however, applies equally to quite a number of Type strains, particularly monotypes of which there are, and will continue to be, several. It seemed more appropriate that names appearing in the *Approved Lists of Bacterial Names*, which constitutes a new base for future nomenclature, should have Type status or be omitted.

5. For some names included in the Lists no strains were available. These names were retained to preserve the status of

A. some microorganisms for which habitats are well known, which have distinct morphological characters but which have never been isolated. In most cases only the Type Species has been retained to preserve the status of the genus.

B. a genus which contained well described species for which representative strains were available for all but the Type Species of the genus itself.

Exclusion of the Type Species would have necessitated the exclusion of the genus as a whole under Rule 20c of the Code of Nomenclature. There were several of these. It is hoped that early action will be taken to request the Judicial Commission to conserve these genera with new Type Species in order that each species within these genera will be represented by a Type strain in a recognised culture collection.

6. The Ad Hoc Committee has repeatedly stressed that its task was nomenclatural and not taxonomic; further that Subcommittees and others were not required to solve taxonomic problems before advising on retention of names. They were requested to omit names of doubtful species as such species could be revived (see 8 below).

Because there are some differences of opinion regarding the generic position of some species it has been necessary to include the same microorganism under two names, each with the same specific epithet and the same nomenclatural type strain. In such instances cross-reference has been made to the alternate name. This applied specifically to the species in the genus *Beneckea* and the genus *Vibrio* and to a few instances in the *Enterobacteriaceae*. For this reason it is necessary here to reaffirm the statement made previously that no name in the Approved Lists of Bacterial Names has been conserved. Names in the Lists may later be conserved, rejected, merged with other names or subjected to any other valid nomenclatural act.

7. The names of some genera, for which there are no available strains for the Type Species, have been omitted from the Lists in order to permit the resolution of a very difficult nomenclatural situation arising from the recent publication of provisional names which have no standing in nomenclature but which have been cited by subsequent authors as though they were valid. Addition of new species, with nomenclatural types, to an invalidly published generic name renders the new names equally invalid. This refers specifically to the methane oxidising bacteria, where the otherwise valid name *Methanomonas* has been omitted in the hope that by so doing the impasse caused by the illegitimate substitution of the name *Methylomonas* may be resolved. Specialists in this field are now urged to publish a fully validated list of appropriate species.

8. Reuse and revival of names which do not appear in the Approved Lists of Bacterial Names is authorized by Rule 28a. In addition, the Code of Nomenclature (1976 Revision) contains a number of Provisional Rules. At the time of publication of this List these Rules still have only provisional status. It will require a specific act on the part of the Judicial Commission at a formally constituted meeting to raise these Provisional Rules to Rule status. Meanwhile they continue to be inapplicable.

Revival of Names: A name which has not appeared in the Approved Lists of Bacterial Names and which has not been listed as a *nomen rejiciendum* by the Judicial Commission may be revived (*nomen revictum*) if it is to be used for the same taxon to which (in the author's opinion) it was originally applied. For citation of such names see Rule 28a and Provisional Rules B2 and B3.

As most names which have not been included in the Approved Lists of Bacterial Names have been omitted because of uncertainty of the validity of the taxa to which they apply, the revival of names should be practised very conservatively.

Reuse of names – Specific and Subspecific epithets: There never has been any rule which forbids the use of the same specific epithet for taxa *within different genera*.

Many contributors to the Approved Lists of Bacterial Names have voiced considerable concern at the possibility that a specific epithet may be used *within the same genus* as that in which it was originally used but for the naming of a taxon to which it was not originally applied.

Unless the Judicial Commission takes action to prevent such usage, the Ad Hoc Committee can only urge taxonomists to avoid such reusage as may lead to considerable confusion in future nomenclature.

For the same reason taxonomists are urged not to use as a specific epithet within a genus a name which has been used for an infrasubspecific subdivision of a species within that genus. This applies particularly to several genera of predominantly plant pathogens, where previously cited species have been relegated to the status of pathovars within species listed in the *Approved Lists of Bacterial Names*. As such infrasubspecific pathovars may later be elevated to the status of subspecies or species, preemption of the pathovar name as a specific or subspecific epithet of a different taxon would obviously cause confusion.

The International Society for Plant Pathology is publishing, in the Review of Plant Pathology, a list of pathovars of species which appear in the *Approved Lists of Bacterial Names*. Taxonomists are urged to consult this list before proposing new specific epithets or reusing or reviving old epithets for new species within the relevant genera.

Reuse of generic names: The reuse of a generic name which has not appeared in the *Approved Lists of Bacterial Names* and which has not been listed as a *nomen rejiciendum* by the Judicial Commission does not appear to be fraught with the same difficulties as those associated with specific and subspecific epithets. Taxonomists are never-theless asked to seriously consider the possibility of confusion arising from the use of such names before taking such action.

The correct form of citation for reused names is given in Provisional Rules B1 and B4.

9.   Omissions from *Approved Lists of Bacterial Names*. No names will be added to or removed from the *Approved Lists of Bacterial Names*. Attention may be drawn to errors in nomenclature or to errors in spelling or citations of references and such communications should be directed to the Executive Secretary, ICSB, for transmission to the appropriate body. Please note that the omission of diacritical signs was intentional and dictated by the limitations of the computers used in setting up the type. These omissions do not constitute 'errors' in the above sense.

Every effort has been made to obviate errors by reference of the computer printouts of the final information to the original advisers for correction and also for insertion of some missing information. The final printout prior to production of the bromide copy for printing has been checked by the Chairman but the magnitude of the task allowed only of a search for the more glaring errors of which there were fortunately few.

APPENDIX I
Reconciliation of approaches to bacterial systematics

In Section 8.4 we discussed briefly the impact of numerical taxonomy and the newer genetic techniques for measuring bacterial relatedness and evolutionary divergence on traditional classification and nomenclature as used in this *Manual*. Because of their fundamental significance for taxonomy in the future we reproduce in full, with permission from the International Committee on Systematic Bacteriology, the report of the *ad hoc* committee set up to consider the various approaches to bacterial systematics and their relationship to each other published in the *International Journal of Systematic Bacteriology* by Wayne *et al.* (1987) on behalf of the International Union [formerly Association] of Microbiological Societies.

Report of the Ad Hoc Committee on Reconciliation of Approaches to Bacterial Systematics

L. G. WAYNE,[1]* D. J. BRENNER,[2] R. R. COLWELL,[3] P. A. D. GRIMONT,[4] O. KANDLER,[5] M. I. KRICHEVSKY,[6] L. H. MOORE,[7] W. E. C. MOORE,[7] R. G. E. MURRAY,[8] E. STACKEBRANDT,[9] M. P. STARR,[10] AND H. G. TRUPER[11].

Veterans Administration Medical Center, Long Beach, California[1]; Centers for Disease Control, Atlanta, Georgia[2]; University of Maryland, College Park, Maryland[3]; Institut Pasteur, Paris, France[4]; University of Munich, Munich, Federal Republic of Germany[5]; National Institute of Dental Research, Bethesda, Maryland[6]; Virginia Polytechnic Institute and State University, Blacksburg, Virginia[7]; University of Western Ontario, London, Ontario, Canada[8]; University of Kiel, Federal Republic of Germany[9]; University of California, Davis, California[10]; University of Bonn, Bonn, Federal Republic of Germany[11]

Bacterial taxonomy, which began as a largely intuitive process, has become increasingly objective with the advent of numerical taxonomy and techniques for the measurement of evolutionary divergence in the structure of semantides, i.e., large, information-bearing molecules such as nucleic acids and proteins. These developments have forced the adoption of changes in nomenclature, sometimes with disruptive or even perilous consequences (2). Since the present nomenclatural system evolved during a period when hierarchial taxonomic divisions were only vaguely defined, it has become important to reexamine that system in the light of newer taxonomic understanding. Accordingly, an ad hoc committee of the International Committee for Systematic Bacteriology was convened for a Workshop on Reconciliation of Approaches to Bacterial Systematics at the Institut Pasteur, Paris, on 14 to 16 May 1987.

Perspectives. To arrive at a common ground of understanding, the committee reviewed the current state of bacterial systematics from the following perspectives:

(i) **Phylogenetic**. Phylogenetic studies are directed at a basic understanding of pathways through which taxa have evolved from primordial and recent ancestors, calculated from analyses of evolutionary distances between selected semantides.

(ii) **Descriptive**. Descriptive research represents the bridge between semantide-based phylogenetic taxonomy and traditional phenotype-based bacterial systematics. Organisms are described in phenotypic terms, and the descriptions help define a taxonomic group that may also be recognized at the phylogenetic level.

(iii) **Diagnostic**. Diagnosis involves the selection of features from those in a phenotypic description, or of probes derived from phylogenetic analyses, in a way that permits the recognition of an unknown strain and the assignment of a label to it. The most useful labels for applied purposes are names at the genus, species, and subspecies levels; infra-

---

* Comments on the conclusions and recommendations included in this report are welcome and should be sent to Lawrence G. Wayne, Tuberculosis Research Laboratory (151), Veterans Administrations Medical Center, 5901 East Seventh St., Long Beach, CA 90822.

subspecific categories that are not governed by the Bacteriological Code (1) may be useful for recognition of special attributes.

(iv) Associative. Associative studies use a name to evoke practical information about a strain, such as its medical, industrial, or ecologic significance.

The committee offers the following conclusions and recommendations.

HIERARCHICAL TAXONOMY

An ideal taxonomy would involve one system. A single formal overall system appears to be adequate, and a second system is not needed if vernacular grouping is retained for diagnostic purposes.

There was general agreement that the complete deoxyribonucleic acid (DNA) sequence would be the reference standard to determine phylogeny and that phylogeny should determine taxonomy. Furthermore, nomenclature should agree with (and reflect) genomic information.

The group agreed that hierarchical consistency is essential but recognized that the depth in a ribonucleic acid (RNA) dendrogram at which a given hierarchical line is to be drawn may vary along different major branches of the dendrogram and will be strongly influenced by phenotypic consistency at each level. This is a consequence of differences in ages of the different branches and the recognition that older branches will exhibit greater nucleic acid structural genetic drift, even as environmental constraints tend to limit phenotypic drift.

A cautionary note about hierarchical interpretation was expressed with the recommendation that active searches continue for additional powerful semantides independent of the ribosomal RNA cistrons.

The chemotaxonomic approach has two sets of derivative data: structural phenetic (including "signatures") and phylogenetic (evolutionary). There should not be further designation of hierarchical levels without substantial chemotaxonomic and sequence data to support the proposal.

Species, subspecies, and infrasubspecific categories. At present, the species is the only taxonomic unit that can be defined in phylogenetic terms. In practice, DNA reassociation approaches the sequence standard and represents the best applicable procedure at the present time. *The phylogenetic definition of a species generally would include strains with approximately 70% or greater DNA-DNA relatedness and with 5°C or less ΔT_m. Both values must be considered.* Phenotypic characteristics should agree with this definition and would be allowed to override the phylogenetic concept of species only in a few exceptional cases.

It is recommended that a distinct genospecies that cannot be differentiated from another genospecies on the basis of *any known phenotypic property not be named until they can be differentiated by some phenotypic property.*

Subspecies designations can be used for genetically close organisms that diverge in phenotype. There is some evidence, based on frequency distribution of ΔT_m values in DNA hybridization, that the subspecies concept is phylogenetically valid and can be distinguished from the infra-subspecific variety concept, which is based solely on selected "utility" attributes, but not demonstrable by DNA reassociation. *There is a need for further guidelines for designation of subspecies.*

Genera. Genera form the essential basis of bacterial systematics, and each genus must remain subject to continuing assessment. A degree of flexibility in circumscription is necessary. Unfortunately, there is currently no satisfactory phylogenetic definition of a genus. *The scope of the definition may differ among genera,* as for any other higher taxa.

Families. Families can be retained as long as they are consistent in terms of chemotaxonomic and hybridization or sequence data. Any other hierarchical level established between family and division must also be consistent in terms of supporting taxonomic data.

Divisions. It is clear that there are at least 15 clearly separated lineages of great antiquity in evolutionary terms at the level of division or greater.

Kingdom. There is no need at this time for more than one kingdom, but there may be need for a term to describe major primary lineages. A rank such as phylum may be needed in the future.

NOMENCLATURE

After a review of alternative approaches to the occasional conflict between binomials based on strict phylogenetic relationships at the species level and the practical application of the binomials, the following recommendations were made.

Nomenclature should reflect genomic relationships to the greatest extent possible. Rare exceptions are sanctioned under the emendation to Rule 56a embodied in Minute 7i of the Judicial Commission (Int. J. Syst. Bacteriol. 37:85–87, 1987), introducing the concept of a "nomen periculosum". It is anticipated that this concept need be applied in only a limited number of cases and hoped that this type of problem will disappear as new taxonomic methods and interpretations are more universally applied. *A mechanism is needed for broad dissemination of information about those cases where such nomenclatural discrepancies have been sanctioned.*

As needed, various vernacular appendices that pertain to needs for special purposes (medical, veterinary, agriculture, industry, etc.) including information about traits coded by plasmids, phages, and other extrachromosomal agents should be applied. These infrasubspecific "utility" categories are not governed by the Bacteriological Code. In certain medical situations, identification of the presence of certain virulence factors may be more important than the species name.

Regarding inadequate nomenclature, it is recommended that formal nomenclature is needed for the major divisional groupings. "Gram positives" should be Firmicutes as presently defined. The term "purple bacteria" causes confusion because it includes more than phototrophic bacteria, which is good reason for a formal name to be established.

OTHER CONCERNS

Special difficulties are expected in accomplishing the taxonomic reorganization of the major phylogenetic taxon listed as "the purple photosynthetic bacteria and their relatives" (3), and this includes most of the classically defined gram-negative genera, both photosynthetic and chemosynthetic, in the alpha, beta, gamma, and delta groups of the purple bacteria. Thus, the major task of the greatest practical importance is the development of a taxonomic and nomenclatural approach to resolving the linked phylogenetic lineages of the remarkably diverse metabolic types of organisms within each of the groupings. Urgency is dictated by the large number of bacteria involved and by the many species that are crucial in ecological and diagnostic bacteriology. A number of genera must be reassessed, although many will persist in part, if not as a whole. There are gaps in our knowledge because the molecular/genetic surveys are incomplete. The first task is the definition and phylogenetic circumscription of the genera in this phylogenetic taxon, with inclusion of type strains of species in the genera. *It is recommended that this problem be assigned for special study by an ad hoc subcommittee of the International Committee on Systematic Bacteriology.*

Research should be directed toward solving the growth and diagnostic problems of noncultivable or hardly cultivable organisms, e.g., cholera somnicells, nongerminable endospores, and organisms not cultivable axenically but cultivable in multiorganism systems, such as representatives of consortia, *Pasteuria, Planctomyces,* etc. The Code may have to be emended to clarify the status of multiorganism cultures as type material; e.g., see Rule 18a and Advisory Note C, Chapter 4(1).

A whole base line of bacterial taxonomy of various ecosystems is urgently needed, as is a broader knowledge of species distribution in ecosystems and improved knowledge of little known bacteria. ("Less than 20% of the bacteria are known.") Encouragement must be given to systematic studies and the search for new chemotaxonomic markers. Recognition of the importance of effective taxonomic understanding to all fields, basic and applied, and especially to biotechnology has been slow to develop, although the need is great. The group recognized, also, that ecologically relevant characterization of the members of complex bacterial populations requires the identification of these characters in a burgeoning field of biochemical/molecular/genetic research.

An overall concern of members of the Committee was that any phylogenetically based taxonomic schemes that result must also show phenotypic consistency.

ACKNOWLEDGMENTS

The International Committee on Systematic Bacteriology and the members of the Ad Hoc committee are grateful to the Bacteriology Division of the International Union of Microbiological Societies, to the International Council of Scientific Unions, and to the Bergey's Manual Board of Trustees for the provision of funds supporting the meeting, and to the Institut Pasteur (Paris) for its hospitality.

LITERATURE CITED

1. **Lapage, S. P., P. H. A. Sneath, E. F. Lessel, V. B. D. Skerman, H. P. R. Seeliger, and W. A. Clark (ed.).** 1975. International code of nomenclature of bacteria. 1976 Revision. American Society for Microbiology, Washington, D.C.

2. **Williams, J. E. 1983.** Warnings on a potential for laboratory-acquired infections as a result of the new nomenclature for the plague bacillus. Bull. WHO **61:**545–546.

3. **Woese, C. R., E. Stackebrandt, T. J. Macke, and G. E. Fox.** 1985. A phylogenetic definition of the major eubacterial taxa. System. Appl. Microbiol. **6:**143–151.

APPENDIX J
Glossary

J1 Taxonomic terms
J2 Abbreviations and Acronyms

J1 TAXONOMIC TERMS

We have been unable to avoid the use of some taxonomic terms in this *Manual*, and short notes on some of those more commonly used are given below. Those who would like more help or greater detail should consult *A Dictionary of Microbial Taxonomy* by Cowan (1978).

Accession number. The number allotted to a culture when it is accessioned (accepted) into a permanently established culture collection. Even if the classification (and the name) of the organism changes, the accession number remains the same.

Antibiogram. A record of the sensitivity or resistance of an organism to the different antibiotics listed. It is often an essential part of the bacteriological report made to the clinician who sent the specimen. Sometimes the sensitivity or resistance to particular antibiotics can aid in identification although the possibility of changes during antibiotic therapy should always be remembered. Non-therapeutic substances such as lysozyme or O/129 may also assist in the identification of an organism.

Carboxyphilic; capnophilic. Used to describe an organism whose growth is improved, or made possible, by an increase in the CO_2 content of the atmosphere.

Category. Used in taxonomy to indicate RANK in a hierarchical system of classification: genus, species, and so on. Often also used with the ordinary meaning of 'kind'.

Chemotaxonomy. A term used to describe the chemical nature of the structure and functions of organisms as applied to their taxonomy.

Conserved Name is one which the Judicial Comission, with reasons, has ruled must be used instead of all earlier synonyms for that taxon.

D_r Value. A term used in numerical taxonomy to express the total difference between two strains, taking into account the growth rates and the temperature and duration of incubation.

Dendrogram. A tree-like figure used to represent a hierarchy (and lines of descent) of organisms or a diagram showing the different levels of similarity among organisms.

Description. The characters of a taxon. When a description has been well written and includes all the essential information, it should enable future workers to recognize the taxon, should they meet it in practice. Descriptions vary greatly in value; older ones, because of the limited knowledge at the time they were written, are often inadequate by present standards, and the taxa may not now be recognizable.

Diagnosis in systematic bacteriology (and taxonomy) is a brief statement of characters that distinguish an organism from its neighbours. It is the equivalent of the term 'differential diagnosis' in clinical medicine.

Diagnostician. In a medical bacteriology laboratory this means the person(s) responsible for identifying an organism. It does *not* mean the person(s) responsible for making a clinical diagnosis or the clinician who sent the specimen to the laboratory.

Effective publication is the term used in the Bacteriological Code for the kind of publication authorized by it. Effective publication consists of publishing relevant information in printed form for distribution to the public and scientific institutions by sale or gift. Reading a paper at a meeting of a learned society does not constitute effective publication for names of bacteria, but publication in the Proceedings (or Transactions) of the Society concerned may well do so. Publication in the IJSB constitutes effective publication for new species (see valid publication).

Family (and **subfamily**) represent biological ranks between those of Order and Genus.

Genus (genera). One of the basic ranks in hierarchical systems of biological classification between families and species. A genus represents a collection of species with many characters in common though the actual limits are a matter of individual judgement.

G+C ratio. The proportions of the four DNA bases guanine (G), cytosine (C), adenine (A) and thymine (T). Because of the molecular equivalence of G+C to A+T, the ratio is usually expressed as the percentage of G+C to the total of bases (% G+C; moles % G+C).

Genotype, –ic. The hereditary potential of an organism. A theoretical unit from which existing organisms have developed under the influence of their surroundings and possibly changed character to become the PHENOTYPE.

Group. A common term for a collection of similar objects or biological entities. It is used in taxonomy for a collection of strains not yet allocated to a particular RANK; it may be a collection of strains (eventually they may form a species) or a collection of species (perhaps a potential genus). In serology it may be a collection of serotypes. It preferably is written or printed (in English) with the lower case letter g so as not to be confused with defined Groups.

Halophil(e) describes an organism that can tolerate and grow in a medium with a salt concentration greater than 0.85%; strictly it should be applied only to organisms with a requirement for a concentration of salt greater than 3%.

Homology. A term used to describe the extent of hybridizing capability between the DNA of microorganisms as a percentage.

Hybridization describes the extent of reassociation of single-stranded DNA derived from different strains to form double stranded DNA. A high degree of hybridization indicates genetic relatedness.

Hyperspace. A term used in numerical taxonomy to represent the dimensions needed to plot the distances between characters in an imaginary space. The closer the points are together, the more characters the organisms share in common.

Hypersphere. A term used in numerical taxonomy to represent a cluster of points (OTUs) defined in a hyperspace and distributed in the form of an imaginary theoretical sphere.

Illegitimate name of an organism is one that has not been formed or published in accordance with the rules of the Bacteriological Code.

Incertae sedis. A term used for named organisms of uncertain taxonomic position and applied to species and genera.

Infrasubspecific. A name given to a taxon below the rank of subspecies but which is not subject to the rules of the Bacteriological Code.

Legitimate name applied to an organism is one that has been formed and published in accordance with the rules of the Bacteriological Code.

Mesophil(e). A term used for organisms that are able to grow over a wide temperature range though not below 8 °C or above 45 °C. Many psychrophilic organisms can grow at temperatures within this range, but mesophiles are not tolerant of cold.

Neotype. The author of a new name (of a bacterium) should designate a nomenclatural type strain (see TYPE). If this is not done, a subsequent author may designate a type strain; a neotype is such a designated strain provided it is not one of the strains used by the original author of the name.

There are official recommendations for the choice, proposal, and designation of type strains; the old Recommendations in rule 12e of the 1958 edition of the Bacteriological Code were unintentionally omitted from the 1966 version printed in the *International Journal of Systematic Bacteriology* (IJSB), **16**, 459–90. They are now dealt with fully in the revised Bacteriological Code (1976 revision) in Rule 18e. The most important points for an author who intends to propose a neotype are (i) the proposal must be published in the IJSB; (ii) it must be accompanied by a description (or a reference to a published description) of the proposed strain; and (iii) it must include a record of the deposition of the strain in a permanently established culture collection so that it is readily available. These requirements, however, together with the *Approved Lists of Bacterial Names* and with the methods currently available for the preservation of bacteria make it unlikely that there will be much need for neotype strains in future.

Nomen periculosum. The term for a name validly proposed and taxonomically correct for a species or taxon but which, if accepted, could cause uncertainty, confusion or danger in practice. For example, the proposed name *Yersinia tuberculosis* subsp. *pestis* for the plague organism was overruled because it could be medically misleading; the correct name accordingly remains *Yersinia pestis*.

Operational Taxonomic Unit (OTU). A term used in relation to work in progress embracing an individual organism, a population of organisms, a taxon, a species or even a genus. In microbiology it is used by numerical taxonomists as a useful substitute for strain(s).

Phase should be reserved for phenomena with cyclical or to-and-fro variation, as for example the phases of *Salmonella* H antigens.

Phenon. A term used for a group of organisms in which the extent of their similarity is established by taxonomic methods. Instead of referring to species and genera, the bacterial groups are defined as phenons with a particular percentage of similarity (e.g. the 85% phenon).

Phenotype, –ic. The characters of an organism that can be determined now; cf. the GENOTYPE, which is the theoretical starting point that contains the hereditary potential of the taxon.

Phylogeny. A term used to describe the expression of evolutionary relationships between organisms.

Plasmid. A particle of genetic material (DNA) which contains recognizable genes which can be transferred to another organism. Antibiotic resistance, for example, may be 'plasmid-mediated' thus signifying that the gene for such resistance can be transferred from one bacterium to another. A wide range of biochemical characteristics may be plasmid-borne.

Probes for DNA or RNA are pieces of nucleic acids, derived from known organisms and labelled in some identifiable way, which are used to seek and bind to stretches of DNA or RNA that have complementary molecular base sequences. The proportion of labelled probe thus hybridizing gives a measure of the extent of genetic relatedness, which itself can be used as a taxonomic tool.

Psychrophil(e) describes an organism that grows at temperatures below those used in most medical laboratories; the optimal temperature for psychrophils is usually about 20 °C. Organisms able to grow below 5 °C may be described as psychrotrophic.

Rank. In a hierarchical system of classification organisms are arranged in a series of ranks (or CATEGORIES) each of which includes all members of the ranks immediately below. A taxon with the rank of family includes the lower taxa with the rank of genus, and each genus is made up of taxa with the rank of species; thus a family consists of the genera of that family and the species of those genera. And as in an army, the species are subordinate to taxa of higher rank. An alternative analogy is to the shelves of a bookstack; families near the top, genera in the middle, and species lower down.

Similarity coefficient (S value) is a measure, usually expressed as a percentage, of the overall similarity of two strains.

Subspecies. A category of rank immediately below that of species. It is the lowest rank to which the rules of the Bacteriological Code apply.

Sphere (see also **Hypersphere**). A term used in numerical taxonomy to represent the concept of a spherical cluster of organisms with an operational taxonomic unit (OTU) close to or at the geometrical centre of the cluster.

Symbiosis. Often used to mean two organisms living together for mutual benefit. Strictly, symbiosis means physical contact between organisms, each of which is a symbiont. Examples of symbiosis are *Rickettsia prowazekii* and *Pediculus corporis*. See also SYNERGISM.

Synergism. The state in which two or more organisms form an organization, sometimes called an ecosystem, for mutual benefit (often called SYMBIOSIS, q.v.). The satellitism shown by colonies of *Haemophilus influenzae* near colonies of *Staphylococcus aureus* growing on blood agar is a one-sided form of synergism.

Synonym. A word with the same meaning as another; synonyms are different words for the same thing. In nomenclature, synonyms are different names applied to the same taxon, but this does not mean that the individual units or organisms making up the taxon are identical. Strictly, synonymy applies only to the names; taxa and individual bacteria cannot be synonymous.

Systematics. A term used to embrace the many different approaches to the characterization, differentiation, labelling and orderly arrangement of organisms so that the information can be communicated succinctly.

T_m Value. The temperature at which a dilute solution of double stranded nucleic acid melts as indicated by increased light absorbance at a wavelength of 260 nm.

Taxon (pl. Taxa). A taxonomic group of any size greater than a single strain. Two or more similar strains can form a taxon; its RANK may be that of a serotype, species, genus, or even a kingdom, with numerous intermediate ranks between kingdom and genus, none of which may have practical significance.

Thermophil(e). A descriptive term applied to organisms capable of growing at temperatures above that of animals, usually not below 40 °C.

Type. This common English word meaning 'kind' has a special use in taxonomy for the nomenclatural type of a taxon. The nomenclatural type of a species is a strain (the type strain); of a genus it is a species (type species), and of a family or higher taxon the type is a genus (type genus).

The nomenclatural type is a means of attaching a name to a taxon; strictly it refers to a particular strain for which that name is published, but other strains that are regarded as similar (and that may be a matter of opinion) are entitled to bear the same name. It is a purely nomenclatural device and it is naive to think that the word type should be used only in its strict taxonomic sense. On the other hand it is reasonable to expect that, in papers on taxonomic subjects, the word will be used only in that strict sense.

Valid publication is publication (of a bacterial name) in accordance with certain requirements laid down in the Bacteriological Code.

Variant. A strain that shows one or more differences in characters from the parent; largely replaced by the word mutant when the change is believed to be due to a genetic change.

Variety (var.) is a term used for a variant that has become stabilized as a regular form. A category of rank below that of species. It equated previously with subspecies but it cannot be applied to new bacterial names published after 1976. It can, however, be used to indicate an infrasubspecific taxon and is then subject to the rules of the Bacteriological Code.

J2 ABBREVIATIONS AND ACRONYMS

An expansion of some less well-known abbreviations and acronyms may be useful to readers of this *Manual*. The list is based partly on queries raised by the proof-readers for this edition and is not exhaustive.

ACES	**buffer** – N-2-acetamido-2-aminoethanesulphonic acid
ADC	albumin + glucose (dextrose) + catalase
AFB	Acid fast bacilli
ALM	Anaerobe Laboratory Manual, Virginia Polytechnic Institute, Blacksburg, Virginia, USA
ANSI	American National Standards Institute
API	Identification kit system as originally described by Buissière & Nardon (1968)
ASB	Aerobic spore-bearing organisms *(Bacillus)*
ASS	Ammonium salt sugars media
ATCC	American Type Culture Collection, 12301 Parklawn Drive, Rockville, Maryland 20852, USA
BASIC	Beginners' All-purpose Symbolic Instruction Code (computer language)
BCG	Bacillus Calmette-Guerin
BCYE	Buffered charcoal yeast-extract medium
BIP	Bacterial Identification Profile
BSS	Buffered single substrate media
CAMP	Test described by Christie, Atkins & Munch-Petersen (1944)
CDC	Centers for Disease Control, Atlanta, Georgia, USA
CDSC	Communicable Disease Surveillance Centre, PHLS
CLED	Cystine-lactose-electrolyte deficient medium
COBOL	Common Business Oriented Language (computer language)
CSU	Carbon source utilization tests
CYLG	Casein yeast lactate glucose medium
DCA	De(s)oxycholate Citrate agar medium
DMRQC	Division of Microbiological Reagents and Quality Control, PHLS
DOS	Disk operating system
EDTA	Ethylenediaminetetra-acetic acid (also known as Sequestric acid)
EHC	Ethylhydrocuprein (optochin)
FEMS	Federation of European Microbiological Societies
FN	Fluorescence–denitrification medium of Pickett & Pedersen (1968)
HTST	High temperature, short time heat-treatment
IAMS	International Association of Microbiological Societies
IATS	International Antigenic Typing Scheme
ICSB	International Committee for Systematic Bacteriology
IJSB	International Journal of Systematic Bacteriology
IMViC	Indole, methyl red, Voges-Proskaüer, and citrate utilization tests
IUMS	International Union of Microbiological Societies (formerly IAMS)
KIA	Kligler iron Agar medium

LJ	Lowenstein-Jensen medium
LV	Lecithovitellin
MR	Methyl Red test
MUMPS	Massachusetts General Hospital Utility Multi-programming System (computer language)
NAD	Nicotinamide adenine dinucleotide (V factor)
NAG	non-agglutinable vibrio
NCTC	National Collection of Type Cultures, PHLS
NCV	non-cholera vibrio
NLF	Non-lactose fermenter
OF	Oxidation-Fermentation test of Hugh & Leifson (1953)
ONPG	o-nitrophenyl-β-D-galactopyranoside
OTU	Operational Taxonomic Unit
PHB	Poly-ß-hydroxybutyrate (used in agar medium)
PHBA	Poly-ß-hydroxybutyric acid (characteristic build-up in *Pseudomonas* cells)
PHLS	Public Health Laboratory Service, 61 Colindale Avenue, London NW9 5DF, UK
PPLO	Pleuropneumonia-like organisms
PRAS	Pre-reduced anaerobically sterilized media
PV	Panton–Valentine leucocidin
PWS	Peptone water sugar media
QAL	Quality Assessment Laboratory, DMRQC
SLM	Single Linkage Method (cluster analysis)
SQL	Structured query language (computer language)
SS	Salmonella-Shigella medium
STAA	Streptomycin Thallous Acetate agar medium
TCH	Thiophane carboxylic acid hydrazide
TSI	Triple sugar iron medium
TTC	2,3,5-triphenyltetrazolium chloride
UKNEQAS	UK National External Quality Assessment Scheme
UPGMA	Unweighted Pair Group Method by Averages (cluster analysis)
VDU	Visual display unit
VP	Voges-Proskaüer test

Codes used for various organisms

Biogroup 3A	*Yersinia enterolitica* biogroup 3A = *Yersinia mollaretti*
Biogroup 3B	*Yersinia enterolitica* biogroup 3B = *Yersinia bercovieri*
B5W	*Acinetobacter calcoaceticus*
C27	*Plesiomonas shigelloides*
CNW	*Campylobacter* (catalase negative/weak) group
Group IIf	*Weeksella virosa*
Group IIj	*Weeksella zoohelcum*
Group IIk2	*Sphingobacterium multivorum*
Group IIb	contains *Flavobacterium indologenes*
Group IVe	*Alcaligenes*-like organism (*Oligella* gen. nov. proposed to include also *Moraxella urethralis*)
Group Vd1	*Achromobacter* biotype 1 = *Ochrobactrum anthropi*
Group Vd2	*Achromobacter* biotype 2 = *Ochrobactrum anthropi*
Group Ve1	*Chryseomonas luteola*
Group Ve2	*Flavimonas oryzihabitans*
Group F	*Vibrio fluvialis* (also known as CDC group EF6)
Group JK	*Corynebacterium jeikeium*
Group M-4f	*Flavobacterium odoratum*
HB-1	*Eikenella corrodens* (Jackson & Goodman, 1972)
29911	group or biotype = *Providencia alcalifaciens*
32011	group or biotype = *Hafnia alvei*

267

REFERENCES

Abbot, J. D. & Shannon, R. (1958). A method for typing *Shigella sonnei*, using colicine production as a marker. *J. clin. Path.* **11**, 71.

Abd-el-Malek, Y. & Gibson, T. (1948*a*). Studies in the bacteriology of milk. I. The streptococci of milk. *J. Dairy Res.* **15**, 233.

Abd-el-Malek, Y. & Gibson, T. (1948*b*). Studies in the bacteriology of milk. II. The staphylococci and micrococci of milk. *J. Dairy Res.* **15**, 249.

Abrams, E., Zierdt, C. H. & Brown, J. A. (1971). Observations on *Aeromonas hydrophila* septicaemia in a patient with leukaemia. *J. clin. Path.* **24**, 49.

Advisory Committee (1990). Advisory Committee on Dangerous Pathogens. *Categorisation of Pathogens according to Hazard and Categories of Containment.* Edn 2. London: HMSO.

Advisory Committee (1991). Health & Safety Commission: Safety in Health Service Laboratories. *Safe working and the prevention of infection in clinical laboratories.* London: HMSO.

Aevaliotis, A., Belle, A. M., Chanione, J. P. & Serruys, E. (1985). *Kluyvera ascorbata* isolated from a baby with diarrhea. *Clin. Microbiol. Newsl.* **7**, 51.

Akiyama, S., Takizawa, K., Ichinoe, H., Enemoto, H., Kobayashi, T. & Sakazaki, R. (1963). Application of teepol to isolation for *Vibrio parahaemolyticus. Jap. J. Bacteriol.* **18**, 255. (In Japanese.)

Albert, H. (1921). Modification of stain for diphtheria bacilli. *J. Am. med. Ass.* **76**, 240.

Albritton, W. L., Penner, S., Staney, L. & Brunton, J. (1978). Biochemical characteristics of *Haemophilus influenzae* in relationship to source of isolation and antibiotic resistance. *J. clin. Microbiol.* **7**, 519.

Alderson, G. (1985). The current taxonomic status of the genus *Micrococcus. Zbl. Bakt. Suppl.* **14**, 117.

Aldová, E., Hausner, O., Brenner, D. J., Kocmoud, Z., Schindler, J., Potuzníková, B & Petrás, P. (1988). *Pragia fontium* gen. nov., sp. nov. of the family *Enterobacteriaceae*, isolated from water. *Int. J. syst. Bact.* **38**, 193.

Aleksić, S., Steigerwalt, A. G., Bockemühl, J., Huntley-

Carter, G. P. & Brenner, D. J. (1987). *Yersinia rohdei* sp. nov. isolated from human and dog feces and surface water. *Int. J. syst. Bact.* **37**, 327.

Allen, D. A., Austin, B. & Colwell, R. R. (1983). *Aeromonas media*, a new species isolated from river water. *Int J. syst. Bact.* **33**, 599.

Allen, L. A., Pasley, S. M. & Pierce, M. S. F. (1952). Conditions affecting the growth of *Bacterium coli* on bile salts media. Enumeration of this organism in polluted waters. *J. gen. Microbiol.* **7**, 257.

Anderhub, B., Pitt, T.L., Erdman Y. J. & Willcox, W. R. (1977). A comparison of typing methods for *Serratia marcescens. J. Hyg., Camb.* **79**, 89.

Anderson, J. S., Cooper, K. E., Happold, F. C. & McLeod, J. W. (1933). Incidence and correlation with clinical severity of gravis, mitis, and intermediate types of diphtheria bacillus in a series of 500 cases at Leeds. *J. Path. Bact.* **36**, 169.

Anderson, J. S., Happold, F. C., McLeod, J. W. & Thomson, J. G. (1931). On the existence of two forms of diphtheria bacillus – *B. diphtheriae gravis* and *B. diphtheriae mitis* – and a new medium for their differentiation and for the bacteriological diagnosis of diphtheria. *J. Path. Bact.* **34**, 667.

Ando, K., Moriya, Y. & Kuwahara, S. (1959). Studies on the effect of Tween 80 on the growth of *Erysipelothrix insidiosa. Jap. J. Microbiol.* **3**, 85.

Andrade, E. (1906). Influence of glycerin in differentiating certain bacteria. *J. med. Res.* **14**, 551.

Andrewes, F. W. (1918). Dysentery bacilli: the differentiation of the true dysentery bacilli from allied species. *Lancet*, i, 560.

Andrewes, F. W. & Inman, A. C. (1919). A study of the serological races of the Flexner group i of dysentery bacilli. *Spec. Rep. Ser. med. Res. Coun.* no. 42.

Approved Lists of Bacterial Names (1980). Ed. V. B. D. Skerman, V. McGowan & P. H. A. Sneath. *Int. J. syst. Bact.* **30**, 225. Printed in book form, 1980. Washington, D. C.: American Society for Microbiology.

Arnold, W. M., Jr & Weaver, R. H. (1948). Quick microtechniques for the identification of cultures. I.

Indole production. *J. Lab. clin. Med.* **33**, 1334.

Asai, T., Iizuka, H. & Komagata, K. (1962). The flagellation of genus *Kluyvera*. *J. gen. appl. Microbiol.* **8**, 187.

Asai, T., Okumura, S. & Tsunoda, T. (1956). On a new genus, *Kluyvera. Proc. Japn. Acad.* **32**, 488.

Asai, T., Okumura, S. & Tsunoda, T. (1957). On the classification of the α-ketoglutaric acid accumulating bacteria in aerobic fermentation. *J. gen. appl. Microbiol.* **3**, 13.

Asheshov, E. H. & Rountree, P. M. (1975). Report (1970–1974) of the Subcommittee on Phage-Typing of Staphylococci to the International Committee on Systematic Bacteriology. *Int. J. syst. Bact.* **25**, 241.

Ashley, D. J. B. & Kwantes, W. (1961). Four cases of human infection with *Achromobacter anitratus. J. clin. Path.* **14**, 670.

Aubert, E. (1950). 'Cold ' stain for acid-fast bacteria. *Can. J. publ. Hlth,* **41**, 31.

Audurier, A., Chatelain, R., Chalons, F. & Piechaud, M. (1979). Lysotypie de 823 souches de *Listeria monocytogenes* isolées en France de 1958 à 1978. *Annls Microbiol. Inst. Pasteur, Paris* **130** B, 179.

Austrian, R. & Collins, P. (1966). Importance of carbon dioxide in the isolation of pneumococci. *J. Bact.* **92**, 1281.

Ayers, S. H. & Rupp, P. (1922). Differentiation of hemolytic streptococci from human and bovine sources by the hydrolysis of sodium hippurate. *J. infect. Dis.* **30**, 388.

Ayres, P. A. & Barrow, G. I. (1978). The distribution of *Vibrio parahaemolyticus* in British coastal waters: report of a collaborative study 1975–6. *J. Hyg., Camb.* **80**, 281.

Baber, K. G. (1969). A selective medium for the isolation of *Haemophilus* from sputum. *J. med. Lab. Technol.* **26**, 391.

Bachmann, B. & Weaver, R. H. (1951). Rapid microtechnics for identification of cultures. V. Reduction of nitrates to nitrites. *Am. J. clin. Path.* **21**, 195.

Bacteriological Code – see *International Code of Nomenclature of Bacteria.*

Baer, H. & Washington, L. (1972). Numerical diagnostic key for the identification of *Enterobacteriaceae. Appl. Microbiol.* **23**, 108.

Bagley, S. T., Seidler, R. J. & Brenner, D. J. (1981). *Klebsiella planticola* sp. nov.: a new species of Enterobacteriaceae found primarily in nonclinical environments. *Curr. Microbiol.* **6**, 105.

Bailey, J. H. (1933). A medium for the isolation of *Bacillus pertussis. J. infect. Dis.* **52**, 94.

Bailey, R. B., Voss, J. L. & Smith, R. F. (1979). Factors affecting isolation and identification of *Haemophilus vaginalis (Corynebacterium vaginale). J. clin. Microbiol.* **9**, 65.

Bailie, W. E., Coles, E.H. & Weide, K. D. (1973). Deoxyribonucleic acid characterization of a microorganism isolated from infectious thromboembolic meningoencephalomyelitis of cattle. *Int. J. syst. Bact.* **23**, 231.

Bain, N. & Shewan, J. M. (1968). Identification of *Aeromonas, Vibrio* and related organisms. In *Identification Methods for Microbiologists*, Part B (ed. B. Gibbs & D.A. Shapton). p.79. London: Academic Press.

Baine, W. B., Rasheed, J. K. & Feeley, J. C. (1978). Effect of supplemental L-tyrosine on pigment production in cultures of the Legionnaires' disease bacterium. *Curr. Microbiol.* **1**, 93.

Baird-Parker, A. C. (1962). An improved diagnostic and selective medium for isolating coagulase positive staphylococci. *J. appl. Bact.* **25**, 12.

Baird-Parker, A. C. (1963). A classification of micrococci and staphylococci based on physiological and biochemical tests. *J. gen. Microbiol.* **30**, 409.

Baird-Parker, A. C. (1965a). The classification of staphylococci and micrococci from world-wide sources. *J. gen. Microbiol.* **38**, 363.

Baird-Parker, A. C. (1965b). Staphylococci and their classification. *Ann. N.Y. Acad. Sci.* **128**, 4.

Baker, J. S. (1986). Differentiation of micrococci from coagulase - negative staphylococci. *In Coagulase negative staphylococci* (ed. P.-A. Mardh & K. H. Schleifer), p.27. Stockholm:Almquist & Wicksell International.

Ball, L. C. (1985). Serological identification of *Streptococcus sanguis* and *Str. mitior. J. clin. Path.* **38**, 452.

Ball, L. C. & Parker, M. T. (1979). The cultural and biochemical characters of *Streptococcus milleri* strains isolated from human sources. *J. Hyg., Camb.* **82**, 63.

Balsdon, M. J., Taylor, G. E., Pead, L. and Maskell, R. (1980). *Corynebacterium vaginale* and vaginitis: A controlled trial of treatment. *Lancet,* **i**, 501.

Baptist, J. N., Mandel, M. & Gherna, R. L. (1978). Comparative zone electrophoresis of enzymes in the genus *Bacillus. Int. J. syst. Bact.* **28**, 299.

Barakat, M. Z. & Abd El-Wahab, M.E. (1951). The differentiation of monosaccharides from disaccharides and polysacchaarides and identification of fructose. *J. Pharm. Pharmac.* **3**, 511.

Barber, M. (1939). A comparative study of *Listerella* and *Erysipelothrix. J. Path. Bact.* **48**, 11.

Barber, M. & Kuper, S. W. A. (1951). Identification of *Staphylococcus pyogenes* by the phosphatase reaction. *J. Path. Bact.* **63**, 65.

Barksdale, L. (1981). The genus *Corynebacterium*. In *The Prokaryotes: A Handbook of Habitats, Isolation and Identification of Bacteria* (ed. M. P. Starr, H. Stolp, H.

G. Trüper, A. Balows & Schlegel). p.1827. Berlin: Springer-Verlag.

Barnham, M., Cole, G., Efstratiou, A., Tagg, J. R. & Skjold, S. A. (1987). Characterization of *Streptococcus zooepidemicus* (Lancefield group C) from human and selected animal infections. *Epidemiol. Inf.* **98**, 171.

Barrett, T. J. & Blake, P. A. (1981). Epidemiological usefulness of changes in hemolytic activity of *Vibrio cholerae* biotype el tor during the seventh pandemic. *J. clin. Microbiol.* **13**, 126.

Barritt, M. M. (1936). The intensification of the Voges-Proskaüer reaction by the addition of α-naphthol. *J. Path. Bact.* **42**, 441.

Barrow, G. I. & Miller, D. C. (1976). *Vibrio parahaemolyticus* and seafood. In *Microbiology in Agriculture, Fisheries and Food* (ed. F. A. Skinner & J. G. Carr), p. 181. (Society for Applied Bacteriology Symposium Series no. 4). London: Academic Press.

Bascomb, S., Lapage, S. P., Curtis, M. A. & Willcox, W. R. (1973). Identification of bacteria by computer. Identification of reference strains. *J. gen. Microbiol.* **77**, 291.

Bascomb, S., Lapage, S. P., Willcox, W. R. & Curtis, M. A. (1971). Numerical classification of the tribe Klebsielleae. *J. gen. Microbiol.* **66**, 279.

Basu, S. & Mukerjee, S. (1968). Bacteriophage typing of *Vibrio eltor. Experimentia*, **24**, 299.

Batty-Smith, C. G. (1941). The detection of acetyl-methyl-carbinol in bacterial cultures. A comparative study of the methods of O'Meara and of Barritt. *J. Hyg., Camb.* **41**, 521.

Baumann, L., Bowditch, R. D. & Baumann, P. (1983). Description of *Deleya* gen. nov. created to accommodate the marine species *Alcaligenes aestus, A. pacificus, A. cupidus, A. venustus* and *Pseudomonas marina. Int. J. syst. Bact.* **33**, 793.

Baumann, P., Doudoroff, M. & Stanier, R. Y. (1968a). Study of the *Moraxella* group. I. Genus *Moraxella* and the *Neisseria catarrhalis* group. *J. Bact.* **95**, 58.

Baumann, P., Doudoroff, M. & Stanier, R. Y. (1968b). A study of the *Moraxella* group. II. Oxidative [sic]-negative species (genus *Acinetobacter*). *J. Bact.* **95**, 1520.

Bayer, S. S., Chow, A. W., Betts, D. & Guze, L. B. (1978). Lactobacillemia – report of nine cases. Important clinical and therapeutic considerations. *Am. J. Med.* **64**, 808.

Beighton, D. (1985). *Streptococcus mutans* and other streptococci from the oral cavity. In *Isolation and Identification of Microorganisms of Medical and Veterinary Importance* (ed. C. H. Collins & J. M. Grange), p.177. (Society for Applied Bacteriology, Technical Series no. 21.) London: Academic Press.

Beijerinck, M. W. (1900). Schwefelwasserstoff bildung in den Stadtgräben und Aufstellung der Gattung Aërobacter. *Zentbl. Bakt. ParasitKde Abt. II* **6**, 193.

Benito, R., Vazquez, J. A., Berron, S. Fenoll, A. & Saez-Nieto, J. A. (1986). A modified scheme for biotyping *Gardnerella vaginalis. J. med. Microbiol.* **21**, 357.

Benjamin, J., Leaper, S., Owen, R. J. & Skirrow, M. B., (1983). Description of *Campylobacter laridis*, a new species comprising the Nalidixic Acid Resistant Thermophilic *Campylobacter* (NARTC) group. *Curr. Microbiol.* **8**, 231.

Bennett, K. W. & Duerden, B. I. (1985). Identification of Fusobacteria in a routine laboratory. *J. appl. Bact.* **59**, 171.

Benson, R. F., Thacker, W. L., Quinlivan, P. A., Mayberry, R., Brenner, D. J. & Wilkinson, H. W. (1989). *Legionella quinlivanii* sp. nov. isolated from water. *Curr. Microbiol.* **18**, 195.

Bercovier, H., Brenner, D.J., Ursing, J., Steigerwalt, A. G, Fanning, G. R., Alonso, J. M., Carter, G. P. & Mollaret, H. H. (1980a). Characterization of *Yersinia enterocolitica sensu stricto. Curr. Microbiol.* **4**, 201.

Bercovier, H., Mollaret, H. H., Alonso, J.M., Brault, J., Fanning, G. R., Steigerwalt, A. G. & Brenner, D. J. (1980b). Intra- and interspecies relatedness of *Yersinia pestis* by DNA hybridization and its relationship to *Yersinia pseudotuberculosis. Curr. Microbiol.* **4**, 225.

Bercovier, H., Steigerwalt, A. G., Guiyoule, A., Huntley-Carter, G. & Brenner, D.J. (1984). *Yersinia aldovae* (formerly *Yersinia enterocolitica*-like Group X2): a new species of *Enterobacteriaceae* isolated from aquatic ecosystems. *Int. J. syst. Bact.* **34**, 166.

Bercovier, H., Ursing, J., Brenner, D.J., Steigerwalt, A. G., Fanning, G.R., Carter, G.P. & Mollaret, H.H. (1980c). *Yersinia kristensenii*: a new species of *Enterobacteriaceae* composed of sucrose-negative strains (formerly called atypical Y*ersinia enterocolitica* or *Yersinia enterocolitica*-like). *Curr. Microbiol.* **4**, 219.

Berdal, B. P. & Søderlund, E. (1977). Cultivation and isolation of *Francisella tularensis* on selective chocolate agar as used routinely for the isolation of gonococci. *Acta path. microbiol. scand.* **B. 85**, 108.

Bergan, T. (1978). Phage typing of *Pseudomonas aeruginosa.* In *Methods in Microbiology* (ed. T. Bergan & J. R. Norris), vol. 10, pp. 169. London: Academic Press.

Bergan, T. & Kocur, M. (1982). *Stomatococcus mucilaginosus* gen. nov., sp. nov., ep. rev., a member of the family Micrococcaceae. *Int. J. syst. Bact.* **32**, 374.

Berger, U. (1960a). *Neisseria haemolysans* (Thjötta und Böe, 1938): Untersuchungen zur Stellung im System. *Z. Hyg. InfektKrankh.* **146**, 253.

Berger, U. (1960b). *Neisseria animalis* nov. spec. *Z. Hyg. InfektKrankh.* **147**, 158.

Berger, U. (1961). A proposed new genus of Gram negative cocci: *Gemella. Int. Bull. bact. Nomencl. Taxon.* **11**, 17.

Berger, U. (1962). Über das Vorkommen von Neisserien bei einigen Tieren. *Z. Hyg. InfektKrankh.* **148**, 445.

Berger, U. (1974). Pathogenicity of lactobacilli. *Dt. med. Wochenschr.* **99**, 1200.

Berger, U. & Pervanidis, A. (1986). Differentiation of *Gemella haemolysans* (Thjötta & Böe, 1938) Berger 1960, from *Streptococcus morbillorum* (Prevot 1933) Holdeman & Moore, 1974. *Zbl. Bakt. Mikrobiol. Hyg.* **261**, 311.

Bergey's Manual of Determinative Bacteriology (1923–74). Eight edns: **1**, 1923; **2**, 1925; **3**, 1930; **4**, 1934; **5**, 1939; **6**, 1948; **7**, 1957; **8**, 1974. Baltimore: The Williams & Wilkins Co.

Bergey's Manual of Systematic Bacteriology. Vol. 1, 1984: *The Gram-negatives of general, medical, or industrial importance* (ed. N. R. Krieg & J. G. Holt); Vol. 2, 1986: *The Gram-positives other than actinomycetes* (ed. P. H. A. Sneath, N. S. Mair, M. E. Sharpe & J. G. Holt): Vol. 3, 1989: *The archaebacteria, cyanobacteria and remaining Gram-negatives* (ed. J. T. Staley, M. P. Bryant, N. Pfennig & J. G. Holt); Vol. 4, 1989: *The actinomycetes* (ed. S. T. Williams, M. E. Sharpe & J. G. Holt). Baltimore: Williams & Wilkins.

Berkeley, R. C. W., Logan, N. A., Shute, L. A. & Capey, A. G. (1984). Identification of *Bacillus* species. In *Methods in Microbiology*, vol. 16 (ed. T. Bergan), p. 291. London: Academic Press.

Bernaerts, M. J. & DeLey, J. (1963). A biochemical test for crown gall bacteria. *Nature, Lond.* **197**, 406.

Biberstein, E. L. & Gills, M. (1961). Catalase activity of *Haemophilus* species grown with graded amounts of haemin. *J. Bact.* **81**, 380.

Biberstein, E. L. & Gills, M. G. (1962). The relation of the antigenic types to the A and T types of *Pasteurella haemolytica. J. comp. Path. Ther.* **72**, 316.

Biberstein, E. L., Gills, M. & Knight, H. (1960). Serological types of *Pasteurella haemolytica. Cornell Vet.* **50**, 283.

Biberstein, E. L. & White, D. C. (1969). A proposal for the establishment of two new *Haemophilus* species. *J. med. Microbiol.* **2**, 75.

Billing, E. (1955). Studies on a soap tolerant organism: a new variety of *Bacterium anitratum. J. gen. Microbiol.* **13**, 252.

Billing, E. & Luckhurst, E. R. (1957). A simplified method for the preparation of egg yolk media. *J. appl. Bact.* **20**, 90.

Black, W. A., Hodgson, R. & McKechnie, A. (1971). Evaluation of three methods using deoxyribonuclease production as a screening test for *Serratia marcescens. J. clin. Path.* **24**, 313.

Blackall, P. J. (1988). Biochemical properties of catalase-positive avian haemophili. *J. gen. Microbiol.* **134**, 2801.

Blaser, M. J., Hickman, F.W., Farmer, J. J., Brenner, D. J., Balows, A. & Feldman, R.A. (1980). *Salmonella typhi*: the laboratory as a reservoir of infection. *J. inf. Dis.* **142**, 934.

Board, R. G. & Holding, A. J. (1960). The utilization of glucose by aerobic Gram-negative bacteria. *J. appl. Bact.* **23**, xi.

Bolton, F.J., Holt, A. V. & Hutchinson, D. N. (1984). Campylobacter biotyping scheme of epidemiological value. *J. clin. Path.* **37**, 677.

Bolton, F. J., Holt, A. V. & Hutchinson, D. N. (1985). Urease-positive thermophilic campylobacters. Lancet, i, 1217.

Bolton, F. J., Hutchinson, D. N. & Parker, G. (1988). Reassessment of selective agars and filtration techniques for isolation of *Campylobacter* species from faeces. *Eur. J. clin. Microbiol. inf. Dis.* **7**, 155.

Bordet, J. & Gengou, O. (1906). Le microbe de la coqueluche. *Annls Inst. Pasteur, Paris,* **20**, 731.

Borman, E. K., Stuart, C. A. & Wheeler, K. M. (1944). Taxonomy or the family Enterobacteriaceae. *J. Bact.* **48**, 351.

Bornstein, R. F., Marmet, D., Nowicki, M., Meugnier, H., Fleurette, J., Ageron, E., Grimont, F., Grimont, P. A. D., Thacker, W. L., Benson, R. F. & Brenner, D. J. (1989). *Legionella gratiana* sp. nov. isolated from French spa water. *Res. Microbiol.* **140**, 541.

Boswell, P. A., Batstone, G. F. & Mitchell, R. G. (1972). The oxidase reaction in the classification of the Micrococcaceae. *J. med. Microbiol.* **5**, 267.

Bouley, G. (1965). Épreuve de C.A.M.P. et distinction rapide entre *Pasteurella multocida* et *Pasteurella haemolytica. Annls Inst. Pasteur, Paris,* **108**, 129.

Bourke, A. T. C., Cossins, Y. N., Gray, B. R. W., Lunney, T. J., Rostron, N.A., Holmes, R. V., Griggs, E. R., Larsen, D. J. & Kelk, V. R. (1986). Investigation of cholera acquired from the riverine environment in Queensland. *Med. J. Australia.* **144**, 229.

Bourne, K.A., Beebe, J. L., Lue, Y. A. & Ellner, P. D. (1978). Bacteremia due to *Bifidobacterium, Eubacterium* or *Lactobacillus*: twenty-one cases and review of the literature. *Yale J. Biol. Med.* **51**, 505.

Bouvet, A., Villeroy, F., Cheng, F., Lamesch, C., Williamson, R. & Gutmann, L. (1985). Characterization of nutritionally variant streptococci by biochemical tests and penicillin-binding proteins. *J. clin. Microbiol.* **22**, 1030.

Bouvet, O. M. M., Grimont, P. A. D., Richard, C., Aldová,

E., Hausner, O. & Gabrhelova, M. (1985). *Budvicia aquatica* gen. nov., sp. nov.: a hydrogen sulfide-producing member of the Enterobacteriaceae. *Int. J. syst. Bact.* **35**, 60.

Bouvet, P. J. M. & Grimont, P. A. D. (1986). Taxonomy of the genus *Acinetobacter* with the recognition of *Acinetobacter baumannii* sp. nov., *Acinetobacter haemolyticus* sp. nov., *Acinetobacter johnsonii* sp. nov., and *Acinetobacter junii* sp. nov. and emended descriptions of *Acinetobacter calcoaceticus* and *Acinetobacter lwoffii*. *Int. J. syst. Bact.* **36**, 228.

Bouvet, P. J. M. & Grimont, P. A. \D. (1987). Identification and biotyping of clinical isolates of *Acinetobacter*. *Annls Inst. Pasteur, Paris*, **138**, 569.

Bowen, M. K., Thiele, L. C., Stearman, B. D. & Schaub, I. G. (1957). The optochin sensitivity test: a reliable method for identification of pneumococci. *J. Lab. clin. Med.* **49**, 641.

Bowers, E. F. & Jeffries, L. R. (1955). Optochin in the identification of *Str. pneumoniae*. *J. clin. Path.* **8**, 58.

Boyce, J. M. H., Frazer, J. & Zinnemann, K. (1969). The growth requirements of *Haemophilus aphrophilus*. *J. med. Microbiol.* **2**, 55.

Boyd, J. S. K. (1938). The antigenic structure of the mannitol-fermenting dysentery bacilli. *J. Hyg., Camb.* **38**, 477.

Branham, S. E. (1930). A new meningococcus-like organism (*Neisseria .flavescens*, n. sp.) from epidemic meningitis. *Publ. Hlth Rep., Wash.* **45**, 845.

Bray, J. (1945). A method of suppressing *Proteus* and coliform bacteria on routine blood agar plates. *J. Path. Bact.* **57**, 395.

Brayton, B. R., Bode, R. B., Colwell, R. R., MacDonell, M. T., Hall, H. L., Grimes, D. J., West, P. A. & Bryant, T. (1986). *Vibrio cincinnatiensis* sp. nov., a new human pathogen. *J. clin. Microbiol.* **23**, 104.

Brenner, D. J. (1973). Deoxyribonucleic acid reassociation in the taxonomy of enteric bacteria. *Int. J. syst. Bact.* **23**, 298.

Brenner, D. J. (1978). Characterization and clinical identification of Enterobacteriaceae by DNA hybridization. *Progress in Clinical Pathology*, vol. 7, p. 71.

Brenner, D. J. (1986). Classification of Legionellaceae. *Israel J. med. Sci.* **22**, 620.

Brenner, D. J., Steigerwalt, A. G. & Fanning, G. R. (1972). Differentiation of *Enterobacter aerogenes* from klebsiellae by deoxyribonucleic acid reassociation. *Int. J. syst. Bact.* **22**, 193.

Brenner, D. J., Steigerwalt, A. G. & McDade, J. E. (1979). Classification of the Legionnaire's disease bacterium: *Legionella pneumophila* genus novum, species nova of the family *Legionellaceae* familia nova. *Annls intern. Med.* **90**, 656.

Brenner, D. J., McWhorter, A. C., Knutson, J. K. L. & Steigerwalt, A. G. (1982*b*). *Escherichia vulneris*: a new species of *Enterobacteriaceae* associated with human wounds. *J. clin. Microbiol.* **15**, 1133.

Brenner, D. J., Bercovier, H., Ursing, J., Alonso, J. M., Steigerwalt, A. G., Fanning, G. R., Carter, G. P. & Mollaret, H. H. (1980*a*). *Yersinia intermedia*: a new species of *Enterobacteriaceae* composed of rhamnose-positive, melibiose-positive, raffinose-positive strains (formerly called *Yersinia enterocolitica* or *Yersinia enterocolitica*-like). *Curr. Microbiol.* **4**, 207.

Brenner, D. J., Davis, B. R., Steigerwalt, A. G., Riddle C.F. McWhorter, A.C., Allen, S.D., Farmer, J.J. III, Saitoh, Y. & Fanning, G.R. (1982*a*). Atypical biogroups of *Escherichia coli* found in clinical specimens and description of *Escherichia hermannii* sp. nov. *J. clin. Microbiol.* **15**, 703.

Brenner, D. J., Fanning, G. R., Knutson, J. K. L., Steigerwalt, A. G. & Krichevsky, M. I. (1984). Attempts to classify herbicola group – *Enterobacter agglomerans* strains by deoxyribonucleic acid hybridization and phenotypic tests. *Int. J. syst. Bact.* **34**, 45.

Brenner, D. J., Farmer, J. J. III, Fanning, G. R., Steigerwalt, A. G., Klykken, P., Wathen, H. G., Hickman, F. W. & Ewing, W. H. (1978). Deoxyribonucleic acid relatedness of *Proteus* and *Providencia* species. *Int. J. syst. Bact.* **28**, 269.

Brenner, D. J., Hickman-Brenner, F. W., Lee, J. V., Steigerwalt, A. G., Fanning, G. R., Hollis, D. G., Farmer J.J. III, Weaver, R. E., Joseph, S. W. & Seidler, R. J. (1983). *Vibrio furnissii* (formerly aerogenic biogroup of *Vibrio fluvialis*), a new species isolated from human faeces and the environment. *J. clin. Microbiol.* **18**, 816.

Brenner, D. J., Mayer, L. W., Carlone, G. M., Harrison, L. H., Bibb, W. F., de Cunto Brandileone, M. C., Sottnek, F. O. *et al.* (1988). Biochemical, genetic and epidemiologic characterization of *Haemophilus influenzae* biogroup Aegyptius (*Haemophilus aegyptius*) strains associated with Brazilian Purpuric Fever. *J. clin. Microbiol.* **26**, 1524.

Brenner, D. J., Richard, C., Steigerwalt, A. G., Asbury, M. A. & Mandel, M. (1980*b*). *Enterobacter gergoviae* sp. nov.: a new species of *Enterobacteriaceae* found in clinical specimens and the environment. *Int. J. syst. Bact.* **30**, 1.

Brenner, D. J., Steigerwalt, A. G., Gorman, G. W., Wilkinson, H. W., Bibb, W. F., Hackell, M., Tyndall, R. *et. al.* (1985). Ten new species of *Legionella*. *Int. J. syst. Bact.* **35**, 50.

Brenner, D. J., Steigerwalt, A. G., Wathen, H. G., Gross, R. J. & Rowe, B. (1982*c*). Confirmation of aerogenic strains of *Shigella boydii* 13 and further study of *Shigella* serotypes by DNA relatedness. *J. clin. Microbiol.* **16**, 432.

Brewer, J. H. (1940). Clear liquid mediums for the 'aerobic' cultivation of anaerobes. *J. Am. med. Ass.* **115**, 598.

Bridge, P. D. & Sneath, P. H. A. (1982). *Streptococcus gallinarum* sp. nov. and *Streptococcus oralis* sp. nov. *Int. J. syst. Bact* **32**, 410.

Bridge, P. D. & Sneath, P. H. A (1983). Numerical taxonomy of *Streptoccus. J. gen. Microbiol.* **129**, 565.

Bridson, E. Y. & Brecker, A. (1970). Design and formulation of microbial culture media. In *Methods in Microbiology*, vol. 3A. (Ed. J. R. Norris & D. W. Ribbons), p. 229. London: Academic Press.

Brindle, C. S. & Cowan, S. T. (1951). Flagellation and taxonomy of Whitmore's bacillus. *J. Path. Bact.* **63**, 571 .

Brisou, J. (1953). Essai sur la systématique du genre *Achromobacter. Annls Inst. Pasteur, Paris*, **84**, 812.

Brisou, J. & Morichau-Beauchant, R. (1952). Identité biochimique entre certaines souches de *B. anitratum* et *Moraxella lwoffi. Annls Inst. Pasteur, Paris*, **82**, 640.

Brisou, J. & Prévot, A. R. (1954). Étude de systématique bactérienne. X. Révision des espèces réunies dans le genre *Achromobacter. Annls Inst. Pasteur, Paris*, **86**, 722.

Brisou, J., Tysset, C., Rautlin de la Roy, Y. de & Jarriault, J. (1962). Intérêt taxinomique des oxydases et cytochromeoxydases microbiennes. *C. r. Séanc. Soc. Biol., Paris*, **156**, 1904.

British Pharmacopoeia (1963). London: The Pharmaceutical Press.

British Standard (1959). B.S. 757:1959. Methods of sampling and testing gelatines. London: British Standards Institution.

British Standard (1978). B.S. 611: Part 1: 1978. Petri dishes: Specification for glass Petri dishes. London: British Standards Institution.

British Standard (1982). B.S. 611: Part 2: 1982. Petri dishes: Specification for plastics Petri dishes for single use. London: British Standards Institution.

Brock, T. D. (1961). *Milestones in Microbiology.* London: Prentice-Hall International Inc.

Brooks, H. J. L., Chambers, T. J. & Tabaqchali, S. (1979). The increasing isolation of *Serratia* species from clinical specimens. *J. Hyg., Camb.* **82**, 31.

Brooks, M. E., Sterne, M. & Warrack, G. H. (1957). A reassessment of the criteria used for type differentiation of *Clostridium perfringens. J. Path. Bact.* **74**,185.

Brough, F. K. (1950). A rapid microtechnique for the determination of nitrate reduction by micro-organisms. *J. Bact.* **60**, 365.

Brouillard, J. A., Hansen, W. & Compete, A. (1984). Isolation of *Serratia ficaria* from human clinical specimens. *J. clin. Microbiol.* **19**, 902.

Brown, A. E. (1961). A simple and efficient method of filtering agar. J. *med. Lab. Technol.* **18**,109.

Brown, A., Garrity, G. M. & Vickers, R. M. (1981). *Fluoribacter dumoffi* (Brenner *et al.*) *comb. nov.* and *Fluoribacter gormanii* (Morris *et al.*) *comb. nov. Int. J. syst. Bact.* **31**, 111.

Brown, E. R., Moody, M. D., Treece, E. L. & Smith, C. W. (1958). Differential diagnosis of *Bacillus cereus, Bacillus anthracis* and *Bacillus cereus* var. *mycoides. J. Bact.* **75**, 499.

Brown, J. A. (1959). Preparing egg base media for tubercle bacilli in the autoclave. *Am. J. med. Technol.* **25**, 53.

Brown, J. H. (1919).The use of blood agar for the study of streptococci. *Monogr. Rockefeller Inst. med. Res.* no. 9.

Brown, R. L. & Evans, J. B. (1963). Comparative physiology of antibiotic-resistant strains of *Staphylococcus aureus. J. Bact.* **85**, 1409.

Brown, V. I. & Lowbury, J. L. (1965). Use of an improved cetrimide agar medium and other culture methods for *Pseudomonas aeruginosa. J. clin.Path.* **18**, 752.

Brown, W. R. L. & Ridout, C. W. (1960). An investigation of some sterilization indicators. *Pharm. J.* **184**, 5.

Brumfitt, W. (1959). Some growth requirements of *Haemophilus influenzae* and *Haemophilus pertussis. J. Path. Bact.* **77**, 95.

Bryant, T., Lee, J. V., West, P. A. & Colwell, R. R. (1986*a*). Numerical classification of species of *Vibrio* and related genera. *J. appl. Bact.* **61**, 437.

Bryant, T., Lee, J. V., West, P. A. & Colwell, R. R. (1986*b*). A probability matrix for the identification of species of *Vibrio* and related genera. *J. appl. Bact.* **61**, 469.

Bryce, D. M. (1956). The design and interpretation of sterility tests. *J. Pharm. Pharmac.* **8**, 561.

Brzin, B. (1965). Spheroplasty effect of the temperature of incubation on the cells of *Bacterium anitratum. Acta path. microbiol. scand.* **63**, 404.

Buchanan, A. M., Scott, J. L., Gerencser, M. A., Beaman, B. L., Jang, S. & Biberstein, E. L. (1984). *Actinomyces hordeovulneris* sp. nov., an agent of canine actinomycosis. *Int. J. syst. Bact.* **34**, 439.

Buchanan, B. B. & Pine, L. (1962). Characterization of a propionic acid producing actinomycete, *Actinomyces propionicus,* sp. nov. *J. gen. Microbiol.* **28**, 305.

Buchanan, R. E., Cowan, S. T., Wiken, T. & Clark, W. A. (1958). *International Code of Nomenclature of Bacteria and Viruses.* Ames, Iowa: State College Press. Reprinted with corrections 1959: Iowa State University Press.

Buchanan, R. E., St John-Brooks, R. & Breed, R. S. (1948). *International bacteriological code of nomenclature. J. Bact.* **55**, 287. Reprinted 1949, *J. gen. Microbiol.* **3**, 444.

Buissière, J. & Nardon, P. (1968). Microméthode d'identification des bactéries. I. Intérêt de la quantification des caractères biochimiques. *Annls Inst. Pasteur, Paris,* **115**, 218.

Bulloch, W. (1938). *The history of Bacteriology.* London: Oxford University Press.

Bulmash, J. M., Fulton, M. & Jiron, J. (1965). Lactose and sulfide reactions of an aberrant *Salmonella* strain. *J. Bat.* **89**, 259.

Burdon, K. L. (1956). Useful criteria for the identification of *Bacillus anthracis* and related species. *J. Bact.* **71**, 25.

Burdon, K. L. & Wende, R. D. (1960). On the differentiation of anthrax bacilli from *Bacillus cereus. J. infect. Dis.* **107**, 224.

Burgess, N. R. H., McDermott, S. N. & Whiting, J. (1973). Laboratory transmission of Enterobacteriaceae by the oriental cockroach, *Blatta orientalis. J. Hyg., Camb.* **71**, 9.

Burke, V., Robinson, J., Beaman, J., Gracey, M., Lesmana, M., Rockhill, R., Echeverria, P. & Janda, J. M. (1983). Correlation of enterotoxicity with biotype in *Aeromonas* sp. *J. clin. Microbiol* **18**, 1196.

Burman, N. P. (1955). The standardisation and selection of bile salt and peptone for culture media used in the bacteriological examination of water. *Proc. Soc. Wat. Treat. Exam.* **4**, 10.

Burrows, T. W., Farrell, J. M. F. & Gillett, W. A. (1964). The catalase activities of *Pasteurella pestis* and other bacteria. *Br. J. exp. Path.* **45**, 579.

Butter, M. N. W. & de Moor, C. E. (1967). *Streptococcus agalactiae* as a cause of meningitis in the newborn, and of bacteraemia in adults. Differentiation of human and animal varieties. *Antonie van Leeuwenhoek* , **33**, 439.

Buttiaux, R., Osteux, R., Fresnoy, R. & Moriamez, J. (1954). Les propriétés biochimiques caractéristiques du genre *Proteus*. Inclusion souhaitable des *Providencia* dans celui-ci. *Annls Inst. Pasteur, Paris,* **87**, 375.

Buu-Höi, A., Branger, C. & Acar, J. F. (1985). Vancomycin-resistant streptococcoi or *Leuconostoc* sp. *Antimicrob. Agents Chemother.* **28**, 458.

Bøvre, K. (1979). Proposal to divide the genus *Moraxella* Lwoff 1939 emend. Henriksen and Bøvre 1968 into two subgenera, subgenus *Moraxella* (Lwoff 1939) Bøvre 1979 and subgenus *Branhamella* (Catlin 1970) Bøvre 1979. *Int. J. syst. Bact.* **29**, 403.

Bøvre, K. (1980). Progress in classification and identification of Neisseriaceae based on genetic affinity. In *Microbiological Classification and Identification* (ed. M. Goodfellow & R. G. Board), p.55. London: Academic Press.

Bøvre, K. (1984). *Moraxella*. In *Bergey's Manual of Systematic Bacteriology*, vol. 1 (ed. N. R. Krieg & J. G. Holt), p.296. Baltimore: Williams & Wilkins.

Bøvre, K., Fiandt, M. & Szybalski, W. (1969). DNA-base composition of *Neisseria, Moraxella, and Acinetobacter,* as determined by measurement of buoyant-density in CsCl gradients. *Can. J. Microbiol.* **15**, 335.

Bøvre, K. & Hagen, N. (1981). The family Neisseriaceae: rod-shaped species of the genera *Moraxella, Acinetobacter, Kingella* and *Neisseria*, and the *Branhamella* group of cocci. In *The Prokaryotes: A Handbook on Habitats, Isolation and Identification of Bacteria* (ed. M. Starr *et al.*), vol. 2, p. 1506. Berlin: Springer-Verlag.

Bøvre, K. & Henriksen, S. D. (1967). A revised description of *Moraxella polymorpha* Flamm 1957, with a proposal of a new name, *Moraxella phenylpyruvica* for the species. *Int. J. syst. Bact.* **17**, 343.

Bøvre, K. & Holten, E. (1970). *Neisseria elongata* sp. nov., a rod-shaped member of the genus *Neisseria.* Re-evaluation of cell shape as a criterion in classification. *J. gen. Microbiol.* **60**, 67.

Cadness-Graves, B., Williams, R., Harper, G. J. & Miles, A. A. (1943). Slide-test for coagulase-positive staphylococci. *Lancet,* i, 736.

Carlone, G. M., Sottnek, F. O. & Plikaytis, B. D. (1985). Comparison of outer membrane protein and biochemical profiles of *Haemophilus aegyptius* and *Haemophilus influenzae* biotype III. *J. clin. Microbiol.* **22**, 708.

Carlone, G. M., Schalla, W. O., Moss, C. W., Ashley, D. L., Fast, D. M., Holler, J. S. & Plikaytis, B. D. (1988). *Haemophilus ducreyi* and other *Haemophilus* species. *Int. J. Syst. Bact.* **38**, 249.

Carpenter, K. P. (1961). The relationship of the enterobacterium A 12 (Sachs) to *Shigella boydii* 14. *J. gen. Microbiol.* **26**, 535.

Carpenter, K. P., Cowan, S. T., Lapage, S. P., Lautrop, H., Le Minor, L., Ørskov, F., Ørskov, I., Rohde, R., Sakazaki, R., Sedlak, J., Taylor, J., Thal, E., Floyd, T. M., Mollaret, H. H., Makela, P. H., Seeliger, H., Lachowicz, K., Rauss, K. & van Oye, E. (1970). Request to the Judicial Commission that *Aerobacter* Beijerinck 1900 and *Aerobacter* Hormaeche and Edwards 1958 be declared rejected generic names. *Int. J. syst. Bact.* **20**, 221.

Carpenter, K. P. & Lachowicz, K. (1959). The catalase activity of *Shigella flexneri. J. Path. Bact.* **77**, 645.

Carpenter, K. P., Lapage, S. P. & Steel, K. J. (1966). Biochemical identification of Enterobacteriaceae. In *Identification Methods for Microbiologists,* Part A, (ed. B. M. Gibbs & F. A. Skinner) p. 21. London: Academic Press.

Carson, F., Kingsley, W. B., Haberman, S. & Race, G. J. (1964). Unclassified mycobacteria contaminating acid-fast stains of tissue sections. *Am. J. clin. Path.* **41**, 561.

Carter, L. & Huzman, E. (1985). *Computers and their Use.* (Teach Yourself series.) Sevenoaks, Kent: Hodder & Stoughton.

Carter, L. & Huzman, E. (1987). *Computer Programming in BASIC.* (Teach Yourself series.) Sevenoaks, Kent: Hodder & Stoughton.

Casin, L., Grimont, F. & Grimont, P. A. D. (1986). Deoxyribonucleic acid relatedness between *Haemophilus aegyptius* and *Haemophilus influenzae.* *Annls Microbiol. Inst. Pasteur, Paris,* **137B**, 155.

Casin, I., Grimont, F., Grimont, P. A. D. & Sanson - Le Pors, M. -J. (1985). Lack of deoxyribonucleic acid relatedness between *Haemophilus ducreyi* and other *Haemophilus* species. *Int. J. sys. Bact.* **35**, 23.

Castellani, A. & Chalmers, A. J. (1919). *Manual of Tropical Medicine* edn 3. London: Baillière, Tindall & Cox.

Catlin, B. W. (1970). Transfer of the organism named *Neisseria catarrhalis* to *Branhamella* gen. nov. *Int. J. syst. Bact.* **20**, 155.

Cato, E. P., Moore, W. E. C., Nygaard, G. & Holdeman, L. V. (1984). *Actinomyces meyeri* sp. nov., specific epithet rev. *Int. J. syst. Bact.* **34**, 487.

Catsaras, M. & Buttiaux, R. (1963). Au sujet de quelques réactions biochimiques pour l'identification des Enterobacteriaceae. *Annls Inst. Pasteur, Lille,* **14**,111.

Chapin, K. C. & Doern, G. V. (1983). Selective media for recovery of *Haemophilus influenzae* from specimens contaminated with upper respiratory tract microbial flora. *J. clin. Microbiol.* **17**, 1163.

Chapman, G. H. (1946). A single culture medium for selective isolation of plasma-coagulating staphylococci and for improved testing of chromogenesis, plasma coagulation, mannite fermentation, and the Stone reaction. *J. Bact.* **51**, 409.

Chapman, G. H. (1952). A simple method for making multiple tests of a microorganism. *J. Bact.* **63**,147.

Cheeseman, G. C. & Fuller, R. (1966). A study by high voltage electrophoresis of the amino acid decarboxylases and arginine dihydrolase of bacteria isolated from the alimentary tract of pigs. *J. appl. Bact.* **29**, 596.

Cherry, W. B. & Moody, M. D. (1965). Fluorescent-antibody techniques in diagnostic bacteriology. *Bact. Rev.* **29**, 222.

Chester, F. D. (1901). *A Manual of Determinative Bacteriology.* New York: The Macmillan Co.

Childs, E. & Allen, L. A. (1953). Improved methods for determining the most probable number of *Bacterium coli* and of *Streptococcus faecalis. J. Hyg. Camb.* **51**, 468.

Chilton, M. L. & Fulton, M. (1946). A presumptive medium for differentiating paracolon from Salmonella organisms. *J. Lab. clin. Med.* **31**, 824.

Christensen, W. B. (1946). Urea decomposition as a means of differentiating Proteus and paracolon cultures from each other and from Salmonella and Shigella. *J. Bact.* **52**, 461.

Christensen, W. B. (1949). Hydrogen sulfide production and citrate utilization in the differentiation of the enteric pathogens and the coliform bacteria. *Res. Bull., Weld County Hlth Dept.* **1**, 3.

Christie, R., Atkins, N. E. & Munch-Petersen, E. (1944). A note on a lytic phenomenon shown by group B streptococci. *Austral. J. exp. Biol. med. Sci.* **22**, 197.

Clark, R. B., Berrafati, J. F., Janda, J. M. & Bottone, E. J. (1984). Biotyping and exoenzyme profiling as an aid in the differentiation of human from bovine group G streptococci. *J. clin. Microbiol.* **20**, 706.

Clark, R. B. & Janda, J. M. (1985). Isolation of *Serratia plymuthica* from a human burn site. *J. clin. Microbiol.* **21**, 656.

Clark, W. M. & Lubs, H. A. (1915). The differentiation of bacteria of the colon-aerogenes family by the use of indicators. *J. infect. Dis.* **17**, 160.

Clark, W. A., Hollis, D. G., Weaver, R. E. & Riley, P. (1984). *Identification of Unusual Pathogenic Gram-negative Aerobic and Facultatively Anaerobic Bacteria.* Atlanta, Georgia: U.S. Department of Health and Human Services.

Clarke, P. H. (1953a). Hydrogen sulphide production by bacteria. *J. gen. Microbiol.* **8**, 397.

Clarke, P. H. (1953b). Growth of streptococci in a glucose phenolphthalein broth. *J. gen. Microbiol.* **9**, 350.

Clarke, P. H. & Cowan, S. T. (1952). Biochemical methods for bacteriology. *J. gen. Microbiol.* **6**, 187.

Claus, D. & Berkeley, R. C. W. (1986). Genus *Bacillus* Cohn, 1872, 1974[AL]. In *Bergey's Manual of Systematic Bacteriology,* vol. 2, (ed. P. H. A. Sneath, N. S. Mair, M. E. Sharpe & J. G. Holt), p. 1105. Baltimore: Williams & Wilkins.

Clayton, P., Feltham, R.K.A., Mitchell, C. J. & Sneath, P. H. A. (1986). Constructing a database for low cost identification of Gram negative rods in clinical laboratories. *J. clin. Path.* **39**, 798.

Clyde, W. A. Jr (1983a). Serological identification of mycoplasmas from humans. In *Methods in Mycoplasmology,* vol. 2 (ed. J. G. Tully & S. Razin), p. 37. New York: Academic Press.

Clyde, W. A. Jr (1983b). Recovery of mycoplasmas from the respiratory tract. In *Methods in Mycoplasmology,* vol. 2 (ed. J. G. Tully & S. Razin), p. 9. New York: Academic Press.

Cobb, R. W. (1966). *Corynebacterium bovis:* fermentation of sugars in the presence of serum or Tween 80. *Vet. Rec.* **78**, 33.

Cohen, R. L., Wittler, R. G. & Faber, J. E. (1968). Modified biochemical tests for characterization of L-phase variants of bacteria. *Appl. Microbiol.* **16**, 1655.

Colbeck, J. C. & Proom, H. (1944). Use of dried rabbit plasma for the staphylococcus coagulase test. *Br. med. J.* ii, 471.

Cole, S. W. & Onslow, H. (1916). On a substitute for peptone and a standard nutrient medium for bacteriological purposes. *Lancet,* ii, 9.

Collins, C. H., Grange, J. M. & Yates, M. D. (1985). *Organisation and Practices in Tuberculosis Bacteriology.* London: Butterworth.

Collins, C. H., Lyne, P. M. & Grange, J. M. (1989). In *Collins & Lyne's Microbiological Methods* (ed. C. H. Collins, P. N. Lyne & J. M. Grange), p. 347. London: Butterworth.

Collins, C. H., Yates, M. D. & Grange, J. M. (1982). Subdivision of *Mycobacterium tuberculosis* into five variants for epidemiological purposes: methods and nomenclature. *J. Hyg. Camb.* **89**, 235.

Collins, M. D. (1982*a*). Reclassification of *Bacterionema matruchotii* (Gilmour, Howell and Bibby) in the genus *Corynebacterium* as *Corynebacterium matruchotii* comb. nov. *Zbl. Bakt. Mikrobiol. Hyg. I. Abt. Orig. C.* **3**, p. 364.

Collins, M. D. (1982*b*). *Corynebacterium mycetoides* sp. nov. nom. rev. *Zbl. Bakt. Mikrobiol. Hyg. I. Abt. Orig. C.* **3**, p. 399.

Collins, M. D. (1987). Transfer of *Brevibacterium ammoniagenes* (Cooke and Keith) to the genus *Corynebacterium* as *Corynebacterium ammoniagenes* comb. nov. *Int. J. syst. Bact.* **37**, 442.

Collins, M. D. & Cummins, C. S. (1986). The genus *Corynebacterium*. In *Bergey's Manual of Systematic Bacteriology*, vol. 2 (ed. P. H. A. Sneath, N. S. Mair, M. E.Sharpe & J. G. Holt), p.1266. New York: Williams & Wilkins.

Collins, M. D. & Jones, D. (1982). Reclassification of *Corynebacterium pyogenes* (Glage) in the genus *Actinomyces*, as *Actinomyces pyogenes* comb. nov. *J. gen. Microbiol.* **128**, 901.

Collins, M. D. & Jones, D. (1983). *Corynebacterium minutissimum* sp. nov. nom. rev. *Int. J. Syst. Bact.* **33**, 870.

Collins, M. D., Burton, R. A. & Jones, D. (1988). *Corynebacterium amycolatum* sp. nov. a new mycolic acid-less *Corynebacterium* species from human skins. *FEMS Microbiol. Lett.* **49**, 349.

Collins, M. D., Farrow, J. A. E. & Jones, D. (1986). *Enterococcus mundtii* sp. nov. *Int. J. syst. Bact.* **36**, 8.

Collins, M. D., Farrow, J. A. E., Phillips, B. A., Feresu, S. B. & Jones, D. (1987). Classification of *Lactobacillus divergens*, *Lactobacillus piscicola* and some catalase-negative asporogenous, rod-shaped bacteria from poultry in a new genus, *Carnobacterium*. *Int. J. syst. Bact.* **37**, 310.

Collins, M. D., Jones, D. and Schofield, G. (1982). Reclassification of *Corynebacterium haemolyticum* (Maclean, Liebow and Rosenburg) in the genus *Arcanobacterium* gen. nov. as *Arcanobacterium haemolyticum* nom. rev. comb. nov. *J. gen. Microbiol.* **128**, 901.

Collins, M. D., Jones, D., Kroppenstedt, R. M. & Schleifer, K. H. (1982). Chemical studies as a guide to the classification of *Corynebacterium pyogenes* and '*Corynebacterium haemolyticum*'. *J. gen. Microbiol.* **128**, 335.

Collins, M. D., Jones, D., Farrow, J. A. E., Kilpper-Bälz, R. & Schleifer, K. H. (1984). *Enterococcus avium* nom. rev., comb. nov.: *E. casseliflavus* nom. rev., comb. nov.: *E. durans* nom. rev., comb. nov.: *E. gallinarum* comb. nov.: and *E. malodoratus* sp. nov. *Int. J. syst. Bact.* **34**, 220.

Colman, G. (1967). Aerococcus-like organisms isolated from human infections. *J. clin. Path.* **20**, 294.

Colman, G. & Ball, L. C. (1984). Identification of streptococci in a medical laboratory. *J. appl. Bact.* **57**, 1.

Colman, G. & Efstratiou, A. (1987). Vancomycin-resistant leuconostocs, lactobacilli and now pediococci. *J. Hosp. Inf.* **10**, 1.

Colman, G. & Williams, R. E. O. (1965). The cell walls of streptococci. *J. gen. Microbiol.* **41**, 375.

Colman, G. & Williams, R. E. O. (1972). Taxonomy of some human viridans streptococci. In *Streptococci and Streptococcal Diseases: Recognition, Understanding and Management*, (ed. L. W. Wannamaker & J. M. Matsen) p. 281. New York: Academic Press.

Colwell, R. R., MacDonell, M. T. & DeLey, J. (1986). Proposal to recognize the family Aeromonadaceae *fam. nov. Int. J. syst. Bact.* **36**, 473.

Conn, H. J. (1936). On the detection of nitrate reduction. *J. Bact.* **31**, 225.

Conn, H. W. (1900). Classification of dairy bacteria. *Twelfth Ann. Rep. Storrs Agric. Exp. Sta., Storrs, Conn. 1899*, 13.

Conn, H. J., Darrow, M. A. & Emmel, V. M. (1960). *Staining Procedures used by the Biological Stain Commission*, edn. 2. Baltimore: The Williams & Wilkins Co.

Conn, H. W., Esten, W. M. & Stocking, W. A. (1907). A classification of dairy bacteria. *Ann. Rep. Storrs Agric. Exp. Sta., Storrs, Conn. 1906*, 91.

Cook, A. M. & Steel, K. J. (1959*a*). The stability of thioglycollate solutions. Part I. Effects of method of preparation of solutions, pH and temperature upon the oxidation of thioglycollate. *J. Pharm. Pharmac.* **11**, 216.

Cook, A. M. & Steel, K. J. (1959*b*). The stability of thioglycollate solutions. Part II. Miscellaneous factors associated with oxidation and stability. *J. Pharm. Pharmac.* **11**, 434.

Cook, G. T. (1950). A plate test for nitrate reduction. *J. clin. Path.* **3**, 359.

Cooper, G. L., Grange, J.M., McGregor, J. A. & McFadden, J. J. (1989). The potential use of DNA probes to identify and type strains within the *Mycobacterium tuberculosis* complex. *Lett. appl. Microbiol.* **8**, 127.

Cornelis, G., Luke, R. K. J. & Richmond, M. H. (1978). Fermentation of raffinose by lactose-fermenting strains of *Yersinia enterocolitica* and by sucrose-fermenting strains of *Escherichia coli. J. clin. Microbiol.* **7**, 180.

Corper, H. J. (1928). The certified diagnosis of tuberculosis. Practical evaluation of a new method for cultivating tubercle bacilli for diagnostic purposes. *J. Am. med. Ass.* **91**, 371.

Cowan, S. T. (1938). The classification of staphylococci by precipitation and biological reactions. *J. Path. Bact.* **46**, 31.

Cowan, S. T. (1956*a*). 'Ordnung in das Chaos' Migula. *Can. J. Microbiol.* **2**, 212.

Cowan, S. T. (1956*b*). Taxonomic rank of Enterobacteriaceae 'groups'. *J. gen Microbiol.* **15**, 345.

Cowan, S. T. (1962*a*). The microbial species – a macromyth? *Symp. Soc. gen. Microbiol.* **12**, 433.

Cowan, S. T. (1962*b*). An introduction to chaos, or the classification of micrococci and staphylococci. *J. appl. Bact.* **25**, 324.

Cowan, S.T. (1965*a*). Principles and practice of bacterial taxonomy – a forward look. *J. gen Micobiol.* **39**, 143.

Cowan, S.T. 1965*b*). Development of coding schemes for microbial taxonomy. *Adv. appl. Microbiol.* **7**, 139.

Cowan, S. T. (1968). An assessment of the value of biochemical and serological techniques in microbial taxonomy. In *Chemotaxonomy and Serotaxonomy.* (ed. J. G. Hawkes), p. 269. London: Academic Press.

Cowan, S. T. (1970*a*). Heretical taxonomy for bacteriologists. *J. gen. Microbiol.* **61**, 145.

Cowan, S. T. (1970*b*). Are some characters more equal than others? *Int. J. syst. Bact.* **20**, 541.

Cowan, S. T. (1971). Sense and nonsense in bacterial taxonomy. *J. gen. Microbiol.* **67**, 1.

Cowan, S. T. (1974). *Cowan and Steel's Manual for the Identification of Medical Bacteria*, Edn. 2. Cambridge University Press.

Cowan, S. T. (1978). *A dictionary of microbial taxonomy.* (ed. L. R. Hill). Cambridge University Press.

Cowan, S. T. & Steel, K. J. (1960). A device for the identification of microorganisms. *Lancet*, i, 1172.

Cowan, S. T. & Steel, K. J. (1961). Diagnostic tables for the common medical bacteria. *J. Hyg., Camb.* **59**, 357.

Cowan, S. T. & Steel, K. J. (1964). Comparison of differentiating criteria for staphylococci and micrococci. *J. Bact.* **88**, 804.

Cowan, S. T., Steel, K. J., Shaw, C. & Duguid, J. P. (1960). A classification of the *Klebsiella* group. *J. gen. Microbiol.* **23**, 601.

Coykendall, A. L. (1977). Proposal to elevate the subspecies of *Streptococcus mutans* to species status, based on their molecular composition. *Int. J. syst. Bact.* **27**, 26.

Coykendall, A. L. & Specht, P. A. (1975). DNA base sequence homologies among strains of *Streptococcus sanguis. J. gen. Microbiol.* **91**, 92.

Coykendall, A. L., Wesbecher, P. M. & Gustafson, K. B. (1987). 'Streptococcus milleri', Streptococcus constellatus, and Streptococcus intermedius are later synonyms of Streptococcus anginosus. Int. J. syst. Bact. **37**, 222.

Craigie, J. (1931). Studies on the serological reactions of the flagella of *B. typhosus. J. Immun.* **21**, 417.

Criswell, B. S., Marston, J. H., Stenback, W. A., Black, S. H. & Gardner, H. L. (1971). *Haemophilus vaginalis* 594, a Gram-negative organism? *Can. J. Microbiol.* **17**, 865.

Criswell, B. S., Stenback, W. A., Black, S. H. & Gardner, H. L. (1972). Fine structure of *Haemophilus vaginalis. J. Bact.* **109**, 930.

Cross, T. (1970). The diversity of bacterial spores. *J. appl. Bact.* **33**, 95.

Cruickshank, J. C. (1935). *A* study of the so-called *Bacterium typhiflavum. J. Hyg., Camb.* **35**, 354.

Cruickshank, R. (1937). Staphylocoagulase. *J. Path. Bact.* **45**, 295.

Cullen, G. A. (1969). *Streptococcus uberis*: a review. *Vet. Bull.* **39**, 155.

Cummins, C. S. & Johnson, J. L. (1974). *Corynebacterium parvum*: a synonym for *Propionibacterium acnes? J. gen. Microbiol.* **80**, 433.

Cummins, C. S. & Johnson, J. L. (1981). The genus *Propionibacterium*. In *The Prokaryotes: A Handbook on Habitats, Isolation and Identification of Bacteria*, vol. 2, (ed. M. P. Starr *et al.*) p. 1864 New York: Springer.

Cummins, C. S. & Johnson, J. L. (1986). The genus *Propionibacterium*. In *Bergey's Manual of Systematic Bacteriology*, vol. 2, (ed. P. H. A. Sneath *et al.*) p. 1346 Baltimore: Williams & Wilkins.

Cure, G. L. & Keddie, R. M. (1973). Methods for the morphological examination of aerobic coryneform bacteria. In *Sampling – Microbiological Monitoring of Environments*, (ed. R. G. Board & D. W. Lovelock), p. 123. London: Academic Press.

Curry, J. C. & Borovian, G. E. (1976). Selective medium for distinguishing micrococci from staphylococci in the clinical laboratory. *J. clin. Microbiol.* **4**, 455.

Curtis, G. D. W., Mitchell, R. G., King, A. F. & Griffin, E. J. (1989). A selective differential medium for the isolation of *Listeria monocytogenes*. *Lett. appl. Microbiol.* **8**, 95.

D'Amato, R. F., Eriquez, L. A., Tomfohrde, K. M. & Singerman, E. (1978). Rapid identification of *Neisseria gonorrhoeae* and *Neisseria meningitidis* by using enzymatic profiles. *J clin. Microbiol.* **7**, 77.

D'Amato, R. F., Holmes, B. & Bottone, E. J. (1981). The systems approach to diagnostic microbiology. *CRC Critical Reviews in Microbiology* **9**, 1.

Dacre, J. C. & Sharpe, M. E. (1956). Catalase production by lactobacilli. *Nature, Lond.* **178**, 700.

Darmady, E. M., Hughes, K. E. A. & Jones, J. D. (1958). Thermal death-time of spores in dry heat in relation to sterilisation of instruments and syringes. *Lancet*, ii, 766.

Daubner, I. (1962) Die Reduktion der Nitrate durch Bakterien der Familie Enterobacteriaceae. *Arch. Hyg. Bakt.* **146**, 147.

Davidson, C. M., Mobbs, P. & Stubbs, J. M. (1968). Some morphological and physiological properties of *Microbacterium thermosphactum*. *J. appl. Bact.* **31**, 551.

Davis, B. R., Fanning, G. R., Madden, J. M., Steigerwalt, A. G., Bradford, H. B., Smith, H. L. & Brenner, D. J. (1981). Characterization of biochemically atypical *Vibrio cholerae* strains and designation of a new pathogenic species, *Vibrio mimicus*. *J. clin. Microbiol.* **14**, 631.

Davis, C. P., Cleven, D., Brown, J. & Balish, E. (1976). *Anaerobiospirillum*, a new genus of spiral-shaped bacteria. *Int. J. syst. Bact.* **26**, 498.

Davis, D. H., Doudoroff, M., Stanier, R. Y. & Mandel, M. (1969). Proposal to reject the genus *Hydrogenomonas*: taxonomic implications. *Int. J. syst. Bact.* **19**, 375.

Davis, G. H. G. & Newton, K. G. (1969). Numerical taxonomy of some named coryneform bacteria. *J. gen. Microbiol.* **56**, 195.

Davis, G. H. G., Fomin, L., Wilson, E. & Newton, K. G. (1969). Numerical taxonomy of *Listeria*, streptococci and possibly related bacteria. *J. gen. Microbiol.* **57**, 333.

Davis, G. H. G. & Park, R. W. A. (1962). A taxonomic study of certain bacteria currently classified as *Vibrio* species. *J. gen. Microbiol.* **27**, 101.

Davis, J. G. (1939). A rapid, simple and reproducible

method for the determination of bacterial sugar fermentations. *Zentbl. Bakt. ParasitKde Abt. II*, **101**, 97.

Davis, M. J., Gillespie, A. G., Vidaver, A. K. & Harris, R. W. (1984). *Clavibacter*: a new genus containing some phytopathogenic coryneform bacteria, including *Clavibacter xyli* subsp. *xyli* sp. nov., subsp. nov. and *Clavibacter xyli* subsp. *cynodontis* subsp. nov., pathogens that cause ratoon stunting disease of sugar cane and Bermuda grass stunting disease. *Int. J. syst. Bact.* **34**, 107.

Dawson, B., Farnworth, E. H., McLeod, J. W. & Nicholson, D. E. (1951). Observations on the value of Bordet-Gengou medium for the cultivation of *Haemophilus pertussis*. *J. gen. Microbiol.* **5**, 408.

De Blieck, L. (1932). A haemoglobinophilic bacterium as the cause of contagious catarrh of the fowl (*Coryza infectiosa gallinarum*). *Vet. J.* **88**, 9.

De Bord, G. G. (1939). Organisms invalidating the diagnosis of gonorrhoea by the smear method. *J. Bact.* **38**, 119.

De Bord, G. G. (1942). Descriptions of Mimeae Trib. nov. with three genera and three species and two new species of *Neisseria* from conjunctivitis and vaginitis. *Iowa St. Coll. J. Sci.* **16**, 471.

De Bord, G. G. (1943). Species of the tribes Mimeae Neisseriae, and Streptococceae which confuse the diagnosis of gonorrhoea by smears. *J. Lab. clin. Med.* **28**, 710.

De Bord, G. G. (1948). *Mima polymorpha* meningitis, *J. Bact.* **55**, 764.

De Vos, P., Kersters, K., Falsen, E., Pot, B., Gillis, M., Segers, P. & DeLey, J. (1985). *Comamonas* Davis and Park 1962 gen. nov., nom. rev. emend., and *Comamonas terrigena* Hugh 1962 sp. nov., nom. rev. *Int. J. syst. Bact.* **35**, 443.

Deibel, R. H. & Niven, C. F., Jr (1960). Comparative study of *Gaffkya homari*, *Aerococcus viridans*, tetrad-forming cocci from meat curing brines, and the genus *Pediococcus*. *J. Bact.* **79**, 175.

Delaplane, J. P., Erwin, L. E. & Stuart, H. O. (1938). The effect of the X factor, of sodium chloride, and of the composition of the nutrient media upon the growth of the fowl coryza bacillus, *Haemophilus gallinarum*. *J. agric. Res.* **56**, 919.

DeLey, J., Segers, P. & Gillis. M. (1978). Intra- and intergeneric similarities of *Chromobacterium* and *Janthinobacterium* ribosomal ribonucleic acid cistrons. *Int. J. syst. Bact.* **28**, 154.

DeMello, J. V. & Snell, J. J. S. (1985). Preparation of simulated clinical material for bacteriological examination. *J. appl. Bact.* **59**, 421.

Dennis, P. J. L. (1988). Isolation of Legionellae from environmental specimens. In: *A laboratory manual for legionella.* (ed. Harrison, T. G. & Taylor, A. G.), p.31. Chichester: Wiley.

Dennis, P. J. L., Bartlett, C. L. R. & Wright, A. E. (1984). Comparison of isolation methods for *Legionella* species. In *Legionella: Proceedings of second International Symposium* (ed. C. Thornsberry, A. Balows, J. C. Feeley & W. Jakubowski). Washington D.C.: American Society for Microbiology.

Dent, V. E. & Williams, R. A. D. (1984*a*) *Actinomyces denticolens* Dent & Williams sp. nov. : a new species from the dental plaque of cattle. *J. appl. Bact.* **56**, 183.

Dent, V. E. & Williams, R. A. D. (1984*b*). *Actinomyces howellii*, a new species from the dental plaque of dairy cattle. *Int. J. syst. Bact.* **34**, 316.

Devriese, L. A., Poutrel, B., Kilpper-Bälz, R. & Schleifer, K. H. (1983). *Staphylococcus gallinarum* and *Staphylococcus caprae*, two species from animals. *Int. J. syst. Bact.* **33**, 480.

Devriese, L. A., Hájek, V., Oeding, P., Meyer, S. A. & Schleifer, K. H. (1978). *Staphylococcus hyicus* (Sompolinsky 1953) comb. nov. and *Staphylococcus hyicus* subsp *chromogenes* subsp. nov. *Int. J. syst. Bact.* **28**, 482.

Devriese, L. A., Hommez, J., Kilpper-Bälz, R. & Schliefer, K.H. (1986). *Streptococcus canis* sp. nov.: a species of group G streptococci from animals. *Int. J. syst. Bact.* **36**, 422.

Dickgiesser, U., Weiss, N. & Fritsche, D. (1984). *Lactobacillus gasseri* as the cause of septic urinary infections. *Infection*, **12**, 14.

Dickson, J. I. S. & Marples R. R. (1986). Coagulase production by strains of *Staphylococcus aureus* of differing resistance characters: a comparison of two traditional methods with a latex agglutination system, detecting both clumping factor and protein A. *J. clin. Path.* **39**, 371.

Difco Manual of Dehydrated Culture Media and Reagents for Microbiological and Clinical Laboratory Procedures (1953). Anonymous, edn 9. Detroit: Difco Laboratories Inc. (Edn. 10: 1984.)

Doern, G. V. & Chapin, K. C. (1984). Laboratory identification of *Haemophilus influenzae*: Effects of basal media on the results of the satellitism test and evaluation of the RapID N. H. System. *J. clin. Microbiol.* **20**, 599.

Donovan, T. J. (1984). Serology and serotyping of *Vibrio cholerae*. In *Vibrios in the Environment* (ed. R. R. Colwell), p.83. New York: John Wiley & Sons.

Donta, S. T. (1988). Mechanism of action of *Clostridium difficile* toxins. In *Clostridium difficile: its Role in Intestinal Disease* (ed. R. D. Rolfe & S. M. Finegold), p.169. New York: Academic Press.

Douglas, H. C. & Gunter, S. E. (1946). The taxonomic position of *Corynebacterium acnes. J. Bact.* **52**, 15.

Douglas, S. R. (1922). A new medium for the isolation *of B. diphtheriae. Br. J. exp. Path.* **3**, 263.

Downie, A. W., Stent, L. & White, S. M. (1931). The bile solubility of pneumococcus, with special reference to the chemical structure of various bile salts. *Br. J. exp. Path.* **12**, 1.

Downie, A. W., Wade, E. & Young, J. A. (1933). An organism resembling the Newcastle type of dysentery bacillus associated with cases of dysentery. *J. Hyg., Camb.* **33**, 196.

Drea, W. F. (1942). Growth of small numbers of tubercle bacilli, H 37, in Long's liquid synthetic medium and some interfering factors. *J. Bact.* **44**,149.

Duguid, J. P. (1951). The demonstration of bacterial capsules and slime. *J. Path. Bact.* **63**, 673.

Dunkelberg, W. E., Jr & McVeigh, I. (1969). Growth requirements of *Haemophilus vaginalis. Antonie van Leeuwenhoek*, **35**, 129.

Dunkelberg, W. E., Skaggs, R. & Kellogg, D. S. (1970). Method for isolation and identification of *Corynebacterium vaginale (Haemophilus vaginalis). Appl. Microbiol.* **19**, 47.

Durham, H. E. (1898). A simple method for demonstrating the production of gas by bacteria. *Br. med. J.* i, 1387.

Dybowski, W. & Franklin, D. A. (1968). Conditional probability and the identification of bacteria: a pilot study. *J. gen. Microbiol.* **54**, 215.

Easmon, C. S. F. & Ison, C. A. (1984). *Gardnerella vaginalis* and bacterial vaginosis. In *Medical Microbiology*, vol. 4 (ed. C. S. F. Easmon), p. 53. London: Academic Press.

Eddy, B. P. (1960). Cephalotrichous, fermentative Gram-negative bacteria: the genus *Aeromonas. J. appl. Bact.* **23**, 216.

Eddy, B. P. (1961). The Voges-Proskaüer reaction and its significance: a review. *J. appl. Bact.* **24**, 27.

Eddy, B. P. (1962). Further studies on *Aeromonas.* I. Additional strains and supplementary biochemical tests. *J. appl. Bact.* **25**,137.

Eddy, B. P. & Carpenter, K. P. (1964). Further studies on *Aeromonas.* II. Taxonomy of *Aeromonas* and C 27 strains. *J. appl. Bact.* **27**, 96.

Edelstein, P. H. (1981). Improved semiselective medium for isolation of *Legionella pneumophila* from contaminated clinical and environmental specimens. *J. clin. Microbiol.* **14**, 298.

Edelstein, P. H. (1982). Comparative study of selective media for isolation of *Legionella pneumophila* from potable water. *J. clin. Microbiol.* **16**, 697.

Edelstein, P. H., Snitzer, J. B. & Bridge, J. A. (1982).

Enhancement of recovery of *Legionella pneumophila* from contaminated respiratory tract specimens by heat. *J. clin. Microbiol.* **16**, 1061.

Edmonds, P., Patton, C. M., Griffin, P. M., Barrett, T. J., Schmid, G. P., Baker, C. N., Lambert, M. A. & Brenner, D. J. (1987). *Campylobacter hyointestinalis* associated with human gastrointestinal disease in the United States. *J. clin. Microbiol.* **25**, 685.

Edmunds, P. N. (1962). The biochemical, serological and haemagglutinating reactions of 'Haemophilus vaginalis'. *J. Path. Bact.* **83**, 411.

Edward, D. G. ff. & Freundt, E. A. (1967). Proposal for Mollicutes as name of the class established for the order Mycoplasmatales. *Int. J. syst. Bact.* **17**, 267.

Edwards, P. R. & Bruner, D. W. (1942). Serological identification of salmonella cultures. *Circ. Ky agric. Exp. Sta.* no. 54.

Edwards, P. R. & Ewing, W. H. (1962, 1972). *Identification of Enterobacteriaceae*, edn 2, 1962; edn 3, 1972. Minneapolis: Burgess Publishing Co.

Edwards, P. R. & Kauffmann, F. (1952). A simplification of the Kauffmann-White schema. *Am. J. clin. Path.* **22**, 692.

Efstratiou, A. (1983). The serotyping of hospital strains of streptococci belonging to Lancefield group C and group G. *J. Hyg., Camb.* **90**, 71.

Eigelsbach, H. T. & McGann, V. G. (1984). Genus *Francisella* Dorofe'ev 1947, 176[AL]. In *Bergey's Manual of Systematic Bacteriology*, Vol. 1 (ed. N. R. Krieg & J. G. Holt), p. 394. Baltimore: Williams & Wilkins.

Eiken, M. (1958). Studies on an anaerobic, rod-shaped, Gram-negative microorganism: *Bacteroides corrodens* n. sp. *Acta path. microbiol. scand.* **43**, 404.

Elek, S. D. (1948). Rapid identification of Proteus. *J. Path. Bact.* **60**, 183.

Elek, S. D. & Levy, E. (1954). The nature of discrepancies between haemolysins in culture filtrates and plate haemolysin patterns of staphylococci. *J. Path. Bact.* **68**, 31.

Elliott, S. D. (1945). A proteolytic enzyme produced by group A streptococci with special reference to its effect on the type-specific M antigen. *J. exp. Med.* **81**, 573.

Ellis, G. (1971). *Units, Symbols and Abbreviations. A Guide for Biological and Medical Editors and Authors.* London: Royal Society of Medicine.

Elston, H. R. & Fitch, D. M. (1964). Determination of potential pathogenicity of staphylococci. *Am. J. clin. Path.* **42**, 346.

Eltinge, E. T. (1956). Nitrate reduction in the genus *Chromobacterium. Antonie van Leeuwenhoek*, **22**, 139.

Eltinge, E. T. (1957). Status of the genus *Chromobacterium. Int. Bull. bact. Nomencl. Taxon.* **7**, 37.

Ensminger, P. W., Culbertson, C. G. & Powell, H. M. (1953). Antigenic *Haemophilus pertussis* vaccines grown on charcoal agar. *J. infect. Dis.* **93**, 266.

Ersgaard, H. & Justensen, T. (1984). Multi-resistant lipophilic corynebacteria from clinical specimens. *Acta path. microbiol. immun. scand.*, B**92**, 39.

Estevez, E. G. (1980). A program for in-house proficiency testing in clinical microbiology. *Am. J. med. Tech.* **46**, 102.

Evans, J. B., Buettner, L. G. & Niven, C. F., Jr (1952). Occurrence of streptococci that give a false-positive coagulase test. *J. Bact.* **64**, 433.

Everall, P. H. & Morris, C. A. (1975). Some observations on cooling in laboratory autoclaves. *J. clin. Path.* **28**, 664.

Ewing, W. H. (1949a). The relationship of *Bacterium anitratum* and members of the tribe Mimeae (de Bord). *J. Bact.* **57**, 659.

Ewing, W. H. (1949b). The relationship of *Shigella dispar* to certain coliform bacteria. *J. Bact.* **58**, 497.

Ewing, W. H. (1953). Serological relationships between shigella and coliform cultures. *J. Bact.* **66**, 333.

Ewing, W. H. (1962). The tribe Proteeae: its nomenclature and taxonomy. *Int. Bull. bact. Nomencl. Taxon.* **12**, 93.

Ewing, W. H. (1963). An outline of nomenclature for the family Enterobacteriaceae. *Int. Bull. bact. Nomencl. Taxon.* **13**, 95.

Ewing, W. H. (1986). Edward and Ewing's *Identification of Enterobacteriaceae*. Edn. 4. New York: Elsevier.

Ewing, W. H. & Davis, B. R. (1972a). Biochemical characterization of *Citrobacter diversus* (Burkey) Werkman and Gillen and designation of the neotype strain. *Int. J. syst. Bact.* **22**, 12.

Ewing, W. H. & Davis, B. R. (1972b). Biochemical characterization of *Serratia marcescens. Publ. Hlth Lab.* **30**, 211.

Ewing, W. H. & Fife, M. A. (1972). *Enterobacter agglomerans* (Beijerinck) comb. nov. (the herbicola-lathyri bacteria). *Int. J. syst. Bact.* **22**, 4.

Ewing, W. H. & Johnson, J. G. (1960). The differentiation of *Aeromonas* and C 27 cultures from Enterobacteriaceae. *Int. Bull. bact. Nomencl. Taxon.* **10**, 223.

Ewing, W. H., Davis, B. R. & Reavis, R. W. (1957). Phenylalanine and malonate media and their use in enteric bacteriology. *Publ. Hlth Lab.* **15**, 153.

Ewing, W. H., Davis, B. R. & Reavis, R. W. (1959). *Studies on the Serratia Group*. Atlanta, Georgia: U.S. Department of Health, Education and Welfare, Communicable Disease Center.

Ewing, W. H., Hugh, R. & Johnson, J. C. (1961). *Studies*

on the Aeromonas Group. Atlanta, Georgia: U.S. Department of Health, Education and Welfare, Communicable Disease Center.

Ewing, W. H., McWhorter, A. C., Escobar, M. R. & Lubin, A. H. (1965). *Edwardsiella,* a new genus of Enterobacteriaceae based on a new species, *E. tarda. Int. Bull. bact. Nomencl. Taxon.* **15**, 33.

Ewing, W. H., Ross, A. J., Brenner, D. J. & Fanning, G. R. (1978). *Yersinia ruckeri* sp. nov., the redmouth (R M) bacterium. *Int. J. syst. Bact.* **28**, 37.

Extra Pharmacopoeia (Martindale). (1955). Vol. II, edn 23. London: The Pharmaceutical Press.

Ezaki, T. & Yabuuchi, E. (1985). Oligopeptidase activity of Gram-positive anaerobic cocci used for rapid identification. *J. gen. appl. Microbiol.* **31**, 255.

Ezaki, T., Yamamoto, N., Ninomiya, K., Suzuki, S. & Yabuuchi, E. (1983). Transfer of *Peptococcus indolicus, Peptococcus asaccharolyticus, Peptococcus prevoti* and *Peptococcus magnus* to the Genus *Peptostreptococcus* and proposal of *Peptostreptococcus tetradius* sp. nov. *Int. J. syst. Bact.* **33**, 683.

Facklam, R. R. (1972). Recognition of group D streptococcal species of human origin by biochemical and physiological tests. *Appl. Microbiol.* **23**, 1131.

Facklam, R. R. (1977). Physiological differentiation of viridans streptococci. *J. clin. Microbiol.* **5**, 184.

Facklam, R. R. (1984). The major differences in the American and British *Streptococcus* taxonomy schemes with special reference to *Streptococcus milleri. Eur. J. clin. Microbiol.* **3**, 91.

Facklam, R. R. & Wilkinson, H. W. (1981). The family Streptococcaceae (medical aspects). In *The Prokaryotes,* vol. 2 (ed. M.P. Starr *et al.*), p.1572. Berlin: Springer-Verlag.

Fainstein, V., Hopfer, R. L., Mills, K. & Bodey, G. P. (1982). Colonization by or diarrhea due to *Kluyvera* species. *J. infect. Dis.* **145**, 127.

Falk, D. & Guering, S. J. (1983). Differentiation of *Staphylococcus* and *Micrococcus* spp with the taxo A bacitracin disk. *J. clin. Microbiol.* **18**, 719.

Falkow, S. (1958). Activity of lysine decarboxylase as an aid in the identification of salmonellae and shigellae. *Am. J. clin. Path.* **29**, 598.

Faller, A. & Schleifer, K. (1981). Modified oxidase and benzidine tests for separation of staphylococci from micrococci. *J. clin. Microbiol.* **13**, 1031.

Fallon, R. J. (1973). The relationship between the biotype of Klebsiella species and their pathogenicity. *J. clin. Path.* **26**, 523.

Farmer, J. J. III (1979). *Vibrio ('Beneckea') vulnificus,* the bacterium associated with sepsis, septicaemia and the sea. *Lancet,* ii, 903.

Farmer, J. J. III, Asbury, M. A., Hickman, F. W., Brenner, D. J. and the *Enterobacteriaceae* Study Group (1980). *Enterobacter sakazakii*: a new species of 'Enterobacteriaceae' isolated from clinical specimens. *Int. J. syst. Bact.* **30**, 569.

Farmer, J. J. III, Davis, B. R., Hickman-Brenner, F. W., McWhorter, A., Huntley-Carter, G. P., Asbury, M. A., Riddle, C., Wathen-Grady, H. G., Elias, C., Fanning, G. R., Steigerwalt, A. G., O'Hara, C. M., Morris, G. K., Smith, P. B. & Brenner, D. J. (1985a). Biochemical identification of new species and biogroups of *Enterobacteriaceae* isolated from clinical specimens. *J. clin. Microbiol.* **21**, 46.

Farmer, J. J. III, Fanning, G. R., Davis, B. R., O'Hara, C. M., Riddle, C., Hickman-Brenner, F. W., Asbury, M. A., Lowery, V. A. III & Brenner D. J. (1985b). *Escherichia fergusonii* and *Enterobacter taylorae,* two new species of *Enterobacteriaceae* isolated from clinical specimens. *J. clin. Microbiol.* **21**, 77.

Farmer, J. J. III, Fanning, G. R., Huntley-Carter, G. P., Holmes, B., Hickman, F. W., Richard, C. & Brenner, D. J. (1981). *Kluyvera,* a new (redefined) genus in the family *Enterobacteriaceae*: identification of *Kluyvera ascorbata* sp. nov. and *Kluyvera cryocrescens* sp. nov. in clinical specimens. *J. clin. Microbiol.* **13**, 919.

Farmer, J. J. III, Hickman-Brenner, F. W. & Kelly, M. T. (1985). *Vibrio*. In *Manual of Clinical Microbiology,* 4th edn, (ed. E. H. Linette, A. Balows, W. J. Hausler & H. J. Shadomy), p. 282. Washington: American Society for Microbiology.

Farmer, J. J. III, Sheth, N. K., Hudzinski, J. A., Rose, H. D. & Asbury, M. F. (1982). Bacteremia due to *Cedecea neteri* sp. nov. *J. clin. Microbiol.* **16**, 775.

Farrow, J. A. E. & Collins, M. D. (1984a). DNA base composition, DNA–DNA homology and long-chain fatty acid studies on *Streptococcus thermophilus* and *Streptococcus salivarius. J. gen. Microbiol.* **130**, 357.

Farrow, J. A. E. & Collins, M. D. (1984b). Taxonomic studies on streptococci of serological groups C, G and L and possibly related taxa. *Syst. appl. Microbiol.* **5**, 483.

Farrow, J. A. E., Jones, D., Phillips, B. A. & Collins, M. D. (1983). Taxonomic studies on some group D streptococci. *J. gen. Microbiol.* **129**, 1428.

Feeley, J. C. & Pittman, M. (1963). Studies on the haemolytic activity of El Tor vibrios. *Bull. Wld Hlth Org.* **28**, 347.

Feltham, R. K. A. (1979). A taxonomic study of the micrococcaceae. *J. appl. Bact.* **47**, 243.

Feltham, R. K. A. & Sneath, P.H.A. (1982). Construction of matrices for computer-assisted identification of aerobic Gram-positive cocci. *J. gen. Microbiol.* **128**, 713.

Feltham, R. K. A. & Stevens, M. (1983). A taxonomic

study of the genus *Serratia*, with particular attention to the position of *Serratia fonticola*. In *Gram-negative bacteria of medical and public health imprtance: Taxonomy – Identification – Applications* (ed. H. Leclerc), p. 143. Paris: L'Institut National de la Santé et de la Récherche Médicale.

Feltham, R. K. A., Wood, P. A. & Sneath, P. H. A. (1984). A general-purpose system for characterising medically important bacteria to genus level. *J. appl. Bact.* **57**, 279.

Feltham, R. K. A., Power, A. K., Pell, P. A. & Sneath, P. H. A. (1978). A simple method for storage of bacteria at –76°C. *J. appl. Bact.* **44**, 313.

Ferguson, W. W. & Henderson, N. D. (1947). Description of strain C 27: a motile organism with the major antigen of *Shigella sonnei* phase I. *J. Bact.* **54**, 179.

Ferragut, C., Izard, D., Gavini, F., Kersters, K., De Ley, J. & Leclerc, H. (1983). *Klebsiella trevisanii*: a new species from water and soil. *Int. J. syst. Bact.* **33**, 133.

Ferragut, C., Izard, D., Gavini, F., Lefebvre, B. & Leclerc, H. (1981). *Buttiauxella*, a new genus of the family *Enterobacteraceae*. *Zbl. Bakt. Hyg. C*, **2**, 33.

Fey, H. (1959). Differenzierungsschema für gramnegative aerobe Stäbchen. *Schweiz. Z. allg. Path. Bakt.* **22**, 641.

Fildes, P. (1920). A new medium for the growth of *B. influenzae*. *Br. J. exp. Path.* **1**, 129.

Finkelstein, R. A. & Mukerjee, S. (1963). Haemagglutination: a rapid method for differentiating *Vibrio cholerae* and *El Tor* vibrios. *Proc. Soc. exp. Biol. Med.* **112**, 355.

Fischer, S., Tsugita, A., Kreutz, B. & Schleifer, K. H. (1983). Immunochemical and protein-chemical studies of class I fructose 1,6 diphosphate aldolases from staphylococci. *Int. J. syst. Bact.* **33**, 443.

Fitts, R., Diamond, M., Hamilton, C. & Neri, M. (1983). DNA-DNA hybridization assay for detection of *Salmonella* spp. in foods. *Appl. environ. Microbiol.* **46**, 1146.

Fleming, A. (1922). On a remarkable bacteriolytic element found in tissues and secretions. *Proc. R. Soc. Lond.* B**93**, 306.

Fleurette, J., Brun, Y., Bes, M., Coulet, M. & Forey, F. (1987). Infections caused by coagulase-negative staphylococci other than *S. epidermidis* and *S. saprophyticus*. *Zbl. Bakt. Suppl.* **16**, 195.

Fliermans, C. B., Cherry, W. B., Orrison, L. H., Smith, S. J., Tison, D. L. & Pope, D. H. (1981). Ecological distribution of *Legionella pneumophila*. *Appl. environ. Microbiol.* **41**, 9.

Floch, H. (1953). Étude comparative des genres *Moraxella, Achromobacter et Alcaligenes*. *Annls Inst. Pasteur, Paris*, **85**, 675.

Floodgate, G. D. [printed C. D.] (1962). Some comments on the Adansonian taxonomic method. *Int. Bull. bact. Nomencl. Taxon.* **12**, 171.

Focht, D. D. & Lockhart, W. R. (1965). Numerical survey of some bacterial taxa. *J. Bact.* **90**, 1314.

Forsdike, J. L. (1950). A comparative study of agars from various geographical sources. *J. Pharm. Pharmac.* **2**, 796.

Foster, A. R. & Cohn, C. (1945). A method for the rapid preparation of Loeffler's and Petroff's media. *J. Bact.* **50**, 561.

Foster, W. D. & Bragg, J. (1962). Biochemical classification of Klebsiella correlated with the severity of the associated disease. *J. clin. Path.* **15**, 478.

Francis, J., Macturk, H.M., Madinaveitia, J. & Snow, G.A. (1953). Mycobactin, growth factor for *Mycobacterium johnei*; isolation from *Mycobacterium phlei*. *Biochem. J.* **55**, 596.

Fraser, G. (1961). Haemolytic activity of *Corynebacterium ovis*. *Nature, Lond.* **189**, 246.

Frazer, J., Zinnemann, K. & Boyce, J. M. H. (1969). The effect of different environmental conditions on some characters of *Haemophilus paraphrophilus*. *J. med. Microbiol.* **2**, 563.

Frazier, W. C. (1926). A method for the detection of changes in gelatin due to bacteria. *J. infect. Dis.* **39**, 302.

Frederiksen, W. (1970). *Citrobacter koseri* (n. sp.) a new species within the genus *Citrobacter*, with a comment on the taxonomic position of *Citrobacter intermedius* (Werkman and Gillen). *Publ. Fac. Sci. J. E. Purkyne, Brno*, **47**, 89.

Frederiksen, W. (1971). A taxonomic study of *Pasteurella* and *Actinobacillus* strains. *J. gen. Microbiol.* **69**, viii .

Freney, J., Brun, Y., Bes, M., Meughier, H., Grimont, F., Grimont, P. A. D., Nervi, C. & Fleurette, J. (1988). *Staphylococcus lugdunensis* sp. nov. and *Staphylococcus schleiferi* sp. nov., two species from human clinical specimens. *Int. J. syst. Bact.* **38**, 168.

Freney, J., Gavini, F., Alexandre, H., Madier, S., Izard, D., Leclerc, H. & Fleurette, J. (1986). Nosocomial infection and colonization by *Klebsiella trevisanii*. *J. clin. Microbiol.* **23**, 948.

Freney, J., Gruer, L. D., Bornstein, N., Kiredjian, M., Guilvout, I., Letouzey, M. N., Combe, C. & Fleurette, J. (1985). Septicemia caused by *Agrobacterium* sp. *J. clin. Microbiol.* **22**, 683.

Fricker, C. R. (1987). A review of the isolation of salmonellae and compylobacters. *J. appl. Bact.* **63**, 99.

Friedman, R. B., Bruce, D., MacLowry, J. & Brenner, V. (1973). Computer-assisted identification of bacteria. *Am. J. clin. Path.* **60**, 395.

Fujino, T. (1974). Discovery of *Vibrio parahaemolyticus*. In *International Symposium on Vibrio parahaemolyticus* (ed. T. Fujino, G. Sakaguchi, R. Sakazaki & Y. Takeda), p. 1. Tokyo: Saikon Publishing Company.

Fujino, T., Miwatani, T., Yasuda, J., Kondo, M., Takeda, Y., Akita, Y., Kotera, K., Okada, M., Nishume, H., Shimizu, T., Tamura, T. & Tamura, Y. (1965). Taxonomic studies on the bacterial strains isolated from cases of 'shirasu' food poisoning (*Pasteurella parahaemolytica* and related organisms). *Biken J.* **8**, 63.

Fuller, A. T. (1938). The formamide method for the extraction of polysaccharides from haemolytic streptococci. *Br. J. exp. Path.* **19**, 130.

Fuller, A. T. & Maxted, W. R. (1939). The production of haemolysins and peroxide by haemolytic streptococci in relation to the non-haemolytic variants of group A. *J. Path. Bact.* **49**, 83.

Fulton, M. (1943). The identity of *Bacterium columbensis* Castellani. *J. Bact.* **46**, 79.

Fulton, M., Halkias, D. & Yarashus, D. A. (1960). Voges-Proskaüer test using α-naphthol purified by steam distillation. *Appl. Microbiol.* **8**, 361.

Furniss, A. L., Lee, J. V. & Donovan, T. J. (1978). *The Vibrios.* (Public Health Laboratory Service Monograph Series no. 11). London: HMSO.

Fyfe, J. A. M., Harris, G. & Govan, J. R. W. (1984). Revised pyocin typing method for *Pseudomonas aeruginosa. J. clin. Microbiol.* **20**, 47.

Gaby, W. L. & Hadley, C. (1957). Practical laboratory test for the identification of *Pseudomonas aeruginosa. J. Bact.* **74**, 356.

Gadberry, J. L. & Amos, M. A. (1986). Comparison of a new commercially prepared porphyrin test and the conventional satellite test for the identification of *Haemophilus* species that require the X factor. *J. clin. Microbiol.* **23**, 637.

Gagnon, M., Hunting, W. M. & Esselen, W. B. (1959). New method for catalase determination. *Analyt. Chem.* **31**, 144.

Gan, G. K. & Tija, S. K. (1963). A new method for differentiation of *Vibrio comma* and *Vibrio eltor. Am. J. Hyg.* **77**, 184.

Gardner, G. A. (1966). A selective medium for the enumeration of *Microbacterium thermosphactum* in meat and meat products. *J. appl. Bact.* **29**, 455.

Gardner, G. A. (1981). *Brochothrix thermosphacta* in the spoilage of meats. In *Psychrotrophic Microorganisms in Spoilage and Pathogenicity* (ed. T. A. Roberts, G. Hobbs, J. H. B. Christian & N. Skovgaard), p. 141. London: Academic Press.

Gardner, H. L. & Dukes, C. D. (1954). New etiologic agent in nonspecific bacterial vaginitis. *Science,* **120**, 853.

Gardner, H. L. & Dukes, C. D. (1955). *Haemophilus vaginalis* vaginitis: a newly defined specific infection previ-

ously classified 'nonspecific' vaginitis. *Am. J. Obstet. Gynecol.* **69**, 962.

Garrity, G. M., Brown, A. & Vickers, R. M. (1980). *Tatlockia* and *Fluoribacter:* Two new genera of organisms resembling *Legionella pneumophila. Int. J. syst. Bact.* **30**, 609.

Garrod, L. P., Lambert, H. P. & O'Grady, F. (1981). *Antibiotics and chemotherapy.* Edn 5. Edinburgh: Churchill Livingstone.

Garvie, E. I. (1960). The genus *Leuconostoc* and its nomenclature. *J. Dairy Res.* **27**, 283.

Garvie, E. I. (1984). Separation of species of the genus *Leuconostoc* and differentiation of the leuconostocs from other lactic acid bacteria. In *Methods in Microbiology,* vol. 16 (ed. T. Bergan), p. 147. London: Academic Press.

Gaughran, E. R. L. (1969). From superstition to science: the history of a bacterium. *Trans. N.Y. Acad. Sci.* **31**, 3.

Gavini, F., Ferragut, C., Izard, D., Trinel, P. A., Leclerc, H., Lefebvre, B. & Mossel, D. A. A. (1979). *Serratia fonticola,* a new species from water. *Int. J. syst. Bact.* **29**, 92.

Gavini, F., Izard, D., Ferragut, C., Farmer, J. J. III & Leclerc, H. (1983). Separation of *Kluyvera* and *Buttiauxella* by biochemical and nucleic acid methods. *Int. J. syst. Bact.* **33**, 880.

Gavini, F., Lefebure, B., Hauze, M. & Izard, D. (1990). Development of an expert system for bacterial identification. *J. appl. Bact.* **68**, 93.

Gaworzewska, E. & Colman, G. (1988). Changes in the pattern of infection caused by *Streptococcus pyogenes. Epidemiol. Inf.* **100**, 257.

Gebhart, C. J., Edmonds, P., Ward, G. E., Kurtz, H. J. & Brenner, D. J. (1985). '*Campylobacter hyointestinalis*' sp.nov.; a new species of *Campylobacter* found in the intestines of pigs and other animals. *J. clin. Microbiol.* **21**, 715.

Gebhart, C. J., Fennell, C. L., Murtaugh, M. P. & Stamm, W. E. (1989). *Campylobacter cinaedi* is normal intestinal flora in hamsters. *J. clin. Microbiol.* **27**, 1692.

Georg, L. K. & Brown, J. M. (1967). *Rothia,* gen. nov. an aerobic genus of the family *Actinomycetaceae. Int. J. syst. Bact.* **17**, 79.

Georgala, D. L. & Boothroyd, M. (1965). A system for detecting salmonellae in meat and meat products. *J. appl. Bact.* **28**, 206.

Georgala, D. L. & Boothroyd, M. (1968). Immunofluorescence – a useful technique for microbial identification. In *Identification Methods for Microbiologists,* part B, (ed. B. M. Gibbs & D. A. Shapton) p. 187. London: Academic Press.

George, H. A., Hoffman, P. S., Smibert, R. M. & Krieg, N.

R. (1978). Improved media for growth and aerotolerance of *Campylobacter fetus. J. clin. Microbiol.* **8**, 36.

Gerencser, M. A. & Bowden, G. H. (1986). The genus *Rothia.* In *Bergey's Manual of Systematic Bacteriology,* vol. 2, (ed. P. H. A. Sneath *et al.*) p. 1342. Baltimore: Williams & Wilkins.

Gershman, M. (1961). Use of a tetrazolium salt for an easily discernible KCN reaction. *Can. J. Microbiol.* **7**, 286.

Gibson, T. & Abd-el-Malek, Y. (1945). The formation of carbon dioxide by lactic acid bacteria and *Bacillus licheniformis* and a cultural method of detecting the process. *J. Dairy Res.* **14**, 35.

Gilardi, G. L. (1971*a*). Characterization of nonfermentative nonfastidious Gram-negative bacteria encountered in medical bacteriology. *J. appl. Bact.* **34**, 623.

Gilardi, G. L. (1971*b*). Characterization of *Pseudomonas* species isolated from clinical specimens. *Appl. Microbiol.* **21**, 414.

Gilardi, G. L. (1971*c*). Antimicrobial susceptibility as a diagnostic aid in the identification of nonfermenting Gram-negative bacteria. *Appl. Microbiol.* 22, 821.

Gilardi, G. L. (1978). Identification of *Pseudomonas* and related bacteria. In *Glucose Nonfermenting Gram-Negative Bacteria in Clinical Microbiology* (ed. G. Gilardi), p.15. West Palm Beach. Florida: CRC Press.

Gilardi, G. (1985*a*). Cultural and biochemical aspects for identification of glucose-nonfermenting Gram-negative rods. In *Nonfermentative Gram-Negative Rods: Laboratory Identification and Clinical Aspects* (ed. G. Gilardi), p. 17. New York: Marcel Dekker.

Gilardi, G. L. (1985*b*). *Pseudomonas.* In *Manual of clinical Microbiology,* Edn 4 (ed. E. H. Lennette, A. Balows, W. J. Hausler & H. J. Shadomy), p. 350. Washington, D. C.: American Society for Microbiology.

Gilardi, G. L. & Hirschl, S. (1969). Morphological and biochemical characterization of *Alcaligenes odorans* var. *viridans. Int. J. syst. Bact.* **19**, 167.

Gilardi, G. L., Bottone, E. & Birnbaum, M. (1970*a*). Unusual fermentative, Gram-negative bacilli isolated from clinical specimens. I. Characterization of *Erwinia* strains of the 'lathyri-herbicola group'. *Appl. Microbiol.* **20**, 151.

Gilardi, G. L., Bottone, E. & Birnbaum, M. (1970*b*). Unusual fermentative, Gram-negative bacilli isolated from clinical specimens. II. Characterization of *Aeromonas* species. *Appl. Microbiol.* **20**, 156.

Gilbert, R. J., Turnbull, P. C. B., Parry, J. M. & Kramer, J. M. (1981). *Bacillus cereus* and other *Bacillus* species: their part in food-poisoning and other clinical infections. In *The aerobic endospore forming bacteria: classification and identification* (ed. R. C. W. Berkeley & M. Goodfellow), p. 297. London: Academic Press.

Gill, V. J., Farmer, J. J. III, Grimont, P. A. D., Asbury, M. A. & McIntosh, C. L. (1981). *Serratia ficaria* isolated from a human clinical specimen. *J. clin. Microbiol.* **14**, 234.

Gillespie, E. H. (1943). The routine use of the coagulase test for staphylococci. *Mon. Bull. Emerg. publ. Hlth Lab. Serv.* **2**, 19.

Gillespie, E. H. (1948). Chloral hydrate plates for the inhibition of swarming of proteus. *J. clin. Path.* **1**, 99.

Gillies, R. R. (1956). An evaluation of two composite media for preliminary identification of Shigella and Salmonella. *J. clin. Path.* **9**, 368.

Gillies, R. R. & Govan, J. R. W. (1966). Typing of *Pseudomonas pyocyanea* by pyocine production. *J. Path. Bact.* **91**, 339.

Gitter, M., Bradley, R. & Blampied, P. H. (1980). *Listeria monocytogenes* infection in bovine mastitis. *Vet. Record* **107**, 390.

Gnezda, J. (1899). Sur des réactions nouvelles des bases indoliques et des corps albuminoides. *C. r. hebd. Séanc. Acad. Sci., Paris*, **128**, 1584.

Goldin, M. & Glenn, A. (1962). A simple phenylalanine paper strip method for identification of *Proteus* strains. *J. Bact.* **84**, 870.

Goldsworthy, N. E. & Still, J. L. (1936). The effect of meat extract and other substances upon pigment production. *J. Path. Bact.* **43**, 555.

Goldsworthy, N. E. & Still, J. L. (1938). The effect of various meat extracts on pigment production by *B. prodigiosus. J. Path. Bact.* **46**, 634.

Goldsworthy, N. E., Still, J. L. & Dumaresq, J. A. (1938). Some sources of error in the interpretation of fermentation reactions, with special reference to the effects of serum enzymes. *J. Path. Bact.* **46**, 253.

Goodfellow, M. (1986). Genus *Rhodococcus* Zopf 1981. In *Bergey's Manual of Systematic Bacteriology,* Vol 2. (ed. P. H. A. Sneath *et al*) p. 1472. Baltimore: Williams & Wilkins.

Goodfellow, M. (1985). Staphylococcal systematics: past, present and future. *Zbl. Bakt. Suppl.* **14**, 69.

Goodfellow, M. (1987). Taxonomy of coagulase-negative staphylococci. Problems and perspectives. *Zbl. Bakt. Suppl.* **16**, 1.

Goodfellow, M. & Cross, T. (1984). Classification. In *The Biology of the Actinomycetes* (ed. M. Goodfellow, H. Mordarski & S.T. Williams), p. 7. London: Academic Press.

Goodfellow, M. & Lechevalier, P. (1986). Genus *Nocardia* Trevisan 1889. In *Bergey's Manual of Systematic Bacteriology,* vol. 2 (ed. P.H.A. Sneath *et al.*), p. 1459. Baltimore: Williams & Wilkins.

Goodfellow, M. & Minnikin, D.E. (eds) (1985). *Chemical*

Methods in Bacterial Systematics (Society for Applied Bacteriology Technical Series No. 20.) London: Academic Press.

Goodfellow, M., Alderson, G., Nahaie, M. R., Peters, G., Schumacher-Perdreau, F., Pulverer, G., Heczko, P. B. & Mordarski, M. (1983). Numerical taxonomy of staphylococci. *Zbl. Bakt. Hyg.* A**256**, 7.

Goodwin, C. S., Armstrong, J. A., Chilvers, T., Peters, M., Collins, M. D., Sly, L., McConnell, W. & Harper, W. E. S. (1989). Transfer of *Campylobacter pylori* and *Campylobacter mustelae* to *Helicobacter* gen. nov. as *Helicobacter pylori* comb. nov., and *Helicobacter mustelae* comb. nov. respectivley. *Int. J. syst. Bact.* **39**, 397.

Goosens, H., Vlaes, L., De Boeck, M., Pot, B., Kersters, K., Levy, J., DeMol, P., Butzler, J. P. & Vandamme, P. (1990). Is *'Campylobacter upsaliensis'* an unrecognized cause of human diarrhoea? *Lancet*, i, 355, 584.

Gordon, R. E. (1967). The taxonomy of soil bacteria. In *The Ecology of Soil Bacteria*. (ed. T. R. G. Gray & D. Parkinson), p. 293. Liverpool University Press.

Gordon, J. & McLeod, J. W. (1928). The practical application of the direct oxidase reaction in bacteriology. *J. Path. Bact.* **31**, 185.

Gordon, R. E. & Mihm, J. M. (1957). A comparative study of some strains received as nocardiae. *J. Bact.* **73**, 15.

Gordon, R. E., Hyde, J. L. & Moore, J. A., Jr (1977). *Bacillus firmus – Bacillus lentus*: a series or one species? *Int. J. syst. Bact.* **27**, 256.

Gordon, R. E. & Smith, M. M. (1953). Rapidly growing, acid fast bacteria. I. Species' descriptions of *Mycobacterium phlei* Lehmann and Neumann and *Mycobacterium smegmatis* (Trevisan) Lehmann and Neumann. *J. Bact.* **66**, 41.

Gordon, R. E. & Smith, M. M. (1955). Rapidly growing, acid fast bacteria. II. Species' description of *Mycobacterium fortuitum* Cruz. *J. Bact.* **69**, 502.

Gordon, R. E., Haynes, W. C. & Pang, C. H.-N. (1973). The genus *Bacillus*. Agriculture Handbook no. 427. Washington, D.C.: US Dept Agriculture.

Gottschalk, G. (ed.) (1985). *Methods in Microbiology*, vol. 18. Society for Applied Bacteriology. London: Academic Press.

von Graevenitz, A. & Bucher, C. (1983). Evaluation of differential and selective media for the isolation of *Aeromonas* and *Plesiomonas* spp. from human faeces. *J. clin. Microbiol.* **17**, 16.

Graham, D. C. & Hodgkiss, W. (1967). Identity of Gram negative, yellow pigmented, fermentative bacteria isolated from plants and animals. *J. appl. Bact.* **30**, 175.

Granato, P. A. Jurek, E.A. & Weiner, L. B. (1983). Biotypes of *Haemophilus influenzae*: relationship to clinical source of isolation, serotype and antibiotic susceptibility. *Am. J. Clin. Path.* **80**, 73.

Gratia, A. (1920). Nature et genèse de l'agent coagulant du Staphylocoque ou 'Staphylocoagulase'. *C. r. Séanc. Soc. Biol.* **83**, 584.

Gratten, M. (1983). *Haemophilus influenzae* biotype VII. *J. clin. Microbiol.* **18**, 1015.

Greene, R. A. & Larks, G. G. (1955). A quick method for the detection of gelatin liquefying bacteria. *J. Bact.* **69**, 224.

Greenwood, J. R. & Pickett, M. J. (1979). Salient features of *Haemophilus vaginalis*. *J. clin. Microbiol.* **9**, 200.

Greenwood, J. R. & Pickett, M. J. (1980). Transfer of *Haemophilus vaginalis* Gardner and Dukes to a new genus. *Gardnerella* : *G. vaginalis* (Gardner and Dukes) comb.nov. *Int. J. syst. Bact.* **30**, 170.

Greenwood, J. R. & Pickett, M. J. (1984, 1986). Genus *Gardnerella*. In *Bergey's Manual of Systematic Bacteriology*, vol. 1, (1984), p. 587; vol. 2, (1986), p. 1283. Baltimore: Williams & Wilkins.

Greenwood, J. R., Pickett, M. J., Martin, W. J. & Mack, E. G. (1977). *Haemophilus vaginalis* (*Corynebacterium vaginale*): Method for isolation and rapid biochemical identification. *Health Lab. Sci.* **14**, 102.

Grimont, P. A. D., & Dulong de Rosnay, H. L. C. (1972). Numerical study of 60 strains of *Serratia*. *J. gen. Microbiol.* **72**, 259.

Grimont, P. A. D. & Grimont, F. (1978*a*). Biotyping of *Serratia marcescens* and its use in epidemiological studies. *J. clin. Microbiol.* **8**, 73.

Grimont, P. A. D. & Grimont, F. (1978*b*). The genus *Serratia*. *Ann. Rev. Microbiol.* **32**, 226.

Grimont, P. A. D., Farmer, J. J. III, Grimont, F., Asbury, M. A., Brenner, D. J. & Deval, C. (1983). *Ewingella americana* gen. nov., sp. nov., a new *Enterobacteriaceae* isolated from clinical specimens. *Ann. Microbiol. Inst. Pasteur*, Paris, **134** A, 39.

Grimont, P. A. D., Grimont, F., Dulong de Rosnay, H. L. C. & Sneath, P. H. A. (1977). Taxonomy of the genus *Serratia*. *J. gen. Microbiol.* **98**, 39.

Grimont, P. A. D., Grimont, F., Farmer, J. J. III & Asbury, M. A. (1981). *Cedecea davisae* gen. nov., sp. nov. and *Cedecea lapagei* sp. nov., new *Enterobacteriaceae* from clinical specimens. *Int. J. syst. Bact.* **31**, 317.

Grimont, P. A. D., Grimont, F., Richard, C., Davis, B. R., Steigerwalt, A. G. & Brenner, D. J. (1978). Deoxyribonucleic acid relatedness between *Serratia plymuthica* and other *Serratia* species, with a description of *Serratia odorifera* sp. nov. *Int. J. syst. Bact.* **28** , 453.

Gross, K. C., Houghton, M. P. & Senterfit, L. B. (1975). Presumptive speciation of *Streptococcus bovis* and other group D streptococci from human sources by using arginine and pyruvate tests. *J. clin. Microbiol.* **1**, 54.

Gross, R. J. & Rowe, B. (1985). *Escherichia coli* diarrhoea. *J. Hyg., Camb.* **95**, 531.

Grov, A., Myklestad, B. & Oeding, J. (1964). Immunochemical studies on antigen preparations from *Staphylococcus aureus*. I. Isolation and chemical characterization of antigen A. *Acta path. microbiol. scand.* **61**, 588.

Gubash, S. M. (1978). Synergistic haemolysis phenomenon shown by an alpha-toxin-producing *Clostridium perfringens* and streptococcal CAMP factor in presumptive streptococcal grouping. *J. clin. Microbiol.* **8**, 480.

Gubash, S. M. (1980). Synergistic haemolysis test for presumptive identification and differentiation of *Clostridium perfringens*, *C. bifermentans*, *C. sordellii*, and *C. paraperfringens*. *J. clin. Path.* **33**, 395.

Gurr, E. (1956). *A Practical Manual of Medical and Biological Staining Techniques*, edn 2. London: Leonard Hill Ltd.

Gurr, G. T. (1963). *Biological Staining Methods*, edn 7. London: George T. Gurr Ltd.

Gutekunst, R. R., Delwiche, E. A. & Seeley, H. W. (1957). Catalase activity in *Pediococcus cerevisiae* as related to hydrogen ion activity. *J. Bact.* **74**, 693.

Gutiérrez-Vázquez, J. M. (1960). Further studies on the spot test for the differentiation of tubercle bacilli of human origin from other mycobacteria. *Am. Rev. resp. Dis.* **81**, 412.

Habeeb, A. F. S. A. (1960*a*). A study of bacteriological media. The examination of Proteose-Peptone. *J. Pharm. Pharmac.* **12**, 119.

Habeeb, A. F. S. A. (1960*b*). A study of bacteriological media: the examination of peptides in Casamin E. *Can. J. Microbiol.* **6**, 237.

Habs, H. & Schubert, R. H. W. (1962). Über die biochemischen Merkmale und die taxonomische Steelung von *Pseudomonas shigelloides* (Bader). *Zentbl. Bakt. ParasitKde Abt. II*, **186**, 316.

Hájek, V. & Marsálek, E. (1971). The differentiation of pathogenic staphylococci and a suggestion for their taxonomic classification. *Zentbl. Bakt. ParasitKde Abt I, A* **217**, 176.

Hajna, A. A. & Damon, S. R. (1934). Differentiation of *Aerobacter aerogenes* and *A. cloacae* on the basis of the hydrolysis of sodium hippurate. *Am. J. Hyg.* **19**, 545.

Hajna, A. A. (1950). A semi-solid medium suitable for both motility and hydrogen sulfide tests. *Publ. Hlth Lab.* **8**, 36.

Hajna, A. A (1955). A new enrichment medium for Gram-negative organisms of the intestinal group. *Publ. Hlth Lab.* **13**, 83.

Halvorsen, J. F. (1963). Gliding motility in the organisms *Bacterium anitratum* (B5W), *Moraxella lwoffii* and *Alkaligenes haemolysans,* as compared to *Moraxella nonliquefaciens. Acta path. microbiol. scand.* **59**, 200.

Hammond, G. W., Lian, C.-J., Wilt, J. C. & Ronald, A. R. (1978). Comparison of specimen collection and laboratory techniques for the isolation of *Haemophilus ducreyi. J. clin. Microbiol.* **7**, 39.

Hansen, M. W. & Glupczynski, G. Y. (1984). Isolation of an unusual *Cedecea* species from a cutaneous ulcer. *Eur. J. clin. Microbiol.* **3**, 152.

Harden, A. & Norris, D. (1912). The bacterial production of acetylmethylcarbinol and 2,3-butylene glycol from various substances. *Proc. R. Soc.* B. **84**, 492.

Hare, R. & Colebrook, L. (1934). The biochemical reactions of haemolytic streptococci from the vagina of febrile and afebrile parturient women. *J. Path. Bact.* **39**, 429.

Harper, E. M. & Conway, N. S. (1948). Clotting of human citrated plasma by Gram-negative organisms. *J. Path. Bact.* **60**, 247.

Harper, J. J. & Davis, G. H. G. (1982). Cell wall analysis of *Gardnerella vaginalis* (*Haemophilus vaginalis*). *Int. J. syst. Bact.* **32**, 48.

Harrison, T. G. & Taylor, A. G. (eds) (1988). *A laboratory manual for Legionella.* Chichester: John Wiley.

Hartley, P. (1922).The value of Douglas's medium for the production of diphtheria toxin. *J. Path. Bact.* **25**, 479.

Harvey, R. W. S. & Thomson, S. (1953). Optimum temperature of incubation for isolation of salmonellae. *Mon. Bull. Minist. Hlth Lab. Serv.*, **12**,149.

Hastings, E. G. (1903). Milchagar als Medium zur Demonstration der Erzeugung proteolytischer Enzyme. *Zentbl. Bakt. ParasitKde Abt.* II, **10**, 384.

Hastings, E. G. (1904). The action of various classes of bacteria on casein as shown by milk-agar plates. *Zentbl. Bakt. ParasitKde Abt.* II, **12**, 590.

Hawn, C. V. Z. & Beebe, E. (1965). Rapid method for demonstrating bile solubility of *Diplococcus pneumoniae. J. Bact.* **90**, 549.

Haynes, W. C. (1951). *Pseudomonas aeruginosa* - its characterization and identification. *J. gen. Microbiol.* **5**, 939.

Haynes, W. C. (1957). *Pseudomonas* Migula, 1894. In *Bergey's Manual of Determinative Bacteriology*, 7th edn (ed. R. S. Breed, E. G. D. Murray & N. R. Smith), p. 89. Baltimore: Williams & Wilkins.

Hayward, N. J. & Miles, A. A. (1943). Inhibition of Proteus in cultures from wounds. *Lancet*, ii, 116.

Hébert, G. A. (1981), Hippurate hydrolysis by *Legionella pneumophila. J. clin. Microbiol.* **13**, 240.

Heiberg, B. (1936). The biochemical reactions of vibrios. *J. Hyg., Camb.* **36**, 114.

Henderson, A. (1967). The urease activity of *Acinetobacter lwoffii* and *A. anitratus. J. gen. Microbiol.* **46**, 399.

Hendry, C. B. (1938). The effect of serum maltase on fermentation reactions with gonococci. *J. Path. Bact.* **46**, 383.

Henriksen, S. D. (1950). A comparison of the phenyl-pyruvic acid reaction and the urease test in the differentiation of Proteus from other enteric organisms. *J. Bact.* **60**, 225.

Henriksen, S. D. (1952). *Moraxella:* classification and taxonomy. *J. gen. Microbiol.* **6**, 318.

Henriksen, S. D. (1960). *Moraxella.* Some problems of taxonomy and nomenclature. *Int. Bull. bact. Nomencl. Taxon.* **10**, 23.

Henriksen, S. D. (1962). Some *Pasteurella* strains from the human respiratory tract. A correction and supplement. *Acta path. microbiol. scand.* **55**, 355.

Henriksen, S. D. (1963). Mimae. The standing in nomenclature of the names of this tribus and of its genera and species. *Int. Bull. bact. Nomencl. Taxon.* **13**, 51.

Henriksen, S. D. & Bøvre, K. (1968a). *Moraxella kingii* sp. nov., a haemolytic, saccharolytic species of the genus *Moraxella. J. gen. Microbiol.* **51**, 377.

Henriksen, S. D. & Bøvre, K. (1968b). The taxonomy of the genera *Moraxella* and *Neisseria. J. gen. Microbiol.* **51**, 387.

Henriksen, S. D. & Closs, K. (1938). The production of phenylpyruvic acid by bacteria. *Acta path. microbiol. scand.* **15**, 101.

Henriksen, S. D. & Jyssum, K. (1960). A new variety of *Pasteurella haemolytica* from the human respiratory tract. *Acta path. microbiol. scand.* **50**, 443.

Henriksen, S. D. & Bøvre, K. (1976). Transfer of *Moraxella kingae* Henriksen and Bøvre to the genus *Kingella* gen. nov. in the family *Neisseriaceae. Int. J. syst. Bact.* **26**, 447.

Hermann, G. J. (1961). The laboratory recognition of *Corynebacterium haemolyticum. Am. J. med. Technol.*, **27**, 61.

Hickman, F. W., Farmer, J. J. III, Hollis, D. G., Fanning, G. R., Steigerwalt, A. G., Weaver, R. E. & Brenner, D. J. (1982). Identification of *Vibrio hollisae* sp. nov. from patients with diarrhoea. *J. clin. Microbiol.* **15**, 395.

Hickman, F. W., Steigerwalt, A. G., Farmer, J. J. III & Brenner, D. J. (1982). Identification of *Proteus penneri* sp. nov., formerly known as *Proteus vulgaris* indole negative or as *Proteus vulgaris* biogroup 1. *J. clin. Microbiol.* **15**, 1097.

Hickman-Brenner, F. W., Farmer, J. J. III, Steigerwalt, A. G. & Brenner, D. J. (1983). *Providencia rustigianii:* a new species in the family *Enterobacteriaceae* formerly known as *Providencia alcalifaciens* biogroup 3. *J. clin. Microbiol.* **17**, 1057.

Hickman-Brenner, F. W., Huntley-Carter, G. P., Fanning, G. R., Brenner, D. J. & Farmer, J. J. III (1985a). *Koserella trabulsii*, a new genus and species of *Enterobacteriaceae* formerly known as Enteric Group 45. *J. clin. Microbiol.* **21**, 39.

Hickman-Brenner, F. W., Huntley-Carter, G. P., Saitoh, Y., Steigerwalt, A. G., Farmer, J. J. III & Brenner, D. J. (1984). *Moellerella wisconsensis*, a new genus and species of *Enterobacteriaceae* found in human stool specimens. *J. clin. Microbiol.* **19**, 460.

Hickman-Brenner, F. W., Vohra, M. P., Huntley-Carter, G. P., Fanning, G. R., Lowery, V. A. III, Brenner, D. J. & Farmer, J. J. III. (1985b). *Leminoarella*, a new genus of *Enterobacteriaceae*: identification of *Leminorella grimontii* sp. nov. and *Leminorella richardii* sp. nov. found in clinical specimens. *J. clin. Microbiol.* **21**, 234.

Hill, L. R. (1959). The Adansonian classification of the staphylococci. *J. gen. Microbiol.* **20**, 277.

Hill, L. R. (1966). An index to deoxyribonucleic acid base compositions of bacterial species. *J. gen. Microbiol.* **44**, 419.

Hill, L. R. (1978) *A dictionary of microbial taxonomy* [by the late S. T. Cowan, edited by L. R. Hill]. Cambridge University Press.

Hill, L. R., Snell, J. J. S. & Lapage, S. P. (1970). Identification and characterisation of *Bacteroides corrodens. J. med. Microbiol.* **3**, 483.

Hill, L. R., Turri, M., Gilardi, E. & Silvestri, L. G. (1961). Quantitative methods in the systematics of Actinomycetales. II. *Giornali Microbiologica.* **9**, 56.

Hinz, K.-H. & Kunjara, C. (1977). *Haemophilus avium*, a new species from chickens. *Int. J. syst. Bact.* **27**, 324.

Hitchens, A. P. & Leikind, M. C. (1939). The introduction of agar-agar into bacteriology. *J. Bact.* **37**, 485.

Hobbs, B. C. & Allison, V. D. (1945). Studies on the isolation of *Bact. typhosum* and *Bact. paratyphosum* B. *Mon. Bull. Minist. Hlth Lab. Serv.* **4**, 63.

Hodgkiss, W. (1960). The interpretation of flagella stains. *J. appl. Bact.* **23**, 398.

Hoffman, P. S., George, H. A., Krieg, N. R. & Smibert, R. M. (1979a). Studies of the microaerophilic nature of *Campylobacter fetus* subsp. *jejuni.* I. Physiological aspects of enhanced aerotolerance. *Can. J. Microbiol.* **25**, 1.

Hoffman, P. S., George, H. A., Krieg, N. R. & Smibert, R. M. (1979b). Studies of the microaerophilic nature of *Campylobacter fetus* subsp. *jejuni.* II. Role of exogenous superoxide anions and hydrogen peroxide. *Can. J. Microbiol.* **25**, 8.

Hofstad, T. (1985). The classification and identification of the anaerobic Gram-positive cocci. *Scand. J. inf. Dis.* (suppl.) **46**, 14.

Hoke, C. & Vedros, N. A. (1982). Taxonomy of the Neisseriae: fatty acid analysis, aminopeptidase activity, and pigment extraction. *Int. J. syst. Bact.* **21**, 51.

Holdeman, L. V. & Moore, W. E. C. (1972). Eds, *Anaerobe Laboratory Manual.* Blacksburg, Virginia: Anaerobe Laboratory, Virginia Polytechnic Institute & State University.

Holdeman, L. V., Cato, E. P. & Moore, W. E. C. (eds) (1977). *Anaerobe Laboratory Manual*, 4th edn Blacksburg, Virginia: V. P. I. Anaerobe Laboratory and State University.

Holdeman-Moore, L. V., Johnson, J. L. & Moore, W. E. C. (1986). Genus *Peptostreptococcus*. In *Bergey's Manual of Systematic Bacteriology*, vol. 2 (ed. P.H.A. Sneath *et al.*), p. 1083. Baltimore: Williams & Wilkins.

Holding, A. J. & Collee, J. G. (1971). Routine biochemical tests. In *Methods in Microbiology,* vol. 6A, (ed. J. R. Norris & D. W. Ribbons) p. 1. London: Academic Press.

Höllander, R. & Mannheim, W. (1975) Characterization of hemophilic and related bacteria by their respiratory quinones and cytochromes. *Int. J. syst. Bact.* **25**, 102.

Höllander, R., Hess-Reihse, A. & Mannheim, W. (1981). Respiratory quinones in *Haemophilus, Pasteurella* and *Actinobacillus*: pattern, function and taxonomic evaluation. In *Haemophilus, Pasteurella and Actinobacillus* (ed. M. Kilian, W. Frederikson & E. L. Biberstein), p. 83. London: Academic Press.

Hollis, D. G., Wiggins, G. L. & Weaver, R. E. (1969). *Neisseria lactamicus* sp. n., a lactose-fermenting species resembling *Neisseria meningitidis. Appl. Microbiol.* **17**, 71.

Hollis, D. G., Hickman, F. W., Fanning, G. R., Farmer, J. J. III, Weaver, R. E. & Brenner, D. J. (1981). *Tatumella ptyseos* gen. nov. sp. nov., a member of the family *Enterobacteriaceae* found in clinical specimens. *J. clin. Microbiol.* **14**, 79.

Hollis, D. G., Weaver, R. E., Steigerwalt, A. G., Wenger, J. D., Moss, C. W. & Brenner, D. J. (1989). *Francisella philomiragia* comb. nov. (formerly *Yersinia philomiragia*) and *Francisella tularensis* biogroup *novicida* (formerly *Francisella novicida*) associated with human disease. *J. clin. Microbiol.* **27**, 1601.

Holman, W. L. & Gonzales, F. L. (1923). A test for indol based on the oxalic reaction of Gnezda. *J. Bact.* **8**, 577.

Holmberg, K. & Höllander, H. O. (1973). Production of bacterial concentrations of hydrogen peroxide by *Streptococcus sanguis. Arch. Oral Biol.* **18**, 423.

Holmberg, K. & Nord, C. E. (1975). Numerical taxonomy and laboratory identification of *Actinomyces* and *Arachnia* and some related bacteria. *J. gen. Microbiol.* **91**, 17.

Holmes, B. & Roberts, P. (1981). The classification, identification and nomenclature of agrobacteria. *J. appl. Bact.* **50**, 443.

Holmes, B. (1986*a*). Identification and distribution of *Pseudomonas stutzeri* in clinical material. *J. appl. Bact.* **60**, 401.

Holmes, B. (1986*b*). The identification of *Pseudomonas cepacia* and its occurrence in clinical material. *J. appl. Bact.* **61**, 299.

Holmes, B. (1987). Identification and distribution of *Flavobacterium meningosepticum* in clinical material. *J. appl. Bact.* **62**, 29.

Holmes, B. & Dawson, C. A. (1983). Numerical taxonomic studies on *Achromobacter* isolates from clinical material. In *Gram Negative Bacteria of Medical and Public Health Importance* (ed. H. Leclerc), *Colloque INSERM,* Vol. 114, p. 331. Paris: Editions INSERM.

Holmes, B. & Dawson, C. A. (1985). Misuse and interlaboratory test reproducibility of API 20E system. *J. clin. Microbiol.* **38**, 937.

Holmes, B. & Gross, R. J. (1990). Coliform bacteria; various other members of the Enterobacteriaceae. In *Topley and Wilson's Principles of Bacteriology, Virology and Immunity*, 8th edn (ed. M. T. Parker and B. I. Duerden), p. 41. Maidenhead: Edward Arnold.

Holmes, B., King, A., Phillips, I. & Lapage, S. P. (1974). Sensitivity of *Citrobacter freundii* and *Citrobacter koseri* to cephalosporins and penicillins. *J. clin. Path.* **27**, 729.

Holmes, B., Lapage, S. P. & Easterling, B. G. (1979). Distribution in clinical material and identification of *Pseudomonas maltophilia. J. clin. Path.* **32**, 66.

Holmes, B., Lapage, S. P. & Malnick, H. (1975). Strains of *Pseudomonas putrefaciens* from clinical material. *J. clin. Path.* **28**, 149.

Holmes, B., Owen, R. J. & McMeekin, T. A. (1984). Genus *Flavobacterium*. In *Bergey's Manual of Systematic Bacteriology*, vol. 1 (ed. N. R. Krieg & J. G. Holt.), p. 353. Baltimore: Williams & Wilkins.

Holmes, B., Owen, R. J., Evans, A., Malnick, H. & Willcox, W. R. (1977). *Pseudomonas paucimobilis*,a new species isolated from human clinical specimens, the hospital environment, and other sources. *Int. J. syst. Bact.* **27**, 133.

Holmes, B., Owen, R.J., Steigerwalt, A. G. & Brenner, D. J. (1984). *Flavobacterium gleum*, a new species found in human clinical specimens. *Int. J. syst. Bact.* **34**, 21.

Holmes, B., Pinning, C. A. & Dawson, C. A. (1986). A probability matrix for the identification of Gram-negative, aerobic, non-fermentative bacteria that grow on nutrient agar. *J. gen. Microbiol.* **132**, 1827.

Holmes, B., Snell, J. J. S. & Lapage, S. P. (1977). Strains of *Achromobacter xylosoxidans* from clinical material. *J. clin. path.* **30**, 595.

Holmes, B., Steigerwalt, A. G., Weaver, R. E. & Brenner, D. J. (1986a). *Weeksella virosa* gen. nov., sp. nov. (formerly Group IIf), found in human clinical specimens. *System. appl. Microbiol.* **8**, 185.

Holmes, B., Steigerwalt, A. G., Weaver, R. E. & Brenner, D. J. (1986b). *Weeksella zoohelcum* sp. nov. (formerly Group IIj), from human clinical specimens. *System. appl. Microbiol.* **8**, 191.

Holmes, B., Steigerwalt, A. G., Weaver, R. E. & Brenner, D. J. (1987). *Chryseomonas luteola* comb. nov. and *Flavimonas oryzihabitans* gen. nov., comb. nov., *Pseudomonas*-like species from human clinical specimens and formerly known, respectively, as Groups Ve-1 and Ve-2. *Int. J. syst. Bact.* **37**, 245.

Hommez, J., Devriese, L. A., Henrichsen, J. & Castryck, F. (1986). Identification and characterization of *Streptococcus suis*. *Vet. Microbiol.* **11**, 349.

Hormaeche, E. & Edwards, P. R. (1958). Observations on the genus *Aerobacter* with a description of two species. *Int. Bull. bact. Nomencl. Taxon.* **8**,111.

Hormaeche, E. & Edwards, P. R. (1960). A proposed genus *Enterobacter*. *Int. Bull. bact. Nomencl. Taxon.* **10**, 71 .

Hormaeche, E. & Munilla, M. (1957). Biochemical tests for the differentiation of *Klebsiella* and *Cloaca*. *Int. Bull. bact. Nomencl. Taxon.* **7**, 1.

Hovelius, B. (1986). Epidemiological and clinical aspects of urinary tract infections caused by *Staphylococcus saprophyticus*. In *Coagulase-negative Staphylococci* (ed. P. A. Mardh & K. H. Schleifer), p. 195. Stockholm: Almqvist & Wiksell International.

Hoyle, L. (1941). A tellurite blood-agar medium for the rapid diagnosis of diphtheria. *Lancet*, i, 175.

Hoyt, R. E. (1951). Tableted substrates in the detection of indol and urease production by bacteria. *Am. J. clin. Path.* **21**, 892.

Hoyt, R. E. & Pickett, M. J. (1957). Use of 'rapid substrate' tablets in the recognition of enteric bacteria. *Am. J. clin. Path.* **27**, 343.

Hsu, S. T., Liu, C. H. & Liao, C. L. (1964). A new differential medium for enteropathogenic vibrios and other Gram-negative intestinal organisms. *Bull. Wld Hlth Org.* **31**, 136.

Hubálek, Z. (1969). Numerical taxonomy of genera *Micrococcus* Cohn and *Sarcina* Goodsir. *J. gen. Microbiol.* **57**, 349.

Hucker, G. J. & Conn, H. J. (1923). Methods of Gram staining. *Tech. Bull. N.Y. St. agric. Exp. Sta.* no. 93.

Hucker, G. J. (1924a). Studies on the Coccaceae. II. A study of the general characters of the micrococci. *Tech. Bull. N. Y. St. agric. Exp. Sta.* no. 100.

Hucker, G. J. (1924b). Studies on the Coccaceae. IV. The classification of the genus *Micrococcus* Cohn. *Tech. Bull. N.Y. St. agric. Exp. Sta.* no. 102.

Hugh, R. (1959). Oxytoca group organisms isolated from the oropharyngeal region. *Canad. J. Microbiol.* **5**, 251 .

Hugh, R. & Leifson, E. (1953). The taxonomic significance of fermentative versus oxidative metabolism of carbohydrates by various Gram negative bacteria. *J. Bact.* **66**, 24.

Hugh, R. & Leifson, E. (1963). A description of the type strain of *Pseudomonas maltophilia*. *Int. Bull. bact. Nomencl. Taxon.* **13**,133.

Hugh, R. & Reese, R. (1968). A comparison of 120 strains of *Bacterium anitratum* Schaub and Hauber with the type strain of this species. *Int. J. syst. Bact.* **18**, 207.

Hugh, R. & Ryschenkow, E. (1961). *Pseudomonas maltophilia*, an Alcaligenes-like species. *J. gen. Microbiol.* **26**, 123.

Hugh, R. & Sakazaki, R. (1972). Minimal number of characters for the identification of *Vibrio* species, *Vibrio cholerae* and *Vibrio parahaemolyticus*. *Publ. Hlth. Lab.* **30**, 133.

Hungate, R. E. (1969). A roll tube method for cultivation of strict anaerobes. In *Methods in Microbiology* vol. 3ʙ, (ed. J. R. Norris & D. W. Ribbons), p. 117. London: Academic Press.

Huq, M.I., Alam, A. K. M. J., Brenner, D. J. & Morris, G.K. (1980). Isolation of *Vibrio*-like group EF-6, from patients with diarrhoea. *J. clin. Microbiol.* **11**, 621.

Hutner, S. H. (1942). Some growth requirements of *Erysipelothrix* and *Listerella*. *J. Bact.* **43**, 629.

Hwang, M-N. & Ederer, G. M. (1975). Rapid hippurate hydrolysis method for presumptive identification of Group B streptococci. *J. clin. Microbiol.* **1**, 114.

International Code of Nomenclature of Bacteria (short title *Bacteriological Code*). Edn. 1, 1948 [known as *International Bacteriological Code of Nomenclature*]; Edn. 2, 1958 [known as *International Code of Nomenclature of Bacteria and Viruses*]; Edn. 3, 1966 [imperfect as some paragraphs unintentionally omitted from text]; Edn. 4, 1975 (1976 revision), (ed. S. P. Lapage, P. H. A. Sneath, E. F. Lessel, V. B. D. Skerman, H. P. R. Seeliger & W. A. Clark). Iowa: State University Press, Ames.

Inzana, T. J. (1983). Electrophoretic heterogeneity and interstrain variation of the lipopolysaccharide of *Haemophilus influenzae*. *J. inf. Dis.* **148**, 492.

Islam, A. K. M. S. (1977). Rapid recognition of group-B streptococci. *Lancet*, i, 256.

Ison, C. A., Dawson, S.G., Hilton, J., Csonka, G. W. & Easmon, C. S. F. (1982). Comparison of culture and microscopy in the diagnosis of *Gardnerella vaginalis* infection. *J. clin. Path.* **35**, 550.

Izard, D., Gavini, F., Trinel, P. A. & Leclerc, H. (1979). *Rahnella aquatilis*, nouveau membre de la famille des *Enterobacteriaceae*. *Annls. Microbiol. Inst. Pasteur, Paris,* **130** A, 163.

Izard, D., Gavini, F., Trinel, P. A., Krubwa, F. & Leclerc, H. (1980). Contribution of DNA-DNA hybridization to the transfer of *Enterobacter aerogenes* to the genus *Klebsiella* as *K. mobilis*. *Zbl. Bakt. Hyg.* C1, 257.

Jackman, P. J. H., Pitcher, D. G., Pelczynska, S.& Borman, P. (1987). Classification of corynebacteria associated with endocarditis (Group JK) as *Corynebacterium jeikeium* sp.nov. *Syst. appl. Microbiol.* **9**, 83.

Jackson, F. L. & Goodman, Y. E. (1972). Transfer of the facultatively anaerobic organism *Bacteroides corrodens* Eiken to a new genus, *Eikenella*. *Int. J. syst. Bact.* **22**, 73.

Jain, K., Radsak, K. & Mannheim, W. (1974). Differentiation of the *Oxytocum* group from *Klebsiella* by deoxyribonucleic acid – deoxyribonucleic acid hybridization. *Int. J. syst. Bact.* **24**, 402.

Jameson, J. E. & Emberley, N. W. (1956). A substitute for bile salts in culture media. *J. gen. Microbiol.* **15**, 198.

Jameson, J. E. (1965). A modified Elek test for toxigenic *Corynebacterium diphtheriae*. *Mon. Bull. Minist. Hlth. Lab. Serv.* **24**, 55.

Jantzen, E., Bergan, T. & Bøvre, K. (1974). Gas chromatography of bacterial whole cell methanolysates. *Acta path. microbiol. scand.* **B 82**, 785.

Jawetz, E. (1950). A pneumotropic pasteurella of laboratory animals. I. Bacteriological and serological characteristics of the organism. *J. infect. Dis.* **86**, 172.

Jayne-Williams, D. J. & Cheeseman, G. C. (1960). The differentiation of bacterial species by paper chromatography. IX. The genus *Bacillus:* a preliminary investigation. *J. appl. Bact.* **23**, 250.

Jayne-Williams, D. J. & Skerman, T. M. (1966). Comparative studies on coryneform bacteria from milk and dairy sources. *J. appl. Bact.* **29**, 72.

Jeffries, C. D., Holtman, D. F. & Guse, D. G. (1957). Rapid method for determining the activity of microorganisms on nucleic acids. *J. Bact.* **73**, 590.

Jeffries, L., Cawthorne, M. A., Harris, M., Cook, B. & Diplock, A. T. (1968). Menaquinone determination in the taxonomy of Micrococcaceae. *J. gen. Microbiol.* **54**, 365.

Jenkins, P. A., Duddridge, L. R., Collins, C. H. & Yates, M. D. (1985). Mycobacteria. In *Isolation and Identification of Microorganisms of Medical and Veterinary importance* (ed. C. H. Collins & J. Grange), p. 275. (Society for Applied Bacteriology Tech. Series No. 21). London: Academic Press.

Jennens, M. G. (1954). The methyl red test in peptone media. *J. gen. Microbiol.* **10**, 121.

Jensen, K. A. (1932). Reinzüchtung und Typenbestimmung von Tuberkelbazillenstämmen. Eine Vereinfachung der Methoden für die Praxis. *Zentbl. Bakt. ParasitKde Abt.* *I,* **125,** 222.

Jensen, W. L., Owen, C. R. & Jellison, W. L. (1969). *Yersinia philomiragia sp.* n., a new member of the Pasteurella group of bacteria, naturally pathogenic for the muskrat (*Ondatra zibethica*) *J. Bact.* **100**, 1237.

Johnson, J. L. & Cummins, C. S. (1972). Cell wall composition and deoxyribonucleic acid similarities among the anaerobic coryneforms, classical propionibacteria, and strains of *Arachnia propionica*. *J. Bact.* **109**, 1047.

Johnson, J. L., Anderson, R. S. & Ordal, E. J. (1970). Nucleic acid homologies among oxidase-negative *Moraxella* species. *J. Bact.* **101**, 568.

Johnson, R. & Sneath, P. H. A. (1973). Taxonomy of *Bordetella* and related organisms of the families *Achromobacteraceae*, *Brucellaceae*, and *Neisseriaceae*. *Int. J. syst. Bact.* **23**, 381.

Johnson, W. M., Disalvo, A. F. & Stener, R. R. (1971). Fatal *Chromobacterium violaceum* septicaemia. *Am. J. clin. Path.* **56**, 400.

Johnston, M. A. & Delwiche, E. A. (1962). Catalase of the Lactobacillaceae. *J. Bact.*, **83**, 936.

Jolly, J. L. S. (1983). Minimal criteria for the identification of *Gardnerella vaginalis* isolated from the vagina. *J. clin. Path.* **36**, 476.

Jones, D. (1986). The genus *Erysipelothrix*. In *Bergey's Manual of Systematic Bacteriology*, vol. 2 (ed. P. H. A. Sneath *et al.*). p. 1245. Baltimore: Williams & Wilkins.

Jones, D. M. (1962). A pasteurella-like organism from the human respiratory tract. *J. Path. Bact.* **83**,143.

Jones, D. & Collins, M. D. (1986). Irregular nonsporing Gram-positive rods. In *Bergey's Manual of Systematic Bacteriology*, vol. 2 (ed. P. H. A. Sneath *et. al.*), p. 1261. Baltimore: Williams & Wilkins.

Jones, D., Pell, P. A. & Sneath, P. H. A. (1984). Maintenance of bacteria on glass beads at −60°C to −76°C. In *Maintenance of microorganisms*, (ed. B.E. Kirsop & J. J. S. Snell), p. 35. London: Academic Press.

Jones, L. M. & Morgan, W. J. B. (1958). A preliminary report on a selective medium for the culture of Brucella, including fastidious types. *Bull. Wld Hlth Org.* **19**, 200.

Jones, L. M. & Wundt, W. (1971). International Committee on Nomenclature of Bacteria. Subcommittee on the taxonomy of *Brucella*. *Int. J. syst. Bact.* **21**, 126.

Jones, N. R. (1956). A tentative method for the determination of the grade strength of agars. *Analyst*, **81**, 243.

Jordan, E. O. (1890). A report on certain species of bacteria observed in sewage. *Rep. Mass. St. Bd Hlth*, part II, 821.

Jordan, E. O., Crawford, R. R. & McBroom, J. (1935). The Morgan bacillus. *J. Bact.* **29**, 131.

Joseph, S. W., Kaper, J. B. & Colwell, R. R. (1982). *Vibrio parahaemolyticus* and related halophilic vibrios. *CRC crit. Rev. Microbiol.* **10**, 77.

Juni, E. (1984). *Acinetobacter*. In *Bergey's Manual of Systematic Bacteriology*, vol. 1 (ed. N. R. Krieg & J. G. Holt), p. 303. Baltimore: Williams & Wilkins.

Kalina, A. P. (1970) The taxonomy and nomenclature of enterococci. *Int. J. syst. Bact.* **20**, 185.

Kalina, G. P., Antonov, A. S., Turova, T. P. & Grafova, T. I. (1984). *Allomonas enterica* gen. nov. sp. nov.: deoxyribonucleic acid homology between *Allomonas* and some other members of the Vibrionaceae. *Int. J. syst. Bact.* **34**, 150.

Kampelmacher, E. H. (1959). On antigenic O-relationships between the groups Salmonella, Arizona, Escherichia and Shigella. *Antonie van Leeuwenhoek*, **25**, 289.

Kandler, O. & Weiss, N. (1986). Regular, nonsporing Gram-positive rods. In *Bergey's Manual of Systematic Bacteriology*, vol. 2 (ed. P.H.A. Sneath *et al.*). p. 1208. Baltimore: Williams & Wilkins.

Kandler, O. (1970). Amino acid sequence of the murein and taxonomy of the genera *Lactobacillus, Bifidobacterium, Leuconostoc* and *Pediococcus*. *Int. J. syst. Bact.* **20**, 491.

Kandler, O. & Weiss, N. (1986). The genus *Lactobacillus*. In *Bergey's Manual of Systematic Bacteriology*, vol. 2 (ed. P. H. A. Sneath *et al.*), p. 1209. Baltimore: Williams & Wilkins.

Karmali, M. A., Allen, A. K. & Fleming, P. C. (1981). Differentiation of catalase-positive campylobacters with special reference to morphology. *Int. J. syst. Bact.* **31**, 64.

Kauffmann, F. (1953). On the classification and nomenclature of Enterobacteriaceae. *Riv. Ist. sieroter. ital.* **28**, 485.

Kauffmann, F. (1954). *Enterobacteriaceae*, edn 2. Copenhagen: Ejnar Munksgaard.

Kauffmann, F. (1959*a*). On the principles of classification and nomenclature of Enterobacteriaceae. *Int. Bull. bact. Nomencl. Taxon.* **9**, 7.

Kauffmann, F. (1959*b*). Definition of genera and species of Enterobacteriaceae. Request for an Opinion. *Int. Bull. bact. Nomencl. Taxon.* **9**, 7.

Kauffmann, F. (1963*a*). Zur Differentialdiagnose der Salmonella-Sub-genera I, II und III. *Acta path. microbiol. scand.* **58**, 109.

Kauffmann, F. (1963*b*). On the species-definition. *Int. Bull. bact. Nomencl. Taxon.* **13**, 181.

Kauffmann, F. & Edwards, P. R. (1952). Classification and nomenclature of Enterobacteriaceae. *Int. Bull. bact. Nomencl. Taxon.* **2**, 2.

Kauffmann, F., Edwards, P. R. & Ewing, W. H. (1956). The principles of group differentiation within the Enterobacteriaceae by biochemical methods. *Int. Bull. bact. Nomencl. Taxon.* **6**, 29.

Keddie, R. M. (1981). The genus *Kurthia*. In *The Prokaryotes: A handbook on habitats, isolation and identification* (ed. M. P. Starr *et al.*), p. 1888. Berlin: Springer-Verlag.

Keddie, R. M. & Cure, G. L. (1978). Cell wall composition of coryneform bacteria. In *Coryneform Bacteria* (ed. I. J. Bousfield & A. G. Calley), p. 47. London: Academic Press.

Keddie, R. M. & Shaw, S. (1986). The genus *Kurthia*. In *Bergey's Manual of Systematic Bacteriology*, vol. 2 (ed. P. H. A. Sneath *et al.*), p.1255. Baltimore: Williams & Wilkins.

Keleti, J., Lüderitz, O., Mlynarcík, D. & Sedlák, J. (1971). Immunochemical studies on *Citrobacter* O antigens (lipopolysaccharides). *Eur. J. Biochem.* **20**, 237.

Kellerman, K. F. & McBeth, I. G. (1912). The fermentation of cellulose. *Zentbl. Bakt. ParasitKde Abt. II*, **34**, 485.

Kelly, A. T. & Fulton, M. (1953). Use of triphenyl tetrazolium in motility test medium. *Am. J. clin. Path.* **23**, 512.

Kelly, K. F. & Evans, J. B. (1974). Deoxyribonucleic acid homology among strains of the lobster pathogen 'Gaffkya homari' and *Aerococcus viridans*. *J. gen. Microbiol.* **81**, 257.

Kelly, R. W. & Kellogg, S. T. (1978). Computer-assisted identification of anaerobic bacteria. *Appl. environ. Microbiol.* **35**, 507.

Kelsey, J. C. (1958). The testing of sterilizers. *Lancet*, i, 306.

Kelsey, J. C. (1961). The testing of sterilizers. 2. Thermophilic spore papers. *J. clin. Path.* **14**, 313.

Kendal, A. I. & Ryan, M. (1919). A double sugar medium for the cultural diagnosis of intestinal and other bacteria. *J. infect. Dis.* **24**, 400.

Kennedy, P. C., Frazier, L. M., Theilen, G. H. & Biberstein, E. L. (1958). A septicaemic disease of lambs caused by *Haemophilus agni. Am. J. vet. Res.* **19**, 645.

Kersters, K. & DeLey, J. (1984*a*). *Agrobacterium*. In *Bergey's Manual of Systematic Bacteriology*, vol. 1 (ed. N. R. Krieg & J. G. Holt), p. 244. Baltimore: Williams & Wilkins.

Kersters, K. & DeLey, J. (1984*b*). Genus *Alcaligenes*. In *Bergey's Manual of Systematic Bacteriology*, vol. 1 (ed.

N. R. Krieg & J. G. Holt), p. 361. Baltimore: Williams & Wilkins.

Khairat, O. (1940). Endocarditis due to a new species of *Haemophilus. J. Path. Bact.* **50**, 497.

Kharasch, M. S., Conway, E. A. & Bloom, W. (1936). Some chemical factors influencing growth and pigmentation of certain microorganisms. *J. Bact.* **32**, 533.

Kielbauch, K. A., Brenner, D. J., Nicholson, M. A., Baker, C. N., Patton, C. M., Steigerwalt, A. G. & Wachsmuth, I. K. (1991). *Campylobacter butzleri* sp. nov. isolated from humans and animals with diarrhoeal illness. *J. clin. Microbiol.* **29**, 376.

Kilian, M. (1974). A rapid method for the differentiation of *Haemophilus* strains – the porphyrin test. *Acta path. microbiol. scand.* B**82**, 835.

Kilian, M. (1976). A taxonomic study of the genus *Haemophilus*, with the proposal of a new species. *J. gen. Microbiol.* **93**, 9.

Kilian, M. & Biberstein, E. L. (1984). *Haemophilus.* In *Bergey's Manual of Systematic Bacteriology,* vol. 1 (ed. N.R. Krieg & J.G. Holt), p. 558. Baltimore: Williams & Wilkins.

Kilian, M., Mordhorst, C.-H., Dawson, C. R. & Lautrop, H. (1976). The taxonomy of haemophili isolated from conjunctivae. *Acta path. microbiol. scand.* B**84**, 132.

Kilpper-Bälz, R. & Schleifer, K. H. (1984). Nucleic acid hybridization and cell wall composition studies of pyogenic streptococci. *FEMS Microbiol. Lett.* **24**, 355.

Kilpper-Bälz, R., Wenzeg, G. & Schleifer, K. H. (1985). Molecular relationships and classification of some viridans streptococci as *Streptococcus oralis* and emended description of *Streptococcus oralis* (Bridge & Sneath 1982). *Int. J. syst. Bact.* **35**, 482.

Kilpper-Bälz, R., Fischer, P. & Schleifer, K. H. (1982). Nucleic acid hybridization of group N and group D streptococci. *Curr. Microbiol.* **7**, 245.

King, E. O. (1962). The laboratory recognition of *Vibrio fetus* and a closely related *Vibrio* isolated from cases of human vibriosis. *Ann. N. Y. Acad. Sci.* **98**, 700.

King E. O. (1964, 1972). *The Identification of Unusual Pathogenic Gram negative Bacteria.* Revised (1972) by Weaver, R. E., Tatum, H. W. & Hollis, D. G. Atlanta, Georgia: Center for Disease Control, US Dept. of Health, Education, and Welfare, Public Health Service.

King, B. M. & Adler, D. L. (1964). A previously undescribed group of Enterobacteriaceae. *Am. J. clin. Path.* **41**, 230.

King E. O. & Tatum, H. W. (1962). *Actinobacillus actinomycetemcomitans* and *Hemophilus aphrophilus. J. infect. Dis.* **111**, 85.

King, E. O., Ward, M. K. & Raney, D. E. (1954). Two sim-

ple media for the demonstration of pyocyanin and fluorescin. *J. Lab. clin. Med.* **44**, 301.

Kingsbury, D. T. (1967). Deoxyribonucleic acid homologies among species of the genus *Neisseria. J. Bact.* **94**, 870.

Kingsbury, D. T., Fanning, G. R., Johnson, K. E. & Brenner, D. J. (1969). Thermal stability of interspecies Neisseria DNA duplexes. *J. gen. Microbiol.* **55**, 201 .

Kirchheimer, W. F. & Storrs, E. E. (1971). Attempts to establish the Armadillo (*Dasypus novemcinctus* Linn) as a model for the study of leprosy. I Report of lepromatoid leprosy in an experimentally infected armadillo. *Int. J. Leprosy*, **39**, 693.

Kiredjian, M. (1979). Le genre *Agrobacterium* peut-il être pathogène pour l'homme? *Méd. Maladies Infect.* **9**, 233.

Kiredjian, M., Holmes, B., Kersters, K., Guilvont, I. & De Ley, J. (1986). *Alcaligenes piechaudii*, a new species from human clinical specimens and the environment. *Int. J. syst. Bact.* **36**, 282.

Kiredjian, M., Popoff, M., Coynault, C., Lefèvre, M. & Lemelin, M. (1981). Taxonomie due genre *Alcaligenes. Annls Microbiol. Inst. Pasteur, Paris*, **132**B, 337.

Kitahara, K. & Suzuki, J. (1963). *Sporolactobacillus* nov. subgen. *J. gen. appl. Microbiol.* **9**, 59.

Kligler, I. J. (1917). A simple medium for the differentiation of members of the typhoid-paratyphoid group. *Am. J. publ. Hlth*, **7**, 1042.

Kligler, I. J. (1918). Modifications of culture media used in the isolation and differentiation of typhoid, dysentery, and allied bacilli. *J. exp. Med.* **28**, 319.

Kligler, I. J. & Defandorf, J. (1918). The Endo medium for the isolation of *B. dysenteriae* and a double sugar medium for the differentiation of *B. dysenteriae,* Shiga and Flexner. *J. Bact.* **3**, 437.

Kloos, W. E. & Schleifer, K. H. (1975*a*). Isolation and characterization of staphylococci from human skin. II. Descriptions of four new species: *Staphylococcus warneri, Staphylococcus capitis, Staphylococcus hominis* and *Staphylococcus simulans. Int. J. syst. Bact.* **25**, 62.

Kloos, W. E. & Schleifer, K. H. (1975*b*). Simplified scheme for routine identification of human *Staphylococcus* species. *J. clin. Microbiol.* **1**, 82.

Kloos, W. E., Schleifer, K. H. & Smith, R. F. (1976). Characterization of *Staphylococcus sciuri* sp. nov. and its subspecies. *Int. J. syst. Bact.* **26**, 22.

Kloos, W. E., Tornabene, T.G. & Schleifer, K. H. (1974). Isolation and characterization of micrococci from human skin, including two new species: *Micrococcus lylae* and *Micrococcus kristinae. Int. J. syst. Bact.* **24**, 79.

Knox, R. (1949). A screening plate for the rapid identification of faecal organisms. *J. Path. Bact.* **61**, 343.

Kobayashi, T., Enomoto, S., Sakazaki, R. & Kuwahara, S. (1963). A new selective medium for pathogenic vibrios, TCBS agar (modified Nakanishi's agar). *Jap. J. Microbiol.* **18**, 387. (In Japanese with an English summary.)

Kocur, M. & Martinec, T. (1962). A contribution to the taxonomy of the genus *Staphylococcus. Publs Fac. Sci. Univ. J. E. Purkyne, Brno,* **28**, 492.

Kocur, M., Bergan, T. & Mortensen, N. (1971). DNA base composition of Gram-positive cocci. *J. gen. Microbiol.* **69**, 167.

Kodaka, H., Armfield, A.Y., Lombard, G. L. & Dowell, V.R. (1982). Practical procedure for demonstrating bacterial flagella. *J. clin. Microbiol.* **16**, 948.

Kodama, K., Kimura, N. & Komagata, K. (1985). Two new species of *Pseudomonas: P. oryzihabitans* isolated from rice paddy and clinical specimens and *P. luteola* isolated from clinical specimens. *Int. J. syst. Bact.* **35**, 467.

Kohler, G. & Milstein, C. (1975). Continuous cultures of fixed cells secreting antibody of predefined specificity. *Nature (London),* **256**, 495.

Kohn, J. (1953). A preliminary report of a new gelatin liquefaction method. *J. clin. Path.* **6**, 249.

Kohn, J. (1954). A two-tube technique for the identification of organisms of the Enterobacteriaceae group. *J. Path. Bact.* **67**, 286.

Koontz, F. B. & Faber, J. E. (1963). A taxonomic study of some Gram-negative, non-fermenting bacteria. *Can. J. Microbiol.* **9**, 499.

Kopper, P. H. (1962). Effect of sodium chloride concentration on the swarming tendency of *Proteus. J. Bact.* **84**, 1119.

Kosako, K., Sakazaki, R. & Yoshizaki, E. (1984). *Yokenella regensburgei* gen. nov., sp. nov.: a new genus and species in the family *Enterobacteriaceae. Jap. J. med. Sci. Biol.* **37**, 117.

Koser, S. A. (1923). Utilization of the salts of organic acids by the colon-aerogenes group. *J. Bact.* **8**, 493.

Kovács, N. (1928). Eine vereinfachte Methode zum Nachweis der Indolbildung durch Bakterien. *Z. ImmunForsch. exp. Ther.* **55**, 311.

Kovács, N. (1956). Identification of *Pseudomonas pyocyanea* by the oxidase reaction. *Nature (London)* **178**, 703.

Kramer, J. M., Turnbull, P.C.B., Munshi, G. & Gilbert, R. J. (1982). Identification and characterization of *Bacillus cereus* and other *Bacillus* species associated with foods and food poisoning. In *Isolation and Identification Methods for Food Poisoning Organisms* (ed. J. E. L. Corry, D. Roberts & F. A. Skinner), p. 261. Society for Applied Bacteriology Tech, series No. 17. London: Academic Press.

Kramer, P. A. & Jones, D. (1969). Media selective for *Listeria monocytogenes. J. appl. Bacteriol.* **32**, 381.

Kriebel, R. M. (1934). A comparative bacteriological study of a group of non-lactose-fermenting bacteria isolated from stools of healthy food-handlers. *J. Bact.* **27**, 357.

Krych, V. K., Johnson, J. L. & Yousten, A. A. (1980). Deoxyribonucleic acid homologies among strains of *Bacillus sphaericus. Int. J. syst. Bact.* **30**, 476.

Kubica, G. P. (1973). Differential identification of mycobacteria. VII. Key features for identification of clinically significant mycobacteria. *Am. Rev. resp. Dis.* **107**, 9.

Kubica, G. P. (1978). The current nomenclature of the mycobacteria. *Bull. int. Un. against Tuberc.* **53**, 192.

Kubica, G. P. & Dye, W. E. (1967). Laboratory methods for clinical and public health mycobacteriology. *Publ. Hlth Ser. Publ.* no. 1547. Washington, DC: US Government Printing Office.

Kulp, W. L. & White, V. (1932). A modified medium for planting *L. acidophilus. Science, N.Y.* **76**, 17.

Kucsera, G. (1973). Proposal for the standardization of the designations used for serotypes of *Erysipelothrix rhusiopathiae* (Migula) Buchanan. *Int. J. syst. Bact.* **23**, 184.

Küster, E. (1972). Simple working key for the classification and identification of named taxa included in the International *Streptomyces* Project. *Int. J. syst. Bact.* **22**, 139.

Lacey, B. W. (1951). Selective media for *Haemophilus pertussis* and *parapertussis. J. gen. Microbiol.* **5**, vi.

Lacey, B. W. (1954). A new selective medium for *Haemophilus pertussis,* containing a diamidine, sodium fluoride and penicillin. *J. Hyg., Camb.* **52**, 18.

Lakso, J. U. & Starr, M. P. (1970). Comparative injuriousness to plants of *Erwinia* spp. and other enterobacteria from plants and animals. *J. appl. Bact.* **33**, 692.

Lambert, M. A., Hollis, D. G., Moss, C. W., Weaver, R. E. & Thomas, M. L. (1971). Cellular fatty acids of non-pathogenic *Neisseria. Can. J. Microbiol.* **17**, 1491.

Lancefield, R. C. (1933). A serological differentiation of human and other groups of hemolytic streptococci. *J. exp. Med.* **57**, 571.

Lancefield, R. C. (1940). The significance of M and T antigens in the cross reactions between certain types of group A hemolytic streptococci. *J. exp. Med.* **71**, 539.

Langenberg, M. L., Tygat, G. N. J., Schipper, M. E. I., Rietra, P. J. G. M. & Zanen, H.C. (1984). *Campylobacter*-like organisms in the stomach of patients and healthy individuals. *Lancet,* i, 1348.

Langham, C. D., Sneath, P. H. A., Williams, S. T. & Mortimer, A. M. (1989). Detecting aberrant strains in bacterial groups as an aid to constructing databases for computer identification. *J. appl. Bact.* **66**, 339.

Lányi, B. & Adám, M. M. (1960). Agar diffusion test and micromethods for the rapid biochemical differentiation of enteric bacteria. *Acta microbiol. Acad. Sci. Hung.* **7**, 313.

Lányi, B. & Bergan, T. (1978). Serological characterization of *Pseudomonas aeruginosa*. In *Methods in Microbiology* vol. 10, (ed. T. Bergan & J. R. Norris), p. 93. London: Academic Press.

Lapage, S. P. (1961). *Haemophilus vaginalis* and its role in vaginitis. *Acta path. microbiol. scand.* **52**, 34.

Lapage, S. P. & Bascomb, S. (1968). Use of selenite reduction in bacterial classification. *J. appl. Bact.* **31**, 568.

Lapage, S. P. & Zinnemann, K. (1971). International Committee on Nomenclature of Bacteria. Subcommittee on the Taxonomy of *Haemophilus*. Minutes of meeting, 11 August, 1970. *Int. J. syst. Bact.* **21**,132.

Lapage, S. P., Bascomb, S., Willcox, W. R. & Curtis, M. A. (1973). Identification of bacteria by computer. General aspects and perspectives. *J. gen. Microbiol.* **77**, 273.

Lapage, S. P., Efstratiou, A. & Hill, L. R. (1973). The ortho-nitrophenol (ONPG) test and acid from lactose in Gram-negative genera. *J. clin. Path.* **26**, 821.

Lapage, S. P., Hill, L. R. & Reeve, J. D. (1968). *Pseudomonas stutzeri* in pathological material. *J. med. Microbiol.* **1**, 195.

Lapage, S. P., Shelton, J. E. & Mitchell, T. G. (1970). Media for the maintenence and preservation of bacteria. In *Methods in Microbiology*, vol. 3A, (ed. J. R. Norris & D. W. Ribbons), p. 1. London: Academic Press.

Lapage, S. P., Clark, W. A., Lessel, E. F., Seeliger, H. P. R. & Sneath, P. H. A. (1973). Proposed revision of the International Code of Nomenclature of Bacteria. *Int. J. syst. Bact.* **23**, 83.

Lapage, S. P., Sneath P. H. A., Lessel, E. F., Skerman, V. B. D., Seeliger, H. P. R. & Clark, W. A. (1975). *International code of nomenclature of bacteria*. Edn. 3. Iowa: State University Press, Ames.

Larkin, J. M. & Stokes, J. L. (1967). Taxonomy of psychrophilic strains of *Bacillus*. *J. Bact.* **94**, 889.

Larson, C. L., Wicht, W. & Jellison, W. L. (1955). An organism resembling *Pasteurella tularensis* from water. *Publ. Hlth. Reports, Washington* **70**, 253.

Lautrop, H. (1956a). A modified Kohn's test for the demonstration of bacterial gelatin liquefaction. *Acta path. microbiol. scand.* **39**, 357.

Lautrop, H. (1956b). Gelatin-liquefying *Klebsiella* strains (*Bacterium oxytocum* (Flügge)). *Acta path. microbiol. scand.* **39**, 375.

Lautrop, H. (1960). Laboratory diagnosis of whooping cough or *Bordetella* infections. *Bull. Wld Hlth Org.* **23**, 15.

Lautrop, H. (1961). *Bacterium anitratum* transferred to the genus *Cytophaga*. *Int. Bull. bact. Nomencl. Taxon.* **11**, 107.

Lautrop, H. (1965). Gliding motility in bacteria as a taxonomic criterion. *Publs Fac. Sci. Univ. J. E. Purkyne, Brno*, **K35**, 322.

Lautrop, H. (1967). *Agrobacterium* spp. isolated from clinical specimens. *Acta path. microbiol. scand.* Suppl. **187**.

Lautrop, H. (1974). *Proteus*. In *Bergey's Manual of Determinative Bacteriology*. Edn. 8. (ed. R. E. Buchan & N. E. Gibbons). p. 327. Baltimore: Williams & Wilkins.

Lautrop, H., Bøvre, K. & Frederiksen, W. (1970). A *Moraxella*-like microorganism isolated from the genitourinary tract of man. *Acta path. microbiol. scand.* **78 B**, 255.

Laybourn, R. L. (1924). A modification of Albert's stain for the diphtheria bacilli. *J. Am. med. Ass.* **83**, 121.

Leclerc, H. (1962). Étude biochimique d'Enterobacteriaceae pigmentées. *Annls Inst. Pasteur, Paris* **102**, 726.

Leclerc, H. & Beerens, H. (1962). Une technique simple de mise en évidence de l'oxydase chez les bactéries. *Annls Inst. Pasteur, Lille*, **13**, 187.

Lederberg, J. (1950). The beta-D-galactosidase of *Escherichia coli*, strain K-12. *J. Bact.* **60**, 381.

Lee, J. V. & Donovan, T. J. (1985). *Vibrio, Aeromonas* and *Plesiomonas*. In *Isolation and Identification of Microorganisms of Medical and Veterinary Importance* (ed. C. H. Collins & J. M. Grange), p.13. Society for Applied Microbiology Tech. series No. 21. London: Academic Press.

Lee, J. V., Gibson, D. M. & Shewan, J. M. (1977). A numerical taxonomic study of some Pseudomonas-like marine bacteria. *J. gen. Microbiol.* **98**, 439.

Lee, J. V., Shread, P., Furniss, A. L. & Bryant, T. (1981). Taxonomy and description of *Vibrio fluvialis* sp. nov. (synonym group F vibrios, group EF6). *J. appl. Bact.* **50**, 73.

Lee, P. C. & Wetherall, B. L. (1987). Cross-reaction between *Streptococcus pneumoniae* and group C streptococcal latex reagent. *J. clin. Microbiol.* **25**, 152.

Leffmann, H. & La Wall, C. H. (1911). Sulphur dioxide in commercial gelatins. *Analyst*, **36**, 271.

Legroux, R. & Genevray, J. (1933). Étude comparative entre le bacille de Whitmore et le bacille pyocyanique. *Annls Inst. Pasteur, Paris*, **51**, 249.

Leidy, G., Hahn, E. & Alexander, H. E. (1959). Interspecific transformation in Haemophilus: a possible index of relationship between *H. influenzae* and *H. aegyptius* (25151). *Proc. Soc. exp. Biol. Med.* **102**, 86.

Leidy, G., Jaffee, I. & Alexander, H. E. (1965). Further evidence of a high degree of genetic homology between *H.*

influenzae and *H. aegyptius. Proc. Soc. exp. Biol. Med.* **118**, 671.

Leifson, E. (1933). The fermentation of sodium malonate as a means of differentiating *Aerobacter* and *Escherichia. J. Bact.* **26**, 329.

Leifson, E. (1935). New culture media based on sodium desoxycholate for the isolation of intestinal pathogens and for the enumeration of colon bacilli in milk and water. *J. Path. Bact.* **40**, 581.

Leifson, E. (1956). Morphological and physiological characteristics of the genus *Chromobacterium. J. Bact.* **71**, 393.

Leifson, E. (1963). Determination of carbohydrate metabolism of marine bacteria. *J. Bact.* **85**, 1183.

Leise, J. M., Carter, C. H., Friedlander, H. & Freed, S. W. (1959). Criteria for the identification of *Bacillus anthracis. J. Bact.* **77**, 655.

LeMinor, L. & Ben Hamida, F. (1962). Avantages de la recherche de la β-galactosidase sur celle de la fermentation du lactose en milieu complexe dans le diagnostic bactériologique, en particulier des Enterobacteriaceae. *Annls Inst. Pasteur, Paris,* **102**, 267.

LeMinor, L. & Piéchaud, M. (1963). Note technique. Une méthode rapide de recherche de la protéolyse de la gélatine. *Annls Inst. Pasteur, Paris,* **105**, 792.

LeMinor, S. & Pigache, F. (1978). Antigenic study of *Serratia marcescens* isolated in France. *Annls. Microbiol. Inst. Pasteur, Paris,* **129**B, 407.

LeMinor, L. & Popoff, M.Y. (1987). Request for an opinion: designation of *Salmonella enterica* sp. nov., nom. rev., as the type and only species of the genus *Salmonella. Int. J. syst. Bact.* **37**, 465.

LeMinor, L., Rhode, R. & Taylor, J. (1970). Nomenclature des *Salmonella. Annls Inst. Pasteur, Paris,* **119**, 206.

LeMinor, L., Popoff, M.Y., Laurent, B. & Hermant, D. (1986). Individualisation d'une septième sous-epèee de *Salmonella: S. choleraesuis* subsp. *indica* subsp. nov. *Annls Inst. Pasteur, Paris,* **137B**, 211.

LeMinor, L., Véron, M. & Popoff, M. (1982). Proposition pour une nomenclature des *Salmonella. Annls Microbiol. Inst. Pasteur, Paris* **133** B, 245.

Leopold, S. (1953). Heretofore undescribed organism isolated from the genito-urinary system. *J.S. Armed Forces Med.* **4**, 263.

Lepper, E. & Martin, C. J. (1929). The chemical mechanisms exploited in the use of meat media for the cultivation of anaerobes. *Br. J. exp. Path.* **10**, 327.

Levett, P. N. (1988). *Clostridium difficile* antibiotic-associated diarrhoea and colitis. In *Anaerobic Infections: Clinical and Laboratory Practice* (ed. A. T. Willis & K. D. Phillips) p. 60. London: Public Health Laboratory Service.

Levin, M. (1943). Two agar-less media for the rapid isolation of *Corynebacterium* and *Neisseria. J. Bact.* **46**, 233.

Levine, M. (1918). A statistical classification of the colon-cloacae group. *J. Bact.* **3**, 253.

Levine, M., Epstein, S. S. & Vaughn, R. H. (1934). Differential reactions in the colon group of bacteria. *Am. J. publ. Hlth,* **24**, 505.

Levinthal, W. (1918). Bakteriologische und serologische Influenzastudien. *Z. Hyg. InfektKrankh.* **86**, 1.

Lewis, B. (1961). Phosphatase production by staphylococci – a comparison of two methods. *J. med. Lab. Technol.* **18**, 112.

Lewis, P. A. & Shope, R. E. (1931). Swine influenza. II. A hemophilic bacillus from the respiratory tract of infected swine. *J. exp. Med.* **54**, 361.

Lillie, R. D. (1928). The Gram stain. I. A quick method for staining Gram-positive organisms in the tissues. *Arch. Path.* **5**, 828.

Lindqvist, K. (1960). A *Neisseria* species associated with infectious kerato-conjunctivitis of sheep, *Neisseria ovis* nov. spec. *J. infect. Dis.* **106**, 162.

Lingappa, Y. & Lockwood, J. L. (1961). A chitin medium for isolation, growth and maintenance of actinomycetes. *Nature, Lond*on **189**, 158.

Linton, C. S. (1925). A note on the Voges-Proskaüer reaction. *J. Am. Wat. Wks Ass.* **13**, 547.

Lior, H. (1984). New, extended biotyping scheme for *Campylobacter jejuni, Campylobacter coli,* and '*Campylobacter laridis'. J. clin. Microbiol.* **20**, 636.

Lior, H. & Patel, A. (1987). Improved toluidine blue-DNA agar for detection of DNA hydrolysis by campylobacters. *J. clin. Microbiol.* **25**, 2030.

Liu, P. V., Matsumoto, H., Kusama, H. & Bergan, T. (1983). Survey of heat-stable, major somatic antigens of *Pseudomonas aeruginosa. Int. J. syst. Bact.* **33**, 256.

Lockhart, W. R. (1967). Factors affecting reproducibility of numerical classifications. *J. Bact.* **94**, 826.

Lockhart, W. R. & Hartman, P. A. (1963). Formation of monothetic groups in quantitative bacterial taxonomy. *J. Bact.* **85**, 68.

Lockwood, D. E., Kreger, A. S. & Richardson, S. H. (1982). Detection of toxins produced by *Vibrio fluvialis. Inf. Immun.* **35**, 702.

Loeb, L. (1903). The influence of certain bacteria on the coagulation of the blood. *J. med. Res.* **10**, 407.

Loeb, M. R. & Smith, D. H. (1980). Outer membrane protein composition in disease isolates of *Haemophilus influenzae*: pathogenic and epidemiological implications. *Inf. Immun.* **30**, 709.

Loesche, W. J., Gibbons, R. J. & Socransky, S. S. (1965). Biochemical characteristics of *Vibrio sputorum* and relationship to *Vibrio bubulus* and *Vibrio fetus*. *J. Bact.* **89**, 1109.

Loeffler, F. (1884). Untersuchungen über Bedeutung der Mikroorganismen für die Entstehung der Diphtherie beim Menschen, bei der Taube und beim Kalbe. *Mitt. Gesundheitsamte* **2**, 421.

Logan, N. A. (1988). *Bacillus* species of medical and veterinary importance. *J. med. Microbiol.* **25**, 157.

Logan, N. A. & Berkeley, R. C. W. (1981). *Bacillus* Taxonomy based on API tests. In *The Aerobic Endospore-forming Bacteria* (ed. R. C. W. Berkeley & M. Goodfellow), p. 104. London: Academic Press.

Logan, N. A. & Berkeley, R. C. W. (1984). Identification of *Bacillus* strains using the API system. *J. gen. Microbiol.* **130**, 1871.

Logan, N. A., Carman, J. A., Melling, J. & Berkeley, R. C. W. (1985). Identification of *Bacillus anthracis* by API tests. *J. med. Microbiol.* **20**, 75.

Lorenz, R. P., Applebaum, P. C., Ward, R. M. & Botti, J. J. (1982). Chorioamnionitis and possible neonatal infection associated with *Lactobacillus* species. *J. clin. Microbiol.* **16**, 558.

Love, M., Teebken-Fisher, D., Hose, J.E., Farmer, J. J. III, Hickman, F. W. & Fanning, G. R. (1981). *Vibrio damsela*, a marine bacterium, causes skin lesions on the damsel fish *Chromis punctipinnis*. *Science* **214**, 1139.

Love, R. M. (1953). A qualitative test for monosaccharides. *Analyst* **78**, 732.

Lowe, G. H. (1962). The rapid detection of lactose fermentation in paracolon organisms by the demonstration of β-D-galactosidase *J. med. Lab. Technol.* **19**, 21.

Lowe, G. H. & Evans, J. H. (1957). A simple medium for the rapid detection of salmonella-like paracolon organisms. *J. clin. Path.* **10**, 318.

Lowenstein, E. (1931). Die Züchtung der Tuberkelbazillen aus dem strömenden Blute. *Zbl. Bakt. ParasitKde Abt. I*, **120**, 127.

Lund, E. (1959). Diagnosis of pneumococci by the optochin and bile tests. *Acta path. microbiol. scand.* **47**, 308.

Lund, M. S. & Blazevic, D. J. (1977). Rapid speciation of *Haemophilus* with the Porphyrin Production Test versus the Satellite Test for X. *J. clin. Microbiol.* **5**, 142.

Lutz, A., Grooten, O. & Wurch, T. (1956). Étude des caracteres culturaux et biochimiques de bacilles de type 'Haemophilus haemolyticus vaginalis': leur sensibilite aux antibiotiques. *Rev. Immunol.* **20**, 132.

Lwoff, A. (1939). Revision et démembrement des Hemophilae, le genre *Moraxella nov. gen. Annls Inst. Pasteur, Paris* **62**, 168.

Lwoff, A. (1958). L'espèce bactérienne. *Annls Inst. Pasteur Paris* **94**, 137.

McAllister, H. A. & Carter, G.R. (1974). An aerogenic *Pasteurella*-like organism recovered from swine. *Am. J. vet. Res.* **35**, 917.

McClung, L. S. & Toabe, R. (1947). Egg-yolk plate reactions for presumptive diagnosis of *Clostridium sporogenes* and certain species of gangrene and botulinum groups. *J. Bact.* **53**, 139.

MacConkey, A. T. (1908). Bile salt media and their advantages in some bacteriological examinations. *J. Hyg., Camb.* **8**, 322.

McCoy, G. W., & Chapin, C. W. (1912). Further observations on a plague-like disease of rodents with a preliminary note on the causative agent *Bacterium tularense*. *J. infec. Dis.* **10**, 61.

MacDonell, M. T. & Colwell, R. R. (1985*a*). The contribution of numerical taxonomy to the systematics of Gram-negative bacteria. In *Computer-Assisted Bacterial Systematics* (ed. M. Goodfellow, D. Jones & F. G. Priest), p. 107. London: Academic Press.

MacDonell, M. T. & Colwell, R. R. (1985*b*). Phylogeny of the *Vibrionaceae*, and recommendation for two new genera, *Listonella* and *Shewanella*. *Syst. appl. Microbiol.* **6**, 171.

Macfarlane, R. G., Oakley, C. L. & Anderson, C. G.(1941). Haemolysis and the production of opalescence in serum and lecitho-vitellin by the α toxin of *Clostridium welchii*. *J. Path. Bact.* **52**, 99.

McIntosh, J. (1920). A litmus solution suitable for bacteriological purposes. *Br. J. exp. Path.* **1**, 70.

McGaughey, C. A. & Chu, H. P. (1948). The egg-yolk reaction of aerobic sporing bacilli. *J. gen. Microbiol.* **2**, 334.

Mackey, J. P. & Sandys, G. H. (1966). Diagnosis of urinary infection. *Br. med. J. i*, 1173.

McLauchlin, J. (1987). *Listeria monocytogenes*, recent advances in the taxonomy and epidemiology of listeriosis in humans. *J. appl. Bact.* **63**, 1.

McLauchlin, J., Black, A., Green, H. T., Nash, J. Q., & Taylor, A. G. (1988). Monoclonal anibodies showing *Listeria monocytogenes* in necropsy tissue samples. *J. clin. Path.* **41**, 983.

McLeod, J. W. (1947). Smear and culture diagnosis in gonorrhoea. *Br. J. vener. Dis.* **23**, 53.

McLeod, J. W., Coates, J. C., Happold, F. C., Priestley, D. P. & Wheatley, B. (1934). Cultivation of the gonococcus as a method in the diagnosis of gonorrhoea with special reference to the oxydase reaction and to the value of air reinforced in its carbon dioxide content. *J. Path. Bact.* **39**, 221.

McNeil, M. M., Martone, W. J. & Dowell, V. R. (1987). Bacteremia with *Anaerobiospirillum succiniciproducens*. *Rev. inf. Dis.* **9**, 737.

Mahl, M. C., Wilson, P. W., Fife, M. A. & Ewing, W. H. (1965). Nitrogen fixation by members of the tribe Klebsielleae. *J. Bact.* **89**, 1482.

Mair, N. S., Fox, E & Thal, E. (1979). Biochemical pathogenicity and toxicity studies of Type III strains of *Yersinia pseudotuberculosis* isolated from the caecal contents of pigs. In *Contributions to Microbiology and Immunology*, vol. 5 (*Yersinia enterocolitica: Biology, Epidemiology and Pathology*), (ed. P. B. Carter, L. Lafleur & S. Toma) p. 359. Basel: Karger.

Mair, W. (1917). The preparation of desoxycholic acid. *Biochem. J.* **11**, 11.

Málek, I., Radochová, M. & Lysenko, 0. (1963). Taxonomy of the species *Pseudomonas odorans. J. gen. Microbiol.* **33**, 349.

Malnick, H., Thomas, M., Lotay, H. & Robbins, M. (1983). *Anaerobiospirillum* species isolated from humans with diarrhoea. *J. clin. Path.* **36**, 1097.

Malone, B. A., Schreiber, M., Schneider, N. H. & Holdeman, L. V. (1975). Obligately anaerobic strains of *Corynebacterium vaginale* (*Haemophilus vaginalis*). *J. clin. Microbiol.* **2**, 272.

Man, J. C. de, Rogosa, M. & Sharpe, M. E. (1960). A medium for the cultivation of lactobacilli. *J. appl. Bact.* **23**, 130.

Manclark, C. R. & Pickett, M. J. (1961). Diagnostic bacteriological screening procedures. *Lab. Wld*, **12**, 446.

Marchette, N. J. & Nicholes, P. S. (1961). Virulence and citrulline ureidase activity of *Pasteurella tularensis. J. Bact.* **82**, 26.

Marcus, S. & Greaves, C. (1950). Danger of false results using screw-capped tubes in diagnostic bacteriology. *J. Lab. clin. Med.* **36**, 134.

Mardy, C. & Holmes, B. (1988). Incidence of vaginal *Weeksella virosa* (formerly group IIf). *J. clin. Path*, **41**, 211.

Marks, J. (1976). A system for the examination of tubercle bacilli and other mycobacteria. *Tubercle* **57**, 207.

Marks, J. & Trollope, D. R. (1960). A study of the 'anonymous' mycobacteria. I. Introduction; colonial characteristics and morphology; growth rates; biochemical tests. *Tubercle, London*, **41**, 51.

Marmur, J., Falkow, S. & Mandel, M. (1963). New approaches to bacterial taxonomy. *Ann. Rev. Microbiol.* **17**, 329.

Marples, R. R. (1969). Violagabriellae variant of *Staphylococcus epidermidis* on normal human skin. *J. Bact.* **100**, 47.

Marples, R. R. & Richardson, J. F. (1980). *Micrococcus* in the blood. *J. med. Microbiol.* **13**, 355.

Marples, R. R. & Richardson, J. F. (1981). Characters of coagulase-negative staphylococci collected for a collaborative phage-typing study. *Zbl. Bakt. Suppl.* **10**, 175.

Marples, R. R. & Richardson, J. F. (1982). Evaluation of a micromethod gallery (API staph) for the identification of staphylococci and micrococci. *J. clin. Path.* **35**, 650.

Marshall, J. H. & Kelsey, J. C. (1960). A standard culture medium for general bacteriology. *J. Hyg., Camb.* **58**, 367.

Marshall, V. M., Cole, W. M. & Phillips, B. A. (1985). Fermentation of milk by *Streptococcus salivarius* and *Streptococcus thermophilus* subspecies *thermophilus* and their use by the yoghurt manufacturer. *J. appl. Bact.* **59**, 147.

Marshall, B. J., Royce, H., Annear, D. I., Goodwin, C. S., Pearman, J. W., Warren, J. R. & Armstrong J. A. (1984). Original isolation of *Campylobacter pyloridis* from human gastric mucosa. *Microbios Lett.* **25**, 83.

Martin, W. J., Mock, W. E. & Ewing, W. H. (1968). Antigenic analysis of *Shigella sonnei* by gel diffusion technics. *Can. J. Microbiol.* **14**, 737.

Maskell, R. M. (1974). Importance of coagulase-negative staphylococci as pathogens in the urinary tract. *Lancet*, i, 1155.

Maslen, L. G. C. (1952). Routine use of liquid urea medium for identifying *Salmonella* and *Shigella* organisms. *Brit. med. J.* **ii**, 545.

Matsen, J. M. (1970). Ten-minute test for differentiating between *Klebsiella* and *Enterobacter* isolates. *Appl. Microbiol.* **19**, 438.

Matsen, J. M., Blazevic, D. J., Ryan, J. A. & Ewing, W. H. (1972). Characterization of indole-positive *Proteus mirabilis. Appl. Microbiol.* **23**, 592.

Matthews, P. R. J. & Pattison, J. H. (1961). The identification of a Haemophilus-like organism associated with pneumonia and pleurisy in the pig. *J. comp. Path. Ther.* **71**, 44.

Maximescu, P., Oprison, A., Pop, A. & Potorac, E. (1974). Further studies on *Corynebacterium* species capable of producing diphtheria toxin (*C. diphtheriae, C. ulcerans, C. ovis*). *J. gen. Microbiol.* **82**, 49.

Maxted, W. R. (1948). Preparation of streptococcal extracts for Lancefield grouping. *Lancet*, ii, 255.

Maxted, W. R. (1953). The use of bacitracin for identifying group A haemolytic streptococci. *J. clin. Path.* **6**, 224.

Mayr, E. (1968). The role of systematics in biology. *Science, N. Y.* **159**, 595.

Mazloum, H. A., Kilian, M., Mohamed, Z. M. & Said, M. D. (1982). Differentiation of *Haemophilus aegyptius* and *Haemophilus influenzae. Acta path. microbiol. immunol. scand.* B**90**, 109.

Mekalinos, J. J. (1985). Cholera toxin: genetic analysis, regulation, and role in pathogenesis. *Curr. Top. Microbiol. Immunol.* **118**, 97.

297

Merkel, J. R., Traganza, E. D., Mukherjee, B. B., Griffin, T. B. & Prescott, J. M. (1964). Proteolytic activity and general characteristics of a marine bacterium, *Aeromonas proteolytica* sp. n. *J. Bact.* **87**, 1227 .

Merlino, C. P. (1924). Bartolomeo Bizio's letter to the most eminent priest, Angelo Bellani, concerning the phenomenon of the red-colored polenta. *J. Bact.* **9**, 527.

Messer, A. I. (1947). Formalin in filter paper. *Mon. Bull. Minist. Hlth. Lab. Serv.* **6**, 94.

Meyer, M. E. & Cameron, H. S. (1961a). Metabolic characterization of the genus *Brucella*. I. Statistical evaluation of the oxidative rates by which type I of each species can be identified. *J. Bact.* **82**, 387.

Meyer, M. E. & Cameron, H. S. (1961b). Metabolic characterization of the genus *Brucella*. II. Oxidative metabolic patterns of the described species. *J. Bact.* **82**, 396.

Meyer, W. (1966). Some possibilities of subdividing the species *Staphylococcus aureus* into subspecies. *Posteky Microbiologii, v*, 435.

Meyer, W. (1967a). *Staphylococcus aureus* strains of phage-group IV. *J. Hyg., Camb.* **65**, 439.

Meyer, W. (1967b). A proposal for subdividing the species *Staphylococcus aureus*. *Int. J. syst. Bact.* **17**, 387.

Meynell, G. G. & Meynell, E. (1965). *Theory and Practice in Experimental Bacteriology,* **1** edn, 1965; **2** edn, 1970. London: Cambridge University Press.

Middleton, G. & Stuckey, R. E. (1951). The standardisation of the digestion process in the Kjeldahl determination of nitrogen. *J. Pharm. Pharmac.* **3**, 829.

Michalcu, F., Vereanu, A., Andronescu, C. & Dumitriu, S. (1982). Group C streptococci, epidemiologic markers and implications in human pathology. *Archs roum. Path. exp. Microbiol.* **41**, 123.

Midgley, J. (1966). The sensitivity to basic dyes of *Pasteurella* and some other Gram-negative genera. *Publs Fac. Sci. Univ. J. E. Purkyne, Brno*, **K 38**, 282.

Miles, A. A. (1965). Introductory essay on microbiological media: Good Food Guide. *Lab. Pract.* **14**, 688.

Miles, A. A. & Misra, S. S. (1938). The estimation of the bactericidal power of the blood. *J. Hyg., Camb.* **38**, 732.

Miller, C. J., Feachem, R. G. & Drasar, B. S. (1985). Cholera epidemiology in developed and developing countries: new thoughts on transmission, seasonality, and control. *Lancet*, i, 261.

Mills, C. K. & Gherna, R. L. (1987). Hydrolysis of indoxyl acetate by *Campylobacter* species. *J. clin. Microbiol.* **25**, 156.

Minnikin, D. E. & O'Donnell, A. G. (1983). Actinomycete envelope lipid and peptidoglycan composition. In *The Biology of the Actinomycetes* (ed. M. Goodfellow, H. Mordarski & S. T. Williams), p. 337. London: Academic Press.

Mitchell, M. S., Rhoden, D. L. & King, E. 0. (1965). Lactose-fermenting organisms resembling *Neisseria meningitidis. J. Bact.* **90**, 560.

Mitchell, R. G. & Clarke, S. K. R. (1965). An Alcaligenes species with distinctive properties isolated from human sources. *J. gen. Microbiol.* **40**, 343.

Miyamoto, Y., Katyo, T., Obara, Y., Akiyama, S., Takizawa, K. & Yamai, S. (1969). In vitro hemolytic characteristic of *Vibrio parahaemolyticus*: Its close correlation with human pathogenicity. *J. Bact.* **100**, 1147.

Moeller, H. (1891). Ueber eine neue Methode der Sporenfärbung. *Zentbl. Bakt. ParasitKde Abt. I*, **10**, 273.

Mollaret, H. H. & Chevalier, A. (1964). Contribution à l'étude d'un nouveau groupe de germes proches du bacille du Malassez et Vignal. I. Caractères culturaux et biochimiques. *Annls Inst. Pasteur, Paris* **107**, 121.

Mollaret, H. H. & Lucas, A. (1965). Sur les particularités biochimiques des souches de *Yersinia enterocolitica* isolées chez les lièvres. *Annls Inst. Pasteur, Paris*, **108**, 121.

Møller, V. (1954a). Activity determination of amino acid decarboxylases in Enterobacteriaceae. *Acta path. microbiol. scand.* **34**, 102.

Møller, V. (1954b). Diagnostic use of the Braun KCN test within the Enterobacteriaceae. *Acta path. microbiol. scand.* **34**, 115.

Møller, V. (1954c) Distribution of amino acid decarboxylases in Enterobacteriaceae. *Acta path. microbiol. scand.* **35**, 259.

Møller, V. (1955). Simplified tests for some amino acid decarboxylases and for the arginine dihydrolase system. *Acta path. microbiol. scand.* **36**, 158.

Moore, H. F. (1915). The action of ethylhydrocuprein (optochin) on type strains of pneumococci in vitro and in vivo, and on some other microorganisms in vitro. *J. exp. Med.* **22**, 269.

Moore, W. E. C. (1966). Techniques for routine culture of fastidious anaerobes. *Int. J. syst. Bact.* **16**, 173.

Moore, W. E. C., Cato, E. P. & Moore, L. V. H. (1985). Index of the bacterial and yeast nomenclatural changes published in the *International Journal of Systematic Bacteriology* since the 1980 Approved Lists of Bacterial Names (1 January 1980 to January 1985). *Int. J. syst. Bact.* **35**, 382.

Morgan, H. de R. (1906). Upon the bacteriology of the summer diarrhoea of infants. *Br. med. J.* i, 908.

Morgan, W. J. B. & Gower, S. G. M. (1966). Techniques in the identification and classification of *Brucella*. In *Identification Methods for Microbiologists,* part A, (ed. by B. M. Gibbs & F. A. Skinner) p. 35. Society for Applied Bacteriology Tech series No. 1. London: Academic Press.

Morris, J. G., Miller, H. G., Wilson, R., Tacket, C. O., Hollis, D. G., Hickman, F. W., Weaver, R. E. & Blake, P. A. (1982). Illness caused by *Vibrio damsela* and *Vibrio hollisae*. *Lancet* i, 1294.

Morris, J. A. & Sojka, W. J. (1985). *Escherichia coli* as a pathogen in animals. In *The virulence* of *Escherichia coli* (ed. M. Sussman), p. 47. London: Academic Press.

Morse, M. L. & Weaver, R. H. (1950). Rapid microtechnics for identification of cultures. III. Hydrogen sulfide production. *Am. J. clin. Path.* **20**, 481.

Morton, H. E. (1945). On the amount of carbon dioxide supplied for the primary isolation of *Neisseria gonorrhoeae*. *J. Bact.* **43**, 651.

Moseley, S. L., Echeverria, P., Seriwatana, J., Tirapat, C., Chaicumpa, W., Sakuldaipeara, T. & Falkow, S. (1982). Identification of enterotoxigenic *Escherichia coli* by colony hybridization using the enterotoxin gene probes. *J. infect. Dis.* **145**, 863.

Moss, C. W., Weaver, R. E., Dees, S. B. & Cherry, W. B. (1977). Cellular fatty acid composition of isolates from Legionnaires' disease. *J. clin. Microbiol.* **6**, 140.

Moss, C. W. & Dunkelberg, W. E. (1969). Volatile and cellular fatty acids of *Haemophilus vaginalis*. *J. Bact.* **100**, 544.

Much, H. (1908). Über eine Vorstufe des Fibrinfermentes in Kulturen von Staphylokokkus aureus. *Biochem. Z.* **14**, 143.

Mudge, C. S. (1917). The effect of sterilization upon sugars in culture media. *J. Bact.* **2**, 403.

Mueller, J. H. & Hinton, J. (1941). A protein-free medium for primary isolation of the gonococcus and meningococcus. *Proc. Soc. exp. Biol. Med.* **48**, 330.

Mukerjee, S. (1963). The bacteriophage-susceptibility test in differentiating *Vibrio cholerae* and *Vibrio el tor*. *Bull. Wld. Hlth. Org.* **28**, 333.

Mukerjee, S., Guha, D. K. & Gua Roy (1957). Studies on typing of cholera by bacteriophage. 1. Phage type of *Vibrio cholerae* from Culcutta epidemics. *Annls Biochem. exp. Med.* **17**, 161.

Mulligan, M. E. (1988). General epidemiology, potential reservoirs, and typing procedures. In *Clostridium difficile: its Role in Intestinal Diseases* (ed. R. D. Rolfe & S. M. Finegold), p. 229. New York: Academic Press.

Murray, E. G. D. (1918). An attempt at classification of *Bacillus dysenteriae*, based upon an examination of the agglutinating properties of fifty-three strains. *J.R. Army med. Cps*, **31**, 257, 353.

Murray, E. G. D., Webb, R. A. & Swann, M. B. R. (1926). A disease of rabbits characterized by a large mononuclear leucocytosis, caused by a hitherto undescribed bacillus *Bacterium monocytogenes* (n. sp.). *J. Path. Bact.* **29**, 407.

Musser, J. M., Granoff, D. M., Pattison, P. E. & Selander, R. K. (1985). A population genetic framework for the study of invasive diseases caused by serotype b strains of *Haemophilus influenzae*. *Proc. nat. Acad. Sci., USA.* **82**, 5078.

Mutters, R., Piechulla, K., Hinz, K.-H. & Mannheim, W. (1985). *Pasteurella avium* (Hinz and Kunjara 1977) comb. nov. and *Pasteurella volantium* sp. nov. *Int. J. syst. Bact.* **35**, 9.

Nagler, F. P. 0. (1939). Observations on a reaction between the lethal toxin of *Cl. welchii* (type A) and human serum. *Br. J. exp. Path.* **20**, 473.

Nairn, R. C. (1976). *Fluorescent Protein Tracing*, 3rd edn. London: E. & S. Livingstone.

Nakanishi, H. & Murase, M. (1974). Enumeration of *Vibrio parahaemolyticus* in raw fish meat. In *International Symposium on Vibrio parahaemolyticus* (ed. T. Fujino *et al.*), p. 117. Tokyo: Saikon Publishing Company.

Nakhla, L. S. (1973). A serological method for distinguishing coagulase-negative staphylococci from micrococci. *J. clin. Path.* **26**, 511.

Namavar, F., de Graaf, J., de With, C. & MacLaren, D. M. (1978). Novobiocin resistance and virulence of strains of *Staphylococcus saprophyticus* isolated from urine and skin. *J. med. Microbiol.* **11**, 243.

National Collection of Type Cultures. *Catalogue*. Edn. 1, 1972; Edn. 2, 1989. London: Her Majesty's Stationery Office.

Neelsen, F. (1883). Ein casuistischer Beitrag zur Lehre von der Tuberkulose. *Centr. Med. Wisse.* **21**, 497.

Neill, S. D., Campbell, J. N., O'Brien, J. J., Weatherup, S. T. C. & Ellis, W. A. (1985). Taxonomic position of *Campylobacter cryaerophila* sp. nov. *Int. J. syst. Bact.* **35**, 342.

Neisser, M. (1903). Die Untersuchung auf Diptheriebacillen in centralisierten Untersuchungsstationen. *Hyg. Rundschau.*, **13**, 705.

Newsom, I. E. & Cross, F. (1932). Some bipolar organisms found in pneumonia in sheep. *J. Am. vet. med. Ass.* **80**, 715.

Nilehn, B. (1969). Studies on *Yersinia enterocolitica* with special reference to bacterial diagnosis and occurrence in human acute enteric disease. *Acta path. microbiol. scand.* (Suppl.) **206**.

Niven, C. F., Jr, Smiley, K. L. & Sherman, J. M. (1942). The hydrolysis of arginine by streptococci. *J. Bact.* **43**, 651 .

Nord, C. E., Holta-Oie, S., Ljungh, A. & Wadstrom, T. (1976). Characterization of coagulase-negative staphylococcal species from human infections. *Zbl. Bakt. Suppl.* **5**, 105.

Norris, J. R., Berkeley, R. C. W., Logan, N. A. &

O'Donnell, A. G. (1981). The genera *Bacillus* and *Sporolactobacillus*. In *The Prokaryotes: a Handbook on Habitats, Isolation and Identification of Bacteria* vol 2, (ed. M. P. Starr *et al.*), p. 1711. Berlin: Springer-Verlag.

Nørrung, V. (1979). Two new serotypes of *Erysipelothrix rhusiopathiae*. *Nrd. vet. Med.* **34**, 462.

Nowinski, R. C. Tam, M. R., Goldstein, L. C., Strong, L., Kuo, C. G., Corey, L., Stamm, W. E., Handsfield, H. H., Knapp, J. S. & Holmes, K. K. (1983). Monoclonal antibodies for diagnosis of infectious diseases in humans. *Science*, **219**, 637

O'Connor, J. J., Willis, A. T. & Smith, J. A. (1966). Pigmentation of *Staphylococcus aureus*. *J. Path. Bact.* **92**, 585.

O'Donnell, A. G., Norris, J. R., Berkeley, R. C. W., Claus, D., Kaneko, T., Logan, N.A. & Nozaki, R. (1980). Characterization of *Bacillus subtilis, Bacillus pumilus, Bacillus licheniformis* and *Bacillus amyloliquefaciens* by pyrolysis gas-liquid chromatography, deoxyribonucleic acid - deoxyribonucleic acid hybridization, biochemical tests and API systems. *Int. J. syst. Bact.* **30**, 448.

O'Meara, R. A. Q. (1931). A simple delicate and rapid method of detecting the formation of acetylmethylcarbinol by bacteria fermenting carbohydrate. *J. Path. Bact.* **34**, 401.

O'Meara, R. A. Q. & MacSween, J. C. (1936). The failure of staphylococcus to grow from small inocula in routine laboratory media. *J. Path. Bact.* **43**, 373.

O'Meara, R. A. Q. & MacSween, J. C. (1937). The influence of copper in peptones on the growth of certain pathogens in peptone broth. *J. Path. Bact.* **44**, 225.

Oakley, C. L. & Warrack, G. H. (1959). The soluble antigens of *Clostridium oedematiens* type D (*Cl. haemolyticum*). *J. Path. Bact.* **78**, 543.

Oakley, C. L., Warrack, G. H. & Clarke, P. H. (1947). The toxins of *Clostridium oedematiens (Cl. novyi)*. *J. gen. Microbiol.* **1**, 91.

Oberhofer, T. R. & Maddox, L. (1970). Combined medium to determine deoxyribonuclease activity and phenylalanine deamination. *Appl. Microbiol.* **19**, 385.

Oberhofer, T. R. & Back, A. E. (1979). Biotypes of *Haemophilus* encountered in clinical laboratories. *J. clin. Microbiol.* **10**, 168.

Old, D. C. & McNeill, G. P. (1979). Endocarditis due to *Micrococcus sedentarius incertae sedis*. *J. clin. Path.* **32**, 951.

Olds, R. J. (1966). An information sorter for identifying bacteria. In *Identification Methods for Microbiologists*, part A, (ed. B. M. Gibbs & F. A. Skinner). p. 131. Society for Applied Bacteriology Tech series No. 1. London: Academic Press.

Olds, R. J. (1970). Identification of bacteria with the aid of an improved information sorter. In *Automation, Mechanization and Data Handling in Microbiology,* (ed. A. Baillie & R. J. Gilbert). p. 85. Society for Applied Bacteriology Tech. series No. 4. London: Academic Press.

Olsufiev, N. G. (1970). Taxonomy and characteristics of the genus *Francisella* Dorofe'ev, 1947. *J Hyg. Epidemiol. Immunol.* **14**, 67.

Olsufiev, N. G., Emelyanova, O. S. & Dunaeva, T. N. (1959). Comparative studies of strains of *B. tularense* in the old and new world and their taxonomy. *J.Hyg. Epidemiol. Microbiol. Immunol.* **3**, 138.

Olsufiev, N. G. & Meshcheryakova, J. S. (1983). Subspecific taxonomy of *Francisella tularensis* McCoy & Chapin 1912. *Int. J. syst. Bact.* **33**, 872.

Opinion 4 (revised) (1954). Rejection of the generic name *Bacterium. Int. Bull. bact. Nomencl. Taxon.* **4**, 141.

Opinion 32 (1970). Conservation of the specific epithet *rhusiopathiae* in the scientific name of the organism known as *Erysipelothrix rhusiopathiae* (Migula 1900) Buchanan 1918. *Int. J. syst. Bact.* **20**, 9.

Opinion 46 (1971). Rejection of the generic name *Aerobacter* Beijerinck. *Int. J. syst. Bact.* **21**, 110.

Orberg, P. K. & Sandine, W. E. (1984). Common occurrence of plasmid DNA and vancomycin resistance in *Leuconostoc* spp. *Appl. environ. Microbiol.* **48**, 1129.

Orchard, V. A. & Goodfellow, M. (1980). Numerical classification of some strains of *Nocardia asteroides* and related isolates from soil. *J. gen. Microbiol.* **118**, 295.

Orcutt, M. L. & Howe, P. E. (1922). Hemolytic action of a staphylococcus due to a fat-splitting enzyme. *J. exp. Med.* **35**, 409.

Orla-Jensen, S. (1919). *The lactic acid bacteria.* Copenhagen: Andr. Fred. Host & Son.

Orr Ewing, J. & Taylor, J. (1945). Variations in the fermentative reactions of antigenically identical strains of *Bact. newcastle. Mon. Bull. Min.. Hlth Lab. Serv.* **4**, 130.

Ørskov, I. (1955). The biochemical properties of *Klebsiella (Klebsiella-aerogenes)* strains. *Acta path. microbiol. scand.* **37**, 353.

Ørskov, I. (1957). Biochemical types in the *Klebsiella* group. *Acta path. microbiol. scand.* **40**, 155.

Ørskov, I. & Ørskov, F. (1985). *Escherichia coli* in extraintestinal infections. *J. Hyg., Camb.* **95**, 551.

Ortali, V. & Samarani, E. (1955). Micrometodi in microbiologia - I. Determinazione della ureasi. *Rc. Inst. sup. Sanitá, Roma* **18**, 1301.

Owen, C.R. (1974). Genus *Francisella* Dorofe'ev 1947. In *Bergey's Manual of Determinative Bacteriology*, Edn. 8 (ed. R. E. Buchanan & N. E. Gibbons), p. 283. Baltimore: Williams & Wilkins.

Owen, C. R., Barker, E.D., Jellison, W. L., Lackman, D. B. & Bell, J. F. (1964). Comparative studies of *Francisella tularensis* and *Francisella novicida*. *J. Bact.* **87**, 676.

Owen, R. J., Legros, R. M. & Lapage, S. P. (1978). Base composition, size and sequence similarities of genome deoxyribonucleic acids from clinical isolates of *Pseudomonas putrefaciens*. *J. gen. Microbiol.* **104**, 127.

Owens, J. D. & Keddie, R. M. (1968). A note on the vitamin requirements of some coryneform bacteria from soil and herbage. *J. appl. Bact.* **31**, 344.

Owens, J. D. & Keddie, R. M. (1969). The nitrogen nutrition of soil and herbage coryneform bacteria. *J. appl. Bact.* **32**, 338.

Page, L. A. (1962). Haemophilus infections in chickens. 1. Characteristics of 12 *Haemophilus* isolates recovered from diseased chickens. *Am. J. vet. Res.* **23**, 85.

Paine, F. S. (1927). The destruction of acetyl-methyl-carbinol by members of the colon-aerogenes group. *J. Bact.* **13**, 269.

Panton, P. N. & Valentine, F. C. 0. (1932). Staphylococcal toxin. *Lancet* i, 506.

Park, R. W. A. (1967). A comparison of two methods for detecting attack on glucose by pseudomonads and achromobacters. *J. gen. Microbiol.* **46**, 355.

Park, R. W. A. & Billing, E. (1965). Media for *Pseudomonas* and related organisms. *Lab. Pract.* **14**, 702.

Park, C. H., Hixon, D. L., Endlich, J. F., O'Connell, P., Bradd, F. T. & Mount, P. M. (1986). *Anaerobiospirillum succiniciproducens*: two case reports. *Am. J. clin. Path.* **85**, 73.

Parker, M. T. (1981). Infection and colonization by the 'other' staphylococci. In *The Staphylococci* (ed. A. Macdonald & G. Smith), p. 156. Aberdeen: Aberdeen University Press.

Parker, M. T. & Ball, L. C. (1976). Streptococci and aerococci associated with systemic infection in man. *J. med. Microbiol.* **9**, 275.

Parnas, J. (1961). Differentiation of brucellae by the aid of phages. J. *Bact.* **82**, 319.

Parr, L. W. (1936). Sanitary significance of the succession of coli-aerogenes organisms in fresh and stored feces. *Am. J. publ. Hlth*, **26**, 39.

Parry, J. M., Turnbull, P. C. B. & Gibson, J. R. (1983). *A colour atlas of* Bacillus *species*. Wolfe Medical Atlases No. 19. London: Wolfe Medical Publications.

Paster, B. J. & Dewhirst, F. E. (1988). Phylogeny of campylobacters, wolinellas, *Bacteroides gracilis*, and *Bacteroides ureolyticus* by 16S ribosomal ribonucleic acid sequencing. *Int. J. syst. Bact.* **38**, 56.

Pathak, A., Custer, J. R. & Levy, J. (1983). Neonatal sep-ticemia and meningitis due to *Plesiomonas shigelloides*. *Pediatrics*, **71**, 389.

Patton, C. M., Shaffer, N., Edmonds, P., Barrett, T. J., Lambert, M. A., Baker, C., Perlman, D. M. & Brenner, D. J. (1989). Human disease associated with '*Campylobacter upsaliensis*' (catalase-negative or weakly positive *Campylobacter* species) in the United States. *J. clin. Microbiol.* **27**, 66.

Payne, L. C. (1963). Towards medical automation. *Wld med. Electron.* **2**, 6.

Pease, A. A., Douglas, C. W. I. & Spencer, R. C. (1986). Identifying non-capsulate strains of *Streptococcus pneumoniae* isolated from eyes. *J. clin. Path.* **39**, 871.

Peck, G. (1986). A case of septicaemic melioidosis in the U.K. *Med. Lab. Sci.* (suppl.) **1**, 43.

Pedersen, M. M., Marso, E. & Pickett, M. J. (1970). Nonfermentative bacilli associated with man: III. Pathogenicity and antibiotic susceptibility. *Am. J. clin. Path.* **54** 178.

Pederson, C. S. & Breed, R. S. (1928). The fermentation of glucose by organisms of the genus *Serratia*. *J. Bact.* **16**, 163.

Peer, H. G. (1971). Degradation of sugars and their reaction with amino acids. In *Effects of sterilization on components in nutrient media. Symposium 1970* (ed. J. Van Bragt, D. A. A. Mossel, R. L. M. Pietik & H. Veldstra), p. 105. Wageningen: Veeman & Zonen.

Peffers, A. S. R., Bailey, J., Barrow, G. I. & Hobbs, B. C. (1973). *Vibrio parahaemolyticus* gastroenteritis and international air travel. *Lancet*, i, 143.

Pelczar, M. J., Jr (1953). *Neisseria caviae* nov. spec. *J. Bact.* **65**, 744.

Penner, J. L. (1984*a*). *Proteus* Hauser. In *Bergey's Manual of Systematic Bacteriology*, vol. 1 (ed. N. R. Krieg & J. G. Holt), p. 491. Baltimore: Williams & Wilkins.

Penner, J. L. (1984*b*). *Morganella* Fulton. In *Bergey's Manual of Systematic Bacteriology*, vol. 1 (ed. N. R. Krieg & J. G. Holt), p. 497. Baltimore: Williams & Wilkins.

Pennock, C. A. P. & Huddy, R. B. (1967). Phosphatase reaction of coagulase-negative staphylococci and micrococci. *J. Path. Bact.* **93**, 685.

Peny, J. & Buissiere, J. (1970). Micromethode d'identification des bacteries II. Identification du genre *Staphylococcus*. *Annls Inst. Pasteur, Paris*, **118**, 10.

Perch, B., Kjems, E. & Ravn, T. (1974). Biochemical and serological properties of *Streptococcus mutans* from various human and animal sources. *Acta path. microbiol. Scand.* B**82**, 357.

Petrovskaya, V. G. & Khomenko, N. A. (1979). Proposals for improving the classification of members of the genus *Shigella*. *Int. J. syst. Bact.* **29**, 400.

Phillips, J. E. (1960). The characterisation of *Actinobacillus lignieresi. J. Path. Bact.* **79** 331.

Phillips, K. D. (1976). A simple and sensitive technique for determining the fermentation reactions of non-sporing anaerobes. *J. appl. Bact.* **41**, 325.

Pickett, M. J. (1955). Fermentation tests for identification of Brucellae. *Am. J. med. Technol.* **21**, 166.

Pickett, M. J. (1970). Buffered substrates in determinative bacteriology. In *Rapid Diagnostic Methods in Medical Microbiology* (ed. C. D. Graber). p 153. Baltimore: The Williams & Wilkins Co.

Pickett, M. J. & Goodman, R. E. (1966). β-galactosidase for distinguishing between *Citrobacter* and *Salmonella. Appl. Microbiol.* **14**, 178.

Pickett, M. J. & Manclark, C. R. (1965). Tribe Mimeae. An illegitimate epithet. *Am. J. clin. Path.* **43**,161.

Pickett, M. J. & Nelson, E. L. (1955). Speciation within the genus *Brucella*. IV. Fermentation of carbohydrates. *J. Bact.* **69**, 333.

Pickett, M. J. & Pedersen, M. M. (1968). Screening procedure for partial identification of nonfermentative bacilli associated with man. *Appl. Microbiol.* **16**, 1631.

Pickett, M.J. & Pedersen, M. M. (1970*a*). Nonfermentative bacilli associated with man: II. Detection and identification. *Am. J. clin. Path.* **54**, 164.

Pickett, M. J. & Pedersen, M. M. (1970*b*). Characterization of saccharolytic nonfermentative bacteria associated with man. *Can. J. Microbiol.* **16**, 351.

Pickett, M. J. & Pedersen, M. M. (1970*c*). Salient features of nonsaccharolytic and weakly saccharolytic nonfermentative rods. *Can. J. Microbiol.* **16**, 401.

Pickett, M. J. & Scott, M. L. (1955). A medium for rapid VP tests. *Bact. Proc.* p. 110.

Pickford, G. E. & Dorris, F. (1934). Micro-methods for the detection of proteases and amylases. *Science, N. Y.* **80**, 317.

Piéchaud, M. (1963). Mobilité chez les *Moraxella. Annls Inst. Pasteur, Paris*, **104**, 291.

Piéchaud, D. & Szturm-Rubinsten, S. (1963). Étude de quelques entérobactéries n'utilisant pas l'acide citrique. *Annls Inst. Pasteur, Paris*, **105**, 460.

Piechulla, K., Hinz, K.-H. & Manneheim, W. (1985). Genetic and phenotypic comparison of three new avian *Haemophilus*-like taxa and of *Haemophilus paragallinarum* Biberstein and White 1969 with other members of the family Pasteurellaceae Pohl 1981. *Avian Dis.* **29**, 601.

Pien, M. D. & Farmer, J. J. (1983). *Serratia ficaria* isolated from a leg ulcer. *Southern med. J.* **76**, 1591.

Pillet, J. & Orta, B. (1977). Analyse sérologique des Staphylocoques coagulase-negatifs études des agglutinogens characteristiques des souches types de neus species individualisés par Schleifer et Kloos. *Annls Microbiol. Inst. Pasteur, Paris* **128B**, 475.

Pine, L. (1970). Classification and phylogenetic relationship of microaerophilic actinomycetes. *Int. J. syst. Bact.* **20**, 445.

Piot, P. (1985). *Gardnerella vaginalis*. In *Manual of Clinical Microbiology*, 4th edn (ed. E. H. Lennette, A. Balows, W. J. Hausler Jr, & H. J. Shadomy), p. 874. Washington, D. C.: American Society for Microbiology.

Piot, P. & van Dyck, E. (1981). *Gardnerella vaginalis*: Neither *Haemophilus* nor *Corynebacterium*. In *Haemophilus, Pasteurella and Actinobacillus* (ed. M. Kilian, W. Frederiksen & E.L. Biberstein), p. 143. London: Academic Press.

Piot, P., van Dyck, E., Goodfellow, M. & Falkow, S. (1980). A taxonomic study of *Gardnerella vaginalis* (*Haemophilus vaginalis*) Gardner and Dukes 1955. *J. gen. Microbiol.* **119**, 373.

Piot, P., van Dyck, E., Totten, P. A. & Holmes, K. K. (1982). Identification of *Gardnerella* (*Haemophilus*) *vaginalis. J. clin. Microbiol.* **15**, 19.

Piot, P., van Dyck, E., Peeters, M., Hale, J., Totten, P. A. & Holmes, K. K. (1984). Biotypes of *Gardnerella vaginalis. J. clin. Microbiol.* **20**, 677.

Pirie, J. H. H. (1940). *Listeria*: change of name for a genus of bacteria. *Nature, Lond.* **145**, 264.

Pitarangsi, C., Echeverria, P., Whitmire, R., Tirapat, C., Formal, S., Dammin, G. J. & Tingtalapong, M. (1982). Enteropathogenicity of *Aeromonas hydrophila* and *Plesiomonas shigelloides*: prevalence among individuals with and without diarrhea in Thailand. *Inf. Imm.* **35**, 666.

Pitt, T. L. (1980*a*). State of the art: typing *Pseudomonas aeruginosa. J. hosp. Inf.* **1**, 193.

Pitt, T. L. (1980*b*). Diphasic variation in the flagellar antigens of *Pseudomonas aeruginosa. FEMS Microbiol. Lett.* **9**, 301.

Pitt, T. L. (1982). State of the art: typing of *Serratia marcescens. J. hosp. Inf.* **3**, 9.

Pitt, T. L. (1988). Epidemiological typing of *Pseudomonas aeruginosa. Eur. J. clin. Microbiol. inf. Dis.* **7**, 238.

Pitt, T. L. & Dey, D. (1970). A method for the detection of gelatinase production by bacteria, *J. appl. Bact.* **33**, 687.

Pitt, T. L. & Erdman, Y. J. (1984). Serological typing of *Serratia marcescens*. In *Methods in Microbiology*, vol. 15 (ed. T. Bergan), p. 173. London: Academic Press.

Pitt, T. L., Erdman, Y. J. & Bucher, C. (1980). The epidemiological type identification of *Serratia marcescens* from outbreaks of infection in hospitals. *J. Hyg., Camb.* **84**, 269.

Pitt, T. L., MacDougall, J. H. S., Penketh, A.R. & Cooke, E. M. (1986). Polyagglutinating and non-typable strains of *Pseudomonas aeruginosa* in cystic fibrosis. *J. med. Microbiol.* **21**, 179.

Pittman, M. (1931). Variation and type specificity in the bacterial species *Haemophilus influenzae. J. exp. Med.* **53**, 471.

Pittman, M. & Davis, D. J. (1950). Identification of the Koch-Weeks bacillus (*Hemophilus aegyptius*). *J. Bact.* **59**, 413.

Plimmer, H. G. & Paine, S. G. (1921). A new method for the staining of bacterial flagella. *J. Path. Bact.* **24**, 286.

Plotkin, G. R. (1980). *Agrobacterium radiobacter* prosthetic valve endocarditis. *Ann. internal Med.* **93**, 839.

Pohl, S. (1981). DNA relatedness among members of *Haemophilus, Pasteurella* and *Actinobacillus.* In *Haemophilus, Pasteurella* and *Actinobacillus* (ed. M. Kilian, W. Frederiksen & E. L. Biberstein), p. 245. London: Academic Press.

Pohl, S., Bertrschinger, H. U., Frederiksen, W. & Mannheim, W. (1983). Transfer of *Haemophilus pleuropneumoniae* and the *Pasteurella haemolytica*-like organism causing porcine necrotic pleuropneumonia to the genus *Actinobacillus* (*Actinobacillus pleuropneumoniae* comb. nov.) on the basis of phenotypic and deoxyribonucleic acid relatedness. *Int. J. syst. Bact.* **33**, 510.

Pollock, M. R. (1948). Unsaturated fatty acids in cotton wool plugs. *Nature, Lond.* **161**, 853.

Poole, P. M. & Wilson, G. (1979). Occurrence and cultural features of *Streptococcus milleri* in various body sites. *J. clin. Path.* **32**, 764.

Pope, C. G. & Smith, M. L. (1932). The routine preparation of diphtheria toxin of high value. *J. Path. Bact.* **35**, 573.

Pope, C. G. & Stevens, M. F. (1939). The determination of amino-nitrogen using a copper method. *Biochem. J.* **33**, 1070.

Pope, H. & Smith, D. T. (1946). Synthesis of B-complex vitamins by tubercle bacilli when grown on synthetic media. *Am. Rev. Tuberc.* **54**, 559.

Popoff, M. Y., Coynault, C., Kiredjian, M. & Lemelin, M. (1981). Polynucleotide sequence relatedness among motile *Aeromonas* species. *Curr. Microbiol.* **5**, 109.

Popoff, M. Y. & Véron, M. T. (1976). A taxonomic study of the *Aeromonas hydrophila – Aeromonas punctata* group. *J. gen. Microbiol.* **94**, 11.

Postgate, J. (1969). *Microbes and man.* Edn 1, 1969; Edn 2, 1986. Harmondsworth, England: Penguin Books. Edn 3, 1992 Cambridge University Press.

Potts, T. V. & Berry, E. M. (1983). Deoxyribonucleic acid – deoxyribonucleic acid hybridization analysis of *Actinobacillus actinomycetemcomitans* and *Haemophilus aphrophilus. Int. J. syst. Bact.* **33**, 765.

Potts, T. V., Zambon, J. J. & Genco, R. J. (1985). Reassignment of *Actinobacillus actinomycetemcomitans* to the genus *Haemophilus* as *Haemophilus actinomycetemcomitans* comb. nov. *Int. J. syst. Bact.* **35**, 337.

Potts, T. V., Mitra, T., O'Keefe, T., Zambon, J. J. & Genco, R. J. (1986). Relationships among isolates of oval haemophili as determined by DNA – DNA hybridization. *Arch. Microbiol.* **145**, 136.

Prefontaine, G. & Jackson, F. L. (1972). Cellular fatty acid profiles as an aid to the classification of 'corroding bacilli' and certain other bacteria. *Int. J. syst. Bact.* **22**, 210.

Prentice, A. W. (1957). *Neisseria flavescens* as a cause of meningitis. *Lancet* i, 613.

Preston, N. W. & Maitland, H. B. (1952). The influence of temperature on the motility of *Pasteurella pseudotuberculosis. J. gen. Microbiol.* **7**, 117.

Preston, N. W. & Morrell, A. (1962). Reproducible results with the Gram stain. *J. Path. Bact.* **84**, 241.

Prévot, A.-R. (1961). *Traité de Systematique Bacterienne.* Paris: Dunod.

Price, T., French, G. L., Talsania, H. & Phillips, I. (1986). Differentiation of *Streptococcus sanguis* and *S. mitior* by whole-cell rhamnose content and possession of arginine dihydrolase. *J. med. Microbiol.* **21**, 189.

Priest, F. G. (1981). DNA homology in the genus *Bacillus.* In *The aerobic endospore-forming bacteria: classification and identification* (ed. R. C. W. Berkeley & M. Goodfellow), p. 33. London: Academic Press.

Priest, F. G. & Alexander, B. (1988). A frequency matrix for probabilistic identification of some bacilli. *J. gen. Microbiol.* **134**, 3011.

Priest, F. G., Goodfellow, M., Shute, L. A. & Berkeley, R. C. W. (1987). *Bacillus amyloliquefaciens* sp. nov., nom. rev. *Int. J. syst. Bact.* **37**, 69.

Priest, F. G., Somerville, H. J., Cole, J. A. & Hough, J. S. (1973). The taxonomic position of *Obesumbacterium proteus,* a common brewery contaminant. *J. gen. Microbiol.* **75**, 295.

The Prokaryotes. A Handbook on Habitats, Isolation and Identification of Bacteria. (1981) Eds: M. P. Starr, H. Stolp, H. G. Trüper, A. Balows & H. G. Schlegel. Berlin & New York; Springer-Verlag.

Proom, H. & Knight, B. C. J. G. (1955). The minimal nutritional requirements of some species in the genus *Bacillus. J. gen. Microbiol.* **13**, 474.

Proom, H. & Woiwod, A. J. (1951). Amine production in the genus *Proteus. J. gen. Microbiol.* **5**, 930.

Pugh, G. W., Jr, Hughes, D. E. & McDonald, T. J. (1966). The isolation and characterization of *Moraxella bovis. Am. J. vet. Res.* **27**, 957.

Rahaman, M. M., Morshed, M. G., Aziz, K. M. S. & Munshi, M. M. H. (1986). Improved medium for isolating *Shigella. Lancet* i, 271.

Rahn, O. (1929). Contributions to the classification of bacteria. IV. Intermediate forms. *Zentbl. Bakt. ParasitKde Abt. II,* **78**, 8.

Rahn, O. (1937). New principles for the classification of bacteria. *Zentbl. Bakt. ParasitKde Abt. III,* **96**, 273.

Ralston, E., Palleroni, N. J. & Doudoroff, M. (1973). *Pseudomonas pickettii,* a new species of clinical origin related to *Pseudomonas solanacearum. Int. J. syst. Bact.* **23**, 15.

Rammell, C. G. (1962). Inhibition by citrate of the growth of coagulase-positive staphylococci. *J. Bact.* **84**, 1123.

Rant, J. D., Feltham, R. K. A. & Shepherd, W. (eds) (1987). *Computers in Microbiology.* The proceedings of the 2nd International Workshop on Computers in Microbiology. Leicester: Continuing Education Unit.

Rauss, K. F. (1936). The systematic position of Morgan's bacillus. *J. Path. Bact.* **42**, 183.

Rauss, K. (1962). A proposal for the nomenclature and classification of the Proteus and Providencia groups. *Int. Bull. bact. Nomencl. Taxon.* **12**, 53.

Rauss, K. & Vörös, S. (1959). The biochemical and serological properties of *Proteus morganii. Acta microbiol. Acad. Sci. Hung.* **6**, 233.

Reddy, C. A., Cornell, C. P. & Fraga, A. M. (1982). Transfer of *Corynebacterium pyogenes* (Glage) Eberson to the genus *Actinomyces* as *Actinomyces pyogenes* (Glage) comb. nov. *Int. J. syst. Bact.* **32**, 419.

Redfearn, M. S., Palleroni, N. J. & Stanier, R. Y. (1966). A comparative study of *Pseudomonas pseudomallei* and *Bacillus mallei. J. gen. Microbiol.* **43**, 293.

Reed, R. W. (1942). Nitrate, nitrite and indole reactions of gas gangre... anaerobes. *J. Bact.* **44**, 425.

Regan, J. & Lowe, F. (1977). Enrichment medium for the isolation of *Bordetella. J. clin. Microbiol.* **6**, 303.

Reichelt, J. L., Baumann, P. & Baumann, L. (1976). Study of the genetic relationships among marine species of the genus *Beneckea* and *Photobacterium* by means of *in vitro* DNA/DNA hybridization. *Archs Microbiol.* **110**, 101.

Report (1953). Diphtheria and pertussis vaccination . Report of a conference of heads of laboratories producing diphtheria and pertussis vaccines. *Tech. Rep. Wld Hlth Org.* no. 61.

Report (1954a). Reports of the Enterobacteriaceae Sub-Committee on the groups Salmonella, Shigella, Arizona, Bethesda, Ballerup, Escherichia, Alkalescens Dispar, Klebsiella, and Proteus in Rio de Janeiro, August, 1950. *Int. Bull. bact. Nomencl. Taxon.* **4**, 1 .

Report (1954b). Reports on the groups: Salmonella, Shigella, Arizona, Bethesda, Escherichia, Klebsiella (Aerogenes, Aerobacter), Providence (29911 of Stuart *et al.*). *Int. Bull. bact. Nomencl. Taxon.* **4**, 47.

Report (1956a). *Constituents of Bacteriological Culture Media.* Special report of the Society for General Microbiology. London: Cambridge University Press.

Report (1956b). The nomenclature of coli-aerogenes bacteria. Report of the Coli-aerogenes (1956) Sub-Committee of the Society for Applied Bacteriology. *J. appl. Bact.* **19**, 108.

Report (1956c). The bacteriological examination of [drinking] water supplies. *Reports on Public Health and Medical Subjects, No. 71.* (Revised 1969, 1983.) London: Her Majesty's Stationery Office.

Report (1958). Report of the Enterobacteriaceae Subcommittee of the Nomenclature Committee of the International Association of Microbiological Societies. *Int. Bull. bact. Nomencl. Taxon.* **8**, 25.

Reuter, G. (1971). Designation of type strains for *Bifidobacterium* species. *Int. J. syst. Bact.* **21**, 273.

Reyn, A. (1970). Taxonomic position of *Neisseria haemolysans* (Thjøtta & Bøe, 1938). *Int. J. syst. Bact.* **20**, 19.

Reyn, A., Birch-Anderson, A. & Lapage, S. P. (1966). An electron microscope study of thin sections of *Haemophilus vaginalis* (Gardner and Dukes) and some possibly related species. *Can. J. Microbiol.* **12**, 1125.

Rhodes, M. (1950). Viability of dried bacterial cultures. *J. gen. Microbiol.* **4**, 450.

Rhodes, M. E. (1958). The cytology of *Pseudomonas* spp. as revealed by a silver-plating staining method. *J. gen. Microbiol.* **18**, 639.

Richard, C. (1965). Mesure de l'activité ureasique des *Proteus* au moyen de la réaction phenol-hypochlorite de Berthelot. Intérêt taxinomique. *Annls Inst. Pasteur, Paris* **109**, 516.

Richard, C. (1966). Caractères biochimiques des biotypes de *Providencia;* leurs rapports avec le genre *Rettgerella. Annls Inst. Pasteur, Paris* **110**, 105.

Richard, C. (1968). Techniques rapides de récherche des lysine-décarboxylase, ornithine-décarboxylase et arginine-dihydrolase dans les genres *Pseudomonas, Alcaligenes* et *Moraxella. Annls Inst. Pasteur, Paris* **114**, 425.

Richard, C., Joly, B., Sirot, J., Stoleru, G. H. & Popoff, M. (1976). Study of *Enterobacter* strains belonging to a particular group related to *Enterobacter aerogenes. Annls Microbiol. Inst. Pasteur, Paris* **127**A, 545.

Richardson, J. F. & Marples, R. R. (1980). Differences in antibiotic susceptibility between *Staphylococcus epidermidis* and *Staphylococcus saprophyticus. J. antimicrob. Chemother.* **6**, 499.

Riddle, J. W., Kabler, P. W., Kenner, B. A., Bordner, R. H., Rockwood, S. W. & Stevenson, H. J. R. (1956). Bacterial identification by infrared spectrophotometry. *J. Bact.* **72**, 593.

Rifkind, D. & Cole, R. M. (1962). Non-beta-hemolytic group M-reacting streptococci of human origin. *J. Bact.* **84**, 163.

Riley, P. S., Tatum, H. W. & Weaver, R. E. (1973). Identity of HB-I of King and *Eikenella corrodens* (Eiken) Jackson and Goodman. *Int. J. syst. Bact.* **23**, 75.

Riley, P. S. & Weaver, R. E. (1977). Comparison of thirty-seven strains of Vd-3 bacteria with *Agrobacterium radiobacter*: morphological and physiological observations. *J. clin. Microbiol.* **5**, 172.

Riley, P. S., Hollis, D. G., Utter, G. B., Weaver, R. E. & Baker, C. N. (1979). Characterization and identification of 95 diphtheroid (group JK) cultures isolated from clinical specimens. *J. clin. Microbiol.* **9**, 418.

Rimler, R. B., Shotts, E. B., Brown J. & Davis, R. B. (1977). The effect of sodium chloride and NADH on the growth of 6 strains of *Haemophilus* species pathogenic to chickens. *J. gen. Microbiol.* **98**, 349.

Roberts, D. H., Hanson, B. S. & Timms, L. (1964). Observations in the incidence and significance of *Haemophilus gallinarum* in outbreaks of respiratory disease among poultry in Great Britain. *Vet. Rec.* **76**, 1512.

Roberts, G. A. & Charles, H. P. (1970). Mutants of *Neurospora crassa, Escherichia coli* and *Salmonella typhimurium* specifically inhibited by carbon dioxide. *J. gen. Microbiol.* **63**, 21.

Roberts, R. B., Krieger, A. G., Schiller, N. L. & Gross, K. C. (1979). Viridans streptococcal endocarditis: the role of various species including pyridoxal-dependent streptococci. *Rev. inf. Dis.* **1**, 955.

Robertson, M. (1916). Notes upon certain anaerobes isolated from wounds. *J. Path. Bact.* **20**, 327.

Robinson, W. & Woolley, P. B. (1957). Pseudo-haemoptysis due to *Chromobacterium prodigiosum. Lancet* i, 819.

Roche, A. & Marquet, F. (1935). Récherches sur le vieillissement du sérum. *C. r. Séanc. Soc. Biol. Med.* **119**, 1147.

Rocourt, J., Audurier, A., Courtieu, A. L., Durst, J., Ortel, S., Schrettenbrünner, A. & Taylor, A. G. (1985). A multi-centre study on the phage typing of *Listeria monocytogenes. Zbl. Bakt. Mikrobiol. Hyg., Abt. 1,* Orig. A **259**, 489.

Rocourt, J., Grimont, F., Grimont, P. A. D. & Seeliger, H. P. R. (1982). DNA relatedness among serovars of *Listeria monocytogenes sensu lato. Curr. Microbiol.* **7**, 383.

Rocourt, J., Schrettenbrünner, A. & Seeliger, H. P. R. (1983). Différentiation biochimique des groupes génomique de *Listeria monocytogenes (sensu lato). Annls microbiol. Inst. Pasteur, Paris* , **134**A, 65.

Rocourt, J., Wehmeyer, U. & Stackebrandt, E. (1987a).

Transfer of *Listeria denitrificans* to a new genus *Jonesia* as *Jonesia denitrificans* comb. nov. *Int. J. syst. Bact.* **37**, 266.

Rocourt, J., Wehmeyer, U. & Stackebrandt, E. (1987b). Proposal to retain *Listeria murrayi* and *Listeria grayi* in the genus *Listeria. Int. J. Syst. Bact.* **37**, 298.

Rogers, K. B. & Taylor, J. (1961). Laboratory diagnosis of gastro-enteritis due to *Escherichia coli. Bull. Wld Hlth Org.* **24**, 59.

Rogosa, M. (1970). Characters used in the classification of lactobacilli. *Int. J. syst. Bact.* **20**, 519.

Rogosa, M. (1971). Transfer of *Veillonella* Prevot and *Acidaminococcus* Rogosa from *Neisseriaceae* to *Veillonellaceae* fam. nov., and the inclusion of *Megasphaera* Rugosa in *Veillonellaceae. Int. J. syst. Bact.* **21**, 231.

Rogosa, M. (1984). Anaerobic Gram-negative cocci. In *Bergey's Manual of Systematic Bacteriology,* vol. 1 (ed. N. R. Krieg & J. G. Holt), p. 680. Baltimore: Williams & Wilkins.

Rogosa, M., Fitzgerald, R. J., Mackintosh, M. E. & Beaman, M. J. (1958). Improved medium for selective isolation of *Veillonella. J. Bact.* **76**, 455.

Rogosa, M., Mitchell, J.A. & Wiseman, R. F. (1951). A selective medium for the isolation and enumeration of oral and fecal lactobacilli. *J. Bact.* **62**, 132.

Rogosa, M. & Sharpe, M. E. (1960). Species differentiation of human vaginal lactobacilli. *J. gen. Microbiol.* 23, 197.

Rogosa, M., Wiseman, R. F., Mitchell, J. A. & Disraely, M. (1953). Species differentiation of oral lactobacilli from man including descriptions of *Lactobacillus salivarius* nov. spec. and *Lactobacillus cellobiosus* nov. spec. *J. Bact.* **65**, 681.

Roguinsky, M. (1969). Reactions de *Streptococcus uberis* avec les serums G et P. *Annls Inst. Pasteur, Paris* **117**, 529.

Roguinsky, M. (1971). Caracteres biochimiques et serologiques de *Streptococcus uberis. Annls Inst. Pasteur, Paris* **120**, 154.

Romick, T. L., Lindsay, J. A. & Busta, F.F. (1987). A visual probe for detection of enterotoxigenic *Escherichia coli* by colony hybridization. *Lett. appl. Microbiol.* **5**, 87.

Ross, R. F., Hall, J. E., Orning, A. P. & Dale, S. E. (1972). Characterisation of an *Actinobacillus* isolated from the sow vagina. *Int. J. syst. Bact.* **22**, 39.

Rossau, R., Kersters, K., Falsen, E., Jantzen, E., Segers, P., Union, A., Nehls, L. & DeLey, J. (1987). *Oligella,* a new genus including *Oligella urethralis* comb. nov. (formerly *Moraxella urethralis*) and *Oligella ureolytica* sp. nov. (formerly CDC Group IVe): relationship to

Taylorella equigenitalis and related taxa. *Int. J. syst. Bact.* **37**, 198.

Rossau, R., Van Landschoot, A., Mannheim, W. & DeLey, J. (1986). Inter- and intrageneric similarities of ribosomal ribonucleic acid cistrons of the Neisseriaceae. *Int. J. syst. Bact.* **36**, 323.

Rowatt, E. (1957). The growth of *Bordetella pertussis:* a review. *J. gen. Microbiol.* **17**, 297.

Rowe, B., Gross, R. J. & Guiney, M. (1976). Antigenic relationships between *Escherichia coli* O antigens O149 to O163 and *Shigella* O antigens. *Int. J. syst. Bact.* **26**, 76.

Rubin, F. A., Kopecko, D. J., Noon, K. F. & Baron, L. S. (1985). Development of a DNA probe to detect *Salmonella typhi. J. clin. Microbiol.* **22**, 600.

Rubin, S. J., Granato, P. A. & Wasilauskas, B. L. (1985). Glucose-nonfermenting Gram-negative bacteria. In *Manual of clinical microbiology*, Edn 4 (ed. E. H. Lennette, A. Balows, W.J. Hausler, Jr & H. J. Shadomy). p. 330. Washington, DC: American Society for Microbiology.

Ruchhoft, C. C., Kallas, J. G., Chinn, B. & Coulter, E. W. (1931). Coli-aerogenes differentiation in water analysis. II. The biochemical differential tests and their interpretation. *J. Bact.* **22**,125.

Rüger, H.-J. & Tan, T. L. (1983). Separation of *Alcaligenes denitrificans* sp. nov., nom. rev. from *Alcaligenes faecalis* on the basis of DNA base composition, DNA homology, and nitrate reduction. *Int. J. syst. Bact.* **33**, 85.

Ruoff, K. L. & Ferraro, M. J. (1986). Hydrolytic enzymes of 'Streptococcus milleri'. *J. clin. Microbiol.* **25**, 1645.

Russell, F. F. (1911). The isolation of typhoid bacilli from urine and feces with the description of a new double sugar tube medium. *J. med. Res.* **25**, 217.

Rustigian, R. & Stuart, C. A. (1945). The biochemical and serological relationships of the organisms of the genus *Proteus. J. Bact.* **49**, 419.

Ryan, W. J. (1964). Moraxella commonly present on the conjunctiva of guinea pigs. *J. gen. Microbiol.* **35**, 361.

Sakaguchi, K. & Mori, H. (1969). Comparative study on *Pediococcus halophilus, P. soyae, P. homari, P. urinae-equi* and related species. *J. gen. appl. Microbiol., Tokyo*, **15**, 159.

Sakazaki, R. (1961). Studies on the Hafnia group of Enterobacteriaceae. *Jap. J. med. Sci. Biol.* **14**, 223.

Sakazaki, R. (1965a). *Vibrio parahaemolyticus,* a non-choleragenic enteropathogenic vibrio. *Proc. Cholera Res. Symposiurn,* 24-9 January 1965, Honolulu. Washington, DC: US Government Printing Office.

Sakazaki, R. (1965b). *Vibrio parahaemolyticus. Isolation and Identification.* Toyko: Nihon Eiyo Kagaku (undated).

Sakazaki, R. (1967). Studies on the Asakusa group of Enterobacteriaceae *(Edwardsiella tarda). Jap. J. med. Sci. Biol.* **20**, 205.

Sakazaki, R. (1972). NaCl – colistin bouillon. In *Media for bacteriological examinations*, 2. Tokyo: Kindai Igaku Co. (In Japanese).

Sakazaki, R. & Balows, H. (1981). The genera *Vibrio, Plesiomonas*, and *Aeromonas.* In *The Prokaryotes: A Handbook on Habitats, Isolation and Identification of Bacteria.* Vol. 2 (ed. M.P. Starr *et al.*), p. 1272. Berlin: Springer-Verlag.

Sakazaki, R., Gomez, C. Z. & Sebald, M. (1967). Taxonomical studies of the so-called NAG vibrios. *Jap. J. med. Sci. Biol.* **20**, 265.

Sakazaki, R., Iwanami, S. & Fukumi, H. (1963). Studies on the enteropatogenic, facultatively halophilic bacteria, *Vibrio parahaemolyticus*. I. Morphological, cultural and biochemical properties and its taxonomical position. *Jap. J. med. sci. Biol.*, **16**, 161.

Sakazaki, R. & Murata, Y. (1962). The new group of the Enterobacteriaceae. The Asakusa group. *Jap. J. Bact.* **17**, 616. (Text in Japanese).

Sakazaki, R. & Tamura, K. (1971). Somatic antigen variation in *Vibrio cholerae. Jap. J. med. Sci. Biol.* **24**, 93.

Sakazaki, R. & Tamura, K. (1975). Priority of the specific epithet *anguillimortiferum* over the specific epithet *tarda* in the name of the organism presently known as *Edwardsiella tarda. Int. J. syst. Bact.* **25**, 219.

Sakazaki, R., Tamura, K. & Murase, M. (1971). Determination of the haemolytic activity of *Vibrio cholerae. Jap. J. med. Sci. Biol.* **24**, 83.

Sakazaki, R., Tamura, K., Gomez, C. Z. & Sen, R. (1970). Serological studies on the cholera group of vibrios. *Jap. J. med. Sci. Biol.* **23**, 13.

Sakazaki, R., Tamura, K., Kato, T., Obara, Y., Yamai, S. & Hobo, K. (1968). Studies on the enteropathogenic, facultatively halophilic bacteria, *Vibrio parahaemolyticus*. III. Enteropathogenicity. *Jap. J. med. Sci. Biol.* **21**, 325.

Salmonella Subcommittee of the Nomenclature Committee of the International Society for Microbiology (1934). The genus *Salmonella* Lignières, 1900. *J. Hyg., Camb.* **34**, 333.

Samuels, S. B., Pittman, B., Tatum, H. W. & Cherry, W. B. (1972). Report on a study set of moraxellae and allied bacteria. *Int. J. syst. Bact.* **22**,19.

Sandstedt, K., Ursing, J. & Walder, M. (1983). Thermotolerant *Campylobacter* with no or weak catalase activity isolated from dogs. *Curr. Microbiol.* **8**, 209.

de Saxe, M. J., Crees-Morris, J. A., Marples, R. R. & Richardson, J. F. (1981). Evaluation of current phagetyping systems for coagulase-negative staphylococci. In *Staphylococci and Staphylococcal Infections* (ed. J. Jeljaszewicz), p. 197. Stuttgart: Gustav Fischer Verlag.

Scardovi, V. (1981). The genus *Bifidobacterium*. In *The Prokaryotes: A Handbook on Habitats, Isolation and Identification of Bacteria*, vol. 2, (ed. M. P. Starr *et al.*) p. 1951 New York: Springer.

Scardovi, V. (1986). The genus *Bifidobacterium*. In *Bergey's Manual of Systematic Bacteriology*, vol. 2, (ed. P. H. A. Sneath et al.), p. 1418. Baltimore: Williams & Wilkins.

Scardovi, V., Trovatelli, L. D., Zani, G., Crociani, F. & Matteuzzi, D. (1971). Deoxyribonucleic acid homology relationships among species of the genus *Bifidobacterium*. *Int. J. syst. Bact.* **21**, 276.

Schaal, K. P. (1984). Laboratory diagnosis of actinomycete diseases. In *The Biology of the Actinomycetes* (ed. M. Goodfellow, M. Mordarski & S. T. Williams), p. 425. London: Academic Press.

Schaal, K. P. (1986a). The genus *Actinomyces*. In *Bergey's Manual of Systematic Bacteriology*, vol. 2, (ed. P. H. A. Sneath *et al.*), p. 1383. Baltimore: Williams & Wilkins.

Schaal, K. P. (1986b). The genus *Arachnia*. In *Bergey's Manual of Systematic Bacteriology*, vol. 2, (ed. P. H. A. Sneath *et al.*), p. 1332. Baltimore: Williams & Wilkins.

Schaal, K. P. & Pulverer, G. (1981). The genera *Actinomyces, Agromyces, Arachnia, Bacterionema*, and *Rothia*. In *The Prokaryotes: A Handbook on Habitats, Isolation and Identification of Bacteria* (ed. M. P. Starr *et al.*), p. 1923. Berlin: Springer-Verlag.

Schaeffer, A. B. & Fulton, M. (1933). A simplified method of staining endospores. *Science, N.Y.* **77**, 194.

Schalm, O. W. & Beach, J. R. (1936). Cultural requirements of the fowl-coryza bacillus. *J. Bact.* **31**, 161.

Schaub, I. G. & Hauber, F. D. (1948). A biochemical and serological study of a group of identical unidentifiable Gram-negative bacilli from human sources. *J. Bact.* **56**, 379.

Schindler, C. A. & Schuhardt, V. T. (1964). Lysostaphin: a new bacteriolytic agent for the staphylococcus. *Proc. natn. Acad. Sci. U.S.A.* **51**, 414.

Schleifer, K. H. (1986). Taxonomy of coagulase-negative staphylococci. In *Coagulase-Negative Staphylococci* (ed. P. A. Mardh & K. H. Schleifer), p. 11. Stockholm: Almqvist & Wiksell.

Schleifer, K. H. & Kilpper-Bälz, R. (1984). Transfer of *Streptococcus faecalis* and *Streptococcus faecium* to the genus *Enterococcus* nom. rev. as *Enterococcus faecalis* comb. nov. and *Enterococcus faecium* comb. nov. *Int. J. syst. Bact.* **34**, 31.

Schleifer, K. H. & Kandler, O. (1972). The peptidoglycan types of bacterial cell walls and their taxonomic implications. *Bact. Rev.* **36**, 407.

Schleifer, K. H. & Kloos, W. E. (1975a). Isolation and characterization of staphylococci from human skin. I. Amended description of *Staphylococcus epidermidis* and *Staphylococcus saprophyticus* and descriptions of three new species: *Staphylococcus cohnii*, *Staphylococcus haemolyticus* and *Staphylococcus xylosus*. *Int. J. syst. Bact.* **25**, 50.

Schleifer, K. H. & Kloos, W. E. (1975b). A simple test system for the separation of staphylococci from micrococci. *J. clin. Microbiol.* **1**, 337.

Schleifer, K. H. & Krämer, E. (1980). Selective medium for isolating staphylococci. *Z. Bakt. Infk. Hyg. Abt. 1*, Orig. C, **1**, 270.

Schleifer, K. H., Kraus, J., Dvorak, C., Kilpper-Bälz, R., Collins, M. D. & Fischer, W. (1985). Transfer of *Streptococcus lactis* and related streptococci to the genus *Lactococcus* gen. nov. *Syst. appl. Microbiol.* **6**, 183.

Schleifer, K. H. & Stackebrandt, E. (1983). Molecular systematics of prokaryotes. *Ann. Rev. Microbiol.* **37**, 143.

Schlievert, P. M. (1986). Staphylococcal enterotoxin B and toxic shock syndrome toxin-1 are significantly associated with non-menstrual toxic shock syndrome. *Lancet* i, 1149.

Schneierson, S. S. & Amsterdam, D. (1964). A punch card system for identification of bacteria. *Am. J. clin. Path.* **42**, 328.

Schofield, G. M. & Schaal, K. P. (1981). A numerical taxonomic study of members of the Actinomycetaceae and related taxa. *J. gen. Microbiol.* **127**, 237.

Schreier, J. B. (1969). Modification of deoxyribonuclease test medium for rapid identification of *Serratia marcescens. Am. J. clin. Path.* **51**, 711.

Schubert, R. H. W. (1967a). The taxonomy and nomenclature of the genus *Aeromonas* Kluyver and van Niel 1936. Part I. Suggestions on the taxonomy and nomenclature of the aerogenic *Aeromonas* species. *Int. J. syst. Bact.* **17**, 23.

Schubert, R. H. W. (1967b). The taxonomy and nomenclature of the genus *Aeromonas* Kluyver and van Niel 1936. Part II. Suggestions on the taxonomy and nomenclature of the anaerogenic aeromonads. *Int. J. syst. Bact.* **17**, 273.

Schubert, R. H. W. (1971). Status of the names *Aeromonas* and *Aerobacter liquefaciens* Beijerinck and designation of a neotype strain for *Aeromonas hydrophila* Stanier. Request for an Opinion. *Int. J. syst. Bact.* **21**, 87.

Schutze, H. (1928). *Bacterium pseudotuberculosis rodentium*. Rezeptorenanalyse von *18* Stämmen. *Arch. Hyg. Bakt.* **100**, 181.

Schütze, H. (1932a). *B. pestis* antigens. I. The antigens and immunity reactions of *B. pestis. Br. J. exp. Path.* **13**, 284.

Schütze, H. (1932b). *B. pestis* antigens. II. Antigenic relationship of *B. pestis* and *B. pseudotuberculosis rodentium*. *Br. J. exp. Path.* **13**, 289.

Sebald, M. & Véron, M. (1963). Teneur en bases de l'ADN et classification des vibrions. *Annls Inst. Pasteur, Paris* **105**, 897.

Sedlák, J., Dlabac, V. & Motlikova, M. (1965). The taxonomy of the Serratia genus. *J. Hyg. Epidem. Microbiol. Immun.* **9**, 45.

Sedlák, J., Puchmayerova-Slajsova, M., Keleti, J. & Lüderitz, O. (1971). On the taxonomy, ecology and immunochemistry of genus Citrobacter. *J. Hyg. Epidem. Microbiol. Immun.* **15**, 366.

Seeliger, H. P. R. (1961). *Listeriosis*. Basel: Karger.

Seeliger, H. P. R. & Jones, D. (1986). The genus *Listeria*. In *Bergey's Manual of Systematic Bacteriology*, vol. 2 (ed. P. H. A. Sneath *et al.*), p. 1235. Baltimore: Williams & Wilkins.

Segal, B. (1940). The utilization of acetyl methyl carbinol by *Staphylococcus albus* and *aureus*. *J. Bact.* **39**, 747.

Seki, T., Chung, C.-K., Mikami, H. & Oshima, Y. (1978). Deoxyribonucleic acid homology and taxonomy of the genus *Bacillus*. *Int. J. syst. Bact.* **28**, 182.

Sewell, C. M., Clarridge, J. E., Young, E. J. & Guthrie, R. K. (1982). Clinical significance of coagulase-negative staphylococci. *J. clin. Microbiol.* **16**, 236.

Shah, H. N., Bonnett, R., Mateen, B. & Williams, R. A. D. (1979). The porphyrin pigmentation of subspecies of *Bacteroides melaninogenicus*. *Biochem. J.* **180**, 45.

Shah, H. N., & Collins, M. D. (1989). Proposal to restrict the genus *Bacteroides* (Castellani and Chalmers) to *Bacteroides fragilis* and closely related species. *Int. J. syst. Bact.* **39**, 87.

Shah, H. N. & Collins, M. D. (1990). *Prevotella*, a new genus to include *Bacteroides melaninogenicus* and related species formerly classified in the genus *Bacteroides*. *Int. J. syst. Bact.* **40**, 205.

Shanson, D. C., Midgeley, J. M., Gazzard, B. G., Dixey, J., Gibson, G. L., Stevenson, J., Finch, R. G. & Cheesbrough, J. (1983). *Streptobacillus moniliformis* isolated from blood in four cases of Haverhill fever. *Lancet* ii, 92.

Sharpe, M. E. (1979). Identification of the lactic acid bacteria. In *Identification methods for Microbiologists*, edn 2 (ed. F. A. Skinner & D. W. Lovelock), p. 223. (Society for Applied Bacteriology Technical Series no. 14.) London: Academic Press.

Sharpe, M. E. (1981). The genus *Lactobacillus*. In *The Prokaryotes: A Handbook on Habitats, Isolation and Identification of Bacteria* (ed. M. Starr *et al.*), p. 1653. New York: Springer.

Sharpe, M. E., Hill, L. R. & Lapage, S. P. (1973).

Pathogenic lactobacilli. *J. med. Microbiol.*, **6**, 281.

Shaw, C. (1956). Distinction between Salmonella and Arizona by Leifson's sodium malonate medium. *Int. Bull. bact.Nomencl. Taxon.* **6**, 1.

Shaw, C. & Clarke, P. H. (1955). Biochemical classification of Proteus and Providence cultures. *J. gen. Microbiol.* **13**, 155.

Shaw, S. & Keddie, R. M. (1983). A numerical taxonomic study of the genus *Kurthia* with a revised description of *Kurthia zopfii* and a description of *Kurthia gibsonii* sp.nov. *Syst. appl. Microbiol.* **4**, 253.

Shaw, C., Stitt, J. M. & Cowan, S. T. (1951). Staphylococci and their classification. *J. gen. Microbiol.* **5**, 1010.

Shaw, C. E. Forsyth, M. E., Bowie, W. R. & Black, W. A. (1981). Rapid presumptive identification of *Gardnerella vaginalis* (*Haemophilus vaginalis*) from Human Blood Agar media. *J. clin. Microbiol.* **14**, 108.

Shayegani, M., Parsons, L. M., Gibbons, W. E. & Campbell, D. (1982). Characterization of non-typable *Streptococcus pneumoniae*-like organisms isolated from outbreaks of conjunctivitis. *J. clin. Microbiol.* **16**, 8.

Shepard, C. C. (1960). The experimental disease that follows the infection of human leprosy bacilli into footpads of mice. *J. exp. Med.* **112**, 445.

Shepard, M. C. (1983). Culture medium for ureaplasmas. In *Methods in Mycoplasmology*, vol. 2 (ed. J. G. Tilly & S. Razin) p. 137. New York: Academic Press.

Sherman, J. M. (1937). The streptococci. *Bacteriol. Revs* **1**, 3.

Sherris, I. C., Shoesmith, I. G., Parker, M. T. & Breckon, D. (1959). Tests for the rapid breakdown of arginine by bacteria: their use in the identification of pseudomonads. *J. gen. Microbiol.* **21**, 389.

Shuman, R. D. & Wellman, G. (1966). Status of the species name *Erysipelothrix rhusiopathiae* with request for an Opinion. *Int. J. syst. Bact.* **16**, 195.

Shuman, R. D., Nord, N., Brown, R. W. & Wessman, G. E. (1972). Biochemical and serological characteristics of Lancefield groups E, P, and U streptococci and *Streptococcus uberis*. *Cornell Vet.* **62**, 540.

Shute, L. A., Gutteridge, C. S., Norris, J. R. & Berkeley, R. C. W. (1984). Curie-point pyrolysis mass spectrometry applied to characterization and identification of selected *Bacillus* species. *J. gen. Microbiol.* **130**, 343.

Sierra, G. (1957). A simple method for the detection of lipolytic activity of micro-organisms and some observations on the influence of the contact between cells and fatty substrates. *Antonie van Leeuwenhoek* **23**, 15.

Silvestri, L. G. & Hill, L. R. (1965). Agreement between deoxyribonucleic acid base composition and taxometric classification of Gram-positive cocci. *J. Bact.* **90**, 136.

Simmons, J. S. (1926). A culture medium for differentiating organisms of typhoid-colon aerogenes groups and for isolation of certain fungi. *J. infect. Dis.* **39**, 209.

Sims, W. (1966). The isolation of pediococci from human saliva. *Archs oral Biol.* **11**, 967.

Sims, W. (1970). Oral haemophili. *J. med. Microbiol.* **3**, 615.

Singer, J. & Bar-Chay, J. (1954). Biochemical investigation of Providence strains and their relationship to the Proteus group. *J. Hyg., Camb.* **52**,1.

Singer, J. & Volcani, B. E. (1955). An improved ferric chloride test for differentiating Proteus-Providence group from other Enterobacteriaceae. *J. Bact.* **69**, 303.

Skerman, V. B. D. (1949). A mechanical key for the generic identification of bacteria. *Bact. Rev.* **13**, 175.

Skerman, V. B. D. (1959-67). A *Guide to the Identification of the Genera of Bacteria,* edn 1, 1959; edn 2, 1967. Baltimore: Williams & Wilkins.

Skerman, V. B. D., McGowan, V. & Sneath, P. H. A. (1980). *Approved Lists of bacterial names. Int. J. syst. Bact.* **30**, 225. (Printed in book form, 1980: Washington, D. C.: American Society for Microbiology.)

Skirrow, M. B. (1977). Campylobacter enteritis: a 'new' disease. *Br. Med. J.* **2**, 9.

Skirrow, M. B. & Benjamin, J. (1980). Differentiation of enteropathogenic campylobacter. *J. clin. Path.* **33**, 1122.

Slack, J. M. & Gerencser, M. A. (1975). *Actinomyces, filamentous bacteria: Biology and Pathogenicity.* Minneapolis, Minnesota: Burgess Publishing Co.

Slotnick, I. J. & Dougherty, M. (1964). Further characterization of an unclassified group of bacteria causing endocarditis in man: *Cardiobacterium hominis* gen. et sp. n. *Antonie van Leeuwenhoek* **30**, 261.

Smith, D. G. & Shattock, P. M. F. (1962). The serological grouping of *Streptococcus equinus. J. gen. Microbiol.* **29,** 731.

Smith, F. R. & Sherman, J. M. (1938). The hemolytic streptococci of human feces. *J. inf. Dis.* **62,** 186.

Smith, G. R. (1961). The characteristics of two types of *Pasteurella haemolytica* associated with different pathological conditions in sheep. *J. Path. Bact.* **81,** 431.

Smith, I. W. (1963). The classification of 'Bacterium salmonicida'. *J. gen. Microbiol.* **33**, 263.

Smith, J. E. & Thal, E. (1965). A taxonomic study of the genus *Pasteurella* using a numerical technique. *Acta path. microbiol. scand.* **64**, 213.

Smith, L. DS. (1977). *Botulism. The organism, its toxins, the disease.* Springfield: Thomas.

Smith, L. DS. & King, E. O. (1962). Occurrence of *Clostridium difficile* in infections of man. *J. Bact.* **84**, 65.

Smith, M. G. (1982). A simple disc technique for the pre-sumptive identification of *Legionella pneumophila. J. clin. Path.* **35**, 1353.

Smith, M. L. (1932). The effect of heat on sugar solutions used for culture media. *Biochem. J.* **26**, 1467.

Smith, N. R., Gordon, R. E. & Clark, F. E. (1946). Aerobic mesophilic sporeforming bacteria. Misc. Publ. no. 559. Washington, D.C.: U.S. Dep. Agriculture.

Smith, N. R., Gordon, R. E. & Clark, F. E. (1952). Aerobic sporeforming bacteria. Monograph no. 16. Washington, D. C.: U.S. Dep. Agriculture

Smith, R. F. (1969). A medium for the study of the ecology of human cutaneous diphtheroids. *J. gen. Microbiol.* **57**, 411.

Smith, R. F. (1979). Comparison of two media for isolation of *Haemophilus vaginalis. J. clin. Microbiol.* **9**, 729.

Smith, R. F., Rogers, R. R. & Bettge, C. L. (1972). Inhibition of the indole test reaction by sodium nitrite. *Appl. Microbiol.* **23**, 423.

Sneath, P. H. A. (1956). Cultural and biochemical characteristics of the genus *Chromobacterium. J. gen. Microbiol.* **15**, 70.

Sneath, P. H. A. (1957a). Some thoughts on bacterial classification. *J. gen. Microbiol.* **17**, 184.

Sneath, P. H. A. (1957b). The application of computers to taxonomy. *J. gen. Microbiol.* **17**, 201.

Sneath, P. H. A. (1960). A study of the bacterial genus *Chromobacterium. Iowa St. J. Sci.* **34**, 243.

Sneath, P. H. A. (1972). Computer taxonomy. In *Methods in Microbiology,* vol. 7A. (ed. J. R. Norris & D. W. Ribbons). p. 29. London: Academic Press.

Sneath, P. H. A. (1974). Test reproducibility in relation to identification. *Int. J. syst. Bact.* **24**, 508.

Sneath, P. H. A. (1978). Identification of microorganisms. In *Essays in Microbiology 10* (ed. J. R. Norris & M. A. Richmond), p. 1. Chichester: John Wiley.

Sneath, P. H. A. (1979a). Basic program for identification of an unknown with presence-absence data against an identification matrix of percent positive characters. *Comp. Geosci.* **5**, 195.

Sneath, P. H. A. (1979b). Basic program for character separation indices from an identification matrix of percent positive characters. *Comp. Geosci.* **5**, 349.

Sneath, P. H. A. (1980a). Basic program for the most diagnostic properties of groups from an identification matrix of percent positive characters. *Comp. Geosci.* **6**, 21.

Sneath, P. H. A. (1980b). Basic program for determining the best identification scores possible from the most typical examples when compared with an identification matrix of percent positive characters. *Comp. Geosci.* **6**, 27.

Sneath, P. H. A. (1980c). Basic program for determining overlap between groups in an identification matrix of percent positive characters. *Comp. Geosci.* **6**, 267.

Sneath, P. H. A. & Collins, V.G. (1974). A study in test reproducibility between laboratories: Report of a Pseudomonas working party. *Antonie van Leeuwenhoek.* **40**, 481.

Sneath, P. H. A. & Cowan, S. T. (1958). An electrotaxonomic survey of bacteria. *J. gen. Microbiol.* **19**, 551

Sneath, P. H. A. & Johnson, R. (1972). The influence on numerical taxonomic similarities of errors in microbiological tests. *J. gen. Microbiol.* **72**, 377.

Sneath, P. H. A. & Johnson, R. (1973). Numerical taxonomy of *Haemophilus* and related bacteria. *Int. J. syst. Bact.* **23**, 405.

Snell, J. J. S. (1973). The distribution and identification of non-fermenting bacteria. *Publ. Hlth Lab. Serv. Techn. Mon.* no. 4. London: HMSO.

Snell, J. J. S. (1984a). Maintenance of bacteria in gelatin discs. In *Maintenance of Microorganisms: a Manual of Laboratory Methods* (ed B. E. Kirsop & J. J. S. Snell), p.41. London: Academic Press.

Snell, J. J. S. (1984b). General introduction to maintenance methods. In *Maintenance of Microorganisms: a Manual of Laboratory Methods* (ed B. E. Kirsop & J. J. S. Snell), p.11. London: Academic Press.

Snell, J. J. S. (1984c). United Kingdom national external quality assessment scheme for microbiology. *Eur. J. clin. Microbiol.* **4**, 464.

Snell, J. J. S. & Davey, P. (1971). A comparison of methods for the detection of phenylalanine deamination by Moraxella species. *J. gen. Microbiol.* **66**, 371.

Snell, J. J. S. & Lapage, S. P. (1971). Comparison of four methods for demonstrating glucose breakdown by bacteria. *J. gen. Microbiol.* **68**, 221.

Snell, J. J. S. & Lapage, S. P. (1973). Carbon source utilization tests as an aid to the classification of nonfermenting Gram-negative bacteria. *J. gen. Microbiol.* **74**, 9.

Snell, J. J. S. & Lapage, S. P. (1976). Transfer of some saccharolytic *Moraxella species to Kingella* Henriksen and Bøvre 1976, with descriptions of *Kingella indologenes* sp. nov. and *Kingella denitrificans* sp. nov. *Int. J. syst. Bact.* **26**, 451.

Snell, J. J. S., DeMello, J. V. & Gardner, P. S. (1982). The United Kingdom national microbiological quality assessment scheme. *J. clin. Path.* **35**, 82.

Snell, J. J. S., DeMello, J. V. & Phua, T. J. (1986). Errors in bacteriological techniques: results from the United Kingdom national external quality assessment scheme for microbiology. *Med. Lab. Sciences* **43**, 344.

Snell, J. J. S., Hill, L. R., Lapage, S. P. & Curtis, M. A. (1972). Identification of *Pseudomonas cepacia* Burkholder and its synonymy with *Pseudomonas kingii* Jonsson. *Int. J. syst. Bact.* **22**, 127.

Sokal, R. R. (1965). Statistical methods in systematics. *Biol. Rev.* **40**, 337.

Soltys, M. A. (1948). Anthrax in a laboratory worker, with observations on the possible source of infection. *J. Path. Bact.* **60**, 253.

Sottnek, F. O. & Albritton, W. L. (1984). *Haemophilus infuenzae* biotype VIII. *J. clin. Microbiol.* **20**, 815.

Spicer, C. C. (1956). A quick method of identifying Salmonella H antigens. *J. clin. Path.* **9**, 378.

Spiegel, C. A. & Roberts, M. (1984). *Mobiluncus* gen. nov., *Mobiluncus curtisii* subsp. *curtisii* sp. nov., *Mobiluncus curtisii* subsp. *holmesii* subsp. nov., and *Mobiluncus mulieris* sp. nov., curved rods from the human vagina. *Int. J. syst. Bact.* **34**, 177.

Spray, R. S. & Johnson, E. J. (1946). The preparation of Loeffler's serum and similar coagulable mediums. *J. Bact.* **52**, 141.

Stableforth, A. W. & Jones, L. M. (1963). Report of the Subcommittee on taxonomy of the genus *Brucella*. *Int. Bull. bact. Nomencl. Taxon.* **13**, 145.

Stackebrandt, E. & Woese, C. R. (1981). The evolution of prokaryotes. In *Molecular and cellular aspects of microbial evolution* (ed. M. J. Carlisle, J. F. Collins & B. E. B. Moseley), *Symp. Soc. gen. Microbiol.* No. **32**, 1.

Stackebrandt, E. & Woese, C. R. (1979). A phylogenetic dissection of the family Micrococcaceae. *Curr. Microbiol.* **2**, 317.

Stackebrandt, E., Wittek, B., Seewaldt, E. & Schleifer, K.H. (1982). Physiological, biochemical and phylogenetic studies on *Gemella haemolysans*. *FEMS Microbiol. Lett.* **13**, 361.

Stanford, J. L., Pattyn, S. R., Portaels, F. & Gunthorpe, W. J. (1972). Studies on *Mycobacterium chelonei*. *J. med. Microbiol.* **5**, 177.

Stanier, R. Y., Palleroni, N. J. & Doudoroff, M. (1966). The aerobic pseudomonads: a taxonomic study. *J. gen. Microbiol.* **43**, 159.

Starr, M. P. & Mandel, M. (1969). DNA base composition and taxonomy of phytopathogenic and other enterobacteria. *J. gen. Microbiol.* **56**, 113.

Steel, K. J. (1958). A note on the assay of some sulphydryl compounds. *J. Pharm. Pharmac.* **10**, 574.

Steel, K. J. (1961). The oxidase reaction as a taxonomic tool. *J. gen. Microbiol.* **25**, 297.

Steel, K. J. (1962a). The practice of bacterial identification. *Symp. Soc. gen. Microbiol.* **12**, 405.

Steel, K. J. (1962b). The oxidase activity of *staphylococci*. *J. appl. Bact.* **25**, 445.

Steel, K. J. (1963). Serological classification of *Pasteurella pseudotuberculosis* and *Pasteurella septica*. *Mon. Bull. Minist. Hlth Lab. Serv.* **22**, 176.

310

Steel, K. J. (1965). Microbial identification. *J. gen. Microbiol.* **40**, 143.

Steel, K. J. (1964). *Micrococcus violagabriellae* Castellani. *J. gen. Microbiol.* **36**, 133.

Steel, K. J. & Cowan, S. T. (1964). Le rattachement de *Bacterium anitratum, Moraxella lwoffi, Bacillus mallei* et *Haemophilus parapertussis* au genre *Acinetobacter* Brisou et Prévot. *Annls Inst. Pasteur, Paris* **106**, 479.

Steel, K. J. & Fisher, P. J. (1961). A fallacy of the nitrate reduction test. *Mon. Bull. Minist. Hlth Lab. Serv.* **20**, 63.

Steele, K. J. & Midgley, J. (1962). Decarboxylase and other reactions of some Gram-negative rods. *J. gen. Microbiol.* **29**, 171.

Steele, T. W. & Owen, R. J. (1988). *Campylobacter jejuni* subsp. *doylei* subsp. nov., a subspecies of nitrate-negative campylobacters isolated from human clinical specimens. *Int. J. syst. Bact.* **38**, 316.

Sterne, M. & Warrack, G. H. (1964). The types of *Clostridium perfringens. J. Path. Bact.* **88**, 279.

Sterzik, B. & Fehrenbach, F. J. (1985). Reaction components influencing CAMP factor induced lysis. *J. gen. Microbiol.* **131**, 817.

Stevens, M. (1980). Computer assisted bacterial identification. *Med. Lab. Sciences* **37**, 223.

Stewart, D. J. (1965). The urease activity of fluorescent pseudomonads. *J. gen. Microbiol.* **41**, 169.

Stokes, E. J. & Ridgway, G. L. (1980). *Clinical Bacteriology*, 5th edn. London: Edward Arnold.

Stonebrink, B.. (1961). A new medium for the cultivation of *Mycobacterium tuberculosis. Select. Pap. R. Neth. Tuberculosis Ass.* **2**, 1.

Stuart, C. A., Formal, S. & McGann, V. (1949). Further studies on B5W, an anaerogenic group in the Enterobacteriaceae. *J. infect. Dis.* **84**, 235.

Stuart, C. A. & Rustigian, R. (1943*a*). Further studies on one type of paracolon organism. *Am. J. publ. Hlth,* **33**, 1323.

Stuart, C. A. & Rustigian, R. (1943*b*). Further studies on the Eijkman reactions of Shigella cultures. *J. Bact.* **46**, 105.

Stuart, C. A., van Stratum, E. & Rustigian, R. (1945). Further studies on urease production by Proteus and related organisms. *J. Bact.* **49**, 437.

Stuart, C. A., Wheeler, K. M. & McGann, V. (1946). Further studies on one anaerogenic paracolon organism, type 29911. *J. Bact.* **52**, 431.

Stuart, M. R. & Pease, P. E. (1972). A numerical study on the relationships of *Listeria* and *Erysipelothrix. J. gen. Microbiol.* **73**, 551.

Stuart, R. D. (1959). Transport medium for specimens in public health bacteriology. *Publ. Hlth Rep., Wash.* **74**, 431 .

Stumbo, C. R. (1973). Death of bacteria subjected to moist heat. In *Thermobacteriology in food processing*, 2nd edn, (ed. C. R. Stumbo), p. 70. New York & London: Academic Press.

Sturm, A. W. (1986). Isolation of *Haemophilus influenzae* and *Haemophilus parainfluenzae* from genital-tract specimens with a selective culture medium. *J. med. Microbiol.* **21**, 349.

Subcommittee on Taxonomy of staphylococci and micrococci [of the International Committee on Bacteriological Nomenclature] (1965). Recommendations. *Int. Bull. bact. Nomencl. Taxon.* **15**, 109. (1976). Minutes and Appendix. *Int. J. syst. Bact.* **26**, 323.

Sulkin, S. E. & Willett, J. C. (1940). A triple sugar-ferrous sulfate medium for use in identification of enteric organisms. *J. Lab. clin. Med.* **25**, 649.

Sutter, V. L. & Foecking, F. J. (1962). Biochemical characteristics of lactose-fermenting *Proteus rettgeri* from clinical specimens. *J. Bact.* **83**, 933.

Sutter, V. L., Citron, D. M. & Finegold, S. M. (1980). *Wadsworth Anaerobic Bacteriology Manual*, 3rd edn. St. Louis: C.V. Mosby Company.

Swan, A. (1954). The use of a bile-aesculin medium and of Maxted's technique of Lancefield grouping in the identification of enterococci (group D streptococci). *J. clin. Path.* **7**, 160.

Swann, R. A., Foulkes, S. J., Holmes, B., Young, J. B., Mitchell, R. G. & Reeders, S. T. (1985). 'Agrobacterium yellow group' and *Pseudomonas paucimobilis* causing peritonitis in patients receiving continuous ambulatory peritoneal dialysis. *J. clin. Path.* **38**, 1293.

Szturm-Rubinsten, S. (1963). Les biotypes de *Shigella sonnei. Annls Inst. Pasteur, Paris* **104**, 423.

Szturm-Rubinsten, S. & Piéchaud, D. (1963). Observations sur la recherche de la β-galactosidase dans le genre *Shigella. Annls Inst. Pasteur, Paris* **104**, 284.

Takahashi, T., Fujisawa, T., Benno, Y., Tamura, Y., Sawada, T., Suzuki, S., Muramatsu, M. & Mitsuoka, T. (1987). *Erysipelothrix tonsillarum* sp. nov. isolated from tonsils of apparently healthy pigs. *Int. J. syst. Bact.* **37**, 166.

Talley, A. J. (1968). Bacteriophage for the recognition of Salmonella and Arizona. *Am. J. med. Technol.* **34**, 542.

Talon, R., Grimont, P.A.D., Grimont, F., Gasser, F. & Boeufgras, J.M. (1988). *Brochothrix campestris* sp.nov. *Int. J. syst. Bact.* **38**, 99.

Tamaoka, J., Ha, D.-M. & Komagata, K. (1987). Reclassification of *Pseudomonas acidovorans* den Dooren de Jong 1926 and *Pseudomonas testosteroni* Marcus and Talalay 1956 as *Comamonas acidovorans* comb. nov. and *Comamonas testosteroni* comb. nov., with an emended description of the genus *Comamonas*. *Int. J. syst. Bact.* **37**, 52.

Tamura, K., Sakazaki, R., Kosako, Y. & Yoshizaki, E. (1986). *Leclercia adecarboxylata* gen. nov., comb. nov., formerly known as *Escherichia adecarboxylata*. *Curr. Microbiol.* **13**, 179.

Tanner, A. C. R., Badger, S., Lai, C.-H., Listgarten, M. A., Visconti, R. A. & Socransky, S.S. (1981). *Wolinella* gen. nov., *Wolinella succinogenes* (*Vibrio succinogenes* Wolin *et al.*) comb. nov., and description of *Bacteroides gracilis* sp. nov., *Wolinella recta* sp. nov., *Campylobacter concisus* sp. nov., and *Eikenella corrodens* from humans with periodontal disease. *Int. J. syst. Bact.* **31**, 432.

Tanner, A. C. R., Listgarten, M. A. & Ebersole, J. L. (1984). *Wolinella curva* sp. nov.: '*Vibrio succinogenes*' of human origin. *Int. J. syst. Bact.* **34**, 275.

Tapsall, J. W. (1987). Pigment production by Lancefield-group B streptococci (*Streptococcus agalactiae*). *J. med. Microbiol.* **21**, 75.

Targowski, S. & Targowski, X. (1979). Characterisation of a *Haemophilus paracuniculus* isolated from gastrointestinal tracts of rabbits with mucoid enteritis. *J. clin. Microbiol.* **9**, 33.

Tarrand, J. J. & Gröschel, D. H. M. (1982). Rapid, modified oxidase test for oxidase-variable bacterial isolates. *J. clin. Microbiol.* **16**, 772.

Taylor, C. B. (1945-6). The effect of temperature of incubation on the results of tests for differentiating species of coliform bacteria. *J. Hyg., Camb.* **44**, 109.

Taylor, C. B. (1951). The soft-rot bacteria of the coli-aerogenes group. *Proc. Soc. appl. Bact.* **14**, 95.

Taylor, C. E. D., Lea, D. J., Heimer, G . V. & Tomlinson, A. J. H. (1964). A comparison of a fluorescent antibody technique with a cultural method in the detection of infections with *Shigella sonnei*. *J. clin. Path.* **17**, 225.

Taylor, C. E. D., Rosenthal, R. O., Brown, D. F. J., Lapage, S.P., Hill, L. R. & Legros, R. M. (1978). The causative organism of contagious equine metritis 1977: Proposal for a new species to be known as *Haemophilus equigenitalis*. *Equine vet. J.* **10**, 136.

Taylor, D. N., Kiehlbauch, J. A., Tee, W., Pitarangsi, C. & Echeveria, P. (1991). Isolation of Group 2 aero-tolerant *Campylobacter* species from Thai children with diarrhoea. *J. inf. Dis.* **163**, 1062.

Taylor, E. & Phillips, I. (1983). The identification of *Gardnerella vaginalis*. *J. med. Microbiol.* **16**, 83.

Taylor, J. A. & Barrow, G. I. (1981). A non-pathogenic vibrio for routine quality control of TCBS cholera medium. *J. clin. Path.* **34**, 208.

Taylor, J. A., Miller, D. C., Barrow, G. I., Cann, D. C. & Taylor, L. Y, (1982). The isolation and identification of *Vibrio parahaemolyticus*. In *Isolation and Identification Methods for Food Poisoning Organisms* (ed. J. E. L. Corry, D. Roberts & F. A. Skinner), p. 287. (Society for Applied Bacteriology Technical Series no. 17). London: Academic Press.

Taylor-Robinson, D. (1983). Recovery of mycoplasmas from the genitourinary tract. In *Methods in Mycoplasmology*, vol. 2 (ed. J. G. Tully & S. Razin), p. 19. New York: Academic Press.

Tazir, M., David, H. L. & Boulahbal, F. (1979). Evaluation of the chloride and bromide salts of cetylpyridinium for the transportation of sputum in tuberculosis bacteriology. *Tubercle* **60**, 31.

Tebbutt, G. M. (1983). Evaluation of some methods for the laboratory identification of *Haemophilus influenzae*. *J. clin. Path.* **36**, 991.

Tee, W., Baird, R., Dyall-Smith, M. & Dwyer, B. (1988). *Campylobacter cryaerophila* isolated from a human. *J. clin. Microbiol.* **26**, 2469.

Thacker, W. L., Benson, R. F., Schifman, R. B., Pugh, E., Steigerwalt, A. G., Mayberry, W. R., Brenner, D. J. & Wilkinson, H. W. (1989). *Legionella tucsonensis* sp. nov. isolated from a renal transplant recipient. *J. clin. Microbiol.* **27**, 1831.

Thiércelin, E. & Jouhaud, L. (1903). Reproduction de l'entercoque: taches centrales: granulations peripheriques et microblastes. *C.R. Seanc. Soc. Biol., Paris* **55**, 686.

Thirst, M. L. (1957*a*). Hippurate hydrolysis in Klebsiella-Cloaca classification. *J. gen. Microbiol.* **17**, 390.

Thirst, M. L. (1957*b*). Gelatin liquefaction – a microtest. *J. gen. Microbiol.* **17**, 396.

Thjøtta, Th. (1920). On the bacillus of Morgan No. 1 - a metacolon-bacillus. *J. Bact.* **5**, 67.

Thjøtta, Th. & Bøe, J. (1938). *Neisseria hemolysans*. A hemolytic species of *Neisseria* Trevisan. *Acta path. microbiol. Scand.* Suppl. **37**, 527.

Thom, A. R., Stephens, M. E., Gillespie, W. A. & Alder, V. G. (1971). Nitrofurantin media for the isolation of *Pseudomonas aeruginosa*. *J. appl. Bact.* **34**, 611.

Thomas, G. M. & Poinar, G. O. Jr. (1979). *Xenorhabdus* gen. nov., a genus of enteropathogenic, nematophilic bacteria of the family *Enterobacteriaceae*. *Int. J. syst. Bact.* **29**, 352.

Thompson, L. M., Smibert, R. M., Johnson, J. L. & Krieg, N. R. (1988). Phylogenetic study of the genus *Campylobacter*. *Int. J. syst. Bact.* **38**, 190.

Thompson, R. E. M. & Knudsen, A. (1958). A reliable fermentation medium for *Neisseria gonorrhoeae:* a comparative study. *J. Path. Bact.* **76**, 501.

Thornley, M. J. (1960). The differentiation of *Pseudomonas* from other Gram-negative bacteria on the basis of arginine metabolism. *J. appl. Bact.* **23**, 37.

Thornley, M. J. (1967). A taxonomic study of *Acinetobacter* and related genera. *J. gen. Microbiol.* **49**, 211.

Threlfall, E. J., Hall, M. L. M. & Rowe, B. (1983). Lactose-fermenting salmonellae in Britain. *FEMS Microbiol. Lett.* **17**, 127.

Tison, D. L. & Kelly, M. T. (1984). *Vibrio* species of medical importance. *Diagnostic Microbiol. inf. Dis.* **2**, 263.

Tittsler, R. P. (1938). The fermentation of acetylmethylcarbinol by the Escherichia-Aerobacter group and its significance in the Voges-Proskaüer reaction. *J. Bact.* **35**, 157.

Tittsler, R. P. & Sandholzer, L. A. (1936). The use of semisolid agar for the detection of bacterial motility. *J. Bact.* **31**, 575.

Todd, E. W. & Hewitt, L. F. (1932). A new culture medium for the production of antigenic streptococcal haemolysin. *J. Path. Bact.* **35**, 973.

Topley & Wilson's Principles of Bacteriology and Immunity. Eight edns: **1**, 1929; **2**, 1936; **3**, 1946; **4**, 1955; **5**, 1964; **6**, 1975; **7**, 1983; **8**, 1990 [*Bacteriology, Virology and Immunity*], 5 volumes (ed. M. T. Parker & L. H. Collier). London: Edward Arnold.

Totten, P. A., Amsel, R., Hale, J., Piot, P. & Holmes, K. K. (1982). Selective differential human blood bilayer media for isolation of *Gardnerella* (*Haemophilus*) *vaginalis*. *J. clin. Microbiol.* **15**, 141.

Totten, P. A., Holmes, K. K., Handsfield, H. H., Knapp, J. S., Perine, P. & Falkow, S. (1983). DNA hybridization technique for the detection of *Neisseria gonorrhoeae* in men with urethritis. *J. inf. Dis.* **148**, 462.

Totten, P. A., Fennell, C. L., Tenover, F. C., Wezenberg, J. M., Perine, P. L., Stamm, W. E. & Holmes, K. K. (1985). *Campylobacter cinaedi* (sp. nov.) and *Campylobacter fennelliae* (sp. nov.): two new *Campylobacter* species associated with enteric disease in homosexual men. *J. inf. Dis.* **151**, 131.

Traub, W. H. (1980). Bacteriocin and phage typing of *Serratia*. In *The Genus Serratia* (ed. A. von Graevenitz & S. J. Rubin), p. 79. Boca Raton, Florida: CRC Press.

Traub, W. H. (1985). Serotyping of *Serratia marcescens*: identification of a new O-antigen (O24). *Zbl. Bakt. Hyg.* A**259**, 485.

Tucker, D. N., Slotnick, I. J., King, E. O., Tynes, B., Nicholson, J. & Crevasse, L. (1962). Endocarditis caused by a Pasteurella-like organism. Report of four cases. *New Engl. J. Med.* **267**, 913.

Tulloch, W. J. (1939). Observations concerning bacillary food infection in Dundee during the period 1923-38. *J. Hyg., Camb.* **39**, 324.

Turk, D. C. (1963). Naso-pharyngeal carriage of *Haemophilus influenzae* type b. *J. Hyg., Camb.* **61**, 247.

Turner, G. C. (1961). Cultivation of *Bordetella pertussis* on agar media. *J. Path. Bact.* **81**, 15.

Tønjum, T., Bukholm, G. & Bøvre, K. (1990). Identification of *Haemophilus aphrophilus* and *Actinobacillus actinomycetemcomitans* by DNA – DNA hybridization and genetic transformation. *J. clin. Microbiol.* **28**, 1994.

Ulrich, J. A. (1944). New indicators to replace litmus in milk. *Science, N. Y.*, **99**, 352.

Ursing, J., Brenner, D. J., Bercovier, H., Fanning, G. R., Steigerwalt, A. G. Brault, J. & Mollaret, H.H. (1980). *Yersinia frederiksenii*: a new species of *Enterobacteriaceae* composed of rhamnose-positive strains (formerly called atypical *Yersinia enterocolitica* or *Yersinia enterocolitica*-like). *Curr. Microbiol.* **4**, 213.

Ursing, J., Steigerwalt, A. G. & Brenner, D. J. (1980). Lack of genetic relatedness between *Yersinia philomiragia* (the 'philomiragia' bacterium) and *Yersinia* species. *Curr. Microbiol.* **4**, 231.

Van der Auwera, P. (1985). Clinical significance of *Streptococcus milleri*. *Eur. J. clin. Microbiol.* **4**, 386.

Valder, J., Schindler, J. & Matusek, J. (1987). VEX – an expert system for microcomputer in the identification of bacteria. *2nd Conference on Taxonomy and Automatic Identification of Bacteria, Prague, Czechoslovakia*, Abstract 109.

Vandamme, P., Falsen, E., Rossau, R., Hoste, B., Seegers, P., Tygat, R. & DeLey, J. (1991). Revision of *Campylobacter, Helicobacter* and *Wolinella* taxonomy: emendation of generic descriptions and proposal of *Arcobacter* gen. nov. *Int. J. syst. Bact.* **41**, 88.

van Loghen, J. J. (1944–5). The classification of the plague-bacillus. *Antonie van Leeuwenhoek* **10**, 15.

Varney, P. L. (1961). A new closure for bacteriologic culture tubes. *Am. J. clin. Path.* **35**, 475.

Vaughn, R. H., Osborne, J. T., Wedding, G. T., Tabachnick, J., Beisel, C. G. & Braxton, T. (1950). The utilization of citrate by *Escherichia coli*. *J. Bact.* **60**, 119.

Vedros, N. A. (1978). Serology of the meningococcus. In *Methods in Microbiology*, vol. 10 (ed. T. Bergan & J. R. Norris), p. 293. London: Academic Press.

Vendrely, R. (1958). La notion d'espèce bactérienne à la lumière des découvertes récentes. La notion d'espèce a travers quelques données biochimiques récentes et le cycle L. *Annls Inst Pasteur, Paris* **94**, 142.

Vera, H. D. (1971). Quality control in diagnostic microbiology. *Hlth Lab. Sci.* **8**, 176.

Verger, J.-M., Grimont, F., Grimont, P. A. D. & Grayon, M. (1985). *Brucella*, a monospecific genus as shown by deoxyribonucleic acid hybridization. *Int. J. syst. Bact.* **35**, 292.

Véron, M. (1966). Taxonomie numérique des vibrions et de certaines bactéries comparables. II. - Corrélation entre similitudes phénétiques et la composition en bases de l'ADN. *Annls Inst. Pasteur, Paris*, **111**, 671 .

Véron, M. & Chatelain, R. (1973). Taxonomic study of the genus *Campylobacter* Sebald and Véron and designation of the neotype strain for the type species, *Campylobacter fetus* (Smith and Taylor) Sebald and Véron. *Int. J. syst. Bact.* **23**, 122.

Vesey, G., Dennis, P. J., Lee, J. V. & West, A. A. (1988). Further development of simple tests to differentiate the legionellas. *J. appl. Bact.* **65**, 339.

Vörös, S. (1969). Les nucléases exocellulaires chez les bactéries Gram négatives en particulier les Enterobacteriaceae. *Annls Inst. Pasteur, Paris*, **116**, 292.

Vörös, S., Angyal, T., Németh, V. & Kontrohr, T. (1961). The occurrence and significance of phosphatase in enteric bacteria. *Acta microbiol. Hung.* **8**, 405.

Voss, J. G. (1970). Differentiation of two groups of *Corynebacterium acnes. J. Bact.* **101**, 392.

Walker, P. D. & Wolf, J. (1971). The taxonomy of *Bacillus stearothermophilus*. In *Spore Research,* (Ed. A. N. Barker, G. W. Gould & J. Wolf) p. 247. London: Academic Press.

Waterworth, P. M. (1980). An evaluation of the replireader in the identification of enterobacteriaceae isolated from urine and in the recording of sensitivity tests performed by an agar dilution method. *J. clin. Path.* **33**, 571.

Watkins, I. D., Tobin, J. O'H., Dennis, P. J., Brown, W., Newnham, R. S. & Kurtz, J. B. (1985). *Legionella pneumophila* serogroup 1 subgrouping by monoclonal antibodies - an epidemiological tool. *J. Hyg., Camb.* **95**, 211.

Wauters, G., Janssens, M., Steigerwalt, A. G. & Brenner, D. J. (1988). *Yersinia mollaretii* sp. nov. and *Yersinia bercovieri* sp. nov., formerly called *Yersinia enterocolitica* biogroups 3A and 3B. *Int. J. syst. Bact.* **38**, 424.

Watt, B. & Brown, F. V. (1983). The *in-vitro* activity of bicozamycin against anaerobic bacteria of clinical interest. *J. antimicrob. Chemother.* **12**, 549.

Watt, B. & Jack, E. P. (1977). What are anaerobic cocci? *J. med. Microbiol.* **10**, 461.

Watt, B., Bushell, A. C. & Wallace, E. T. (1984). Characterization of anaerobic cocci in the diagnostic laboratory. *J. clin. Path.* **37**, 1197.

Watt, B., Wallace, E.T. & Bushell, A. C. (1986). Characterization of anaerobic cocci. In *Anaerobic bacteria in habitats other than man* (ed. E. M. Barnes & G. C. Mead), p. 61. Society for Applied Bacteriology Symposium No. 13. London: Blackwell Scientific Publications.

Wayne, L. G. (1962). Differentiation of mycobacteria by their effect on Tween 80. *Am. Rev. resp. Dis.* **86**, 579.

Wayne, L. G., Brenner, D. J., Colwell, R. R., Grimont, P. A. D., Kandler, O., Krichevsky, M. I., Moore, L. H., Moore, W. E. C., Murray, R. G. E., Starr, M. P.& Truper, H. G. (1987). Report of the ad hoc committee on reconciliation of approaches to bacterial systematics. *Int. J. syst. Bact.* **37,** 463.

Wayne, L. G., Krichevsky, E. J., Love, L. L., Johnson, R. & Krichevsky, M. I. (1980). Taxonomic probability matrix for use with slow growing mycobacteria. *Int. J. syst. Bact.* **30**, 528.

Weaver, R. E. & Feeley, R. M. (1979). Cultural and biochemical characterization of the Legionnaire's disease bacterium. In *Legionnaire's: the Disease, the Bacterium and the Methodology* (ed. G. L. Jones & G. A. Hébert), p. 19. Atlanta, Georgia: Centers for Disease Control.

Weaver, R. E., Tatum, H. W. & Hollis, D. G. (1972). Revision of King, E. O. (1964). Atlanta, Georgia: Center for Disease Control.

Werkman, C. H. & Gillen, G. F. (1932). Bacteria producing trimethylene glycol. *J. Bact.* **23**, 167.

Wertlake, P. T. & Williams, T. W. (1968). Septicaemia caused by *Neisseria flavescens. J. clin. Path.* **21**, 437.

Wessman, G. E. (1986). Biology of the group E streptococci: a review. *Vet. Microbiol.* **12**, 297.

Wetmore, P. & Gochenour, W. S., Jr (1956). Comparative studies of the genus *Malleomyces* and selected *Pseudomonas* species. I. Morphological and cultural characteristics. *J. Bact.* **72**, 79.

Wetmore, P. W., Thiel, J. F., Herman, Y. F. & Harr, J. R. (1963). Comparison of selected *Actinobacillus* species with a hemolytic variety of *Actinobacillus* from irradiated swine. *J. infect. Dis.* **113**, 186.

White, D. C. & Garrick, S. (1963). Hemin biosynthesis in *Haemophilus. J. Bact.* **85**, 842.

White, J. N. & Starr, M. (1971). Glucose fermentation endproducts of *Erwinia* spp. and other enterobacteria. *J. appl. Bact.* **34**, 459.

White, M. L. & Pickett, M. J. (1953). A rapid phosphatase test for *Micrococcus pyogenes* var. *aureus* for detection of potentially pathogentic strains. *Am. J. clin. Path.* **23**, 1181.

White, T. G. & Shuman, R. D. (1961). Fermentation reactions of *Erysipelothrix rhusiopathiae. J. Bact.,* **82**, 595.

Whittenbury, R. (1963). The use of soft agar in the study of conditions affecting the utilization of fermentable substrates by lactic acid bacteria. *J. gen. Microbiol.* **32**, 375.

Whittenbury, R. (1964). Hydrogen peroxide formation and catalase activity in the lactic acid bacteria. *J. gen. Microbiol.* **35**, 13.

Whittenbury, R. (1965a). The differentiation of *Streptococcus faecalis* and *S. faecium. J. gen. Microbiol.* **38**, 279.

Whittenbury, R. (1965*b*). A study of some pediococci and their relationship to *Aerococcus viridans* and the enterococci. *J. gen. Microbiol.* **40**, 97.

Wideman, P. A., Vargo, V. L., Citronbaum, D. & Finegold, S. M. (1976). Evaluation of the sodium polyanethol sulfonate disk test for the identification of *Peptostreptococcus anaerobius. J. clin. Microbiol.* **4**, 330.

Wildhack, W. A. & Stern, J. (1958). The Peek-a-boo system - optical coincidence subject cards in information searching. In *Punched Cards: their Applications to Science and Industry*, 2 edn. (ed. R. S. Casey, J. W. Perry, M. M. Berry & A. Kent), p. 125. New York: Reinhold Publ. Corp.

Wilfert, J. N., Barrett, F. F., Ewing, W. H., Finland, M. & Kass, E. H. (1970). *Serratia marcescens*: biochemical, serological, and epidemiological characteristics and antibiotic susceptibility of strains isolated at Boston City Hospital. *Appl. Microbiol.* **19**, 345.

Willcox, W. R., Lapage, S. P. & Holmes, B. (1980). A review of numerical methods in bacterial identification. *Ant. van Leeuwenhoek* **46**, 233.

Wilkinson, A. E. (1962). Notes on the bacteriological diagnosis of gonorrhoea. *Br. J. vener. Dis.* **38**,145.

Wilkinson, H. W., Drasar, V., Thacker, W. L., Benson, R. F., Schindler, J., Potuznikova, B., Mayberry, W. R. & Brenner, D. J. (1988). *Legionella moravica* sp. nov. and *Legionella brunensis* sp. nov. isolated from cooling-tower water. *Annls Inst. Pasteur, Paris* **139**, 393.

Wilkinson, H. W., Thacker, W. L., Benson, R. F., Polt, S.S. Brookings, E., Mayberry, W. R., Brenner, D. J., Gilley, R. G. & Kirklin, J. K. (1987). *Legionella birminghamensis* sp. nov. isolated from a cardiac transplant recipient. *J. clin. Microbiol.* **25**, 2120.

Williams, J. E. (1983). Warnings on a potential for laboratory-acquired infections as a result of the new nomenclature for the plague bacillus. *Bull. Wld Hlth Org.* **61**, 545.

Williams, O. B. & Morrow, M. B. (1928). The bacterial destruction of acetyl-methyl-carbinol. *J. Bact.* **16**, 43.

Williams, R. E. O. (1958). Laboratory diagnosis of streptococcal infections. *Bull. Wld Hlth Org.* **19**, 153.

Williams, R. E. O. & Harper, G. J. (1946). Determination of coagulase and alpha-haemolysin production by staphylococci. *Br. J. exp. Path.* **27**, 72.

Williams, R. E. O. & Hirch, A. (1950). The detection of streptococci in air. *J. Hyg., Camb.* **48**, 504.

Williams, R. E. O., Hirch, A. & Cowan, S. T. (1953). *Aerococcus,* a new bacterial genus. *J. gen. Microbiol.* **8**, 475.

Williams, S. T. & Davies, F. L. (1967). Use of a scanning electron microscope for the examination of actinomycetes. *J. gen. Microbiol.* **48**, 171.

Williams, S. T., Goodfellow, M., Wellington, E. M. H., Vickers, J. C., Alderson, G., Sneath, P. H. A., Sackin, M. J. & Mortimer, A. M. (1983). A probability matrix for identification of some streptomycetes. *J. gen. Microbiol.* **129**, 1815.

Williamson, D. H. & Wilkinson, J. F. (1958). The isolation and estimation of the poly-β-hydroxybutyrate inclusions of *Bacillus* species. *J. gen. Microbiol.* **19**, 198.

Willis, A. T. (1960). The lipolytic activity of some clostridia. *J. Path. Bact.* **80**, 379.

Willis, A. T. (1962). Some diagnostic reactions of clostridia. *Lab. Pract.* **11**, 526.

Willis, A. T. (1964). *Anaerobic Bacteriology in Clinical Medicine*, 2 edn. London: Butterworths.

Willis, A. T. (1969). *Clostridia of Wound Infection.* London: Butterworths.

Willis, A. T. (1977). *Anaerobic Bacteriology: Clinical and Laboratory Practice*, 3rd edn. London: Butterworths.

Willis, A. T. & Gowland, G. (1962). Some observations on the mechanism of the Nagler reaction. *J. Path. Bact.* **83**, 219.

Willis, A. T. & Phillips, K. D. (1983). *Anaerobic Infections*, 2nd edn. (Public Health Laboratory Service Monograph Series, no. 3). London: Her Majesty's Stationery Office.

Willis, A. T. & Phillips, K. D. (1988). *Anaerobic infections: Clinical and Laboratory Practice.* London: Public Health Laboratory Service.

Willis, A. T., O'Connor, J. J. & Smith, J. A. (1966). Some observations on staphylococcal pigmentation. *Nature, Lond.* **210**, 653.

Wilson, W. J. (1934). A blood agar tellurite arsenite selective medium for *B. diphtheriae. J. Path. Bact.* **38**, 114.

Wilson, W. J. & Blair, E. M. McV. (1927). Use of a glucose bismuth sulphite iron medium for the isolation of *B. typhosus* and *B. proteus. J. Hyg., Camb.* **26**, 374.

Wilson, W. J. & Blair, E. M. McV. (1931). Further experience of the bismuth sulphite media in the isloation of *Bacillus typhosus* and *B. paratyphosus* B from faeces, sewage and water. *J. Hyg., Camb.* **31**, 138.

Wilson, W. J., & Blair, E. M. McV. (1941). A tellurite-iron-rosolic acid medium selective for *B. dysenteriae* (Flexner). *Br. med. J.* ii, 501.

Winslow, C.-E. A., Broadhurst, J., Buchanan, R. E., Krumwiede, C., Jr, Rogers, L. A. & Smith, G. H. (1917). The families and genera of the bacteria: preliminary report of the Committee of the Society of American Bacteriologists on characterization and classification of bacterial types. *J. Bact.* **2**, 505.

Winslow, C.-E. A., Broadhurst, J., Buchanan, R. E., Krumwiede, C., Jr, Rogers, L. A. & Smith, G. H. (1920). The families and genera of bacteria. Final report of the Committee of the Society of American Bacteriologists on characterization and classification of bacterial types. *J. Bact.* **5**,191.

Woese, C. R., Stackebrandt, E., Macke, T. J. & Fox, G. E. (1985). A phylogenetic definition of the major enbacterial taxa. *Appl. Microbiol.* **6**, 141.

Wolf, J. & Barker, A. N. (1968). The genus *Bacillus:* aids to the identification of its species. In *Identification Methods for Microbiologists,* part B, (Ed. B. M. Gibbs & D. A. Shapton). p. *93.* London: Academic Press.

Wolin, M. J., Wolin, E.A. & Jacobs, N. J. (1961). Cytochrome-producing anaerobic vibrio, *Vibrio succinogenes,* sp. n. *J. Bact.* **81**, 911.

Wood, M. (1959). The clotting of rabbit plasma by group D streptococci. *J. gen. Microbiol.* **21**, 385.

Wood, R. D. (1957). Hand-sorted punched cards in taxonomic research. *Brittonia,* **9**, 65.

Wood, R. L. (1970). *Erysipelothrix.* In *Manual of Clinical Microbiology.* Edn 1 (ed. J. E. Blair, E. H. Lennette & J. R. Truant), p. 101. Bethesda, Maryland: American Society for Microbiology.

Wood, R. L., Haubrich, D. R. & Harrington, R. (1978). Isolation of previously unreported serotypes of *Erysipelothrix rhusiopathiae* from swine. *Am. J. vet. Res.* **39**, 1958.

Wormser, R. E. & Bottone, E. J. (1983). *Cardiobacterium hominis*: a review of microbiological and clinical features. *Rev. inf. Dis.* **5**, 680.

Wright, H. D. (1933). The importance of adequate reduction of peptone in the preparation of media for the pneumococcus and other organisms. *J. Path. Bact.* **37**, 257.

Wright, H. D. (1934*a*). A substance in cotton-wool inhibitory to the growth of the pneumococcus. *J. Path. Bact.* **38**, 499.

Wright, H. D. (1934*b*). The preparation of nutrient agar with special reference to pneumococci, streptococci and other Gram-positive organisms. *J. Path. Bact.* **39**, 359.

Yabuuchi, E. & Yano, I. (1981). *Achromobacter* gen. nov. and *Achromobacter xylosoxidans* (ex Yabuuchi and Ohyama 1971) nom. rev. *Int. J. syst. Bact.* **31**, 477.

Yabuuchi, E., Kaneko, T., Yano, I., Moss, C.W. & Miyoshi, N. (1983). *Sphingobacterium* gen. nov. *Sphingobacterium spiritivorum* comb. nov., *Sphingobacterium multivorum* comb. nov., *Sphingobacterium minutae* sp. nov., and *Flavobacterium indologenes* sp. nov.: glucose-nonfermenting Gram-negative rods in CDC groups IIK-2 and IIb. *Int. J. syst. Bact.* **33**, 580.

Yan, W. K. (1969). Methylene blue sensitivity of *Vibrio* organisms. *Med. Lab. Technol.* **26**, 90.

Yanagawa, R. & Honda, E. (1978). *Corynebacterium pilosum* and *Corynebacterium cystitidis*, two new species from cows. *Int. J. syst. Bact.* **28**, 209.

Yong, D. C. T. & Thompson, J.S. (1982). Rapid microbiochemical method for identification of *Gardnerella* (*Haemophilus*) *vaginalis*. *J. clin. Microbiol.* **16**, 30.

Young, V. M., Kenton, D. M., Hobbs, B. J. & Moody, M. R. (1971). *Levinea,* a new genus in the family Enterobacteriaceae. *Int. J. syst. Bact.* **21**, 58.

Yourassowsky, E., Hansen, W., Labbe, M. & van Molle, J. (1965). Problemes taxinomiques. Orientation mecanographique du diagnostic des espèces microbiennes. *Acta clin. Belg.* **20**, 279.

Ziehl, F. (1882). Zur Färbung des Tuberkebacillus. *Dt. med. Wschr.* **8**, 451.

Zierdt, C. H. (1971). Autolytic nature of iridescent lysis in *Pseudomonas aeruginosa*. *Antonie van Leeuwenhoek,* **37**, 319.

Zierdt, C. H. & Marsh, H. H., III. (1971). Identification of *Pseudomonas pseudomallei*. *Am. J. clin. Path.* **55**, 596.

Zinnemann, K. (1960). *Haemophilus influenzae* and its pathogenicity. *Ergebn. Mikrobiol. ImmunForsch. exp. Ther.* **33**, 307.

Zinnemann, K. & Turner, G. C. (1963). The taxonomic position of 'Haemophilus vaginalis' [*Corynebacterium vaginale*]. *J. Path. Bact.* **85**, 213.

ZoBell, C. E. (1932). Factors influencing the reduction of nitrates and nitrites by bacteria in semisolid media. *J. Bact.* **24**, 273.

ZoBell, C. E. & Feltham, C. B. (1934). A comparison of lead, bismuth, and iron as detectors of hydrogen sulfide produced by bacteria. *J. Bact.* **28**, 169.

Index

Species names in brackets have either been transferred into another genus, fallen into disuse, or are in the process of being ratified by the Judicial Commission.